AF714913

Non-Alzheimer's and Atypical Dementia

Non-Alzheimer's and Atypical Dementia

Edited by

Michael D. Geschwind, MD PhD
Memory and Aging Center
Department of Neurology
University of California, San Francisco
San Francisco, CA, USA

Caroline Racine Belkoura, PhD
Department of Neurological Surgery
University of California, San Francisco
San Francisco, CA, USA

WILEY Blackwell

This edition first published 2016 © 2016 by John Wiley & Sons, Ltd

Registered Office
John Wiley & Sons, Ltd, The Atrium, Southern Gate, Chichester, West Sussex, PO19 8SQ, UK

Editorial Offices
9600 Garsington Road, Oxford, OX4 2DQ, UK
The Atrium, Southern Gate, Chichester, West Sussex, PO19 8SQ, UK
111 River Street, Hoboken, NJ 07030-5774, USA

For details of our global editorial offices, for customer services and for information about how to apply for permission to reuse the copyright material in this book please see our website at www.wiley.com/wiley-blackwell

The right of the author to be identified as the author of this work has been asserted in accordance with the UK Copyright, Designs and Patents Act 1988. All rights reserved. No part of this publication may be reproduced, stored in a retrieval system, or transmitted, in any form or by any means, electronic, mechanical, photocopying, recording or otherwise, except as permitted by the UK Copyright, Designs and Patents Act 1988, without the prior permission of the publisher.

Designations used by companies to distinguish their products are often claimed as trademarks. All brand names and product names used in this book are trade names, service marks, trademarks or registered trademarks of their respective owners. The publisher is not associated with any product or vendor mentioned in this book. It is sold on the understanding that the publisher is not engaged in rendering professional services. If professional advice or other expert assistance is required, the services of a competent professional should be sought.

The contents of this work are intended to further general scientific research, understanding, and discussion only and are not intended and should not be relied upon as recommending or promoting a specific method, diagnosis, or treatment by health science practitioners for any particular patient. The publisher and the author make no representations or warranties with respect to the accuracy or completeness of the contents of this work and specifically disclaim all warranties, including without limitation any implied warranties of fitness for a particular purpose. In view of ongoing research, equipment modifications, changes in governmental regulations, and the constant flow of information relating to the use of medicines, equipment, and devices, the reader is urged to review and evaluate the information provided in the package insert or instructions for each medicine, equipment, or device for, among other things, any changes in the instructions or indication of usage and for added warnings and precautions. Readers should consult with a specialist where appropriate. The fact that an organization or Website is referred to in this work as a citation and/or a potential source of further information does not mean that the author or the publisher endorses the information the organization or Website may provide or recommendations it may make. Further, readers should be aware that Internet Websites listed in this work may have changed or disappeared between when this work was written and when it is read. No warranty may be created or extended by any promotional statements for this work. Neither the publisher nor the author shall be liable for any damages arising herefrom.

Library of Congress Cataloging-in-Publication Data

Non-Alzheimer's and atypical dementia / edited by Michael D. Geschwind, Caroline Racine Belkoura.
p. ; cm.
Includes bibliographical references and index.
ISBN 978-1-4443-3624-5 (cloth)
I. Geschwind, Michael D., editor. II. Belkoura, Caroline Racine, editor.
[DNLM: 1. Dementia. 2. Alzheimer Disease. 3. Neurobehavioral Manifestations. WM 220]
RC521
616.8′3–dc23

2015036764

A catalogue record for this book is available from the British Library.

Wiley also publishes its books in a variety of electronic formats. Some content that appears in print may not be available in electronic books.

Set in 9.5/12pt Minion by SPi Global, Pondicherry, India

1 2016

Contents

Notes on contributors

Roger L. Albin, MD
Anne B. Young Collegiate Professor of Neurology
University of Michigan
and
Chief, Neuroscience Research, VAAAHS GRECC
Ann Arbor, MI, USA

Cynthia Barton, RN MSN
Nurse Practitioner
Health Sciences Assistant Clinical Professor
Memory and Aging Center
Department of Neurology
University of California, San Francisco
San Francisco, CA, USA

Caroline Racine Belkoura, PhD
Assistant Professor
Clinical Neuropsychologist
Department of Neurological Surgery
University of California, San Francisco
San Francisco, CA, USA

Helena C. Chui, MD
McCarron Professor and Chair
Department of Neurology
Keck School of Medicine
University of Southern California
Los Angeles, CA, USA

Praveen Dayalu, MD
Assistant Professor
Department of Neurology
University of Michigan
Ann Arbor, MI, USA

Christopher M. Filley, MD
Professor of Neurology and Psychiatry
Director, Behavioral Neurology Section
University of Colorado School of Medicine
and
Neurology Service Chief
Denver VA Medical Center
Denver, CO, USA

Michael D. Geschwind, MD PhD
Professor of Neurology
Michael J. Homer Chair in Neurology
Memory and Aging Center
Department of Neurology
University of California, San Francisco
San Francisco, CA, USA

Liliana Ramirez-Gomez, MD
Adjunct Assistant Professor of Clinical Neurology
Department of Neurology
Keck School of Medicine
University of Southern California
Los Angeles, CA, USA

John Halperin, MD FAAN FACP
Medical Director
Atlantic Neuroscience Institute
Summit, NJ, USA
and
Professor of Neurology & Medicine
Sidney Kimmel Medical College of Thomas Jefferson University
Philadelphia, PA, USA
and
Chair, Department of Neurosciences
Overlook Medical Center
Summit, NJ, USA

Emily L. Ho, MD PhD
Clinical Instructor in Neurology
University of Washington
and
Neurohospitalist
Swedish Neuroscience Institute
Seattle, WA, USA

Cheryl A. Jay, MD
Health Sciences Clinical Professor of Neurology
University of California, San Francisco
and
Neurology Service
San Francisco General Hospital (SFGH)
San Francisco, CA, USA

Laura J. Julian, PhD
Assistant Professor of Medicine
University of California, San Francisco
San Francisco, CA, USA

Robin Ketelle, RN MS
Clinical Nurse Specialist
Health Sciences Assistant Clinical Professor
Memory and Aging Center
Department of Neurology
University of California, San Francisco
San Francisco, CA, USA

Amy Kuo, RN MS GNP-BC
Nurse Practitioner
On Lok Lifeways
San Francisco, CA, USA

Suzee E. Lee, MD
Assistant Professor of Neurology
Memory and Aging Center
Department of Neurology
University of California, San Francisco
San Francisco, CA, USA

Carol F. Lippa, MD
Professor and Interim Chair
Department of Neurology
Director, Memory and Cognitive Disorders Program
Drexel Neurosciences Institute
Drexel University College of Medicine
Philadelphia, PA, USA

Michelle Mattingly, PhD ABPP
Assistant Professor
Departments of Psychiatry and Behavioral Neurosciences and Neurology
University of South Florida College of Medicine
Tampa, FL, USA

Andrew McKeon, MD
Associate Professor of Neurology, and Laboratory Medicine and Pathology
Neurologist, Department of Neurology
Co-Director, Neuroimmunology Laboratory
Mayo Clinic
Rochester, MN, USA

Jennifer Merrilees, RN PhD
Clinical Nurse Specialist
Health Sciences Associate Clinical Professor
Memory and Aging Center
Department of Neurology
University of California, San Francisco
San Francisco, CA, USA

Bruce L. Miller, MD
A.W and Mary Clausen Distinguished Professor of Neurology
Memory and Aging Center
Department of Neurology
University of California, San Francisco
San Francisco, CA, USA

Katie Osborn, MA
Predoctoral Intern
Department of Psychiatry
Geisel School of Medicine at Dartmouth
Hanover, NH, USA

Gregory M. Pastores, MD
Consultant
National Center for Inherited Metabolic Diseases
Department of Medicine
Mater Misericordiae University Hospital
Dublin, Ireland
and
Visiting Professor
Department of Medicine
Yale University School of Medicine
New Haven, CT, USA

Henry Paulson, MD PhD
Lucile Gross Professor of Neurology
University of Michigan
Ann Arbor, MI, USA

David C. Perry, MD
Assistant Professor
Memory and Aging Center
Department of Neurology
University of California, San Francisco
San Francisco, CA, USA

Sean J. Pittock, MD
Professor of Neurology
Director, Neuroimmunology Laboratory
Director, Center for MS and Autoimmune Neurology
Mayo Clinic
Rochester, MN, USA

Katherine L. Possin, PhD
Assistant Professor of Neuropsychology
Memory and Aging Center
Department of Neurology
University of California, San Francisco
San Francisco, CA, USA

Leon Prockop, MD
Department of Neurology
University of South Florida
Tampa, FL, USA

Gil D. Rabinovici, MD
Associate Professor of Neurology
Memory and Aging Center
Department of Neurology
University of California, San Francisco
San Francisco, CA, USA

Howard J. Rosen, MD
Professor of Neurology
Memory and Aging Center
Department of Neurology
University of California, San Francisco
San Francisco, CA, USA

Swati A. Sathe, MD MS
Associate Professor
Department of Neurology
Neurological Institute of New Jersey
Rutgers, The State University of New Jersey
New Jersey Medical School
Newark, NJ, USA

Sharon J. Sha, MD MS
Clinical Assistant Professor
Neurology and Neurological Sciences
Stanford Center for Memory Disorders
Stanford, CA, USA
and
Memory and Aging Center
Department of Neurology
University of California, San Francisco
San Francisco, CA, USA

Leonel T. Takada, MD PhD
Neurologist at Hospital das Clinicas
Department of Neurology
University of Sao Paulo Medical School
Sao Paulo, Brazil

CHAPTER 1

Introduction

Michael D. Geschwind and Caroline Racine Belkoura
University of California, San Francisco, San Francisco, CA, USA

This book was developed in order to provide a clinically relevant review of non-Alzheimer's and atypical dementia syndromes. Specifically, we felt there was a need for a broad but comprehensive overview of the differential diagnoses for atypical dementia that could be utilized by health-care providers who encounter these patients in their clinical practice, including neurologists, primary care providers, psychiatrists, neuropsychologists, nurses, social workers, etc. Where relevant, we have included clinical case studies in each chapter to help illustrate key or unique diagnostic features of each disorder and to provide a "real-world" view of how each disorder might present in the clinic.

Multidisciplinary evaluation of the atypical dementia patient

In this chapter, the editors review a framework for the clinical evaluation of the patient with a suspected atypical dementia syndrome. In particular, we focus on the benefits of a multidisciplinary evaluation with a team that includes a combination of a neurologist, neuropsychologist, psychiatrist, nurse, and social worker. Each team member brings a unique set of skills to the evaluation, which enables an in-depth and comprehensive assessment of a variety of domains, including relevant history, neurological function, cognitive abilities, mood and behavior, and daily function. Obtaining information from both the patient and a close family member or friend is essential as many atypical syndromes lead to loss of insight, and thus, more accurate reporting might come from someone other than the patient themselves. We have found that a case conference approach, where all team members meet after seeing the patient to review all relevant findings and discuss the case in detail, leads to a more accurate differential diagnosis, which can then be relayed to the patient and their family members in a timely fashion.

Atypical Alzheimer's disease

In this chapter, Sharon Sha and Gil Rabinovici review the atypical presentations of Alzheimer's disease (AD), which by definition present with symptoms other than memory loss and therefore might not meet most standard diagnostic criteria for AD. These patients tend to be younger than "typical" AD cases and might present with visuospatial complaints, executive dysfunction, behavioral changes, or language impairment. Additionally, often, patients meet diagnostic criteria for posterior cortical atrophy (PCA, a visual dysfunction syndrome), corticobasal syndrome (CBS, executive dysfunction or behavioral syndrome), and/or primary progressive aphasia (PPA, language syndrome) disorders that have not historically associated with AD pathology; however, recent research has demonstrated that a significant portion of these clinical syndromes are ultimately found to have AD pathology at autopsy. Neuropsychological testing and atrophy patterns on MRI often are very helpful in the differential diagnosis of the clinical syndrome. PET imaging with amyloid binding agents such as Pittsburgh compound B (PiB) or florbetapir F^{18} might provide additional, if not even more convincing, evidence of underlying AD pathology. The recognition of AD pathology as a causative factor in these atypical syndromes is important because of available symptomatic treatments and ongoing clinical trials for AD. Future diagnostic criteria for AD will need to incorporate the possibility of atypical presentations in order to increase sensitivity.

Vascular cognitive impairment: Diagnosis and treatment

In this comprehensive chapter, Helena Chui and Liliana Ramirez Gomez first review the complex history and terminology of vascular contributions to cognitive impairment. They postulate that the physiological effects of vascular brain impairment (VBI) lead to variable vascular cognitive impairment (VCI), depending on the location, extent, and severity of injury. White matter imaging methods including structural (i.e., white matter hyperintensities) and functional (diffusion tensor imaging) techniques provide the most useful information regarding the extent of VBI. VCI usually involves slowed processing speed and executive dysfunction but can vary widely depending on the location of pathology. The effect of VBI is additive and might be worsened by the presence of other underlying neuropathological conditions (i.e., AD). Risk factors for VBI/VCI include hypertension, hyperlipidemia,

Non-Alzheimer's and Atypical Dementia, First Edition. Edited by Michael D. Geschwind and Caroline Racine Belkoura.
© 2016 John Wiley & Sons, Ltd. Published 2016 by John Wiley & Sons, Ltd.

and diabetes, which suggest that the risk profile for cognitive impairment in many individuals could be lowered via lifestyle modifications. Current pharmacological treatments (i.e., cholinesterase inhibitors, NMDA receptor blockers) are symptomatic in nature, and firm evidence regarding their utility is lacking.

Frontotemporal dementia

In this chapter by David Perry and Howard Rosen, the clinical syndrome of frontotemporal dementia (FTD) and its underlying pathological etiologies (frontotemporal lobar degeneration (FTLD)) are reviewed. Newly developed diagnostic criteria for FTD have been developed, which identify three core clinical syndromes: (i) behavioral variant FTD (bvFTD), (ii) semantic variant primary progressive aphasia (svPPA, also called semantic dementia), and (iii) nonfluent variant primary progressive aphasia (nfvPPA). The most common presentation is bvFTD, with initial symptoms that might include apathy, disinhibition, loss of empathy, and other personality changes and MRI revealing relative atrophy of the fronto-insular cortex and underlying white matter. Cognitive testing often reveals relative deficits in executive function, although cognition might be relatively preserved early in the disorder. The hallmark features of svPPA include word-finding deficits and loss of semantic knowledge for words and objects, with MRI usually revealing relative atrophy in the left anterior temporal lobe. Bilateral temporal lobe atrophy becomes more prevalent over the course of the disease with additional frontal lobe involvement and behavioral symptoms including loss of empathy, and compulsions might appear (although they are not usually a presenting feature as in bvFTD). Slow and effortful speech is a classic feature of nfvPPA, with frank mutism being common over the course of the disease. MRI typically reveals asymmetric atrophy of the left inferior frontal cortex. Other clinical syndromes, including motor neuron disease (i.e., amyotrophic lateral sclerosis (ALS), progressive supranuclear palsy (PSP), and corticobasal syndrome (CBS)), can overlap significantly with FTD syndromes and are referred to as FTD spectrum disorders. The underlying neuropathology of FTD is complex, and research in this field is evolving rapidly. As a general guideline, svPPA tends to be associated with TDP-43 pathology, nfvPPA tends to be associated with tau pathology, and bvFTD is associated with a variety of pathologies (TDP-43, tau, FUS, PSP, and CBD). Treatments for these disorders are currently symptomatic, although clinical trials are in development.

Lewy body dementias

In this chapter, dementia with Lewy bodies (DLB) and Parkinson's disease with dementia (PDD) are reviewed by Carol Lippa and Katherine Possin. Both disorders feature a parkinsonian motor syndrome (i.e., rigidity, bradykinesia, tremor), cognitive impairment (visuospatial dysfunction, fluctuations in attention/arousal, and executive dysfunction), and neuropsychiatric symptoms (depression, anxiety, visual hallucinations). DLB is usually associated with relatively simultaneous onset of cognitive and motor symptoms, while PDD is associated with cognitive impairment in the setting of an established PD diagnosis (usually occurring >1 year after motor symptoms). Both syndromes are disorders of alpha-synuclein and are associated with underlying Lewy body pathology. Concomitant AD pathology is often present. Structural MRI findings are often grossly normal for age, while clinical symptoms associated with alpha-synuclein disorders (i.e., REM sleep behavior disorder, anosmia, autonomic dysfunction) might provide additional confirmation of a suspected DLB or PDD diagnosis. The treatment of the motor symptoms is usually with standard dopaminergic therapies utilized in PD, while acetylcholinesterase inhibitors often improve attention deficits and visual hallucinations. Neuropsychiatric symptoms might require SSRIs or low doses of newer antipsychotic agents such as quetiapine. These patients are susceptible to delirium, and exposure to anesthetics, anticholinergics, and antipsychotics should be closely monitored.

Corticobasal degeneration and progressive supranuclear palsy

Suzee Lee and Bruce Miller define the terms in the title of their chapter as reflecting the neuropathological entities of corticobasal degeneration (CBD) and progressive supranuclear palsy (PSP), which are both disorders of tau. They move on to discuss the typical clinical presentations of CBD as (i) nonfluent variant PPA (nfvPPA), (ii) an executive motor (EM) syndrome, and (iii) behavioral variant FTD (bvFTD). The clinical syndromes of nfvPPA and bvFTD have been reviewed in Chapter 5. EM syndrome typically presents with early executive dysfunction and motor impairment, often including axial rigidity and dystonia. MRI findings might include relative atrophy in the left frontal cortex. The clinical syndrome associated with pathological PSP is labeled PSP syndrome (PSP-S), which typically presents with oculomotor abnormalities (reduced saccade velocity and restricted vertical downgaze), axial rigidity and falls, executive dysfunction, and behavioral changes including apathy and disinhibition. Many individuals with PSP-S during life, however, are found to have other neuropathological disorders at autopsy, such as CBD. Conversely, clinical syndromes other than PSP-S are sometimes associated with pathological PSP at autopsy (i.e., CBS, bvFTD). Treatment of both CBD and PSP remains symptomatic, but several anti-tau agents are currently in the early stages of clinical trials.

Repeat expansion diseases and dementia

This chapter by Praveen Dayalu, Roger Albin, and Henry Paulson reviews DNA repeat expansion disorders that cause cognitive impairment, the most common of which is Huntington's disease

(HD). HD is an autosomal dominant, triplet repeat polyglutamine disorder with motor symptoms (chorea, ataxia, dystonia, rigidity), cognitive dysfunction (early executive dysfunction), and neuropsychiatric features (depression, anxiety, obsessive–compulsive symptoms) that progress to profound dementia and eventual death. A careful family history is critical in determining potential underlying genetic contributions to a clinical syndrome. Genetic testing for the HD mutation ensures accurate diagnosis, but involvement of a genetic counselor in this process is recommended, as the information has broad implications for family members. The HD mutation affects the protein huntingtin, although how this leads to neurodegeneration is unknown. MRI often shows relative caudate atrophy on visual assessment, and there is disproportionate pathology in the striatum at autopsy, although changes in cortical and white matter are also present. Pharmacological treatments are currently symptomatic in nature, targeting the motor (dopamine receptor blockers) or neuropsychiatric symptoms (i.e., antidepressants, antipsychotics), whereas social work, physical therapy, speech therapy, and nursing are required as the disease progresses. Other less common triplet repeat disorders that can cause cognitive impairment are presented, including spinocerebellar ataxia type 17 (SCA17), which presents with ataxia and prominent cognitive and behavioral symptoms, and fragile X premutation tremor/ataxia syndrome (FXTAS), which develops late in life and often presents with ataxia, tremor, and cognitive impairment and is more common in men.

Prion disorders

This chapter, written by Leonel Takada and Michael Geschwind, discusses the three basic forms of human prion disease (PrDs): sporadic (spontaneous), genetic, and acquired. PrDs are uniformly fatal, often rapidly progressive, neurodegenerative dementias. They are caused by the transformation of a normal prion protein into a misshapen form called the prion (pree-ahn). Prions then act as templates, causing nearby prion proteins to also change shape into the disease-causing, misshapen form, the prion. As sporadic Creutzfeldt–Jakob disease (sCJD) is by far the most common type of human PrD, much of the chapter focuses on this form, including the importance of diffusion-weighted brain MRI, and the shortcomings of relying on CSF biomarkers alone for diagnosis. The most common clinical features of sCJD are rapid-onset (weeks to months) dementia, ataxia, behavioral/personality changes, and other motor features (parkinsonism, myoclonus, etc.). Although myoclonus sometimes occurs in DLB and CBD, its presence in a patient with rapid progression should suggest CJD. A minority of sCJD patients present with prominent vision and visuospatial abnormalities (Heidenhain variant). Brain MRI should include FLAIR, DWI, and ADC sequences, which have the highest diagnostic utility for sCJD, showing restricted diffusion in the cortex (cortical ribboning) and/or deep nuclei, particularly the striatum. The use of CSF biomarkers, such as 14-3-3, neuron-specific enolase (NSE), and total tau (t-tau), is somewhat controversial. Many feel that these are merely markers of rapid neuronal injury and thus not specific, but sometimes they can be helpful for CJD diagnosis. Several conditions mimic sporadic CJD, some of which are currently untreatable, such as rapid forms of other more common neurodegenerative diseases, such as DLB, AD, CBD, and PSP (discussed in other chapters), and treatable, reversible conditions, such as autoimmune dementias (Chapter 10). Genetic prion diseases (gPrDs), comprising about 15% of human PrDs, are due to autosomal dominant mutations in the prion gene, *PRNP*. These forms may present identically to sCJD with a rapid course or present as other neurodegenerative diseases, with prolonged courses of a few years to more than a decade, sometimes with prominent psychiatric features. Often, patients with gPrDs do not have a known positive family history, although further investigation often reveals neuropsychiatric disorders, which likely were misdiagnosed. Although the most notorious, acquired prion diseases are the least common form of PrD. They can occur from iatrogenic exposure, consumption of bovine spongiform encephalopathy (BSE), blood transfusion from variant CJD (vCJD), or other causes. Despite ongoing research, presently there are no cures or disease-modifying treatments for PrDs.

Autoimmune dementias

This chapter, written by Andrew McKeon and Sean Pittock, reviews autoimmune etiologies of cognitive impairment or encephalopathy. Clinical features suggestive of an autoimmune disorder include acute or subacute presentation with fluctuating symptoms, CSF or laboratory results suggestive of autoimmunity, and positive response to immunotherapy. Past medical and family history is important to review for a history of cancer, familial autoimmune disorders or cancers, smoking history, and constitutional symptoms. Neuropsychological testing sometimes provides evidence of cognitive dysfunction in those with subtle complaints. MRI may demonstrate T2 abnormalities in the mesial temporal lobe, and EEG sometimes demonstrates generalized and/or focal slowing or epileptiform discharges. An elevated CSF protein, oligoclonal bands, and elevated IgG are all potentially suggestive of an autoimmune disorder, although not diagnostic. Antithyroid and antinuclear antibodies (ANA) tend to be nonspecific but should prompt further autoimmune workup, while neural antibodies (i.e., anti-Hu, CV2, NMDAR, VGKC) should prompt further evaluation for cancer as a paraneoplastic etiology should be high on the differential. Acute treatment of suspected autoimmune illness usually involves high-dose corticosteroids, IVIG, or plasma exchange for 6–12 weeks, with subsequent evaluation to determine improvement. If there is a positive response to treatment, an autoimmune diagnosis is more likely. Maintenance therapy may be required, as many individuals will relapse once treatment is discontinued. Unfortunately, long-term treatments can be associated with a variety of negative side effects, and the relative risks and benefits should be weighed accordingly.

Toxic and metabolic dementias

In this chapter, Michelle Mattingly, Katie Osborn and Leon Prockop review toxic and metabolic causes of dementia. Although rare, many of these etiologies are treatable, which emphasizes the need for accurate identification and appropriate intervention. The fluctuating alterations in consciousness associated with delirium can often masquerade as a dementia, but delirium typically is more acute in onset and often associated with toxins or underlying medical illnesses (i.e., cancer, liver disease, thyroid problems). A list of common toxic agents that can cause dementia is provided, with detailed descriptions of the effects of ethanol, carbon monoxide, and lead exposure; these toxins can cause cognitive, neuropsychiatric, and/or movement symptoms that can range from mild to severe with heterogeneous presentations. MRI is not only helpful in some cases of carbon monoxide exposure, with abnormalities in the globus pallidus and white matter, but also may be normal. Treatments include cessation of alcohol intake, hyperbaric oxygen therapy for carbon monoxide, and chelation therapy for lead exposure. Metabolic causes of dementia are broad, and this chapter reviews three common presentations, including thyroid disease, hepatic dysfunction, and disorders of glucose metabolism. Both hypo- and hyperthyroidism can lead to cognitive impairment and psychiatric symptoms, with resolution of symptoms often observed after appropriate medication is administered and euthyroid laboratory values are obtained. Hepatic encephalopathy can range from mild to severe and may be chronic in individuals with severe hepatic disease; treatment involves the use of nonabsorbable disaccharides and antibiotics. Both hypo- and hyperglycemia can lead to cognitive impairment. Individuals with diabetes are at a higher risk for cognitive decline and dementia, which may be due to secondary effects in the vascular system of the brain or may modify the effects of Alzheimer's disease pathology. Consideration of potential toxic or metabolic contributions to cognitive and neuropsychiatric dementia syndromes is important because of the possibility of treatment and reversal of symptoms.

Leukoencephalopathies/leukodystrophies

Authors Gregory Pastores and Swati Sathe review adult-onset leukoencephalopathies, a diverse group of disorders of white matter that cause cognitive decline. A distinction between acquired (i.e., inflammatory, vascular, toxic) causes and hereditary forms is made. The chapter largely focuses on these hereditary causes, termed leukodystrophies. Although many of these disorders have onset in childhood, there are also late-onset presentations that are often misdiagnosed as multiple sclerosis. Symmetric white matter changes on MRI should raise suspicion for leukodystrophy. CADASIL typically presents in the 30s and involves migraine with aura, recurrent strokes, seizures, cognitive impairment, mood changes, and apathy, with progressive episodes of decline over decades. It is an autosomal dominant disorder associated with mutations in the Notch3 gene. Treatment is largely symptomatic for migraine prevention and control of vascular risk factors. Adult-onset leukoencephalopathy with axonal spheroids and pigmented glia (ALSP) is a term that encompasses other syndromes (hereditary diffuse leukoencephalopathy (HDLS) and pigmentary orthochromatic leukodystrophy (POLD)), in which individuals present in their 40s with behavioral changes and motor impairment (i.e., parkinsonism, ataxia) and are often suspected to have a frontotemporal dementia syndrome. In an exciting development, the gene CSF1R has recently been identified as the cause for both POLD and HDLS, further supporting that they are a spectrum of the same disease entity. Several other leukodystrophies are reviewed, including adult-onset autosomal dominant leukodystrophy with autonomic dysfunction, adult polyglucosan body disease, and adult-onset Alexander disease. Mitochondrial disorders that can have significant white matter involvement and can cause dementia are reviewed, including mitochondrial encephalopathy, lactic acidosis, and strokes (MELAS); myoclonic epilepsy with ragged-red fibers (MERRF); Leigh syndrome; Kearns–Sayre syndrome (KSS); neuropathy, ataxia, and retinitis pigmentosa (NARP); Leber hereditary optic neuropathy (LHON); or Muir–Torre syndrome (MTS). Treatment of these disorders may involve ketogenic diet, physiotherapy, metabolite administration, and avoidance of stress. Lysosomal storage disorders are multisystemic, but can have cognitive impairment as a feature, and may include late-onset forms of metachromatic leukodystrophy (MLD) and globoid cell leukodystrophy (Krabbe disease) and Fabry disease. Treatment may involve hematopoietic stem cell transplant, dietary therapy, enzyme replacement therapy, or adrenal hormone replacement therapy. Although often confused with multiple sclerosis, identifying the cause of a leukoencephalopathy or leukodystrophy is important to consider in order to ensure appropriate diagnosis, genetic counseling, and management.

Infectious causes of dementia

This chapter, written by Cheryl Jay, Emily Ho, and John Halperin, reviews the subacute and chronic infections that may lead to a dementia syndrome. HIV-associated dementia is less common in the era of combination antiretroviral therapies (cART) but may involve apathy, slowed thinking, and motor symptoms, along with generalized cognitive dysfunction. The effects of concomitant infections (e.g., hepatitis C, cryptococcal meningitis), substance abuse, and other associated syndromes (e.g., primary CNS lymphoma, progressive multifocal leukoencephalopathy) must be ruled out. Treatment with appropriate cART for HIV and appropriate treatment of any other contributing infections or syndromes is recommended. Subacute sclerosing panencephalitis (SSPE) occurs long after an acute measles infection and is relatively rare in locations with adequate measles vaccination programs. Myoclonus is common, along with cognitive and behavioral impairment and seizures developing over months. Treatment is largely symptomatic with progression to death typically over one to two years from diagnosis. Acute presentations of hepatitis C and viral encephalitis may also cause long-lasting cognitive impairment. Bacterial causes of dementia include neurosyphilis, Lyme disease, and Whipple's disease. Acute bacterial meningitis may also be associated with cognitive impairment, which continues to stabilize or improve over many years. Fungal infections such as cryptococcal meningitis can cause cognitive impairment, most often in the context of concomitant HIV infection. Intensive antifungal treatment is required. Dementia may also occur in the context of parasitic infection such as neurocysticercosis (NCC), related to tapeworm infection. CNS cysts can be observed on MRI or CT. Seizure and neuropsychiatric symptoms are common presentations. Treatment involves cysticidal drugs and steroids. Although many of these disorders are responsive to therapy, many cognitive deficits will be long-lasting, and some cases are, unfortunately, fatal.

Rheumatologic and other autoimmune dementias

In this chapter by Laura Julian and Christopher Filley, the intersection between neurology and rheumatology is discussed, with a particular focus on systemic lupus erythematosus (SLE). SLE is an autoimmune disease that may affect any organ system and is frequently associated with cognitive and neuropsychiatric symptoms. MRI findings are often notable for white matter hyperintensities. Antiphospholipid syndrome (APS) can lead to stroke or transient ischemic attack (TIA) and thus secondary cognitive and neuropsychiatric dysfunction. Sneddon's syndrome also causes early strokes and TIAs that has a more severe clinical course and greater extent of cognitive impairment in comparison to APS. Treatment may involve anticoagulation and immunosuppressive drugs. Sjögren's syndrome can be associated with a variety of CNS manifestations, although the underlying causes are less well understood. Various vasculitides (blood vessel inflammation) can also cause CNS symptoms and frequently require blood vessel biopsy for confirmation. These syndromes include Wegener's granulomatosis, Churg–Strauss syndrome, Behcet's disease, and giant cell arteritis. Systemic sclerosis or scleroderma may have white matter lesions in the absence of severe neurological symptoms or patient's cognitive complaints. Sarcoidosis in the CNS is frequently associated with cranial neuropathy but may also be accompanied by cognitive and behavioral symptoms, depending on brain lesion location. With neurosarcoidosis, there are typically profound MRI abnormalities, often around the brainstem. Immunosuppressive drugs are typically used for treatment. Celiac disease, an inflammatory reaction to wheat, may lead to CNS complications in 10–20% of individuals with this disorder, most typically an ataxia. A gluten-free diet is appropriate for treatment. The link between rheumatological disorders and cognitive impairment is still in its relative infancy, and further studies with large numbers of patients are needed to more fully understand this phenomenon.

Comprehensive management of the patient with an atypical dementia

This chapter, written by Jennifer Merrilees, Cynthia Barton, Robin Ketelle, and Amy Kuo, provides a framework for clinical management of patients with atypical dementia. These patients often have unique challenges relative to older, more typical dementia patients, including younger age, greater behavioral disturbance, inability to work, and increased caregiver strain. These disorders are underrecognized and caregivers and families may have seen multiple health-care providers before being accurately diagnosed, which can lead to high levels of familial stress. Environmental modifications and behavioral strategies are recommended for a first line of defense in managing mood and personality changes, prior to pharmacological intervention. Caregiver training can be a crucial tool in helping keep the patient at home and delay placement within a facility, which can be difficult as many facilities are not equipped or trained to deal with severe behavioral or motor symptoms.

CHAPTER 2

The multidisciplinary evaluation of the atypical dementia patient

Michael D. Geschwind and Caroline Racine Belkoura
University of California, San Francisco, San Francisco, CA, USA

Introduction

The clinical presentation of atypical dementia varies widely and typically involves more than one symptom domain (e.g., cognition, motor function, behavior, autonomic function). This heterogeneity of presentation, in combination with the relative rarity of these disorders, can make accurate diagnosis difficult even for experienced clinicians. In our experience, the evaluation of individuals with suspected atypical dementia is optimal when conducted by a multidisciplinary team (e.g., neurology, neuropsychology, nursing, speech therapy, genetic counseling), allowing for a more comprehensive evaluation and the input of experts from several disciplines.

History

Acquiring a thorough history is one of the most critical features of an atypical dementia evaluation. Because these disorders frequently present with symptoms affecting multiple systems (e.g., gastrointestinal, sleep, autonomic, higher cortical function, etc.), a broad review of systems (ROS) is necessary. A review of previous medical records and the input of family (and sometimes even friends and colleagues) is essential, as patients may not appreciate or be able to accurately report symptoms secondary to their cognitive deficits or lack of insight. Given that the patient has some cognitive impairment, the presence at the interview of an informant who knows the patient well, such as a family member, a close friend, or a caregiver, is very important. If they cannot be present, then the informant should be interviewed by telephone. When possible, try to leave time to interview the informant separately, such as when the patient is undergoing neuropsychological (cognitive) testing. This will allow the informant to discuss topics that might upset the patient or they do not feel comfortable discussing in front of the patient. Specific key elements to be included in the history are discussed in the following paragraphs.

First symptoms

Determining the first symptom of a dementia is often the key to making the correct diagnosis. Encouraging family members to describe the earliest atypical behaviors or actions, even if only noted in retrospect, provides important information regarding the initial underlying neuroanatomy of their disease. For example, in a right-hander, early visuospatial problems might suggest right parietal involvement, early calculation difficulties might suggest left parietal dysfunction, and nonfluent speech might suggest left pre-Broca's area frontal lobe involvement. These early symptom clusters can also assist with differential diagnosis. For example, profound changes in personality or behavior are seen early in behavioral variant frontotemporal dementia (bvFTD), whereas behavioral changes in the context of early falls are more typical of progressive supranuclear palsy (PSP). New-onset psychiatric symptoms (i.e., depression, anxiety, apathy) in someone without a psychiatric history are particularly noteworthy, although family members and patients might not realize they are an early symptom of the dementia. A change in employment status is sometimes an early sign that something is wrong but may initially be attributed to outside factors (e.g., downsizing) rather than patient issues. Determining the first symptoms of a disease is a critical step toward earlier detection, correct diagnosis, and, when available, appropriate treatment.

Memory

Irrespective of what cognitive symptoms the patient presents with, a typical complaint might be, "I can't remember things." When evaluating a possible memory deficit, it is critical to determine if it is truly a primary memory problem. For example, semantic dementia (SD) patients might report, "I can't remember words," which actually reflects semantic loss rather than a primary memory problem. Similarly, posterior cortical atrophy (PCA) patients might describe, "I can't remember where I put things," reflecting their visual difficulties rather than impaired memory. Thus, detailed questioning during the history is required to determine the specific nature and

Non-Alzheimer's and Atypical Dementia, First Edition. Edited by Michael D. Geschwind and Caroline Racine Belkoura.
© 2016 John Wiley & Sons, Ltd. Published 2016 by John Wiley & Sons, Ltd.

etiology of presenting memory complaints. If it is a memory problem, then one must determine if it is an encoding or a retrieval problem. Many patients with frontal-executive deficits, such as due to ischemic vascular disease, report a primary memory problem, but often have problems with retrieval, but not encoding. Patients with frontal-executive function typically are aided in recall when given clues, whereas those with encoding deficits, such as occurs in Alzheimer's disease (AD), usually are not. Other questions to ask the family and patient include "How are short-term and/or long-term memory affected, how long does it take for the patient to forget something they were told, and how has this changed over time?" In AD, short-term memory is often affected early by the illness, and only later is long-term memory (autobiographical and remote memory) affected.

It is important to note how much of the history the patient can provide and in what level of detail, *without* relying on clues and hints provided by their family—thus, part of the neurological examination occurs during the history taking. It is sometimes necessary to explicitly tell family members (who might be used to speaking on behalf of the patient) to allow the patient to answer independently, assuring that they will have an opportunity to provide their input later.

Asking about recent and more remote current major local, regional, national (e.g., "911," "Hurricane Katrina," etc.), or world events (e.g., who was the president during, or which countries were involved in, World War II) or family vacations provides additional opportunities to examine the patient's recall abilities. Additional topics to discuss when asking about for memory difficulties include misplacing objects (e.g., keys, wallet, purse); being overly reliant on lists, post-it notes, or calendars; missing appointments; getting lost or disoriented in new (or old) environments; repeating oneself in conversation; and forgetting recent events (e.g., dinner with friends, movie recently seen).

Word list learning tasks (e.g., *California Verbal Learning Test*-2nd Edition (CVLT-II) [1], Hopkins Verbal Learning Test-Revised (HVLT-R)) [2] are among the most common memory tasks used in neuropsychological testing and require the individual to recall a long series of words across multiple trials (learning) with recall tested again after a 20–30 min delay (delayed recall) followed by yes–no recognition. For younger and relatively high-functioning individuals, it is necessary to use a longer 16-item word list rather than a 9-item list, as ceiling effects are prominent and often mask subtle deficits. Story learning and recall tasks (e.g., *Wechsler Memory Scale*–4th Edition (WMS-IV) Logical Memory [3]) are also helpful tools. Story recall is less dependent on executive function in comparison to word list learning but is often difficult to interpret in the context of semantic and/or auditory comprehension difficulties.

When interpreting the history and neuropsychological test results, it is helpful to think about the pattern of memory deficits, which suggests underlying neuroanatomy, thereby assisting with the differential diagnosis. A simplified view of memory deficits is that they are either hippocampal (medial temporal lobe (MTL)) or frontal executive in origin. Each anatomy generally has a different clinical pattern. Involvement of the MTL leads to anterograde amnesia (i.e., poor new learning and deficits in encoding) and the rapid forgetting of newly learned information. Associated clinical symptoms often include misplacing objects, repeating self in conversation, forgetting appointments, getting lost or disoriented in new environments, and poor memory for recent events. Neuropsychological testing typically reveals reduced learning, poor recall, and poor recognition (suggesting information was not appropriately stored or consolidated) even when provided with clues. These deficits are common in AD, SD (semantic variant (SV) frontotemporal dementia (FTD)), hippocampal sclerosis, limbic encephalopathy, and other disorders that affect MTL structures [4].

A frontal-subcortical pattern of memory loss, on the other hand, is associated with variable learning that is typically due to poor attention, difficulties with self-initiated recall (which typically improves with cues), and relatively spared recognition (suggesting information has been encoded in the MTL, but self-initiated access is difficult). These individuals tend to benefit from multiple learning trials and show progressive learning over time, whereas those with MTL involvement usually have flat learning curves. Clinical symptoms may be more variable (i.e., "he can remember if he pays attention") and are often seen in combination with frontal-executive dysfunction on other tasks. Family members often will note that patients will recognize information when it is presented to them (i.e., "he remembered that we had gone to the movie as soon as I started talking about the plot"). These deficits are more typical of diseases that affect frontal-subcortical circuits, such as bvFTD and related disorders, Huntington's disease (HD), Lewy body disorders, and white matter disorders [4, 5].

Motor

Many atypical dementias have accompanying motor features that help with differential diagnosis. For example, in AD, motor features typically occur very late, although there are motor presentations of AD, such as corticobasal syndrome (CBS) [6]. If the motor problems occur early, other diagnoses must also be considered. Early parkinsonism is a common feature of dementia with Lewy bodies (DLB), corticobasal degeneration (CBD), PSP, and Creutzfeldt–Jakob disease (CJD). Some genetic forms of FTD (i.e., FTD-17) commonly present with parkinsonism. Axial rigidity and early falls are suggestive of PSP, whereas asymmetric progressive apraxia might suggest CBS. Myoclonus is frequently observed in DLB, CBD, CJD, and less commonly in late AD. Ataxia is often present in multiple system atrophy (MSA), fragile X-associated tremor/ataxia syndrome (FXTAS), spinocerebellar ataxias (SCAs), HD, prion disease, paraneoplastic disorders, and metabolic disorders such as Wernicke's. Extraocular motor abnormalities occur in many neurodegenerative conditions and often are nonspecific, but some findings are helpful diagnostically. Gaze-evoked nystagmus is common in cerebellar degenerative disorders. Vertical supranuclear gaze palsy (limitations in downgaze) and slowed velocity of saccades are hallmark features of PSP. Breakdown of saccades can be observed in many disorders, particularly those that affect frontal-subcortical circuits including the frontal eye fields.

Choreiform movements are commonly seen in HD, several HD-like syndromes (including some forms of genetic and variant prion disease, HDL2 due to junctophilin-3 gene mutations, and a few SCAs, particularly SCA17), other genetic disorders (e.g., dentatorubral-pallidoluysian atrophy (DRPLA), neuroferritinopathy, pantothenate kinase-associated neurodegeneration (PKAN), and chorea–acanthocytosis), and autoimmune/paraneoplastic conditions [7, 8]. Muscle wasting and fasciculations in combination with other upper/lower motor neuron signs are suggestive of amyotrophic lateral sclerosis (ALS) and when seen in combination with behavioral symptoms may suggest a combined FTD–ALS syndrome, although many conditions can mimic features of ALS [9]. Isolated, as well as concomitant, vascular disease is a frequent cause of motor symptoms and should always be considered.

Behavior and neuropsychiatric symptoms

Most atypical dementias have prodromal states involving mood or behavior changes that are often recognized only in retrospect (i.e., depression and anxiety in DLB, depression and irritability in HD, apathy in bvFTD). Early changes in mood or behavior are frequently attributed to a psychiatric disorder or life stressors rather than an underlying neurodegenerative disease. A thorough review of the patient's prior psychiatric history (e.g., depression, anxiety, suicidal ideation/attempt, mania) is essential in order to understand and differentiate new behaviors from those which are exacerbations of previous behaviors. Because patients may have limited insight into their own symptoms and behavior, it is crucial to obtain additional information from a reliable informant (i.e., spouse, relative, or close friend) who knows the person well. Important topics to cover in an interview include depression, anxiety, apathy, hallucinations, delusions, illusions, irritability/agitation, disinhibition, personality change, obsessions/compulsions, sleep disturbance, and appetite change; using an instrument such as The Neuropsychiatric Inventory can be helpful [10].

Certain conditions have neuropsychiatric symptoms that can greatly assist with differential diagnosis. Well-formed complex visual hallucinations (i.e., people at the dinner table or small animals) and delusions are common early in DLB but can also occur in late-stage AD. Depression is common in disorders with basal ganglia involvement (i.e., PSP, CBS, HD, vascular disease, and DLB), whereas anxiety is often seen in many disorders, including DLB, MSA, and HD.

Sleep abnormalities such as REM sleep behavior disorder (RBD), restless legs syndrome (RLS), and periodic limb movements of sleep (PLMS) are also common in Lewy body disorders and other synucleinopathies and may predate the onset of the disorder by many years, if not decades [11]. Both central sleep apnea and obstructive sleep apnea (OSA) are relatively common in the general population and may contribute to cognitive deficits and depression if left untreated. The presence of sleep abnormalities should prompt a formal sleep evaluation, including polysomnography, to assess and adequately treat any underlying disorders.

Profound personality changes, including early behavioral disinhibition, early apathy, early loss of empathy, and hyperorality, are hallmark features of bvFTD [12]. Many of these features, particularly apathy, increased appetite (particularly for sweets), and disinhibition, are also seen in SV where they are associated with right hemisphere atrophy [13–16]. Compulsions or obsessions (i.e., compulsive recycling, eating the same meal at the same time every day) become common in semantic variant primary progressive aphasia (svPPA) as the disease progresses [15]. Apathy is very common in PSP [17, 18], CBD [6], and frontal AD and tends to correlate with medial frontal and anterior cingulate involvement [19–21]. Frontal AD is often misdiagnosed as bvFTD because of prominent executive dysfunction and apathy; frontal AD, however, usually does not have prominent early disinhibition and loss of empathy [10, 16, 22].

Behavioral changes and neuropsychiatric symptoms can greatly affect quality of life, including difficulties maintaining employment and caregiver strain. In addition to assisting with diagnosis, the accurate assessment of neuropsychiatric symptoms allows the provider to intervene with appropriate treatment and also to better prepare the family for upcoming changes.

Speech and language

A thorough evaluation of speech and language involves the assessment of motor speech symptoms (i.e., speech apraxia, dysarthria, swallowing) and language (i.e., reading, spelling, comprehension, repetition, fluency). Portions of the Western Aphasia Battery (WAB), the Boston Diagnostic Aphasia Examination (BDAE), the Boston Naming Test (BNT), the Boston Cookie Theft picture description, and the Pyramid and Palm Trees Test are useful in assessing language symptoms [13, 23, 24]. Most language disorders are affected by frequency and regularity effects, with high-frequency, short, and regular words being preserved until relatively late in the disease. Thus, it is very important to utilize relatively complex, unfamiliar, low-frequency stimuli in order to maximize the chance of detecting early, subtle language deficits.

Word-finding difficulties are a common, but nonspecific, symptom associated with several neurodegenerative conditions, particularly progressive aphasias [25]. The types of errors made on naming tasks, however, can provide insight with respect to the underlying anatomy of disease. Patients with frontal deficits may make phonemic paraphasias (i.e., bread for bed) or have frank misarticulation errors but often benefit from phonemic cues and can select the appropriate answer from multiple-choice cues, whereas those with temporal involvement may make semantic paraphasias (i.e., dog for rhinoceros), do not typically benefit from phonemic cues, and may select incorrect answers on multiple-choice testing, suggesting frank semantic loss. Conversational speech should be examined for rate, rhythm, articulation errors, slurring, phonemic substitutions, word-finding pauses, circumlocution, and use of syntax. Verbal fluency tasks, including letter fluency (i.e., "State as many words starting with 'D' that you can think of") and category prompts (i.e., "Tell me all the animals you can think of"), can be beneficial in determining underlying neuroanatomy, with frontal involvement usually leading to relative reductions in letter fluency but preserved category fluency (although as speech becomes more impaired, performance for both tasks declines) and temporal involvement leading to relative reduction in category fluency relative to letter fluency. Semantic knowledge can be tested with the Pyramid and Palm Trees Test, as well as asking general knowledge questions in several categories [23, 24].

There are three main subtypes of primary progressive aphasia. The nonfluent variant primary progressive aphasia (nvPPA) is associated with relative declines in left frontal function and presents with early motor speech abnormalities, including decreased speech output and reduced fluency (i.e., fewer words per minute, slow labored speech), dysarthria, and altered phoneme production, and also typically involves altered use of syntax (i.e., telegraphic speech or writing). Swallowing difficulties may also be present, particularly as the disease progresses, and most often these patients become mute within the first several years of the disorder. Reading, spelling, and comprehension tend to be relatively preserved, while writing may be noteworthy for syntactical errors and reduced output. Repetition may be impaired due to articulation deficits. nfvPPA is most often associated with CBD and PSP at autopsy [23, 26].

The semantic variant primary progressive aphasia (svPPA; formerly called SD) is associated with relative left temporal lobe atrophy and presents with fluent but empty speech, with the frequent use of generic words (i.e., thing, stuff) and relative omission of nouns. Patients may also ask for clarification regarding word meaning (i.e., "what do you mean by banister?"), and they often demonstrate frank difficulties on tasks requiring them to identify body parts (i.e., chin) or choose pictures representing single words (i.e., "primate" on Peabody Picture Vocabulary Test). Errors in the reading and spelling of irregular words (e.g., yacht, gnaw) suggest surface dyslexia, in which a loss of semantic knowledge associated with temporal lobe involvement results in the application of phonetic rules (e.g., knight = kah-nih-ght). Frequency effects are typical, with low-frequency and irregular words being affected early in the disease, while knowledge about high-frequency words may be preserved until late in the disease course [23, 26]. The nfvPPA and svPPA are discussed in more detail in Chapter 5.

The logopenic variant primary progressive aphasia (lvPPA) has relative left temporoparietal atrophy and presents with decreased short-term auditory storage (or echoic memory). These individuals have a reduction in digit span forward, being unable to maintain more than 3–4 bits of information in short-term storage rather than the 7±2 bits that is typical. This reduction affects the ability to comprehend lengthy sentences and also results in reduced sentence repetition, particularly for long, unfamiliar phrases. Speech tends to be slow with long pauses, "uh's and um's"; frequent word-finding difficulties; and circumlocution. This variant is often misdiagnosed as nfPPA because of these speech symptoms; however, relative to nfPPA, there are less frequent articulation errors (although there may be phonemic substitutions for complex words) and fewer syntactical errors in speech. Decreased reading, poor calculation skills, and left–right confusion are often observed in lvPPA due to left parietal involvement and help distinguish these individuals from nfPPA [23, 26]. Chapter 5 discusses lvPPA in more detail.

Visuospatial

Early visuospatial abnormalities are common in DLB and PCS (typically AD pathology) [27] as well as the Heidenhain variant of CJD [28]. Common complaints include difficulties finding specific objects among many (i.e., in the refrigerator or a messy desk), changes in driving (i.e., drifting within the lane, difficulties parallel parking, and recent accidents), getting lost or disoriented in unfamiliar environments, and complaints about vision despite adequate visual acuity. Complex visual-constructional copy tasks (i.e., three-dimensional cube, Rey–Osterrieth Complex Figure, Benson Figure) are typically impaired early in these disorders. Decreased interest in reading and difficulty maintaining one's place while reading or working on the computer (especially common in PSP) might be early symptoms. Difficulties with face or object perception suggest alterations in the ventral visual processing stream within the temporal lobe, whereas difficulties with spatial orientation and location suggest alterations in the dorsal visual processing stream within the parietal lobe [29]. Due to bilateral superior parietal involvement, individuals with PCA often exhibit some degree of Balint's syndrome, including optic ataxia (difficulties integrating visual and motor movements, i.e., reaching for a cup), oculomotor apraxia (volitional eye movements), and simultagnosia (ability to pay attention to more than one item in the visual field) [27, 30]. In DLB, in addition to visuospatial difficulties, visual illusions or hallucinations are common [31]. Individuals with PSP may also report early visual difficulties, although upon testing it becomes obvious that this is secondary to restricted eye movements rather than visual perception per se.

Visuospatial difficulties should prompt an evaluation of driving skills, with appropriate restrictions made (i.e., no night driving, limited freeway use) and, if necessary, early voluntary cessation from driving. In some states, health-care professionals are mandated to report individuals who are diagnosed with dementia or otherwise thought to be unsafe to drive. A home safety evaluation might also be warranted.

Executive function

Executive function is an umbrella term representing many subabilities that allow one to pursue goal-directed action (i.e., working memory, inhibition, organization, rapid processing, multitasking, set-shifting, planning, goal maintenance, and judgment). Patients may have reductions in specific aspects of executive function (i.e., working memory), whereas other aspects remain intact (i.e., inhibition). Executive function is usually associated with the frontal lobe and its links to circuits in the basal ganglia (i.e., frontal-striatal circuits) [32, 33]. Cerebellar dysfunction, however, can also lead to executive function impairment due to connections between the cerebellum and frontal lobe via the thalamus [34].

Poor executive function is one of the strongest predictors of reduced functional abilities and thus is particularly important to assess during neuropsychological testing. The Mini-Mental State Examination (MMSE) is not very sensitive to executive dysfunction [35, 36], whereas the Montreal Cognitive Assessment (MoCA) is a screening measure that is more sensitive to executive dysfunction and includes a set-shifting task, verbal fluency, and digit span backwards (www.mocatest.org) [4]. Some other neuropsychological tasks that measure executive function include the Wisconsin Card Sorting Test (hypothesis testing), Category Booklet Test (hypothesis testing), Trail Making Test (set-shifting), Tower of Hanoi (planning), Digit Span Backwards (working memory), Four Word Short-Term Memory Test (working memory), Stroop Interference, and the Delis–Kaplan Executive Function System (D-KEFS Trail Making Test, Design Fluency Test, Color–Word Interference Test, Tower Test, Sorting Test, Verbal Fluency Test) [4].

Poor performance on executive function tasks can occur for several reasons, particularly slowed processing speed (increased time to perform tasks) and/or making errors (i.e., rule violations, intrusions, perseverations). Errors are often a better predictor of true executive dysfunction than just slowed processing, which can be related to reduced motor function and other more general factors. Qualitative observations of the patient in the clinic, during neuropsychological testing, or in their home/work environment may also provide evidence of difficulties with executive function (i.e., impulsivity, perseveration, tendencies to make errors, poor problem solving, reduced judgment, poor ability to learn new tasks).

Functional history

A functional history involves identifying what activities of daily living (ADLs) a person is capable of, including such tasks as work, finances, cooking, shopping, medication management, and driving. A functional history is critical for determining if an individual has dementia, because significant functional impairment usually is required to make this diagnosis.

Important topics to cover during an interview or via a questionnaire include instrumental activities of daily living (often referred to as iADLs), which are higher-level skills such as management of finances, performance at work, medication management, and driving skills, as well as more basic ADLs such as dressing, bathing, grooming, toileting, and cooking. Detailed questioning regarding each symptom can be particularly helpful. For example, if a patient stopped driving, knowing when or why this occurred would be informative. Did they stop driving due to poor depth perception or reduced night vision (suggesting visuospatial issues)? Were they swerving within the lane or scraping the car on one particular side (suggesting possible neglect)? Were they stopping abruptly, getting too close to cars in front of them, or speeding around corners (suggesting disinhibition)? Were they getting lost because they were forgetting where they were going or how to get to their destination (suggesting memory loss)? Answers to these types of questions can provide useful clues to which areas of the brain are impacted and enhance differential diagnosis.

The timeline of functional changes may also be helpful in determining when the cognitive decline started. For example, many patients in the early stages of a neurodegenerative illness will begin having troubles at work, particularly if their position changes in some way or they are required to learn a new task or system. Their difficulties may initially be attributed to "normal aging" or issues with management but in retrospect may be an early sign of cognitive decline.

In our clinic, nurses and/or social workers participate in the multidisciplinary evaluation by completing the functional history with an informant in a separate interview typically while the patient is undergoing a neuropsychological assessment. Additional functional information is then obtained in the joint patient/informant interview with the physician. There are many questionnaires regarding functional skills that can be utilized either before or during the clinical visit (please see Chapter 15 for a review of these measures).

Review of Systems (ROS)

In evaluating atypical dementias, the ROS is critical and should include not only standard medical systems but also items such as behavior, sensory, sleep, motor, and other changes. A focused review of symptoms can help with not only diagnosis but also treatment. For example, patients with an RBD are more likely to have a synucleinopathy such as DLB, PD, or MSA. If dysautonomia is present, MSA and DLB should be considered among the neurodegenerative causes of cognitive impairment. Patients with depression causing memory impairment may have a positive ROS with many somatic complaints. Neuropathies may suggest a more systemic neurologic problem, including metabolic, autoimmune, or genetic etiologies.

Past medical and surgical history

An examination of the past medical and surgical history can reveal factors that increase the risk of dementia or may exacerbate symptoms, including cardiac issues (e.g., hypertension, coronary artery disease, history of myocardial infarction or arrhythmia or cardiac bypass), metabolic syndromes (e.g., diabetes mellitus, hyperlipidemia, thyroid disease, vitamin B12 deficiency), and previous brain injury (e.g., motor vehicle accidents, concussion, loss of consciousness (LOC), seizures, etc.). When acquiring information on possible LOC, it is important to confirm the LOC and how long the person might have had LOC [37]. Prior chemotherapy or radiation to the head or neck can have both acute and delayed effects on cognition [38], particularly those who received whole-brain radiation treatment [39, 40]. Malabsorption syndromes (i.e., celiac disease, B12 or other vitamin deficiencies) may also have effects on cognition.

With respect to past surgical history or hospitalizations, delirium in response to new medicines, including anesthesia, or even hospitalization alone is often observed in Lewy body disorders [41] but may also be observed in individuals with other dementias as well [42]. Anoxia secondary to extended cardiac or other surgeries may also contribute to cognitive impairment.

Prior and current psychiatric history is also important to obtain in order to determine whether behavioral and personality changes are exacerbations of previous traits or new phenomenon. A subtle enhancement of previous tendencies (i.e., depression, anxiety) is often generally observed in the context of cognitive decline, whereas the onset of new behaviors may be more telling regarding the presence of a specific type of dementia (e.g., compulsions in SD or bvFTD). The development of new-onset psychiatric symptoms in later life should always raise concerns regarding possible underlying neurodegenerative illness [43, 44]. Many individuals with late-onset psychiatric or behavioral changes will be referred to psychiatry clinic first and may be relatively impaired by the time they present to a neurology or dementia clinic. If there has been a history of electroconvulsive therapy (ECT) for depression or bipolar disease, this often leads to significant short-term memory loss, some of which might be transient [45–47], whereas prior treatment with psychiatric medications, particularly first-generation antipsychotics, can lead to movement disorders, including tardive dyskinesia, parkinsonism, or dystonia.

Medications

A thorough medication history can best be obtained by having the patient bring in all of the medications that they are taking, as memory impairment may prevent accurate recollection of medications and their doses. By seeing the bottles and examining the type and number of pills, the medical provider might be able to discern if a patient has indeed been taking all prescribed medications. Details regarding when the medication was started, what specific problem it is prescribed for, and any side effects or benefits experienced should be elicited; this should also apply to past medicines as well. It is also critical to obtain similar information about any over-the-counter medicines, including herbal remedies, vitamins, and other nonprescribed medications; many patients do not consider these "medicines" and might not report these unless specifically questioned about them. Drug allergies or reactions should also be noted. A review of the complete medication list with particular attention to medications that may interact and/or are known to have significant effects on cognition (e.g., anticholinergics, pain medications, lithium) is important as cognitive impairment can be observed due to medication side effects alone. This is particularly true in the elderly who generally require lower doses of medications due to decreased metabolism and thus are more susceptible to medication side effects. Enhanced susceptibility to the effects of neuroleptic medications may be suggestive of underlying DLB, whereas enhanced agitation or delirium in the context of anesthesia or other medications affecting the CNS may be more likely in individuals with underlying cognitive impairment, irrespective of etiology. The review of previous medications might also be important due to long-term side effects; for example, tardive dyskinesia may be secondary to psychotropic use.

Family medical history

The family medical history (FHM) should be relatively comprehensive, generally including information about parents, siblings, grandparents, and children, including age at death, developmental delay, mental retardation, neurological disease, psychiatric disease, autoimmune disorders, cardiovascular risk factors, cancer, "odd" behaviors, and "suspicious" early deaths. Based on the differential or any trends for concern, the history might need to be expanded to include cousins, aunts/uncles, and great aunts/uncles. Issues in younger generations (i.e., autism, polycystic ovary syndrome, mental retardation, spontaneous abortion) may have relevance to older family members (i.e., FXTAS) [48]. If a condition might be genetic in origin, this should prompt consideration of genetic counseling and testing. It is important to recall that many genetic disorders present heterogeneously, even within the same family, despite a common underlying genetic predisposition (i.e., some family members with tau mutations may have CBS, while others have bvFTD or PSP) [49, 50].

Social history

If relevant, social history should include birth history (prematurity, anoxic birth injury) and developmental milestones, particularly for younger patients. Educational history should include the highest level of education obtained, relative strengths and weaknesses, the need to repeat specific classes or grades, and learning disability/attention difficulties (even if not diagnosed as such). A history of childhood illness, trauma, or seizures should be explored. Occupational history should note frequency of job change and any history of being terminated and the reasons, as well as any specific difficulties in the workplace. The history of marriages and relationships can provide important information about personality and behavior. Current use and past history of illicit substance use and abuse, including alcohol, should be established. When inquiring about alcohol, it can be important to determine the precise amount being consumed (i.e., how large are the glasses of alcohol being consumed?).

Neurological examination

General appearance

Level of personal hygiene (neglected vs. well groomed) is an important indicator of self-care abilities. Poor color matching or unusual color/print choice may be seen in bvFTD (particularly right temporal variants) and related disorders [51]. The accuracy of shaving and applying makeup, improper buttoning, or putting clothes on incorrectly may suggest visual-perceptual and/or motor deficits.

Cranial nerve examination

The cranial nerve examination should include a thorough examination of ocular motor function (including smoothness of visual pursuit, velocity and latency of saccades, presence of square wave jerks or nystagmus) [52–54], assessment of gag or swallowing reflex, and an examination of extraneous tongue, palate, or facial movements (for HD, or tongue wasting/fasciculations often observed in ALS). Evidence of asymmetry may suggest focal lesions, such as underlying vascular injury.

Motor examination

The motor examination should include not just strength, but bulk (particularly important for ALS; do not forget to check distal extremities and oropharynx), limb and axial tone (important in PSP and atypical parkinsonian disorders), fine rapid alternating movements, and apraxia testing (both limb (i.e., show me how you would hold a nail in your left hand and hammer with your right), oral buccal (blowing a kiss or out a match), and speech (i.e., repeating multisyllabic words such as "catastrophe" five times and listening for phonemic distortion or frank substitution of syllables)). Slowed rapid movements often suggest pyramidal involvement. Dysdiadochokinesis or irregular movements might suggest cerebellar dysfunction, and small or micro movements are often seen in parkinsonian disorders. Often, focal motor symptom abnormalities can be elicited on gait exam; reduced arm swing (asymmetric or symmetric) and/or focal limb posturing (particularly with distraction maneuvers by having the patient walk on the outside or lateral aspects of their feet) is often seen with basal ganglia abnormalities in atypical parkinsonian syndromes. Postural instability should be tested by retropulsion pull testing, making sure there is adequate room behind the examiner for a proper test. Signs of upper and lower motor neuron involvement should be carefully evaluated, particularly in bvFTD syndromes in which ALS might co-occur; a proper exam for fasciculations should be completed with the patient undressed, such as in a gown. Although myoclonus is classically seen in CJD, it also is common in DLB and CBS [55–58], as well as in some autoimmune and metabolic encephalopathies [59].

Sensory examination

Some dementias, particularly genetic etiologies, including SCAs, leukodystrophies, APBD, and certain prion gene mutations, can be associated with neuropathies. Large fiber neuropathies should raise concern for a B12 deficiency and should prompt looking for other associated features. The effects of long-standing diabetes may also contribute to neuropathy, particularly involving small fiber nerves.

Cerebellar examination

A standard cerebellar examination is warranted in any atypical dementia patient. Examination should include a thorough assessment of eye movements (looking for any restriction of gaze, nystagmus, etc.); dysdiadochokinesia of hands, feet, or speech; limb dysmetria; and gait and balance. Many genetic dementias, including SCAs, Huntington's, lysosomal storage diseases, and prion diseases, are associated with cerebellar involvement. The recently described FTD–ALS syndrome due to the hexanucleotide repeat expansion in C9orf72 has been associated with cerebellar atrophy on MRI [60].

Neuropsychological testing

In our experience, neuropsychological testing (whether a brief or extended battery) optimally is conducted within the context of a same-day clinic visit to allow for integration of a multidisciplinary evaluation including the history, neurological findings, and caregiver assessment, in addition to MRI and laboratory results. Neuropsychological testing provides a quantitative method for assessing the integrity of various cognitive domains (i.e., memory, language, frontal executive, visuospatial, etc.). Results often mirror patient and caregiver complaints but might also suggest additional or more significant impairment that would have been predicted by the history. The pattern of neuropsychological test results can suggest specific underlying diagnoses or at least narrow the differential (i.e., parkinsonism on exam and vague cognitive complaints per history). For example, prominent fluctuations in attention and visuospatial difficulties may suggest DLB, whereas on language assessment, logopenic aphasia might suggest an AD pathology, and a nonfluent aphasia is more suggestive of CBD, PSP, or another tauopathy [23].

Although the scores themselves are important, the behavioral observations associated with performance also are crucial and provide an important source of information regarding the etiology of impairment on a specific test. For example, when performing an object naming task, there may be difficulties secondary to speech apraxia, semantic loss, visual difficulties, and/or an inability to focus on the task secondary to behavioral disturbances, with each finding suggestive of a differing underlying neuroanatomy. Thus, knowing the final score is often not sufficient; it is important to know specifically how a patient has done poorly on a task.

There are several brief cognitive screening measures exist that can be utilized in the clinic [61], including the MMSE [62] and the MoCA (www.mocatest.org) [63]. MMSE scores below 26 have historically been used to identify those with cognitive impairment, and many use a cutoff of less than 24 for dementia [64]. Unfortunately, the MMSE has reduced sensitivity to subtle cognitive impairment, and many patients with prominent behavioral or executive dysfunction will perform normally (i.e., bvFTD, PSP, CBD) [65]. Furthermore, as the MMSE is a very language-based test, patients with language deficits often do substantially worse on it, making them appear to have more clinical and functional impairment than they actually have [65]. The MoCA was developed to include more tests of executive function as well as a more difficult memory task (5-word vs. 3-word recall). A cut-off score below 26 still represents mild cognitive impairment (MCI), and the MoCA has been shown to be more sensitive with less of a ceiling effect than the MMSE particularly for cognitive dysfunction in many disorders, particularly those with prominent frontal-executive dysfunction [66–68]. Unfortunately, although the MMSE and MoCA are beneficial in clinical settings requiring rapid screening and evaluation, they are necessarily limited in their ability to comprehensively assess cognitive impairment and may not detect more subtle dementia or MCI [67].

In our clinic, typically a 1 h "bedside" neuropsychological evaluation is conducted by a trained examiner (physician, neuropsychologist, or even an assistant). This bedside evaluation examines memory using a word list learning task [1] and figure recall, language through naming, verbal fluency, sentence repetition, apraxia of speech and semantic knowledge, visuospatial skills using figure copy and a visual discrimination task, and attention and executive function with the Stroop interference, modified (simplified) trail making tests, design fluency, and digit span forwards and backwards [4]. Mood is assessed with a patient-reported depression screen (i.e., Geriatric Depression Scale (GDS)) and also via informant-rated questionnaires (i.e., Neuropsychiatric Inventory (NPI)) [10, 69]. Informant-rated questionnaires such as the Frontal Systems Behavior Scale (FrSBE) can also be useful for quantifying the level of apathy, disinhibition, and executive dysfunction [70], which may be underrecognized by the patient due to loss of insight. The identification of deficits in a specific cognitive arena (i.e., visuospatial) may prompt the administration of other tests in order to more fully characterize the impairment.

Additionally, it may be appropriate at times to refer patients for more comprehensive neuropsychological testing (i.e., 2–6 h), particularly if complaints are vague and subtle and/or patients are young, for which screening tests are less sensitive. A demonstration of subtle levels of impairment may not be diagnostic early in the course of the disease (i.e., early difficulties with executive function can progress to bvFTD, PSP, CBD, PD, or frontal version of AD, among others); however, at the least, a comprehensive evaluation serves as a useful baseline that can then be used to demonstrate stability versus cognitive decline over successive test sessions. This is particularly important in individuals of high premorbid intellect, as "average" performances in these individuals may actually represent a significant decline with respect to their premorbid level of performance. Comprehensive neuropsychological evaluations are also of benefit in assisting with work accommodations, recommendations for intervention, and disability applications.

Laboratory testing

A basic dementia blood screen is recommended. The American Academy of Neurology (AAN) guidelines recommend the following testing in the routine evaluation of a patient with dementia: complete blood count (CBC), serum electrolytes (we include calcium, magnesium, and phosphorus), creatinine, blood urea nitrogen (BUN), glucose, thyroid function tests (TFTs), liver function tests (LFTs), and vitamin B12 (http://tools.aan.com/professionals/practice/pdfs/dementia_guideline.pdf). Although screening for syphilis is not recommended by current AAN guidelines because of the low positive rate (unless patient has a specific risk factor, e.g., living in a high-incidence region), because it is a treatable disorder, we recommend screening for syphilis with an nontreponemal test, such as with rapid plasma reagin (RPR), although a treponemal-specific test is often preferred and cerebrospinal fluid (CSF) must be analyzed when neurosyphilis is suspected (please refer to Chapter 13 for additional details) [71]. If vascular disease is a potential etiology, include a fasting lipid panel, homocysteine, and possibly methylmalonic acid. For rapidly progressive dementias, additional lab testing is required [72].

CSF

CSF analysis can be very helpful for diagnosis in certain dementias. In most typical dementias, CSF is not tested routinely, but there are certain cases in which CSF testing is helpful or even necessary. If inflammatory etiologies, infections, mitochondrial disorders, neoplasms, prion disease, or other rapid dementias are in the differential, CSF analysis is required. If AD is in the differential but the diagnosis is unclear and/or there are some atypical features, CSF testing for abeta amyloid, total tau (t-tau), and phosphorylated tau (p-tau) levels can be helpful; in AD, there are often very low abeta amyloid and mild to moderately elevated t-tau and p-tau levels. At our center, because of the increasing incidence of autoimmune/inflammatory etiologies for dementia, we routinely test for IgG index and oligoclonal bands in most patients with atypical dementias. For rapidly progressive dementias, in addition to testing for the aforementioned, we recommend testing for t-tau, neuron-specific enolase, and 14-3-3 as markers of rapidly neuronal injury (not because of their utility in diagnosing CJD); as noted in Chapter 9 on prion disease, these CSF biomarkers should be interpreted with caution. A new assay, RT-QuIC, however, seems to have relatively high specificity (as high as 98%) in CSF for diagnosing sCJD. Although not discussed in this text, if normal pressure hydrocephalus (NPH) is in the differential, a large volume tap (~30 or more cc) is recommended with pre- and post-gait and/or balance assessment.

Genetic testing

A positive FMH suggesting autosomal dominant inheritance or the presence of multiple affected family members may suggest a need for genetic testing for confirmation of genetic status (i.e., mutation and/or relevant polymorphism). As many neurogenetic dementias present with great variability even within the same family and often not just cognitive symptoms, the clinician should inquire about a FMH of other symptoms, such as psychiatric illness or peripheral nervous system dysfunction

[73]. For example, a FMH of mental retardation or miscarriage in a patient with cognitive impairment, tremor, and/or ataxia might be indicative of FXTAS [74], or premature ovarian failure in a leukodystrophy might indicate mutations in eIF2B causing vanishing white matter disease [75]. As autosomal recessive disorders can also cause atypical dementia, inquiring about any consanguinity and the ethnic backgrounds of both biological parents is important for consideration of genetic etiologies.

Consideration of genetic testing ideally should be performed with the assistance of a genetic counselor or physician with experience in genetic testing, optimally one with expertise in neurological conditions. Counseling regarding the specific genetic tests being performed, the implications of the test, and the desire of each family member to know the results should be performed prior to initiating the testing. Disclosure of the results ideally should take place with the assistance of a genetic counselor or equivalently trained physician [76]. The Genetic Information Nondiscrimination Act (GINA), passed in 2008 in the United States, has made it illegal for bias or discrimination in health insurance or employment on the basis of genetic testing alone. It is our experience, however, that obtaining specific types of health insurance or long-term care policies may best be done prior to undergoing genetic testing or receiving genetic results [77]. Please refer to each individual chapter regarding appropriate genetic tests for suspected conditions.

Neuroimaging

Brain MRI has largely supplanted head CT as a critical tool in the evaluation of atypical dementia, as the MRI is more sensitive to focal atrophy, neuroanatomy, white matter abnormalities, and abnormalities not detected at all by CT, such as restricted diffusion. There is no "approved" or standard protocol for MRI in dementia. At our center, we generally recommend acquiring at least the following: T1 (axial, coronal, and sagittal if possible), T2 and FLAIR axial (coronal is also helpful for the evaluation of hippocampal MTL pathology, whereas sagittal is helpful for the evaluation of corpus callosum and demyelinating disease), and a hemosiderin sequence, such as gradient echo (GRE) or susceptibility weighted imaging (SWI). If stroke, intravascular processes, demyelination, thiamine deficiency, or prion disease is on the differential, diffusion weighted imaging (DWI) and attenuation diffusion coefficient (ADC) maps are necessary. If there are focal abnormalities on exam or there is concern for a process involving breakdown of the blood–brain barrier (BBB), at least one sequence with contrast should be done. MRI protocols as well as findings supportive of certain conditions will be discussed under each chapter.

Brain positron emission tomography (PET) or SPECT scans can be useful to delineate areas of low glucose utilization or hypoperfusion, which is sometimes helpful for diagnosis, particularly if trying to differentiate between conditions with different anatomical involvement. The advent of ligands for ß-amyloid and tau has increased the clinical utility of PET scans. Certain ligands are only available in research or not widely available due to short radioactive half-lives (but F18-labeled antibodies against ß-amyloid are now clinically approved in the United States with florbetapir (Amyvid)). Florbetapir can be helpful in early-onset dementia patients when trying to distinguish between an AD and FTD etiology.

Body imaging

When antibody-mediated or antibody-associated syndromes are identified or being considered, a neoplasm workup is often required, as some of these are often paraneoplastic. This typically would involve whole-body CT with contrast and/or whole-body PET/CT. More focused examinations such as MRI of the breast, testicular ultrasound, or transvaginal ultrasound might be indicated based on the type of tumor suspected. PET scans may be beneficial in cases in which a paraneoplastic syndrome is suspected and no clear cause (or suspected cause) is identified by other body imaging.

Other tests

Electroencephalogram (EEG) is necessary to rule out seizures or nonconvulsive status epilepticus. EEG also can be helpful in trying to determine if a syndrome is neurological or psychiatric. For example, patients with focal or diffuse cognitive deficits often show commensurate slowing of EEG activity.
Electromyogram (EMG) is essential for the diagnosis of motor neuron disease (MND) or other neuromuscular disorders. It is particularly useful when considering FTD syndromes that often have concurrent MND, such as due to the C9orf72 mutations.

Putting it all together: Multidisciplinary assessment/review

After the multidisciplinary assessment, including patient/caregiver interview(s), neurological exam, and neuropsychological testing, is complete, it is helpful to have a group meeting among all involved staff to discuss the case, develop a differential, determine the likely diagnosis, additional assessments/testing, and propose a treatment and management plan. We have found that it is best to do the assessment and presentation of findings and conclusions to the patient/caregiver on the same day. It is helpful to provide the patient and caregivers additional reading material or resources (e.g., websites, support groups, etc.) to learn more about the diagnosis on their own time. Depending on the diagnosis and/or clinician preference, one might provide suggestions and leave management to the referring or primary care physician or plan a follow-up visit to review any recommended or ordered tests. For detailed description regarding the management of patients with atypical dementia, please refer to Chapter 15. In our clinic, we find that having the family/caregivers interviewed separately from the patient at some point is helpful, as they can provide information that might be comfortable or possible to present in front of the patient. When a diagnosis is made and treatment trials are being considered, a useful website to find out about ongoing studies in the United States (and often internationally) is www.clinicaltrials.gov.

References

1 Delis DC, Kramer JH, Kaplan E, et al. (2000) *California Verbal Learning Test*. 2nd edn., The Psychological Corporation; San Antonio, TX.

2 Brandt J, Benedict R. 2001 *Hopkins Verbal Learning Test-Revised: Professional Manual*. Psychological Assessment Resources (PAR); Odessa, FL.

3 Wechsler D. (2009) *Wechsler Memory Scale*. 4th edn., The Psychological Corporation; San Antonio, TX.

4 Krueger CE, Kramer JH. (2010) Neurocognitive assessment. *Continuum (Minneap Minn)* **16**:2, 176–90.

5 Bonelli RM, Cummings JL. (2008) Frontal-subcortical dementias. *Neurologist* **14**:2, 100–7.

6 Lee SE, Rabinovici GD, Mayo MC, et al. (2011) Clinicopathological correlations in corticobasal degeneration. *Ann Neurol* **70**:2, 327–40.

7 Schneider SA, Walker RH, Bhatia KP. (2007) The Huntington's disease-like syndromes: what to consider in patients with a negative Huntington's disease gene test. *Nat Clin Pract Neurol* **3**:9, 517–25.

8 Lorincz MT. (2006) Geriatric chorea. *Clin Geriatr Med* **22**:4, 879–97, vii.

9 Baek WS, Desai NP. (2007) ALS: pitfalls in the diagnosis. *Pract Neurol* **7**:2, 74–81.

10 Cummings JL. (1997) The Neuropsychiatric Inventory: assessing psychopathology in dementia patients. *Neurology* **48**:5 Suppl 6, S10–S6.

11 Claassen DO, Josephs KA, Ahlskog JE, et al. (2010) REM sleep behavior disorder preceding other aspects of synucleinopathies by up to half a century. *Neurology* **75**:6, 494–9.

12 Rascovsky K, Hodges JR, Knopman D, et al. (2011) Sensitivity of revised diagnostic criteria for the behavioral variant of frontotemporal dementia. *Brain* **134**:Pt 9, 2456–77.

13 Kertesz A, Jesso S, Harciarek M, et al. (2010) What is semantic dementia?: a cohort study of diagnostic features and clinical boundaries. *Arch Neurol* **67**:4, 483–9.

14 Rosen HJ, Allison SC, Ogar JM, et al. (2006) Behavioral features in semantic dementia vs. other forms of progressive aphasias. *Neurology* **67**:10, 1752–6.

15 Seeley WW, Bauer AM, Miller BL, et al. (2005) The natural history of temporal variant frontotemporal dementia. *Neurology* **64**:8, 1384–90.

16 Rankin KP, Gorno-Tempini ML, Allison SC, et al. (2006) Structural anatomy of empathy in neurodegenerative disease. *Brain* **129**:Pt 11, 2945–56.

17 Gerstenecker A, Duff K, Mast B, et al. (2013) Behavioral abnormalities in progressive supranuclear palsy. *Psychiatry Res* **210**:3, 1205–10.

18 Yatabe Y, Hashimoto M, Kaneda K, et al. (2011) Neuropsychiatric symptoms of progressive supranuclear palsy in a dementia clinic. *Psychogeriatrics* **11**:1, 54–9.

19 Stanton BR, Leigh PN, Howard RJ, et al. (2013) Behavioral and emotional symptoms of apathy are associated with distinct patterns of brain atrophy in neurodegenerative disorders. *J Neurol* **260**:10, 2481–90.

20 Rosen HJ, Allison SC, Schauer GF, et al. (2005) Neuroanatomical correlates of behavioral disorders in dementia. *Brain* **128**:11, 2612–25.

21 Landes AM, Sperry SD, Strauss ME, et al. (2001) Apathy in Alzheimer's disease. *J Am Geriatr Soc* **49**:12, 1700–7.

22 Levenson RW, Sturm VE, Haase CM. (2014) Emotional and behavioral symptoms in neurodegenerative disease: a model for studying the neural bases of psychopathology. *Annu Rev Clin Psychol* **10**: 581–606.

23 Gorno-Tempini ML, Dronkers NF, Rankin KP, et al. (2004) Cognition and anatomy in three variants of primary progressive aphasia. *Ann Neurol* **55**:3, 335–46.

24 Gorno-Tempini ML, Brambati SM, Ginex V, et al. (2008) The logopenic/phonological variant of primary progressive aphasia. *Neurology* **71**:16, 1227–34.

25 Rohrer JD, Knight WD, Warren JE, et al. (2008) Word-finding difficulty: a clinical analysis of the progressive aphasias. *Brain* **131**:Pt 1, 8–38.

26 Gorno-Tempini ML, Hillis AE, Weintraub S, et al. (2011) Classification of primary progressive aphasia and its variants. *Neurology* **76**:11, 1006–14.

27 Crutch SJ, Lehmann M, Schott JM, et al. (2012) Posterior cortical atrophy. *Lancet Neurol* **11**:2, 170–8.

28 Jacobs DA, Lesser RL, Mourelatos Z, et al. (2001) The Heidenhain variant of Creutzfeldt-Jakob disease: clinical, pathologic, and neuro-imaging findings. *J Neuroophthalmol* **21**:2, 99–102.

29 McMonagle P, Deering F, Berliner Y, et al. (2006) The cognitive profile of posterior cortical atrophy. *Neurology* **66**:3, 331–8.

30 Zakzanis KK, Boulos MI. (2001) Posterior cortical atrophy. *Neurologist* **7**:6, 341–9.

31 McKeith IG, Dickson DW, Lowe J, et al. (2005) Diagnosis and management of dementia with Lewy bodies: third report of the DLB Consortium. *Neurology* **65**:12, 1863–72.

32 Chow TW, Cummings JL. (2007) Frontal-subcortical circuits. In: Miller B, editor. *The Frontal Lobes*, 2nd edn., The Guilford Press; New York, pp. 3–26.

33 Tekin S, Cummings JL. (2002) Frontal-subcortical neuronal circuits and clinical neuropsychiatry: an update. *J Psychosom Res* **53**:2, 647–54.

34 Koziol LF, Budding D, Andreasen N, et al. (2014) Consensus paper: the cerebellum's role in movement and cognition. *Cerebellum* **13**:1, 151–77.

35 Mioshi E, Kipps CM, Dawson K, et al. (2007) Activities of daily living in frontotemporal dementia and Alzheimer disease. *Neurology* **68**:24, 2077–84.

36 Knopman DS, Kramer JH, Boeve BF, et al. (2008) Development of methodology for conducting clinical trials in frontotemporal lobar degeneration. *Brain* **131**:Pt 11, 2957–68.

37 Mehta KM, Ott A, Kalmijn S, et al. (1999) Head trauma and risk of dementia and Alzheimer's disease: the Rotterdam study. *Neurology* **53**:9, 1959–62.

38 Janelsins MC, Kesler SR, Ahles TA, et al. (2014) Prevalence, mechanisms, and management of cancer-related cognitive impairment. *Int Rev Psychiatry* **26**:1, 102–13.

39 Tallet AV, Azria D, Barlesi F, et al. (2012) Neurocognitive function impairment after whole brain radiotherapy for brain metastases: actual assessment. *Radiat Oncol* **7**, 77.

40 Greene-Schloesser D, Robbins ME. (2012) Radiation-induced cognitive impairment—from bench to bedside. *Neuro Oncol* **14** Suppl 4, iv37–44.

41 Jicha GA, Schmitt FA, Abner E, et al. (2010) Prodromal clinical manifestations of neuropathologically confirmed Lewy body disease. *Neurobiol Aging* **31**:10, 1805–13.

42 Moretti R, Torre P, Antonello RM, et al. (2004) Cholinesterase inhibition as a possible therapy for delirium in vascular dementia: a controlled, open 24-month study of 246 patients. *Am J Alzheimers Dis Other Demen* **19**:6, 333–9.

43 Girard C, Simard M, Noiseux R, et al. (2011) Late-onset-psychosis: cognition. *Int Psychogeriatr* **23**:8, 1301–16.

44 Castle DJ, Murray RM. (1993) The epidemiology of late-onset schizophrenia. *Schizophr Bull* **19**:4, 691–700.

45 Viswanath B, Harihara SN, Nahar A, et al. (2013) Battery for ECT Related Cognitive Deficits (B4ECT-ReCoDe): development and validation. *Asian J Psychiatr* **6**:3, 243–8.

46 Rose D, Fleischmann P, Wykes T, et al. (2003) Patients' perspectives on electroconvulsive therapy: systematic review. *BMJ* **326**: 7403, 1363.

47 Bergsholm P. (2012) Patients' perspectives on electroconvulsive therapy: a reevaluation of the review by Rose et al. on memory loss after electroconvulsive therapy. *J ECT* **28**:1, 27–30.

48 Jacquemont S, Hagerman RJ, Hagerman PJ, et al. (2007) Fragile-X syndrome and fragile X-associated tremor/ataxia syndrome: two faces of FMR1. *Lancet Neurol* **6**:1, 45–55.

49 Bugiani O, Murrell JR, Giaccone G, et al. (1999) Frontotemporal dementia and corticobasal degeneration in a family with a P301S mutation in tau. *J Neuropathol Exp Neurol* **58**:6, 667–77.

50 Rademakers R, Cruts M, van Broeckhoven C. (2004) The role of tau (MAPT) in frontotemporal dementia and related tauopathies. *Hum Mutat* **24**:4, 277–95.

51 Edwards-Lee T, Miller BL, Benson DF, et al. (1997) The temporal variant of frontotemporal dementia. *Brain* **120**:Pt 6, 1027–40.

52 McCarten JR. (2013) Clinical evaluation of early cognitive symptoms. *Clin Geriatr Med* **29**:4, 791–807.

53 Garbutt S, Matlin A, Hellmuth J, et al. (2008) Oculomotor function in frontotemporal lobar degeneration, related disorders and Alzheimer's disease. *Brain* **131**:Pt 5, 1268–81.

54 Hellmuth J, Mirsky J, Heuer HW, et al. (2012) Multicenter validation of a bedside antisaccade task as a measure of executive function. *Neurology* **78**:23, 1824–31.

55 Litvan I, Agid Y, Goetz C, et al. (1997) Accuracy of the clinical diagnosis of corticobasal degeneration: a clinicopathologic study. *Neurology* **48**:1, 119–25.

56 Petersen RC. (1998) Clinical subtypes of Alzheimer's disease. *Dement Geriatr Cogn Disord* **9**:Suppl 3, 16–24.

57 Tartaglia MC, Johnson DY, Thai JN, et al. (2012) Clinical overlap between Jakob-Creutzfeldt disease and Lewy body disease. *Can J Neurol Sci* **39**:3, 304–10.

58 Tschampa HJ, Neumann M, Zerr I, et al. (2001) Patients with Alzheimer's disease and dementia with Lewy bodies mistaken for Creutzfeldt-Jakob disease. *J Neurol Neurosurg Psychiatry* **71**:1, 33–9.

59 Geschwind MD, Tan KM, Lennon VA, et al. (2008) Voltage-gated potassium channel autoimmunity mimicking Creutzfeldt-Jakob disease. *Arch Neurol* **65**:10, 1341–6.

60 Yokoyama JS, Rosen HJ. (2012) Neuroimaging features of C9ORF72 expansion. *Alzheimers Res Ther* **4**:6, 45.

61 Mitchell AJ, Malladi S. (2010) Screening and case finding tools for the detection of dementia. Part I: evidence-based meta-analysis of multidomain tests. *Am J Geriatr Psychiatry* **18**:9, 759–82.

62 Folstein MF, Folstein SE, McHugh PR. (1975) "Mini-mental state." A practical method for grading the cognitive state of patients for the clinician. *J Psychiatr Res* **12**:3, 189–98.

63 Nasreddine ZS, Phillips NA, Bedirian V, et al. (2005) The Montreal Cognitive Assessment, MoCA: a brief screening tool for mild cognitive impairment. *J Am Geriatr Soc* **53**:4, 695–9.

64 Mitchell AJ. (2009) A meta-analysis of the accuracy of the mini-mental state examination in the detection of dementia and mild cognitive impairment. *J Psychiatr Res* **43**:4, 411–31.

65 Tan KS, Libon DJ, Rascovsky K, et al. (2013) Differential longitudinal decline on the mini-mental state examination in frontotemporal lobar degeneration and Alzheimer disease. *Alzheimer Dis Assoc Disord* **27**:4, 310–5.

66 Zadikoff C, Fox SH, Tang-Wai DF, et al. (2008) A comparison of the mini mental state exam to the Montreal cognitive assessment in identifying cognitive deficits in Parkinson's disease. *Mov Disord* **23**:2, 297–9.

67 Hoops S, Nazem S, Siderowf AD, et al. (2009) Validity of the MoCA and MMSE in the detection of MCI and dementia in Parkinson disease. *Neurology* **73**:21, 1738–45.

68 Mickes L, Jacobson M, Peavy G, et al. (2010) A comparison of two brief screening measures of cognitive impairment in Huntington's disease. *Mov Disord* **25**:13, 2229–33.

69 Yesavage JA, Brink TL, Rolse TL, et al. (1983) Development and validity of a Geriatric Depression Scale: a preliminary report. *J Psychiatr Res* **17**, 37–49.

70 Malloy P, Grace J. (2005) A review of rating scales for measuring behavior change due to frontal systems damage. *Cogn Behav Neurol* **18**:1, 18–27.

71 Marra CM. (2014) Neurosyphilis. In: Scheld WM, Whitley RJ, Marra CM, editors. *Infections of the Central Nervous System*, 4th edn., Wolters Kluwer Health; Philadelphia, PA, pp. 659–73.

72 Paterson RW, Takada LT, Geschwind MD. (2012) Diagnosis and treatment of rapidly progressive dementias. *Neurol Clin Pract* **2**:3, 187–200.

73 Goldman JS, Miller BL, Safar J, et al. (2004) When sporadic disease is not sporadic: the potential for genetic etiology. *Arch Neurol* **61**:2, 213–6.

74 Hall DA, Berry-Kravis E, Jacquemont S, et al. (2005) Initial diagnoses given to persons with the fragile X associated tremor/ataxia syndrome (FXTAS). *Neurology* **65**:2, 299–301.

75 Fogli A, Rodriguez D, Eymard-Pierre E, et al. (2003) Ovarian failure related to eukaryotic initiation factor 2B mutations. *Am J Hum Genet* **72**:6, 1544–50.

76 Huntington's Disease Society of America I. Guidelines for genetic testing for Huntington's disease (Revised 1994). 1994 [cited May 8, 2003]; Available from: http://www.hdfoundation.org/html/hdsatest.php.

77 Feldman EA. (2012) The Genetic Information Nondiscrimination Act (GINA): public policy and medical practice in the age of personalized medicine. *J Gen Intern Med* **27**:6, 743–6.

CHAPTER 3

Atypical Alzheimer's disease

Sharon J. Sha[1,2] and Gil D. Rabinovici[1]
[1] University of California, San Francisco, San Francisco, CA, USA
[2] Stanford Center for Memory Disorders, Stanford, CA, USA

Introduction

Alzheimer's disease (AD) is the most common pathologic cause of dementia [1]. Clinically, AD typically presents with early episodic memory loss and visuospatial dysfunction. Less prominent deficits in executive function, attention, and language are common as well. Behavioral disturbances such as psychosis do not typically occur until late disease stages [2]. It is increasingly recognized, however, that AD pathology can be found in patients with nonamnestic clinical presentations [3–5]. AD is the most common cause of posterior cortical atrophy (PCA) [6, 7] and is found to be the causative pathology in 20–50% of patients with corticobasal syndrome (CBS) [3, 8] and in 20–40% of patients with primary progressive aphasia (PPA) [9, 10], focal cortical syndromes that were initially postulated to be pathologically distinct from AD [11–13]. Identifying patients with atypical clinical syndromes who have underlying AD is important clinically as symptomatic therapies are available for AD, but not yet for other degenerative dementias, and disease-specific therapies for AD are on the horizon [14]. Whereas previous criteria for AD included obligatory decline in memory [15], the new criteria propose to include nonamnestic presentations as well [16, 17].

Epidemiology

AD affects 5.2 million people in the United States and 17 million people worldwide [18, 19]. The prevalence of AD is about 1% at age 60–65 and doubles every 5 years, approaching 40% in 85–90-year-olds. The prevalence of atypical presentations of AD is difficult to estimate. Nonamnestic presentations might account for up to 15% of patients seen in dementia referral centers [5]. The average age of onset in patients with atypical syndromes is typically in the 60s [6, 7, 20, 21], and it has been suggested that early age-of-onset AD (EOAD) patients (defined in most studies as under age 65 at symptom onset) are more likely to show nonamnestic presentations [22, 23]. It is not known whether patients with atypical presentations differ from typical patients in disease progression or survival, although rapidly progressive forms of AD recently have been recognized [24].

Diagnosis

In 1984, the National Institute of Neurological Disorders and Stroke–Alzheimer's Disease and Related Disorders Association (NINCDS-ADRDA) working group formulated diagnostic criteria that remained in practice through 2011 (Table 3.1) [15]. The NINCDS-ADRDA criteria had several limitations. First, they were only about 70–80% sensitive and 70% specific compared to pathology [25, 26]. Furthermore, patients with AD who presented with atypical patterns of cognitive impairment often did not meet NINCDS-ADRDA criteria, which require memory impairment as one of the core features. [5] In addition, biomarkers such as molecular, functional, and structural imaging modalities, cerebrospinal fluid (CSF) evaluation, as well as genetic information were not available when these criteria were developed and therefore were not included in the original criteria.

Integrating biomarkers and genetics into diagnostic criteria has been an ongoing process [27]. There are currently two partly overlapping sets of criteria set forth by expert workgroups (Tables 3.1 and 3.2). Both sets of criteria recognize nonamnestic presentations of AD, and both allow the integration of imaging and fluid biomarkers to supplement clinical criteria, but in different ways. The criteria proposed by the US National Institutes of Health National Institute on Aging (NIA) and the Alzheimer's Association (AAS) (NIA-AAS) workgroup allow the diagnosis of probable AD to be made on clinical grounds alone (Table 3.1). If available, biomarkers can be used to supplement the clinical evaluation. Biomarkers are divided into two categories: markers of amyloid beta (Aβ, including CSF $A\beta_{42}$ levels or amyloid positron emission tomography (PET)) and markers of neuronal injury (CSF measures of total or phosphorylated tau, atrophy on MRI or hypometabolism/hypoperfusion on fluorodeoxyglucose

Non-Alzheimer's and Atypical Dementia, First Edition. Edited by Michael D. Geschwind and Caroline Racine Belkoura.
© 2016 John Wiley & Sons, Ltd. Published 2016 by John Wiley & Sons, Ltd.

Table 3.1 1984 NINCDS-ADRDA criteria for probable Alzheimer's disease [15].

1. Insidious onset after age 40 with gradual progression
2. Dementia
3. Deficit in at least 2 areas of cognition (one must include memory) for at least 12 months
4. Progressive worsening of cognition
5. No disturbance of consciousness
6. Other systemic disease or brain disorder does not account for the disease

*Possible AD: atypical onset, presentation, or clinical course of dementia without a systemic disease or brain disorder that could account for the disease

*Definite AD: pathological confirmation by biopsy or autopsy + criteria listed for probable AD

2011 updated clinical criteria for AD [16]

1. Insidious onset with gradual progression
2. Clear-cut history of worsening of cognition by report or observation
3. The initial and most prominent cognitive deficits are evident on history and examination in one of the following categories.
   - Amnestic presentation
   - Nonamnestic presentations:
     - Language presentation
     - Visuospatial presentation
     - Executive dysfunction
4. The diagnosis of probable AD dementia should not be applied when there is evidence of
   - Substantial concomitant cerebrovascular disease
   - Core features of dementia with Lewy bodies
   - Prominent features of behavioral variant frontotemporal dementia
   - Prominent features of semantic variant primary progressive aphasia or nonfluent/ agrammatic variant primary progressive aphasia
   - Other systemic disease or brain disorder accounting for symptoms

Source: Adapted from McKhann et al. [15]. © 2011 by AAN Enterprises, Inc.

Case 1

Mr. M is a 72-year-old right-handed gentleman who has had memory problems for 4 years. He asks repetitive questions, cannot remember plans for business trips, and forgets conversations. Recently, he has had problems with navigation. Executing complex tasks such as cooking has become more difficult. Functionally, he is no longer able to work or drive. His wife has taken over bill paying and assisted him with cooking. He needs reminders to shower but is able to perform all basic activities of daily living (ADLs). Neurological examination is normal. He scores 22/30 on the Mini-Mental Status Examination (MMSE). Neuropsychological testing reveals significant deficits in episodic memory and visuospatial and executive functions. Laboratory tests for thyroid function and B12 are normal. An MRI demonstrates cortical atrophy, primarily in temporoparietal regions, and prominent hippocampal atrophy (Figure 3.1). He passed away at age 77. Autopsy diagnosis is high-likelihood AD (NIA-Reagan; see neuropathology in the following text).

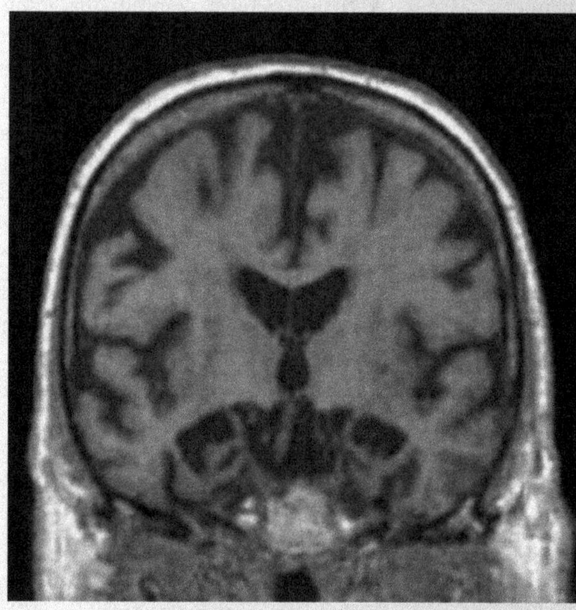

Figure 3.1 Coronal T1-weighted MRI of case 1 showing bilateral hippocampal and less severe frontal and temporal cortical atrophy.

PET (FDG-PET) or single-photon emission computed tomography (SPECT)). Various combinations of these markers modify the likelihood of underlying AD pathophysiology, for example, from low (if biomarkers from both categories are negative) to high (if there are positive markers in both categories) (Table 3.2) [16].

An International Working Group (IWG) has proposed an alternative set of criteria, which require both a suggestive clinical syndrome ("typical" amnestic or "atypical" nonamnestic) and a biomarker evidence of AD pathophysiology by either amyloid PET or CSF $A\beta_{42}$ and tau measures [17]. MRI and FDG-PET/SPECT are conceptualized as "topographical markers" of disease progression, but are not included in the criteria because they are not specific to AD pathophysiology. The IWG criteria are intended to maximize accuracy in research studies but may have limited utility in the clinical setting where access to CSF biomarkers and amyloid PET is limited. Importantly, both sets of criteria also recognize mixed or atypical presentations (which can be distinguished from nonamnestic presentations that are still characteristic of underlying AD, such as PCA or the logopenic variant of PPA).

This case represents a "typical" AD presentation in a patient who developed problems with recent memory in late life. Visuospatial ability, language, and executive function are affected more variably.

Neuropathology

The core neuropathological features of AD are neuritic plaques (NPs) and neurofibrillary tangles (NFTs). NPs are extracellular, florid (flowerlike) appearing structures composed largely of the 42-amino-acid amyloid-beta polypeptide ($A\beta_{1-42}$), a cleavage product of the amyloid precursor protein (APP). Mature NPs have a dense core surrounded by dystrophic neurites; NPs are more specific for AD than the less fibrillar, diffuse plaques often seen in normal aging [28]. Plaques form seemingly simultaneously

Table 3.2 Various criteria for AD incorporating clinical presentation and biomarkers.

Updated AD dementia criteria incorporating biomarkers [16].

Diagnostic Category	**Biomarker probability of AD etiology**	**Aβ (PET or CSF)**	**Neuronal injury (CSF tau, FDG-PET, structural MRI)**
Probable AD dementia			
Based on clinical criteria	Uninformative	Unavailable, conflicting, or indeterminate	Unavailable, conflicting, or indeterminate
With 3 levels of evidence of AD pathophysiological process	Intermediate	Unavailable or indeterminate	Positive
	Intermediate	Positive	Unavailable or indeterminate
	High	Positive	Positive
Possible AD dementia (atypical clinical presentation)			
Based on clinical criteria	Uninformative	Unavailable, conflicting, or indeterminate	Unavailable, conflicting, or indeterminate
With evidence of AD pathophysiological process	High but does not rule out second etiology	Positive	Positive
Dementia unlikely due to AD	Lowest	Negative	Negative

Proposed criteria for typical AD (must have A and B) [17]

A. Presence of early and significant episodic memory impairment that includes:
- Gradual and progressive change in memory function > 6 months
- Objective evidence of an amnestic syndrome of the hippocampal type

B. In vivo evidence of Alzheimer's pathology (one of the following):
- Decreased $A\beta_{1-42}$ together with increased t-tau or p-tau in CSF
- Increased tracer retention on amyloid PET
- AD autosomal dominant mutation present (in *PSEN1*, *PSEN2*, or *APP*)

Exclusion criteria:
- Sudden onset
- Early occurrence of gait disturbances, seizures, and major and prevalent behavioral changes
- Focal neurological signs
- Early extrapyramidal signs
- Early hallucinations
- Cognitive fluctuations
- Non-AD dementia
- Major depression
- Cerebrovascular disease
- Toxic, inflammatory, and metabolic disorders
- MRI FLAIR or T2 signal changes in the medial temporal lobe that are consistent with infectious or vascular insults

Proposed criteria for atypical AD (must have A and B) [17]

A. Specific phenotype (one of the following):
- Posterior variant including an occipitotemporal variant defined by the presence of early, predominant, and progressive impairment of visuoperceptive functions or of visual identification of objects, symbols, words, or faces or a biparietal variant defined by the presence of early, predominant, and progressive difficulty with visuospatial functions, features of Gerstmann's syndrome or Balint's syndrome, limb apraxia, or neglect
- Logopenic variant defined by the presence of early, predominant, and progressive impairment of single-word retrieval and in repetition of sentences in the context of spared semantic, syntactic, and motor speech abilities
- Frontal variant defined by the presence of early, predominant, and progressive behavioral changes including association of primary apathy or behavioral disinhibition or predominant executive dysfunction on cognitive testing
- Down's syndrome variant defined by occurrence of a dementia characterized by early behavioral changes and executive dysfunction in people with Down's syndrome

B. In vivo evidence of Alzheimer's pathology (as noted above)

Exclusion criteria
- Sudden onset
- Early and prevalent episodic memory disorder
- Major depression
- Cerebrovascular disease
- Toxic, inflammatory, or other metabolic disorders

Source: McKhann et al. [16]. Reproduced with permission of Elsevier.

throughout the association isocortex, including parietal, prefrontal, and lateral temporal regions [29, 30]. Primary sensorimotor, visual, and auditory cortices, medial temporal cortex, and hippocampus are relatively spared of plaques in AD. NFTs are flame-shaped, intracellular inclusions composed of hyperphosphorylated species of the microtubule-associated protein tau (MAPT). NFTs first appear in the entorhinal cortex and then spread to limbic and paralimbic regions and to the temporal and parietal neocortex, with later involvement of prefrontal regions. Primary visual and sensorimotor regions are the last to develop pathology [29]. Pathologic criteria for AD include rating the distribution and burden of NPs (using Consortium to Establish a Registry for AD (CERAD) criteria [31]) and NFTs (using Braak staging [29]). Combined CERAD and Braak staging is used to establish NIA-Reagan criteria, which use these pathology ratings to state whether an individual suffered from AD with low, intermediate, or high probability (NIA-Reagan criteria). In 2012, a new set of neuropathological criteria were proposed by the NIA-AAS that integrate Thal Aβ plaque score [30] with traditional CERAD and Braak staging [32].

Genetics

Approximately 1–6% of AD patients present under the age of 65, and 60% of these cases have a positive family history with 13% showing an autosomal dominant pattern [33]. Autosomal dominant AD has been associated with mutations in three genes: -presenilin 1 (PS1, chromosome 14), the most common gene associated with familial AD; presenilin 2 (PS2, chromosome 1), and APP (chromosome 21). Both PS1 and PS2 are components of the gamma-secretase complex that cleaves APP into the toxic species $A\beta_{1-42}$. Mutations in PS1 have been reported to cause early behavioral changes similar to frontotemporal dementia (FTD) [34] and, in some cases, have been associated with Pick bodies, a pathologic feature of FTLD, in addition to AD pathology. Patients with trisomy 21 (Down's syndrome) develop AD pathology in the fourth and fifth decade, likely related to the presence of 3 copies of wild-type APP [35].

APOE, the polymorphic genetic locus for apolipoprotein E on chromosome 19, is the strongest genetic determinant in sporadic AD. There are three allelic variants of APOE: ε3 is the most common, ε2 might decrease the risk of AD, whereas carriers of the ε4 allele are at higher risk for developing the disease [36, 37]. Although the ε3 allele is the most common in the general population, 50–65% of AD patients have at least one ε4 allele [38, 39]. Furthermore, there is a strong gene dose effect, such that ε4 heterozygotes are at approximately threefold greater risk than ε4 noncarriers for developing AD, whereas homozygotes have a 15-fold greater risk [40]. Each ε4 allele is associated with an approximately 10-year younger age of onset [40]. The relationship between APOE genotype and AD phenotype (aside from early age of onset) is not clear. One study found that homozygosity for the ε4 allele was present in 17 of 71 patients presenting with an amnestic phenotype compared to only one patient of 29 patients presenting with nonamnestic phenotype [41]. Another study found a paucity of ε4 carriers (2 out of 10) in patients presenting with PCA [42], but this finding has not been replicated by other groups [6, 43]. A study from our center found no difference in the frequency of APOE ε4 between EOAD patients presenting with typical AD, PCA, or logopenic variant PPA (lvPPA), though the frequency of ε4 carriers was higher in all patient groups compared to controls [20]. Curiously, in European cases of rapidly progressive AD, ε4 carriers were underrepresented [24]. Additional risk factors for sporadic late-onset AD are being uncovered via genome-wide association studies and next-generation sequencing [44].

Structural and functional neuroimaging: MRI, FDG-PET, and SPECT

MRI in typical AD demonstrates atrophy in the areas affected by NFTs, including the hippocampus, medial temporal cortex, lateral temporoparietal cortex, and posterior cingulate/precuneus, with relatively less involvement of dorsolateral prefrontal cortex until advanced disease stages [45, 46]. A similar topographic pattern is seen with FDG-PET (reflecting hypometabolism) and SPECT (reflecting hypoperfusion) [47]. The degree of atrophy correlates with neurofibrillary pathology [48] and with clinical severity and can be used to track clinical progression [49]. It is increasingly recognized that there is a "hippocampal-sparing" endophenotype of AD which deviates from traditional Braak staging in that the medial temporal lobes are spared on imaging and at autopsy. Hippocampal-sparing AD correlates with younger age of onset and a nonamnestic clinical presentation [50, 51].

CSF/amyloid imaging

An exciting recent development in the field has been the emergence and validation of biomarkers for molecular pathology. Patients with AD show decreased levels of $A\beta_{1-42}$ and increased levels of total and phosphorylated tau in the CSF, and a ratio of tau/$A\beta_{1-42}$ can distinguish AD patients from controls with high sensitivity and specificity [52–54]. NPs can be imaged using a variety of PET tracers, including ^{11}C-PIB [55], ^{18}F-florbetapir [56], ^{18}F-flutemetamol [57], ^{18}F-florbetaben [58], and ^{18}F-NAV4694 [59]. Both CSF biomarkers and amyloid PET have been validated against autopsy-confirmed cases [53, 60, 61]. These biomarkers might be helpful for ruling in AD in patients with atypical clinical presentations [45, 62, 63] as will be demonstrated in the vignettes below. More recently, PET tracers specific to NFTs have been developed and used in pilot human studies [64–66]. These tracers will allow us for the first time to see in vivo how amyloid and tau interact with each other and with brain structure and function in aging and AD.

Case 2

Mr. D is a 51-year-old right-handed man with a history of dyslexia who developed word-finding difficulties over the past 4–5 years. When speaking, he loses phonemes (the speech sound in language of which words are represented) at the end of words and occasionally stutters. He has significant problems producing and comprehending long sentences as well as retaining long strings of numbers. Grammar is intact, but spelling is difficult. Memory has started to decline in the past year. He and his family deny any problems with visuospatial or executive function. He has been anxious and irritable. Functionally, he was forced to stop working but remains independent with all basic ADLs. On exam, his speech is hesitant and deliberate with normal syntax. Repetition is significantly impaired—for example, when asked to repeat "the ship crashed into the shore," he states, "the boat crashed into the sand" (video 1). He has word-finding difficulties for which he compensates with circumlocutions (video 2). The remainder of his neurological exam is normal. The MMSE score is 26/30, missing points for repetition and orientation to place. Neuropsychological testing shows significant deficits in naming, repetition, echoic memory (i.e., short-term auditory storage; e.g., digit span forwards), and calculations with only minor deficits in episodic memory and executive functioning. Laboratory studies of vitamin B12 and thyroid function are normal. An MRI demonstrates global atrophy with more prominent atrophy in the left parietal and posterior temporal lobe with normal hippocampal size bilaterally (Figure 3.2). A Pittsburgh compound B PET scan is positive for amyloid. He is started on a trial of donepezil and referred to speech therapy.

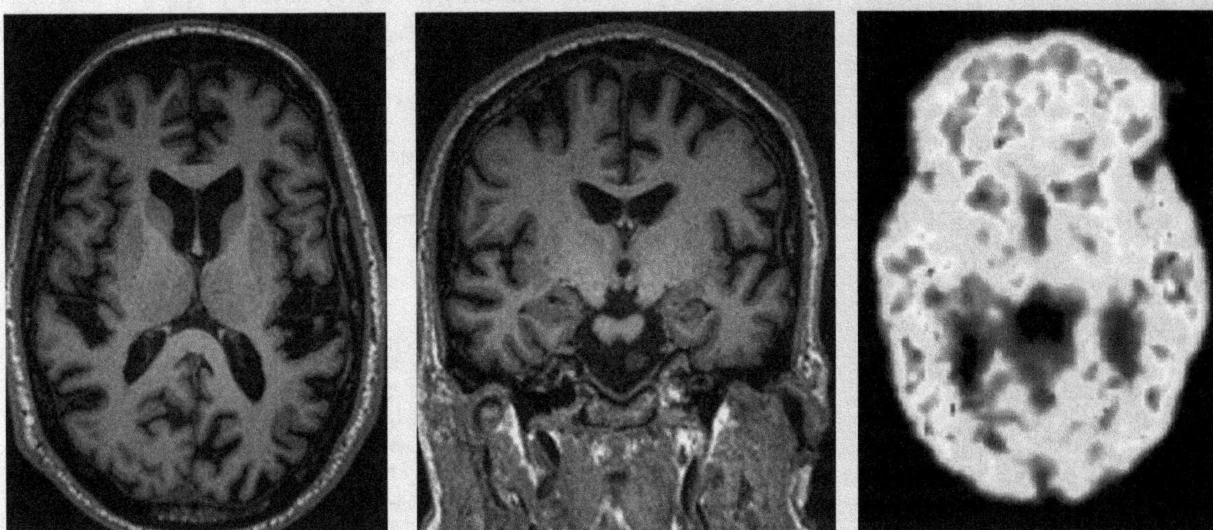

(a) (b) (c)

Figure 3.2 **(a)** Axial T1-weighted MRI of case 2 showing left parietal atrophy. **(b)** Coronal T1-weighted MRI showing normal hippocampal size. **(c)** PIB-PET showing cortical PIB binding (yellow to red indicate increasing spectrum of PIB binding). Orientation of MRIs is radiologic (left is right). Orientation of PET scan is neurological (right is right). (*See insert for color representation of the figure.*)

Table 3.3 Criteria for primary progressive aphasia.

1. Gradual progression of word finding, naming, or comprehension problems
2. No other cognitive domains affected until 2 years after onset with language as the primary deficit (apraxia and acalculia may be present)
3. ADLs limited by language only in the first 2 years
4. No other systemic illness or brain disorder (stroke) accountable for the disease

Source: Adapted from Mesulam [67]. © Wiley.

The patient in case 2 meets Mesulam criteria for PPA as he evolved progressive difficulties with language with relative sparing of other cognitive functions for at least 2 years from symptom onset [67] (Table 3.3). As is often the case, neurodegeneration appears focal and asymmetric. PPA typically is divided into three distinct clinical variants based on the pattern of aphasia: a nonfluent variant (nfvPPA), also referred to as progressive nonfluent aphasia (PNFA), characterized by motor speech deficits and agrammatism; a semantic variant (svPPA), previously referred to as semantic dementia, characterized by fluent speech with loss of meaning for single words; and a logopenic variant (lvPPA), defined by anomia and impaired repetition (especially for long sentences with unpredictable content) with intact grammar, motor speech, and single-word comprehension [69]. Each variant is associated with a selective atrophy pattern with left inferior frontal and perisylvian involvement in nfvPPA, anterior temporal in svPPA, and left temporoparietal junction in lvPPA [21, 62, 68, 69].

Gorno-Tempini and colleagues characterized the language and cognitive deficits in lvPPA in depth and have proposed diagnostic criteria [69] (Table 3.4). Mr. D in case 2 meets core criteria and four supportive features for lvPPA. Furthermore, his MRI and PET qualify for an imaging-supported diagnosis of lvPPA.

Determining the PPA variant can help predict underlying pathology, as AD is frequently the cause of lvPPA, whereas nfvPPA and svPPA are usually associated with FTLD pathology [3, 10].

Table 3.4 Criteria for logopenic variant PPA.

Clinical diagnosis of lvPPA (both core features must be present)
1. Impaired single-word retrieval in spontaneous speech and confrontational naming
2. Impaired repetition of sentences and phrases

At least three of the following other features must be present:
1. Speech (phonological) errors in spontaneous speech and naming
2. Spared single-word comprehension and object knowledge
3. Spared motor speech
4. Absence of frank agrammatism

Imaging-supported diagnosis of lvPPA (both criteria must be present)
1. Clinical diagnosis of lvPPA
2. Imaging must show at least one of the following results:
   - Predominant left posterior perisylvian or parietal atrophy on MRI
   - Predominant left posterior perisylvian or parietal hypoperfusion or hypometabolism on SPECT or PET

lvPPA with definite pathology (clinical diagnosis of LV and 1 or 2 must be present)
1. Histopathological evidence of a specific neurodegenerative pathology (e.g., AD, FTLD-tau, FTLD-TDP, and others)
2. Presence of a known pathogenic mutation

Source: Adapted from Gorno-Tempini 2011 [69]. © 2011 by AAN Enterprises, Inc.

Several studies have shown that the majority of, but not all, lvPPA patients have AD pathology using PIB, autopsy, or CSF biomarkers [62, 70, 71]. Therefore, whereas lvPPA appears to be a marker for AD pathology, the syndrome is pathologically heterogeneous, and both CSF biomarkers and amyloid imaging can be helpful in determining whether AD is the causative pathology. For Mr. D, a positive PIB scan (Figure 3.2) greatly increases the likelihood of AD as the pathologic substrate.

In most studies, PPA patients with pathological AD have been found to have increased NFTs in the left hemisphere [10] compared [72] to the right, though this was not observed in all patients [5]. Results regarding plaque distribution have been more variable, with some studies reporting a left-sided predominance in PPA [5] and others finding a symmetric distribution of plaques indistinguishable from a typical AD pattern [10, 62].

Ms. S meets criteria for the clinical syndrome PCA [73]. Frank Benson and colleagues coined the term describing five patients with deficits in "high visual function" leading to dementia [12].

Case 3

Ms. S is a 62-year-old right-handed woman with a 5-year history of visuospatial dysfunction. She began having difficulty driving at night and found several dents on her car. She began bumping into doors and cabinets on her right side and had difficulty deciding whether to push or pull doors to open them. She became unable to read. Writing has also been difficult, as she tends to write letters on top of one another. She does not get lost in familiar environments but has had problems finding public restrooms on her own. She describes difficulty finding her mascara among her other makeup accessories on the dresser which are right in front of her. She needs more time to plan and organize her activities and, in the past 6 months, has had trouble multitasking. She denies memory or language impairment. Her mood is good, but she describes visual hallucinations of cats or a human figure in her room at night. Functionally, she is still able to perform instrumental ADLs (IADLs), but for the past 6 months, she has asked her husband to verify her management of finances. She has stopped driving. On exam, her MMSE is 26/30. She has difficulty reading words. She focuses on details but has difficulty appreciating the gestalt when describing a picture (i.e., simultagnosia). She has intact visual acuity, full visual fields, and no extinction to simultaneous bilateral visual stimulation. Neuropsychological testing shows significant impairments in visuospatial function and constructional praxis (Figure 3.3a). An MRI shows significant atrophy in the parietal, posterior temporal, and occipital cortex, right greater than left, with slight hippocampal atrophy and scattered white matter disease (Figure 3.3b and c). FDG-PET reveals hypometabolism in the parietal, posterior temporal, and lateral occipital cortex. PIB-PET shows diffuse cortical PIB binding. She is started on donepezil. Occupational therapy for the visually impaired is recommended.

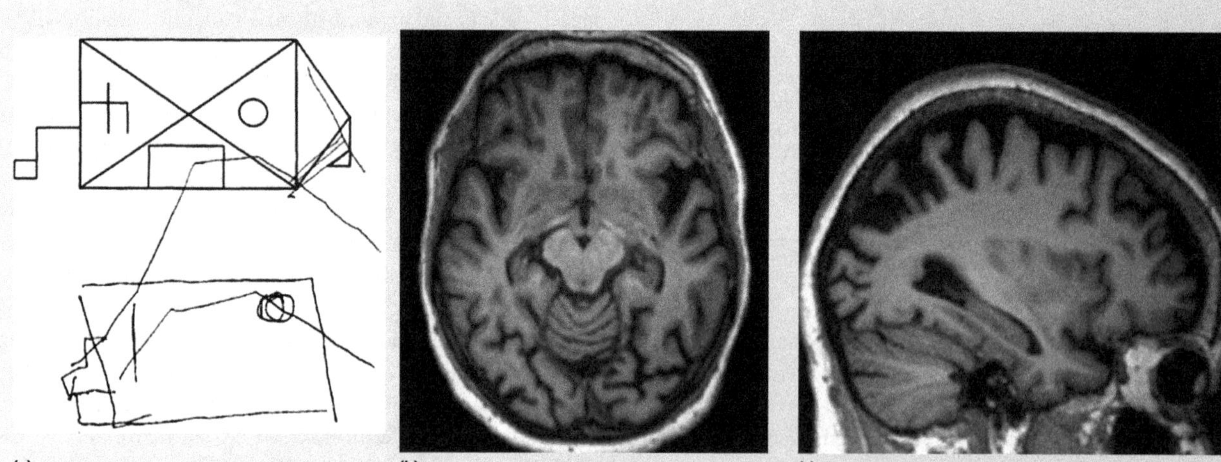

(a) (b) (c)

Figure 3.3 **(a)** Benson Figure (top) with patient copy (bottom). **(b)** Axial T1-weighted MRI showing occipital atrophy. **(c)** Sagittal T1-weighted MRI showing parietal and occipital atrophy. Orientation is radiologic.

All patients had problems with visuospatial function but had intact visual acuity and visual fields. Many patients developed agnosia, alexia, agraphia, anomia, and components of Balint's syndrome (simultanagnosia, optic ataxia, oculomotor apraxia) or Gerstmann's syndrome (agraphia, finger agnosia, right–left confusion, acalculia). Benson noted that memory and judgment were intact until later in the course of the disease. Insight is typically preserved [43, 74]. Later in the course, patients may develop parkinsonism, alien limb, or asymmetric limb apraxia, and these may suggest a non-AD pathologic substrate. The mean age of onset in PCA is in the late 50s/early 60s in most series, with a mean duration from symptom onset to diagnosis of approximately 4 years [6, 43, 75]. One study found a female predominance in PCA compared to AD [6], but this was not replicated in other series [43, 75]. Neuropsychological testing typically shows impairments in visuospatial tasks, spatial memory, alexia, agraphia, and variable performance on construction and calculations compared to AD patients [6, 43, 76]. Memory testing is relatively spared compared to typical AD [43, 75], whereas language function is similar to typical AD patients. There are no consensus clinical criteria for PCA, and we thus list criteria proposed by the two separate groups below (Table 3.5).

In Benson et al.'s original series of five cases, three patients showed PCA on brain imaging as determined by qualitative assessment [12]. Subsequent imaging studies comparing PCA patients to normal controls have demonstrated right-sided predominant atrophy and hypometabolism in the posterior parietal, temporal, and lateral occipital cortex and relative sparing of the hippocampus and medial temporal cortex [20, 43, 63, 77, 78]. Compared to typical AD patients, PCA patients show more atrophy in primary and association visual and right posterior parietal lobe, whereas AD patients have relatively greater left medial and, inferior and middle temporal atrophy and hypometabolism [63, 77].

Although Benson speculated that PCA was likely caused by non-AD pathology [12], subsequent studies have demonstrated that AD is the most common pathologic substrate, accounting for 67–100% of cases [6, 7, 20]. Additional pathologic causes of PCA include DLB and CBD, suggested by characteristic neuropsychiatric and motor features [79], and prion disease, suggested by a rapid course, as well as cortical ribboning on DWI MRI (see Chapter 9). A positive PIB scan supports the notion of underlying AD in Ms. S.'s case, with visual hallucinations suggesting possible comorbid DLB (although visual hallucinations can also occur in individuals with significant visual impairment, including those with glaucoma or macular degeneration).

Patients with PCA generally have higher counts of NFTs in the occipital cortex, posterior parietal, and posterior cingulate cortex and fewer tangles in the prefrontal cortex and hippocampus than typically seen in AD [6, 7]. One study found that amyloid plaques were also elevated in visual regions compared to typical AD [80], but most studies have not found a difference in the distribution of plaques in PCA and AD as assessed at autopsy or using PIB-PET [6, 63, 78].

Table 3.5 Two proposed criteria for PCA.

Mendez 2002 [43]

Core features (all must be present)

1. Insidious onset with gradual progression
2. Presentation with visual complaints with intact primary visual function
3. On examination, evidence of predominant complex visual disorder (Balint's, visual agnosia, dressing apraxia, environmental disorientation)
4. Proportionally less deficits in memory and verbal fluency
5. Relatively preserved insight

Supportive features

1. Presenile onset
2. Alexia
3. Elements of Gerstmann's syndrome
4. Ideomotor apraxia
5. Normal physical examination
6. Investigations: neuropsychology (impaired perceptual deficits), imaging (occipitoparietal abnormality with sparing of frontal and mesiotemporal regions)

McMonagle 2006 [75]

1. Presentation with progressive visual or visuospatial impairment in the absence of ophthalmologic impairment
2. Evidence of complex visual disorder on examination: elements of Balint's syndrome, visual agnosia, dressing apraxia, or environmental disorientation
3. Proportionately less memory loss or reduced verbal fluency

Case 4

Mr. T is a 56-year-old left-handed man presenting with 8 years of progressive behavioral problems. His first symptom was loss of empathy, exemplified by not calling his wife when she was hospitalized for surgery. He developed compulsive recycling and composting, sorting through garbage ritualistically and bagging items for disposal. He began collecting shoes and fruit peels, as well as urine and feces. He became obsessed with having his dog with him at all times and pretended to be blind so that he could bring his dog with him on a train. He became disinhibited, at one point running naked on the beach, inviting a homeless stranger into the home to drink with him, and assisting in the escape of two tenants of a home for cognitively impaired persons. He began overeating and displaying a lack of disgust—eating moldy lemons, apple cores, and sodas left by strangers. Memory problems began 3 years after the onset of behavioral changes, having difficulty remembering his new cell phone number. He became disorganized and developed trouble with household tasks such as making the bed and putting away laundry. He also developed repetitive motor behaviors such as frequent yawning and rubbing the edges of his mouth. Language has been relatively preserved. His navigation skills declined. His personal hygiene worsened, and he had to be encouraged to bathe and change his clothes. On exam, his speech was tangential and perseverative. His behavior was jocular and disinhibited, frequently asking the examiner's age and marital status and speaking out of context. He was found to be hoarding food under the covers of his hospital bed. On neuropsychological testing, he scored 18 of 30 on the MMSE. Cognitive testing revealed impairment in episodic memory and executive and visuospatial function with relative sparing of language. His initial clinical diagnosis was bvFTD. Brain MRI and FDG-PET demonstrated atrophy and hypometabolism in both the frontal and parietal cortex, right greater than left, with prominent involvement of the precuneus (Figure 3.4a and b). PIB-PET scan was positive (Figure 3.4c). Based on his MRI and PIB-PET scan, his diagnosis was changed to frontal variant EOAD.

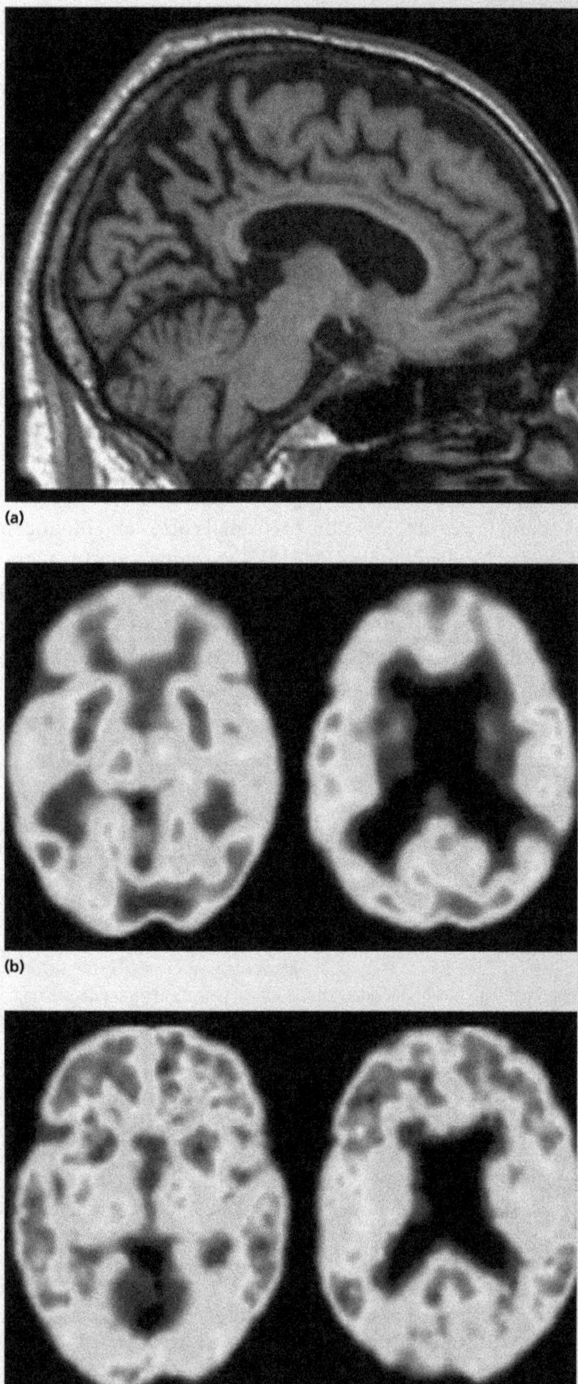

Figure 3.4 (a) Sagittal T1-weighted MRI showing parietal and occipital atrophy. (b) FDG-PET showing hypometabolism in frontal and parietal cortices. (c) PIB-PET showing diffuse cortical binding. Orientation is neurological. (*See insert for color representation of the figure.*)

Mr. T is an example of a patient with very prominent behavioral symptoms suggestive of behavioral variant frontotemporal dementia (bvFTD; see Chapter 5 for additional details) but in whom imaging studies supported an AD pathology (biparietal atrophy and hypometabolism as well as positive PIB). Johnson and colleagues described clinical and pathologic features of three patients with pathological AD who presented with a dysexecutive cognitive profile, coining this presentation "frontal variant AD" (fvAD) [81]. Evidence for a behavioral predominant form of fvAD is provided by the fact that 10–20% of patients clinically diagnosed with bvFTD during life are found to have AD postmortem [3, 82–84]. Differentiating bvFTD due to FTLD and fvAD on clinical grounds often is difficult [85]. Many bvFTD patients met the original NINCDS-ARDA criteria for AD [86], whereas up to one-third of AD patients fulfill clinical criteria for bvFTD [87]. Factors that predispose to fvAD are not known, although PS1 mutation carriers in particular may present with a frontal syndrome [34, 74, 88]. Limited studies comparing the distribution of AD pathology in fvAD and typical AD patients found no difference in the distribution or burden of plaques but greater frontal NFTs in fvAD and greater medial temporal NFTs in typical AD [81]. Notably, Mr. T showed a diffuse pattern of PIB binding, similar to that seen in typical AD (Figure 3.4).

Distinguishing between fvAD and bvFTD based on cognitive testing can be challenging, as both groups show impairment on tests of executive function. Episodic memory can be variably affected in bvFTD, such that the presence of amnesia does not assure that AD is the underlying pathology [89, 90]. Rather, the presence of visuospatial dysfunction might be the most predictive of underlying AD [89], whereas the presence of executive dysfunction in the absence of behavioral changes makes underlying FTLD less likely [91]. Conversely, greater behavioral changes are suggestive of bvFTD [92, 93], though, as illustrated in Mr. T's case, patients with fvAD can have very prominent behavioral disturbances [94–96]. The clinical overlap and distinctions between AD and FTLD are mirrored by neuroimaging studies [97, 98]. Both diseases lead to atrophy in the dorsolateral prefrontal cortex and hippocampus, as suggested by the common findings of executive dysfunction and episodic memory loss. The atrophy patterns diverge in that AD also leads to parietal atrophy, whereas FTLD is associated with medial prefrontal atrophy [45]. Temporoparietal and precuneus involvement on imaging suggests that AD is the underlying disease in patients with behavioral or dysexecutive presentations [98].

Mr. T actually fulfilled research criteria for bvFTD [99]. The presence of visuospatial dysfunction and to a lesser degree memory loss relatively early in the course raised suspicion for AD. Prominent parietal involvement on MRI and FDG-PET supported the diagnosis of fvAD, and this diagnosis was preliminarily confirmed with a positive PIB scan.

Case 5

Mr. Z is a 65-year-old right-handed man presenting with 5 years of memory and movement problems. His family noted 5 years ago that he was misplacing objects and had difficulty remembering recent events. Three years prior to presentation, he developed problems using his left hand and leg, leading to an abnormal gait. Two years later, he evolved difficulty using tools and noticed a tremor and jerks in the left arm. He began running into walls on the left and developed left–right confusion. He was tried on levodopa without a clear response. Language function was unchanged except for less legible handwriting. Visuospatial function declined, with problems recognizing the faces of his grandchildren and difficulty reading one line to the next. He never became lost, but was involved in a motor vehicle accident in which he was at fault. He began having hallucinations, hearing voices, and seeing lights and on one occasion thought a snake was in his bed. He did not act out his dreams nor did he have fluctuations in alertness. He lived in a nursing home for the year prior to presentation. Neurological examination revealed myoclonus in the upper extremities, left greater than right. Tone was increased in the right arm with a tonically contracted left arm. There was extinction on the left with double simultaneous stimulation and ideomotor apraxia of the left arm and leg. His gait was bradykinetic and stooped. His MMSE was 21 of 30. Neuropsychological testing showed deficits in memory, executive function, naming, and visuospatial function. An MRI demonstrated right greater than left parietal and temporal atrophy with some milder atrophy of the bilateral medial perirolandic cortex (Figure 3.5a). PIB-PET was positive. He died 15 months following the evaluation, 6.5 years after onset. Autopsy revealed high-likelihood AD (NIA-Reagan) (Figure 3.5b and c) and intermediate-likelihood DLB [100b].

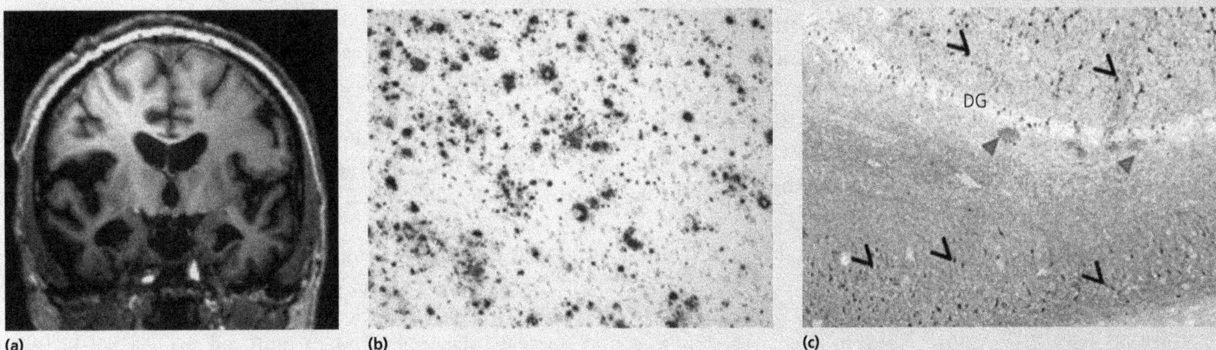

Figure 3.5 **(a)** Coronal T1-weighted MRI showing bilateral (right > left) temporal and right parietal (not shown) atrophy; orientation is radiological. **(b)** His pathology showed AD characteristic amyloid-beta-positive plaques (brown) in the middle frontal gyrus (4G8 (anti-amyloid-beta) immunohistochemistry; 100x). **(c)** AD characteristic tau-positive inclusions in the hippocampus. Neurofibrillary tangles (arrows), neuritic plaques (arrow heads), and neuropil threads (brown background) are present (CP13 (anti-phosphorylated tau) immunohistochemistry; 40x). DG, dentate gyrus. *(See insert for color representation of the figure.)*

Mr. Z's clinical presentation included many features of CBS (see Chapter 7 for additional details). Although CBS is most often associated with FTLD pathology, roughly 15–50% of patients are found to have underlying AD postmortem [8, 98, 100a]. Unfortunately, the core features of CBS do not appear to discriminate patients with underlying AD from those with FTLD [101, 102]. The additional presence of episodic memory loss and visuospatial dysfunction might predict underlying AD, whereas nonfluent aphasia, prominent behavioral symptoms, preferential executive dysfunction, and lower limb apraxia are suggestive of underlying FTLD [101]. Atrophy/ hypometabolism/hypoperfusion in a perirolandic network that includes the pre- and postcentral gyrus, supplementary motor areas, and dorsomedial prefrontal cortex is associated with CBS regardless of underlying neuropathology [46, 103]. Extension of atrophy or hypoperfusion/hypometabolism into the temporoparietal cortex might be a marker for underlying AD, whereas greater frontal or brainstem lesions may indicate FTLD [98, 103]. Mr. Z presented with many of the core features of CBS including cortical sensory loss, ideomotor apraxia, and myoclonus. Extrapyramidal dysfunction was also present with asymmetric increased tone. Early episodic memory loss, visuospatial dysfunction, a posterior-predominant atrophy pattern on MRI, and a positive PIB-PET suggested AD as the underlying pathology, whereas the episode of visual hallucinations hinted at comorbid DLB. Autopsy demonstrated mixed AD/DLB.

Treatment

Two classes of medications are approved in the United States for symptomatic treatment of AD: acetylcholinesterase inhibitors (AChEIs) and memantine, an *N*-methyl-D-aspartic acid (NMDA) receptor antagonist. Both classes of medications show a symptomatic benefit later, followed by a decline in parallel with placebo, with small but statistically significant treatment benefits at study's end on cognitive, behavioral, and functional measures [104–107]. These appear to translate into improved patient and caregiver quality of life and delay the need for custodial care [108–110]. The benefit of AChEIs has been established in patients with mild to severe AD, whereas memantine only has shown benefit in moderate to severe disease [107, 111]. Combined therapy with AChEI and memantine might provide greater benefit than either medication alone [112, 113]. Selective serotonin reuptake inhibitors and serotonin–norepinephrine reuptake inhibitors are often helpful for treating depression, irritability, and perhaps apathy associated with AD [114–116].

There is essentially no data to determine whether AChEIs or memantine is effective in patients with atypical presentations, and in fact, a small study suggested that AChEIs are not beneficial in patients with PCA [43]. A trial of dopaminergic therapy should be considered in patients with CBS with prominent parkinsonism, and botulinum toxin might be helpful for dystonia in these patients. Patients with lvPPA often benefit from speech therapy, and PCA patients benefit from rehabilitative services for the visually impaired. Physical and occupational therapies are often helpful for maximizing function, and a structured exercise program is universally recommended in our clinic. A multidisciplinary clinical approach to treatment is critical, emphasizing the needs of the individual patient and providing caregiver education and support specific to the needs of the particular patient (see Chapter 15).

Conclusion

A century following Alois Alzheimer's initial case report, it has become apparent that AD is the great "mimicker" of other neurodegenerative diseases and can present not only with episodic memory loss but also with language, visuospatial, motor, and behavior predominant syndromes. Each syndrome is associated with a distinct degenerative pattern apparent on structural and functional imaging, though anatomic overlap across syndromes is found in the precuneus/posterior cingulate and lateral temporoparietal cortex [20]. As is the case in typical AD, the distribution of NFTs correlates more strongly with clinical phenotype and degenerative pattern than the distribution of NPs. Developmental, genetic, environmental, and physiologic mechanisms that contribute to phenotypic heterogeneity in AD are at this point largely unknown.

The clinical heterogeneity of AD poses a challenge for clinicians, as the disease overlaps clinically with syndromes previously associated with other neurodegenerative diseases such as FTLD. Fortunately, sensitive molecular biomarkers such as CSF Aβ_{1-42}, tau, and p-tau and amyloid imaging have been developed and will likely be adopted into clinical practice to "rule out" AD in patients with atypical clinical presentations. These patients could then be candidates for emerging biologically specific therapies for this devastating illness.

Acknowledgments

The authors would like to thank Michael WEINER for providing MRI images, Bill Jagust for providing PET images, and William Seeley for assisting with pathology images.

References

1 Plassman BL, Langa KM, Fisher GG, Heeringa SG, Weir DR, Ofstedal MB, et al. Prevalence of dementia in the United States: the aging, demographics, and memory study. *Neuroepidemiology* 2007;**29**(1–2):125–132.

2 Lopez OL, Becker JT, Sweet RA, Klunk W, Kaufer DI, Saxton J, et al. Psychiatric symptoms vary with the severity of dementia in probable Alzheimer's disease. *J Neuropsychiatry Clin Neurosci* 2003 Summer;**15**(3):346–353.

3 Alladi S, Xuereb J, Bak T, Nestor P, Knibb J, Patterson K, et al. Focal cortical presentations of Alzheimer's disease. *Brain* 2007 Oct;**130**(Pt 10):2636–2645.

4 Green RC, Goldstein FC, Mirra SS, Alazraki NP, Baxt JL, Bakay RA. Slowly progressive apraxia in Alzheimer's disease. *J Neurol Neurosurg Psychiatry* 1995 Sep;**59**(3):312–315.

5 Galton CJ, Patterson K, Xuereb JH, Hodges JR. Atypical and typical presentations of Alzheimer's disease: a clinical, neuropsychological, neuroimaging and pathological study of 13 cases. *Brain* 2000 Mar;**123** Pt 3:484–498.

6 Tang-Wai DF, Graff-Radford NR, Boeve BF, Dickson DW, Parisi JE, Crook R, et al. Clinical, genetic, and neuropathologic characteristics of posterior cortical atrophy. *Neurology* 2004 Oct 12;**63**(7): 1168–1174.

7 Renner JA, Burns JM, Hou CE, McKeel DW, Jr, Storandt M, Morris JC. Progressive posterior cortical dysfunction: a clinicopathologic series. *Neurology* 2004 Oct 12;**63**(7):1175–1180.

8 Boeve BF, Maraganore DM, Parisi JE, Ahlskog JE, Graff-Radford N, Caselli RJ, et al. Pathologic heterogeneity in clinically diagnosed corticobasal degeneration. *Neurology* 1999 Sep 11;**53**(4):795–800.

9 Knibb JA, Xuereb JH, Patterson K, Hodges JR. Clinical and pathological characterization of progressive aphasia. *Ann Neurol* 2006 Jan;**59**(1):156–165.

10 Mesulam M, Wicklund A, Johnson N, Rogalski E, Leger GC, Rademaker A, et al. Alzheimer and frontotemporal pathology in subsets of primary progressive aphasia. *Ann Neurol* 2008 Jun;**63**(6):709–719.

11 Rebeiz JJ, Kolodny EH, Richardson EP, Jr. Corticodentatonigral degeneration with neuronal achromasia. *Arch Neurol* 1968 Jan; **18**(1):20–33.

12 Benson DF, Davis RJ, Snyder BD. Posterior cortical atrophy. *Arch Neurol* 1988 Jul;**45**(7):789–793.

13 Mesulam MM. Primary progressive aphasia. *Ann Neurol* 2001 Apr;**49**(4):425–432.

14 Carter MD, Simms GA, Weaver DF. The development of new therapeutics for Alzheimer's disease. *Clin Pharmacol Ther* 2010 Oct;**88**(4):475–486.

15 McKhann G, Drachman D, Folstein M, Katzman R, Price D, Stadlan EM. Clinical diagnosis of Alzheimer's disease: report of the NINCDS-ADRDA work group under the auspices of department of health and human services task force on Alzheimer's Disease. *Neurology* 1984 Jul;**34**(7):939–944.

16 McKhann GM, Knopman DS, Chertkow H, Hyman BT, Jack CR, Jr, Kawas CH, et al. The diagnosis of dementia due to Alzheimer's disease: recommendations from the National Institute on Aging-Alzheimer's Association workgroups on diagnostic guidelines for Alzheimer's disease. *Alzheimers Dement* 2011 May;**7**(3):263–269.

17 Dubois B, Feldman HH, Jacova C, Hampel H, Molinuevo JL, Blennow K, et al. Advancing research diagnostic criteria for

Alzheimer's disease: the IWG-2 criteria. *Lancet Neurol* 2014;**13**(6): 614–629.

18 Ferri CP, Prince M, Brayne C, Brodaty H, Fratiglioni L, Ganguli M, et al. Global prevalence of dementia: a Delphi consensus study. *Lancet* 2005 Dec 17;**366**(9503):2112–2117.

19 Thies W, Bleiler L, Alzheimer's Association. 2013 Alzheimer's disease facts and figures. *Alzheimers Dement* 2013 Mar;**9**(2):208–245.

20 Migliaccio R, Agosta F, Rascovsky K, Karydas A, Bonasera S, Rabinovici GD, et al. Clinical syndromes associated with posterior atrophy: early age at onset AD spectrum. *Neurology* 2009 Nov 10; **73**(19):1571–1578.

21 Gorno-Tempini ML, Dronkers NF, Rankin KP, Ogar JM, Phengrasamy L, Rosen HJ, et al. Cognition and anatomy in three variants of primary progressive aphasia. *Ann Neurol* 2004 Mar;**55**(3): 335–346.

22 Frisoni GB, Pievani M, Testa C, Sabattoli F, Bresciani L, Bonetti M, et al. The topography of grey matter involvement in early and late onset Alzheimer's disease. *Brain* 2007 Mar;**130**(Pt 3):720–730.

23 Rabinovici GD, Furst AJ, Alkalay A, Racine CA, O'Neil JP, Janabi M, et al. Increased metabolic vulnerability in early-onset Alzheimer's disease is not related to amyloid burden. *Brain* 2010 Feb;**133** (Pt 2):512–528.

24 Schmidt C, Redyk K, Meissner B, Krack L, von Ahsen N, Roeber S, et al. Clinical features of rapidly progressive Alzheimer's disease. *Dement Geriatr Cogn Disord* 2010;**29**(4):371–378.

25 Knopman DS, DeKosky ST, Cummings JL, Chui H, Corey-Bloom J, Relkin N, et al. Practice parameter: diagnosis of dementia (an evidence-based review). Report of the Quality Standards Subcommittee of the American Academy of Neurology. *Neurology* 2001 May 8;**56**(9):1143–1153.

26 Beach TG, Monsell SE, Phillips LE, Kukull W. Accuracy of the clinical diagnosis of Alzheimer disease at National Institute on Aging Alzheimer Disease Centers, 2005–2010. *J Neuropathol Exp Neurol* 2012 Apr;**71**(4):266–273.

27 Dubois B, Feldman HH, Jacova C, Dekosky ST, Barberger-Gateau P, Cummings J, et al. Research criteria for the diagnosis of Alzheimer's disease: revising the NINCDS-ADRDA criteria. *Lancet Neurol* 2007 Aug;**6**(8):734–746.

28 Dickson DW, Bergeron C, Chin SS, Duyckaerts C, Horoupian D, Ikeda K, et al. Office of rare diseases neuropathologic criteria for corticobasal degeneration. *J Neuropathol Exp Neurol* 2002 Nov;**61**(11):935–946.

29 Braak H, Braak E. Neuropathological stageing of Alzheimer-related changes. *Acta Neuropathol* 1991;**82**(4):239–259.

30 Thal DR, Rub U, Orantes M, Braak H. Phases of A beta-deposition in the human brain and its relevance for the development of AD. *Neurology* 2002 Jun 25;**58**(12):1791–1800.

31 Mirra SS, Heyman A, McKeel D, Sumi SM, Crain BJ, Brownlee LM, et al. The consortium to establish a registry for Alzheimer's Disease (CERAD). Part II. Standardization of the neuropathologic assessment of Alzheimer's disease. *Neurology* 1991 Apr;**41**(4):479–486.

32 Hyman BT, Phelps CH, Beach TG, Bigio EH, Cairns NJ, Carrillo MC, et al. National institute on aging–Alzheimer's association guidelines for the neuropathologic assessment of Alzheimer's disease. *Alzheimers Dement* 2012;**8**(1):1–13.

33 Campion D, Dumanchin C, Hannequin D, Dubois B, Belliard S, Puel M, et al. Early-onset autosomal dominant Alzheimer disease: prevalence, genetic heterogeneity, and mutation spectrum. *Am J Hum Genet* 1999 Sep;**65**(3):664–670.

34 Mendez MF, McMurtray A. Frontotemporal dementia-like phenotypes associated with presenilin-1 mutations. *Am J Alzheimers Dis Other Demen* 2006 Aug–Sep;**21**(4):281–286.

35 Margallo-Lana M, Morris CM, Gibson AM, Tan AL, Kay DW, Tyrer SP, et al. Influence of the amyloid precursor protein locus on dementia in Down syndrome. *Neurology* 2004 Jun 8;**62**(11):1996–1998.

36 Jarvik G, Larson EB, Goddard K, Schellenberg GD, Wijsman EM. Influence of apolipoprotein E genotype on the transmission of Alzheimer disease in a community-based sample. *Am J Hum Genet* 1996 Jan;**58**(1):191–200.

37 Corder EH, Saunders AM, Risch NJ, Strittmatter WJ, Schmechel DE, Gaskell PC, Jr, et al. Protective effect of apolipoprotein E type 2 allele for late onset Alzheimer disease. *Nat Genet* 1994 Jun;**7**(2): 180–184.

38 Mayeux R, Saunders AM, Shea S, Mirra S, Evans D, Roses AD, et al. Utility of the apolipoprotein E genotype in the diagnosis of Alzheimer's disease. Alzheimer's Disease centers consortium on apolipoprotein E and Alzheimer's Disease. *N Engl J Med* 1998 Feb 19;**338**(8):506–511.

39 Saunders AM, Strittmatter WJ, Schmechel D, George-Hyslop PH, Pericak-Vance MA, Joo SH, et al. Association of apolipoprotein E allele epsilon 4 with late-onset familial and sporadic Alzheimer's disease. *Neurology* 1993 Aug;**43**(8):1467–1472.

40 Corder EH, Saunders AM, Strittmatter WJ, Schmechel DE, Gaskell PC, Small GW, et al. Gene dose of apolipoprotein E type 4 allele and the risk of Alzheimer's disease in late onset families. *Science* 1993 Aug 13;**261**(5123):921–923.

41 van der Flier WM, Schoonenboom SN, Pijnenburg YA, Fox NC, Scheltens P. The effect of APOE genotype on clinical phenotype in Alzheimer disease. *Neurology* 2006 Aug 8;**67**(3):526–527.

42 Schott JM, Ridha BH, Crutch SJ, Healy DG, Uphill JB, Warrington EK, et al. Apolipoprotein E genotype modifies the phenotype of Alzheimer disease. *Arch Neurol* 2006 Jan;**63**(1):155–156.

43 Mendez MF, Ghajarania M, Perryman KM. Posterior cortical atrophy: clinical characteristics and differences compared to Alzheimer's disease. *Dement Geriatr Cogn Disord* 2002;**14**(1):33–40.

44 Karch CM, Goate AM. Alzheimer's disease risk genes and mechanisms of disease pathogenesis. *Biol Psychiatry* 2015; **77**(1): 43–51.

45 Rabinovici GD, Seeley WW, Kim EJ, Gorno-Tempini ML, Rascovsky K, Pagliaro TA, et al. Distinct MRI atrophy patterns in autopsy-proven Alzheimer's disease and frontotemporal lobar degeneration. *Am J Alzheimers Dis Other Demen* 2007 Dec–2008 Jan; **22**(6):474–488.

46 Seeley WW, Crawford RK, Zhou J, Miller BL, Greicius MD. Neurodegenerative diseases target large-scale human brain networks. *Neuron* 2009 Apr 16;**62**(1):42–52.

47 Hoffman JM, Welsh-Bohmer KA, Hanson M, Crain B, Hulette C, Earl N, et al. FDG PET imaging in patients with pathologically verified dementia. *J Nucl Med* 2000 Nov;**41**(11):1920–1928.

48 Whitwell JL, Josephs KA, Murray ME, Kantarci K, Przybelski SA, Weigand SD, et al. MRI correlates of neurofibrillary tangle pathology at autopsy: a voxel-based morphometry study. *Neurology* 2008 Sep 2;**71**(10):743–749.

49 Silbert LC, Quinn JF, Moore MM, Corbridge E, Ball MJ, Murdoch G, et al. Changes in premorbid brain volume predict Alzheimer's disease pathology. *Neurology* 2003 Aug 26;**61**(4):487–492.

50 Whitwell JL, Dickson DW, Murray ME, Weigand SD, Tosakulwong N, Senjem ML, et al. Neuroimaging correlates of pathologically

defined subtypes of Alzheimer's disease: a case–control study. *Lancet Neurol* 2012;**11**(10):868–877.

51 Murray ME, Graff-Radford NR, Ross OA, Petersen RC, Duara R, Dickson DW. Neuropathologically defined subtypes of Alzheimer's disease with distinct clinical characteristics: a retrospective study. *Lancet Neurol* 2011;**10**(9):785–796.

52 Blennow K, Hampel H. CSF markers for incipient Alzheimer's disease. *Lancet Neurol* 2003 Oct;**2**(10):605–613.

53 Shaw LM, Vanderstichele H, Knapik-Czajka M, Clark CM, Aisen PS, Petersen RC, et al. Cerebrospinal fluid biomarker signature in Alzheimer's disease neuroimaging initiative subjects. *Ann Neurol* 2009 Apr;**65**(4):403–413.

54 Tapiola T, Alafuzoff I, Herukka SK, Parkkinen L, Hartikainen P, Soininen H, et al. Cerebrospinal fluid {beta}-amyloid 42 and tau proteins as biomarkers of Alzheimer-type pathologic changes in the brain. *Arch Neurol* 2009 Mar;**66**(3):382–389.

55 Klunk WE, Engler H, Nordberg A, Wang Y, Blomqvist G, Holt DP, et al. Imaging brain amyloid in Alzheimer's disease with Pittsburgh Compound-B. *Ann Neurol* 2004 Mar;**55**(3):306–319.

56 Wong DF, Rosenberg PB, Zhou Y, Kumar A, Raymont V, Ravert HT, et al. In vivo imaging of amyloid deposition in Alzheimer disease using the radioligand 18F-AV-45 (florbetapir [corrected] F 18). *J Nucl Med* 2010 Jun;**51**(6):913–920.

57 Vandenberghe R, Van Laere K, Ivanoiu A, Salmon E, Bastin C, Triau E, et al. 18F-flutemetamol amyloid imaging in Alzheimer disease and mild cognitive impairment: a phase 2 trial. *Ann Neurol* 2010 Sep;**68**(3):319–329.

58 Rowe CC, Ackerman U, Browne W, Mulligan R, Pike KL, O'Keefe G, et al. Imaging of amyloid beta in Alzheimer's disease with 18F-BAY94-9172, a novel PET tracer: proof of mechanism. *Lancet Neurol* 2008 Feb;**7**(2):129–135.

59 Rowe CC, Pejoska S, Mulligan RS, Jones G, Chan JG, Svensson S, et al. Head-to-head comparison of 11C-PiB and 18F-AZD4694 (NAV4694) for beta-amyloid imaging in aging and dementia. *J Nucl Med* 2013 Jun;**54**(6):880–886.

60 Ikonomovic MD, Klunk WE, Abrahamson EE, Mathis CA, Price JC, Tsopelas ND, et al. Post-mortem correlates of in vivo PiB-PET amyloid imaging in a typical case of Alzheimer's disease. *Brain* 2008 Jun;**131**(Pt 6):1630–1645.

61 Clark CM, Schneider JA, Bedell BJ, Beach TG, Bilker WB, Mintun MA, et al. Use of florbetapir-PET for imaging beta-amyloid pathology. *JAMA* 2011 Jan 19;**305**(3):275–283.

62 Rabinovici GD, Jagust WJ, Furst AJ, Ogar JM, Racine CA, Mormino EC, et al. Abeta amyloid and glucose metabolism in three variants of primary progressive aphasia. *Ann Neurol* 2008 Oct;**64**(4):388–401.

63 Rosenbloom MH, Alkalay A, Agarwal N, Baker SL, O'Neil JP, Janabi M, et al. Distinct clinical and metabolic deficits in PCA and AD are not related to amyloid distribution. *Neurology* 2011 May 24;**76**(21):1789–1796.

64 Maruyama M, Shimada H, Suhara T, Shinotoh H, Ji B, Maeda J, et al. Imaging of tau pathology in a tauopathy mouse model and in Alzheimer patients compared to normal controls. *Neuron* 2013;**79**(6):1094–1108.

65 Xia C, Arteaga J, Chen G, Gangadharmath U, Gomez LF, Kasi D, et al. [^{18} F] T807, a novel tau positron emission tomography imaging agent for Alzheimer's disease. *Alzheimer's Dement* 2013 Nov; **9**(6):666–676.

66 Okamura N, Furumoto S, Fodero-Tavoletti MT, Mulligan RS, Harada R, Yates P, et al. Non-invasive assessment of Alzheimer's disease neurofibrillary pathology using ^{18}F-THK5105 PET. *Brain* 2014 Jun;**137**(Pt 6):1762–1771.

67 Mesulam MM. Slowly progressive aphasia without generalized dementia. *Ann Neurol* 1982 Jun;**11**(6):592–598.

68 Rohrer JD, Geser F, Zhou J, Gennatas ED, Sidhu M, Trojanowski JQ, et al. TDP-43 subtypes are associated with distinct atrophy patterns in frontotemporal dementia. *Neurology* 2010 Dec 14;**75**(24):2204–2211.

69 Gorno-Tempini ML, Hillis AE, Weintraub S, Kertesz A, Mendez M, Cappa SF, et al. Classification of primary progressive aphasia and its variants. *Neurology* 2011 Mar 15;**76**(11):1006–1014.

70 Mesulam MM, Weintraub S, Rogalski EJ, Wieneke C, Geula C, Bigio EH. Asymmetry and heterogeneity of Alzheimer's and frontotemporal pathology in primary progressive aphasia. *Brain* 2014 Apr;**137**(Pt 4):1176–1192.

71 Grossman M. Primary progressive aphasia: clinicopathological correlations. *Nat Rev Neurol* 2010 Feb;**6**(2):88–97.

72 Gefen T, Gasho K, Rademaker A, Lalehzari M, Weintraub S, Rogalski E, et al. Clinically concordant variations of Alzheimer pathology in aphasic versus amnestic dementia. *Brain* 2012 May;**135**(Pt 5):1554–1565.

73 Crutch SJ, Lehmann M, Schott JM, Rabinovici GD, Rossor MN, Fox NC. Posterior cortical atrophy. *Lancet Neurol* 2012;**11**(2):170–178.

74 Tang-Wai D, Lewis P, Boeve B, Hutton M, Golde T, Baker M, et al. Familial frontotemporal dementia associated with a novel presenilin-1 mutation. *Dement Geriatr Cogn Disord* 2002;**14**(1):13–21.

75 McMonagle P, Deering F, Berliner Y, Kertesz A. The cognitive profile of posterior cortical atrophy. *Neurology* 2006 Feb 14;**66**(3):331–338.

76 Aresi A, Giovagnoli AR. The role of neuropsychology in distinguishing the posterior cortical atrophy syndrome and Alzheimer's disease. *J Alzheimers Dis* 2009;**18**(1):65–70.

77 Whitwell JL, Jack CR, Jr, Kantarci K, Weigand SD, Boeve BF, Knopman DS, et al. Imaging correlates of posterior cortical atrophy. *Neurobiol Aging* 2007 Jul;**28**(7):1051–1061.

78 Lehmann M, Ghosh PM, Madison C, Laforce R, Corbetta-Rastelli C, Weiner MW, et al. Diverging patterns of amyloid deposition and hypometabolism in clinical variants of probable Alzheimer's disease. *Brain* 2013;**136**(3):844–858.

79 Josephs KA, Whitwell JL, Boeve BF, Knopman DS, Tang-Wai DF, Drubach DA, et al. Visual hallucinations in posterior cortical atrophy. *Arch Neurol* 2006 Oct;**63**(10):1427–1432.

80 Hof PR, Archin N, Osmand AP, Dougherty JH, Wells C, Bouras C, et al. Posterior cortical atrophy in Alzheimer's disease: analysis of a new case and re-evaluation of a historical report. *Acta Neuropathol* 1993;**86**(3):215–223.

81 Johnson JK, Head E, Kim R, Starr A, Cotman CW. Clinical and pathological evidence for a frontal variant of Alzheimer disease. *Arch Neurol* 1999 Oct;**56**(10):1233–1239.

82 Mendez MF, Joshi A, Tassniyom K, Teng E, Shapira JS. Clinicopathologic differences among patients with behavioral variant frontotemporal dementia. *Neurology* 2013 Feb 5;**80**(6): 561–568.

83 Kertesz A, McMonagle P, Blair M, Davidson W, Munoz DG. The evolution and pathology of frontotemporal dementia. *Brain* 2005 Sep;**128**(Pt 9):1996–2005.

84 Forman MS, Farmer J, Johnson JK, Clark CM, Arnold SE, Coslett H, et al. Frontotemporal dementia: clinicopathological correlations. *Ann Neurol* 2006;**59**(6):952–962.

85 Ossenkoppele R, Pijnenburg YA, Perry DC, Cohn-Sheehy BI, Scheltens NM, Vogel JW, et al. The behavioural/dysexecutive variant of Alzheimer's disease: clinical, neuroimaging and pathological features. *Brain J Neurol* 2015 Epub 2015/07/05.

86 Varma AR, Snowden JS, Lloyd JJ, Talbot PR, Mann DM, Neary D. Evaluation of the NINCDS-ADRDA criteria in the differentiation of Alzheimer's disease and frontotemporal dementia. *J Neurol Neurosurg Psychiatry* 1999 Feb;**66**(2):184–188.

87 Ikeda M, Ishikawa T, Tanabe H. Epidemiology of frontotemporal lobar degeneration. *Dement Geriatr Cogn Disord* 2004;**17**(4): 265–268.

88 Raux G, Gantier R, Thomas-Anterion C, Boulliat J, Verpillat P, Hannequin D, et al. Dementia with prominent frontotemporal features associated with L113P presenilin 1 mutation. *Neurology* 2000 Nov 28;**55**(10):1577–1578.

89 Kramer JH, Jurik J, Sha SJ, Rankin KP, Rosen HJ, Johnson JK, et al. Distinctive neuropsychological patterns in frontotemporal dementia, semantic dementia, and Alzheimer disease. *Cogn Behav Neurol* 2003 Dec;**16**(4):211–218.

90 Hodges JR, Davies RR, Xuereb JH, Casey B, Broe M, Bak TH, et al. Clinicopathological correlates in frontotemporal dementia. *Ann Neurol* 2004 Sep;**56**(3):399–406.

91 Woodward M, Jacova C, Black SE, Kertesz A, Mackenzie IR, Feldman H, et al. Differentiating the frontal variant of Alzheimer's disease. *Int J Geriatr Psychiatry* 2010 Jul;**25**(7):732–738.

92 Back-Madruga C, Boone KB, Briere J, Cummings J, McPherson S, Fairbanks L, et al. Functional ability in executive variant Alzheimer's disease and typical Alzheimer's disease. *Clin Neuropsychol* 2002 Aug;**16**(3):331–340.

93 Jenner C, Reali G, Puopolo M, Silveri MC. Can cognitive and behavioral disorders differentiate frontal variant-frontotemporal dementia from Alzheimer's disease at early stages? *Behav Neurol* 2006;**17**(2):89–95.

94 Habek M, Hajnsek S, Zarkovic K, Chudy D, Mubrin Z. Frontal variant of Alzheimer's disease: clinico-CSF-pathological correlation. *Can J Neurol Sci* 2010 Jan;**37**(1):118–120.

95 Taylor KI, Probst A, Miserez AR, Monsch AU, Tolnay M, Clinical course of neuropathologically confirmed frontal-variant Alzheimer's disease. *Nat Clin Pract Neurol* 2008 Apr;**4**(4):226–232.

96 Larner AJ. "Frontal variant Alzheimer's disease": a reappraisal. *Clin Neurol Neurosurg* 2006 Oct;**108**(7):705–708.

97 Rabinovici GD, Furst AJ, O'Neil JP, Racine CA, Mormino EC, Baker SL, et al. 11C-PIB PET imaging in Alzheimer disease and frontotemporal lobar degeneration. *Neurology* 2007 Apr 10;**68**(15):1205–1212.

98 Whitwell JL, Jack CR, Jr, Przybelski SA, Parisi JE, Senjem ML, Boeve BF, et al. Temporoparietal atrophy: A marker of AD pathology independent of clinical diagnosis. *Neurobiol Aging* 2011 Sep;**32**(9):1531–1541.

99 Rascovsky K, Hodges JR, Knopman D, Mendez MF, Kramer JH, Neuhaus J, et al. Sensitivity of revised diagnostic criteria for the behavioural variant of frontotemporal dementia. *Brain* 2011 Sep;**134**(Pt 9):2456–2477.

100 (a) Ling H, O'Sullivan SS, Holton JL, Revesz T, Massey LA, Williams DR, et al. Does corticobasal degeneration exist? A clinicopathological re-evaluation. *Brain* 2010 Jul;**133**(Pt 7):2045–2057; (b) McKeith IG. 2006. Consensus guidelines for the clinical and pathologic diagnosis of dementia with Lewy bodies (DLB): report of the Consortium on DLB International Workshop. *J Alzheimers Dis* **9**:417–423.

101 Shelley BP, Hodges JR, Kipps CM, Xuereb JH, Bak TH. Is the pathology of corticobasal syndrome predictable in life? *Mov Disord* 2009 Aug 15;**24**(11):1593–1599.

102 Hu WT, Rippon GW, Boeve BF, Knopman DS, Petersen RC, Parisi JE, et al. Alzheimer's disease and corticobasal degeneration presenting as corticobasal syndrome. *Mov Disord* 2009 Jul 15; **24**(9):1375–1379.

103 Hu WT, Rippon GW, Boeve BF, Knopman DS, Petersen RC, Parisi JE, et al. Alzheimer's disease and corticobasal degeneration presenting as corticobasal syndrome. *Mov Disord* 2009;**24**(9): 1375–1379.

104 Rosler M, Anand R, Cicin-Sain A, Gauthier S, Agid Y, Dal-Bianco P, et al. Efficacy and safety of rivastigmine in patients with Alzheimer's disease: international randomised controlled trial. *BMJ* 1999 Mar 6;**318**(7184):633–638.

105 Wilcock GK, Lilienfeld S, Gaens E. Efficacy and safety of galantamine in patients with mild to moderate Alzheimer's disease: multicentre randomised controlled trial. Galantamine International-1 study group. *BMJ* 2000 Dec 9;**321**(7274):1445–1449.

106 Winblad B, Wimo A, Engedal K, Soininen H, Verhey F, Waldemar G, et al. 3-year study of donepezil therapy in Alzheimer's disease: effects of early and continuous therapy. *Dement Geriatr Cogn Disord* 2006;**21**(5–6):353–363.

107 Reisberg B, Doody R, Stoffler A, Schmitt F, Ferris S, Mobius HJ, et al. Memantine in moderate-to-severe Alzheimer's disease. *N Engl J Med* 2003 Apr 3;**348**(14):1333–1341.

108 Lingler JH, Martire LM, Schulz R. Caregiver-specific outcomes in antidementia clinical drug trials: a systematic review and meta-analysis. *J Am Geriatr Soc* 2005 Jun;**53**(6):983–990.

109 Beusterien KM, Thomas SK, Gause D, Kimel M, Arcona S, Mirski D. Impact of rivastigmine use on the risk of nursing home placement in a US sample. *CNS Drugs* 2004;**18**(15):1143–1148.

110 Mohs RC, Doody RS, Morris JC, Ieni JR, Rogers SL, Perdomo CA, et al. A 1-year, placebo-controlled preservation of function survival study of donepezil in AD patients. *Neurology* 2001 Aug 14; **57**(3):481–488.

111 Birks J. Cholinesterase inhibitors for Alzheimer's disease. *Cochrane Database Syst Rev* 2006 Jan 25; **1**(1):CD005593.

112 Tariot PN, Farlow MR, Grossberg GT, Graham SM, McDonald S, Gergel I, et al. Memantine treatment in patients with moderate to severe Alzheimer disease already receiving donepezil: a randomized controlled trial. *JAMA* 2004 Jan 21;**291**(3): 317–324.

113 Lopez OL, Becker JT, Wahed AS, Saxton J, Sweet RA, Wolk DA, et al. Long-term effects of the concomitant use of memantine with cholinesterase inhibition in Alzheimer disease. *J Neurol Neurosurg Psychiatry* 2009 Jun;**80**(6):600–607.

114 Nyth AL, Gottfries CG, Lyby K, Smedegaard-Andersen L, Gylding-Sabroe J, Kristensen M, et al. A controlled multicenter clinical study of citalopram and placebo in elderly depressed patients with and without concomitant dementia. *Acta Psychiatr Scand* 1992 Aug;**86**(2):138–145.

115 Lyketsos CG, DelCampo L, Steinberg M, Miles Q, Steele CD, Munro C, et al. Treating depression in Alzheimer disease: efficacy and safety of sertraline therapy, and the benefits of depression reduction: the DIADS. *Arch Gen Psychiatry* 2003 Jul;**60**(7): 737–746.

116 Mizukami K, Tanaka Y, Asada T. Efficacy of milnacipran on the depressive state in patients with Alzheimer's disease. *Prog Neuropsychopharmacol Biol Psychiatry* 2006 Sep 30;**30**(7): 1342–1346.

CHAPTER 4

Vascular cognitive impairment: Diagnosis and treatment

Helena C. Chui and Liliana Ramirez-Gomez
University of Southern California, Los Angeles, CA, USA

Background

History

During the past century, the estimated contribution of vascular factors to cognitive decline has swung like a pendulum from high to low to high again. In the early twentieth century, progressive loss of intellectual function in late life was ascribed to "hardening of the arteries," so-called arteriosclerotic dementia. Alzheimer's disease (AD) was considered a relatively rare early-onset dementia associated with neurofibrillary tangles and senile plaques, as first described by Alois Alzheimer in 1907.

When Tomlinson et al. [1] observed identical tangle and plaque lesions in late-onset dementia cases, AD, not arteriosclerosis, became the ascendant cause. Abrupt onset and stepwise decline in cognition due to cumulative strokes formed the conceptual basis of multi-infarct dementia (MID). Slowly progressive dementia due to severe arteriopathy and demyelination of subcortical white matter, so-called Binswanger's syndrome, was regarded as relatively rare.

The landscape shifted once again with the advent of structural imaging in the 1980s. Asymptomatic white matter hyperintensities (WMH) and silent brain infarcts (SBI) were discovered on brain MRI in 20–30% of nondemented, community-dwelling elderly subjects [2]. The ability to detect early and subclinical vascular disease without overt dementia inspired a broader designation, vascular cognitive impairment (VCI). In the 1990s, epidemiologic studies noted associations between stroke risk factors and cognitive impairment (absent history of symptomatic stroke). This has led to the notion (still unproven) that vascular factors might promote AD, further broadening the saliency of potential adverse downstream effects of hypertension, diabetes, and dyslipidemia.

Concepts

VCI is a syndrome or phenotype, not a disease. At its simplest, VCI embodies the concept that cognitive impairment is due to vascular brain injury (VBI). (See Table 4.1 for terms and abbreviations used in this chapter.) Yet the sequence of underlying events can be incredibly diverse. The pathways leading from risk factors to cerebrovascular disease (CVD) to VBI are widely heterogeneous (Table 4.2). Moreover, the *likelihood* that VBI contributes to cognitive impairment is highly variable. Location within cognitive networks and number and size of lesions are considered to be important determinants of cognitive impairment and dementia.

> **G&E → VRF → CVD → VBI → VCI**
> Genetic and environmental factors → vascular risk factors → cerebrovascular disease → vascular brain injury →vascular cognitive impairment

In order to prevent or reduce VCI, efforts must be directed to preventing CVD and VBI. VBI may result from ischemic, hemorrhage, toxic and inflammatory conditions or oxidative stress [3]. There are several forms of CVD, including atherosclerosis, arteriolosclerosis, cerebral amyloid angiopathy (CAA), cerebral autosomal dominant arteriopathy with subcortical infarcts and leukoencephalopathy (CADASIL), and CARASIL [4]. Risk factors for arteriosclerosis are well known, including hypertension, diabetes mellitus, and dyslipidemia, whereas risk factors for other types of CVD are less well recognized.

To complicate matters further, pathological overlap between VBI and neurodegenerative disorders is frequent, especially with increasing age. The application of "either-or" diagnostic criteria in epidemiologic studies fosters a dichotomous view of VCI and AD. Autopsy studies show a more complex reality. Macro- and microinfarcts are each found in approximately 30% of elderly persons, often combined with AD pathology [5–7]. Converging evidence indicates that ischemic infarcts and neurodegenerative lesions combine in an additive fashion to increase the risk of cognitive impairment and dementia [8–12].

> **Aging + AD + VBI + Lewy bodies – cognitive reserve = cognitive impairment**
> ***Lewy bodies**

Non-Alzheimer's and Atypical Dementia, First Edition. Edited by Michael D. Geschwind and Caroline Racine Belkoura.
© 2016 John Wiley & Sons, Ltd. Published 2016 by John Wiley & Sons, Ltd.

Table 4.1 Terms and abbreviations.

Syndromes
MCI = mild cognitive impairment (cognitive impairment without significant compromise of instrumental or personal activities of daily living)
MCI subtypes: amnestic, amnestic plus other cognitive domain, nonamnestic single domain, nonamnestic plus other cognitive domains
Memory impairment = free recall is below expectations
Amnestic memory impairment = free recall is below expectations and is not attributed to diminished attention or retrieval (i.e., does not improved significantly with cueing)
VCI = vascular cognitive impairment (cognitive impairment ascribed to vascular disease or vascular brain injury)
VaD = vascular dementia (dementia ascribed to vascular disease or vascular brain injury)

Alzheimer disease
AD = Alzheimer's disease (refers to progressive cognitive decline associated with widespread neurofibrillary tangles and neuritic amyloid plaques)
Clinically diagnosed AD (mild cognitive impairment or dementia ascribed to AD, without pathological data)

Cerebrovascular disease
CAA = cerebral amyloid angiopathy
CVD = cerebrovascular disease (disease of blood vessels) (e.g., atherosclerosis, arteriolosclerosis)
Atherosclerosis = disorder affecting endothelial and elastic lamina of larger arteries
Arteriolosclerosis = disorder affecting smooth muscle cell layer of arterioles
Arteriosclerosis = includes atherosclerosis and arteriolosclerosis

Vascular risk factors
VRF = vascular risk factors (refers to known risk factors for stroke (e.g., hypertension, hyperlipidemia, diabetes mellitus, atrial fibrillation))
Vascular factors = included VRF and CVD

Vascular brain injury
Stroke = sudden-onset neurological deficit ascribed to CVD
VBI = vascular brain injury (parenchymal brain injury ascribed to vascular disease)

MRI lesions
MTA = medial temporal atrophy
WMH = white matter hyperintensity on MRI (synonyms include WML (white matter lesion), WMSH (white matter signal hyperintensity), and leukoaraiosis (rarefaction of white matter on CT))
SBI = silent brain infarct on MRI
SI = silent infarct on MRI
SL = silent lacune (may include infarcts and perivascular spaces)

Table 4.2 The pathogenic spectrum of vascular cognitive impairment: RF→ CVD → VBI →VCI.

Risk factors	Vascular phenotype: "Cerebrovascular disease (CVD)"	Vascular distribution	Mechanism of brain injury	Brain pathology phenotype: vascular brain injury (VBI)	Location/neural network	Clinical phenotype or syndrome: "stroke" or vascular cognitive impairment (VCI)
Modifiable	*Cerebrovascular*	*Single artery*	*Ischemia*	Complete infarction	Limbic–diencephalic memory system	Multi-infarct dementia
Hypertension	Atherosclerosis	Large artery	*Acute*	(Symptomatic or silent)		Strategic infarct dementia
Hyperglycemia	Arteriolosclerosis	Small arteriole	thrombosis	Incomplete infarction	Multimodal association areas	Lacunar state
Hyperlipidemia	Amyloid angiopathy	Capillary	Embolism	(demyelination;	Corticobasal ganglia-thalamocortical loops	Subcortical vascular dementia
(Apolipoproteins)	Vasculitis	*Border zone*	*Chronic*	selective neuronal loss)	Deep white matter connections	Binswanger's syndrome
Smoking	Tortuosity	Large arteries	hypoperfusion	Hematoma	(cingulum, superior frontal occipital fasciculus, superior longitudinal fasciculus)	
Obesity	Anomaly	Small arterioles	*Hemorrhage*	Microbleed		
Nonmodifiable	*Cardiac*	Capillaries	*Leaky BBB*	Neuronal loss with gliosis		
Age	Atrial fibrillation	*Vein*	*Anoxia*			
Gender	Endocarditis					
Race	Myopathy					
Heredity	Mural thrombus					
CADASIL	*Blood content*					
CARASIL	Hypoglycemia					
HCHWA-D	Hypoxemia					
HCHWA-I	Hemoglobinopathy					
	Coagulopathy					

Table 4.3 Clinical Criteria for vascular dementia (VaD).

Diagnostic criteria		Dementia	VBI	Evidence of causal relationship
Hachinski Ischemic Score (HIS) (0–17 points) [38]: HIS ≥7 suggests MID HIS 5–6 suggests MIX HIS ≤4 suggests AD		No specific criteria	CVD risk factors (HTN, ASCVD)	Not specifically required
DSM-IV [39]		Memory loss Sufficient to interfere No clouding of consciousness	Sudden onset Stepwise progression Focal neurological signs and symptoms Stepwise deteriorating course and "patchy" distribution of deficits, focal neurologic signs and symptoms	Evidence from the history, physical examination, or laboratory tests of significant cerebrovascular disease that is judged to be etiologically related to the disturbance
ICD-10 [42]		Unequal distribution of deficits in higher cognitive functions with some affected and others relatively spared	There is evidence of focal brain damage, manifest as at least one of the following: unilateral spastic weakness of the limbs, unilaterally increased tendon reflexes, an extensor plantar response, or pseudobulbar palsy	From the history, examination, or test, there is evidence of significant cerebrovascular disease which may reasonably be judged to be etiologically related to the dementia (history of stroke, evidence of cerebral infarction)
ADDTC [41]	Probable	Multifaceted cognitive impairment sufficient to interfere with customary affairs of life	Infarct outside the cerebellum by imaging	Two infarcts or one infarct with temporal relationship to onset of cognitive impairment
	Possible		One infarct outside the cerebellum by imaging OR confluent white matter change	Not required
NINDS-AIREN [40]	Probable	Memory loss Plus impairment in two other cognitive domains	Focal neurological signs Imaging findings	Abrupt onset Stepwise progression Temporal relationship to onset of cognitive impairment
	Possible		Either imaging findings, abrupt onset, stepwise, OR temporal relationship	
AHA/ASA (2011) [43]	Probable	Decline in cognitive function in ≥2 domains sufficient to interfere with ADL At least 4 domains tested (attention/ executive, memory, language, visuospatial) Decline in ADL is independent from motor/ sensory sequelae of the vascular event	Imaging evidence of CVD	Clear temporal relationship between vascular event and cognitive deficit onset Clear relationship between severity and pattern of cognitive impairment and diffuse subcortical CVD No history of gradually progressive cognitive deficits before/ after CVA to suggest nonvascular neurodegenerative etiology
	Possible	Above Severe aphasia precludes cognitive assessment	Imaging findings, but no clear relationship (temporal, severity, or cognitive pattern) with cognitive impairment No imaging available	Evidence of another potential cause for cognitive dysfunction in addition to CVD
DSM-5 [44] Major or mild NCD	Probable	Decline in cognitive function in ≥1 cognitive domains	Imaging findings CT or MRI Temporal relationship Prominent decline in attention and executive function Presence of clinical evidence + genetic disorder (i.e., CADASIL)	Evidence from the history, physical examination, or laboratory tests of significant cerebrovascular disease that is judged to be etiologically related to the neurocognitive deficits
	Possible	Sufficient to interfere with ADL No clouding of consciousness	Evidence of VBI without clear temporal relationship to cognitive deficits	

ADDTC, State of California Alzheimer's Disease Diagnostic and Treatment Centers; ASCVD, asymptomatic cardiovascular disease; DSM, Diagnostic and Statistical Manual of Mental Disorders, Fifth Edition (DSM-5); HTN, hypertension; MID, multi-infarct dementia; MIX, mixed dementia (vascular and Alzheimer's disease (AD); NCD, neurocognitive disorder; NINDS-AIREN, National Institute of Neurological Disorders and Stroke and Association Internationale pour la Recherché et l'Enseignement en Neurosciences; VBI, vascular brain injury.

Epidemiology

From a public health perspective, VCI is the second most common cause of cognitive impairment in late life after AD. One of three persons meets criteria for dementia following first stroke [13]. Persons with stroke who are not initially demented are twice as likely as normal controls to develop dementia over the next 10 years [14]. The incidence of vascular dementia (VaD) increases exponentially after 65 years of age, ranging from 3 to 19 per 1000 persons/year at age 80 years [15–17], approximately half the rate of AD. In the Canadian Study of Health and Aging of persons older than age 65 years, the prevalence of cognitive impairment no dementia (CIND) was similar to (17%) the number of combined persons with dementia or stroke (8% each) [18]. In this study, the relative contributions of VBI to CIND were believed to be considerable.

To minimize survival bias, cohorts at risk should be established in midlife and followed longitudinally. In the Honolulu Heart Program, history of high systolic blood pressure (SBP) [19] and diabetes mellitus [20] was associated with greater risk of dementia in late life (especially among persons with the apolipoprotein E ε4 allele). In the Framingham Heart Study [21], duration of diabetes was related to poorer cognitive performance. In the CAIDE study, higher midlife cholesterol levels were associated with increased risk of dementia [22, 23]. These epidemiologic studies underscore the importance of managing hypertension, diabetes mellitus, and cholesterol beginning in midlife.

MRI scans in longitudinal population-based studies reveal SBI and WMH in approximately one-third of persons over age 65 years [24–26]. These lesions increase with age, are associated with hypertension, and increase the risk of stroke and dementia [27, 28]. In the Framingham Offspring Study of middle-aged adults, SBI and severe WMH were associated with increased risk of stroke and dementia independent of vascular risk factors [29]. These studies identify subclinical VBI on MRI as relevant targets for early detection and primary prevention. Cerebral microbleeds (CMBs) are also present in one-third of persons over age 80 years based on population studies and are associated with increased risk of stroke, cognitive decline, and mortality [30].

Genetic epidemiology

Several forms of CVD are associated with genetic mutations or polymorphisms. CADASIL is caused by mutations or deletions in the Notch3 gene (chromosome 19p13) [31, 32]. A similar autosomal recessive syndrome (CARASIL) results from mutations in the HtrA serine peptidase 1 (HTRA1) [33]. Dutch, Icelandic, and Finnish forms of familial CAA are associated with hereditary cerebral hemorrhage with amyloidosis (HCHWA) [34]. At the population level, the apolipoprotein E ε4 allele increases vascular deposition of abeta in the sporadic form of CAA [35].

Case presentations

The clinical presentation for VCI is highly heterogeneous, varying in onset, progression, and profile of cognitive impairment. In the following case presentations, we illustrate two approaches to diagnosis of VCI: (i) the application of criteria for the clinical diagnosis of VaD (Table 4.3) and (ii) a neurobehavioral approach, which considers location of VBI within memory and cognitive networks (Table 4.4).

Table 4.4 Neurobehavioral approach to diagnosis of VCI, AD, or mixed VCI/AD.

Feature	Favors VCI	Favors AD	Other Differential
Neuropsychological testing			
Amnesic memory disorder?		+++	
Semantic fluency better than phonemic fluency		++	
Executive impairment worse than memory impairment	++		
MRI findings			
Moderate to severe hippocampal atrophy		+++	Hippocampal sclerosis Anoxic injury Herpes simplex Encephalitis
Severe WMH (CHS grade ≥7)	++	+(Can be seen in AD with CAA)	Hypertensive angiopathy Cerebral amyloid angiopathy CADASIL
Infarction within frontal-subcortical loops or other strategic locations	+++		
Acute stroke with temporal relationship to onset of cognitive impairment	+++		
Nonstrategic infarction	+		

AD, Alzheimer's disease; CAA, cerebral amyloid angiopathy; CADASIL, cerebral autosomal dominant arteriopathy with subcortical infarcts and leukoencephalopathy; CHS, Cardiovascular Health Study; VCI, vascular cognitive impairment; WMH, white matter hyperintensities.

Case 1

Four years prior, a 71-year-old Caucasian gentleman sustained a mild stroke with right-sided weakness and slurred speech. Following this, he became quiet and withdrawn, which the family thought was depression. The family noted a gradually progressive cognitive decline over the past 4 years. He now forgets conversations and, events within a few minutes, offers very little spontaneous speech, shows lack of interest, and is quite apathetic.

Past medical history is significant for a 20-year history of hypertension and a 15-year history of type 2 diabetes and hypercholesterolemia, as well as benign prostatic hypertrophy. He takes aspirin, tolazamide, metformin, troglitazone, lisinopril, and lovastatin. He is a retired salesman with 16 years of education.

On physical examination, blood pressure (BP) was 146/92 mmHg. Neurologic examination showed blunted affect, mild right spastic hemiparesis, and bilateral Babinski signs. Mini-Mental State Examination (MMSE) score was 22/30. He had word-finding difficulties, concrete thinking, and mild perseveration. Neuropsychological testing revealed severe impairment in all aspects of verbal list learning, including acquisition, immediate and delayed recall, and recognition. He was severely impaired on confrontation naming and semantic and phonemic fluency. Working memory was mildly impaired. Visuospatial skills and abstract reasoning were low average. A self-reported scale did not suggest depression.

EKG showed left ventricular hypertrophy. MRI revealed cystic infarcts in the right anterior thalamus, left genu of the internal capsule, and left posterior limb of the internal capsule (Figure 4.1). SBI were noted in the right putamen and left frontal white matter. Periventricular white matter changes were mild (grade 1 on the Cardiovascular Health Study (CHS) white matter scale [25]). Coronal T1 MRI showed moderate medial temporal atrophy (MTA) (2+ on MTA scale [36]) and moderate cerebral atrophy (Figure 4.2).

Comment

This patient has significant risk factors for VaD. His Framingham stroke risk profile [37] is calculated at 19 (+5 age 71; +7 treated systolic blood pressure; +2 diabetes; +5 left ventricular hypertrophy). A Framingham profile of 19 is associated with a 33% 10-year probability of first stroke. His history of prior right-sided weakness corresponds with infarct in the left posterior limb of the internal capsule, further increasing the probability of recurrent stroke.

He meets criteria for MID by Hachinski Ischemic Score [38], DSM-IV criteria for VaD [39], National Institute of Neurological Disorders and Stroke and Association Internationale pour la Recherché et l'Enseignement en Neurosciences (NINDS-AIREN) criteria for possible VaD [40], the State of California Alzheimer's Disease Diagnostic and Treatment Centers (ADDTC) criteria for probable ischemic VaD [41], ICD-10 criteria for VaD [42], American Heart Association/American Stroke Association (AHA/ASA) criteria for possible VaD [43], and DSM-5 criteria for possible major vascular neurocognitive disorder [44] (Table 4.3). He meets NINDS-AIREN criteria for possible but not probable VaD, because there was no temporal relationship between a stroke and his gradual cognitive decline.

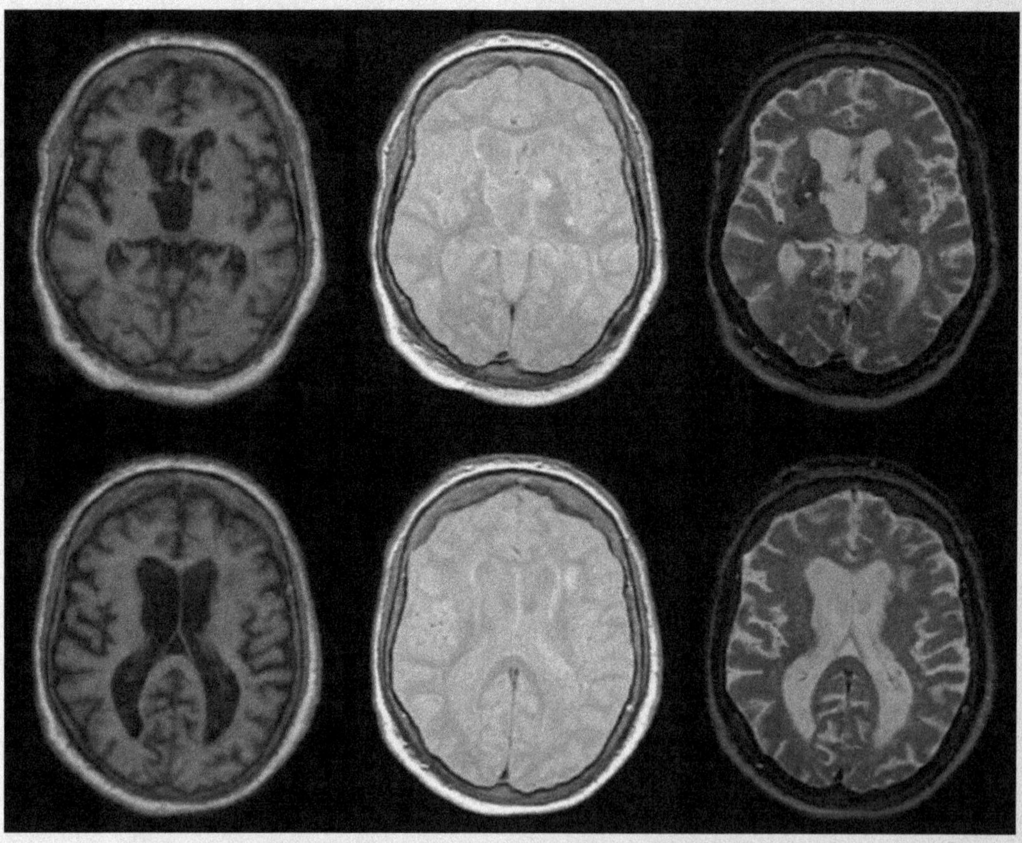

Figure 4.1 Case 1: axial MRI (T1, proton density (PD), and T2 weighted) shows cystic infarcts in the right anterior thalamus and left genu internal capsule. SBI are seen in the right putamen, left posterior limb of the internal capsule (top row), and left frontal white matter (bottom row). Periventricular white matter changes are rated grade 1 on CHS scale.

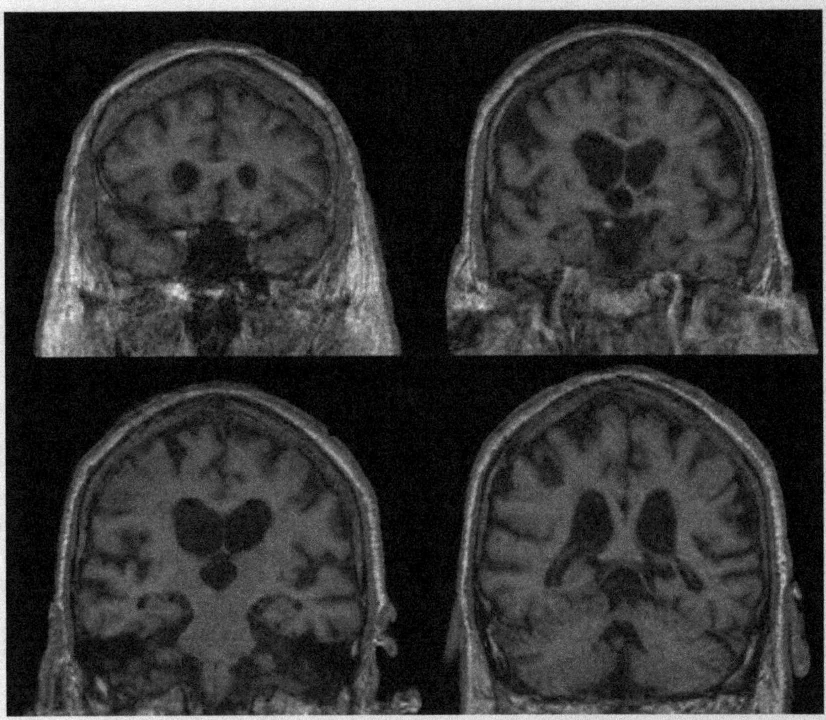

Figure 4.2 Case 1: coronal T1-weighted MRI shows moderate 2+ hippocampal atrophy on Scheltens' rating scale [110, 111] and moderate generalized cerebral atrophy.

Apathy, withdrawal, and slowing are typical in SVD. Severe impairment in verbal memory on neuropsychological testing plus moderate atrophy of the hippocampi suggests the possibility of concomitant AD. Two cystic infarcts, however, are observed in strategic locations for memory: the right anterior thalamus and the left genu of the internal capsule. Anterior thalamic lesions are well known to disturb episodic memory [45], and lesions in the genu of the internal capsule disrupt outflow in the anterior thalamic peduncle [46]. The parsimonious clinical diagnosis is VCI.

Neuropathology

Autopsy revealed severe, complicated atheroma in the basal vessels with 55–70% stenosis and multiple lacunar infarcts in the basal ganglia. No significant AD pathology was present (Braak and Braak stage = 0; the Consortium to Establish a Registry for Alzheimer's Disease (CERAD) criteria neuritic plaque = none). The final clinicopathologic diagnosis is pure VaD with strategic infarcts.

Case 2

An 85-year-old African American gentleman with a history of several old strokes and a combination of stepwise and progressive cognitive decline. The first stroke, 21 years ago, had no significant cognitive or physical sequelae. Eighteen years ago, a more serious stroke caused forgetfulness, mild left hemiparesis, and transient speech disturbance, leading to a right carotid endarterectomy. After this, his memory declined gradually and slowly. He has developed gradual and progressive word-finding difficulty for 5 years. He still manages his activities of daily living, drives locally, and watches television. He complains of poor memory and decreased interest in socializing but denies depression. Past medical history is significant for hypercholesterolemia. He reports no history of hypertension, diabetes, or heart disease. He takes only aspirin.

On physical examination, BP is 148/94 mmHg; pulse is 84 and regular. Spasticity and weakness are present in both upper extremities, left greater than right. Deep tendon reflexes are increased on the left, and Babinski signs are present bilaterally. Snout, glabellar, palmomental, and right grasp reflexes are present. His gait is wide based and paretic (left- greater than right-sided weakness). His MMSE score is 18 of 30. He is friendly but dysarthric and has significant word-finding difficulties. Neuropsychological testing reveals severe impairments in verbal memory, naming, and semantic fluency.

MRI shows moderate hyperintensities in bilateral periventricular white matter, SBI in the right anterior limb of the internal capsule, and prominent perivascular spaces plus encephalomalacia in the right putamen (Figure 4.3). WMH are rated 6–7 on the CHS scale [25]. Coronal sections show 3+ MTA [36] and severe cerebral atrophy (Figure 4.4).

Comment

This patient had two strokes and has a Framingham risk profile score [37] of 15 (+10 age 85; +5 untreated SBP). Left- greater than right-sided spastic hemiparesis is consistent with bilateral lesions and worse in the right hemisphere. The left hemiparesis could be related either to the ischemic events involving the right cortical spinal tract in the white matter or in the posterior limb of the internal capsule. The gradual deterioration

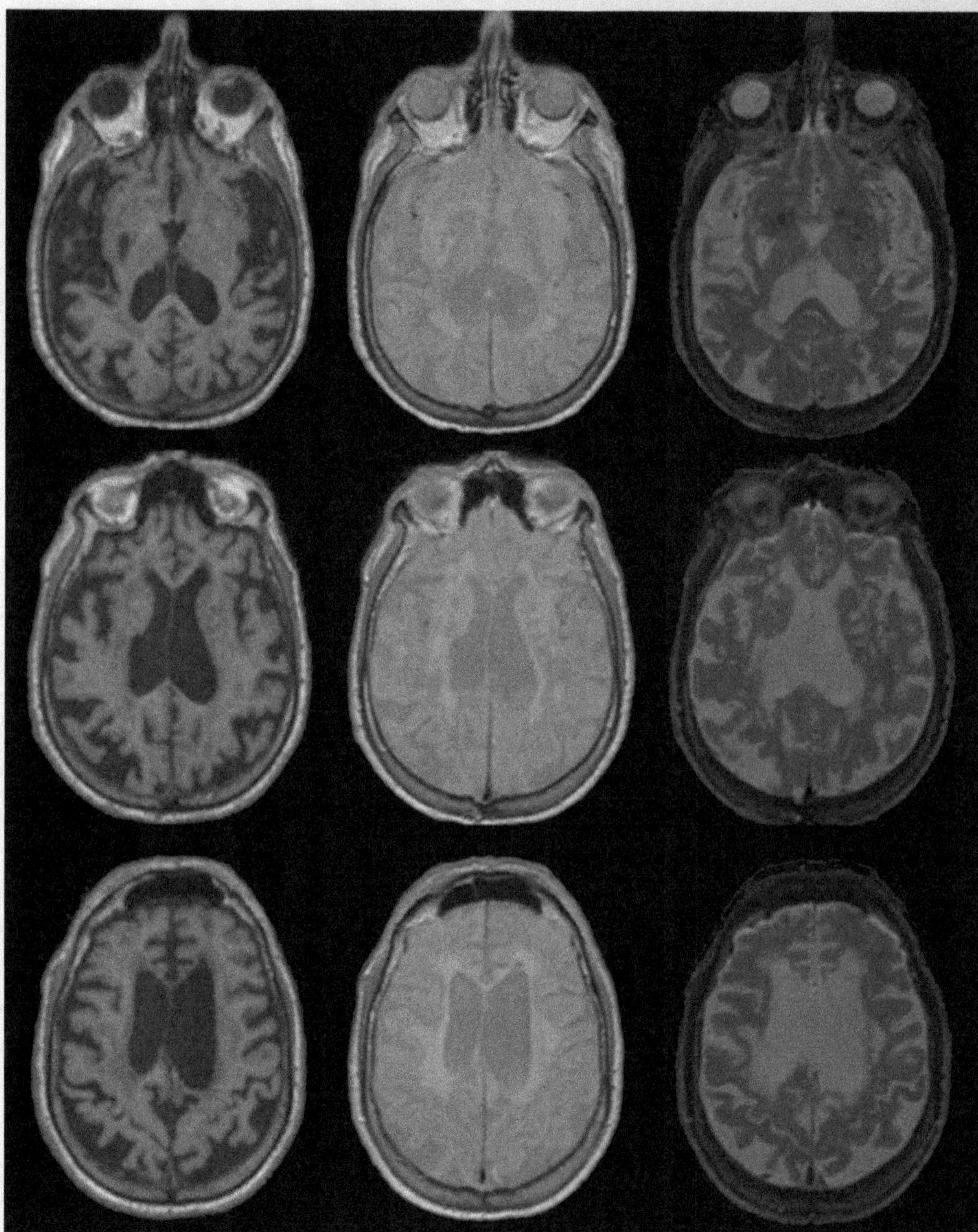

Figure 4.3 Case 2: axial MRI (T1, PD, and T2 weighted) shows T2-weighted hyperintensities in bilateral periventricular white matter, SBI in the right anterior limb of the internal capsule, and prominent perivascular spaces plus encephalomalacia in the right putamen. White matter hyperintensities are rated 6–7 on the CHS scale.

during the past 5 years can be attributed to moderately severe WMH. He meets NINDS-AIREN criteria and AHA/ASA for probable VaD and DSM-IV and DSM-V criteria for VaD (Table 4.3).

The history of two strokes and the presence of infarcts and white matter changes on MRI offer a partial explanation of his cognitive impairment. The second stroke showed a temporal relationship with the onset of forgetfulness. Silent incomplete infarcts (note: incomplete infarct refers to MRI lesions that are hyperintense on T2 or FLAIR and minimally hypointense on T1-weighted sequences) in the right anterior limb of the internal capsule disconnect frontal-subcortical loops and contribute to dysexecutive syndrome and disinhibition. The severity of his verbal memory loss and difficulty with confrontation naming suggests the possibility of a superimposed neurodegenerative process such as AD. This is supported by significant atrophy of the hippocampus and cerebral cortex. Taking a neurobehavioral approach, the clinical diagnosis is mixed dementia due to VCI and possible AD.

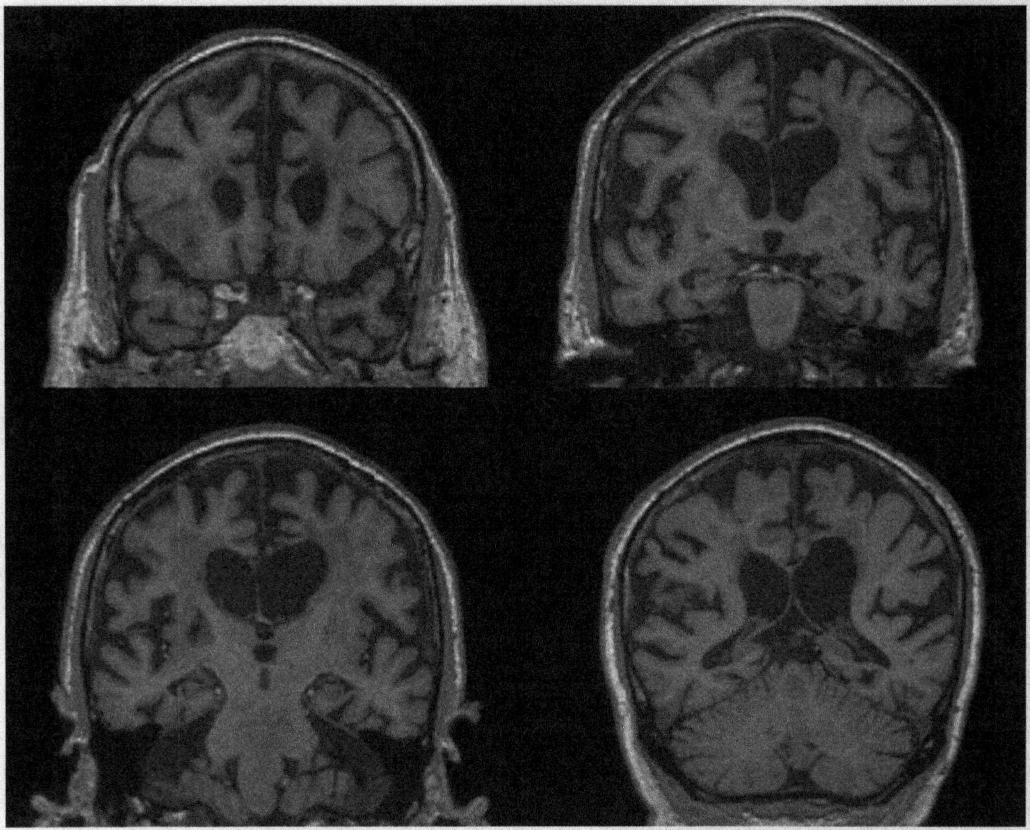

Figure 4.4 Case 2: coronal T1-weighted MRI shows 3+ atrophy by Scheltens' scale [110] of the hippocampus and severe cerebral atrophy.

Neuropathology

Postmortem revealed severe atherosclerosis in the anterior cerebral artery, infarcts in the right putamen and frontal lobe, and deep white matter, with degeneration of the corpus callosum. The white matter demonstrated spongy changes and gliosis. An infarct was noted in the medulla as well. Widespread AD pathology was present (Braak and Braak stage=VI; CERAD neuritic plaque=moderate). Final clinicopathologic diagnosis is dementia due to mixed AD and CVD.

Case 3

A 78-year-old white female gives a 1- to 3-year history of slow decline in memory. She is unable to remember the plots of plays and is using memory aids. For the past year, she has had difficulty with handling her checking account but is otherwise independent in IADL. Her PMH revealed she has a 25-year history of hypertension which is well controlled and takes aldactazide. Her father died following a stroke. Blood pressure was 110/80, MMSE, 27/30, and blessed memory-information-concentration test, 26/33. She has mild difficulty with tandem gait and slowed alternating movements. Neuropsychological testing shows circumscribed verbal and visual memory deficits. Cholesterol was 225; LDL cholesterol was 156. MRI shows severe confluent deep white matter changes (grade 7–8 on the CHS white matter scale), SBI in the right lateral thalamus, and mineralization of the globus pallidi (Figure 4.5). Coronal sections show 3+ atrophy of both hippocampi and moderate cerebral atrophy (Figure 4.6).

Comment

She fits criteria for mild cognitive impairment, amnestic type [47], and AHA/ASA criteria for probable VaMCI [43]. She has a long-standing hypertension. Confluent white matter changes are consistent with small vessel disease, either due to hypertension or to CAA. Neither the WMH nor the SBI in the lateral thalamus explain her amnesic memory impairment.

Neuropathology

The patient died 1 year later at age 79 years. Autopsy showed mild atherosclerosis, moderate arteriolosclerosis, and mild CAA.

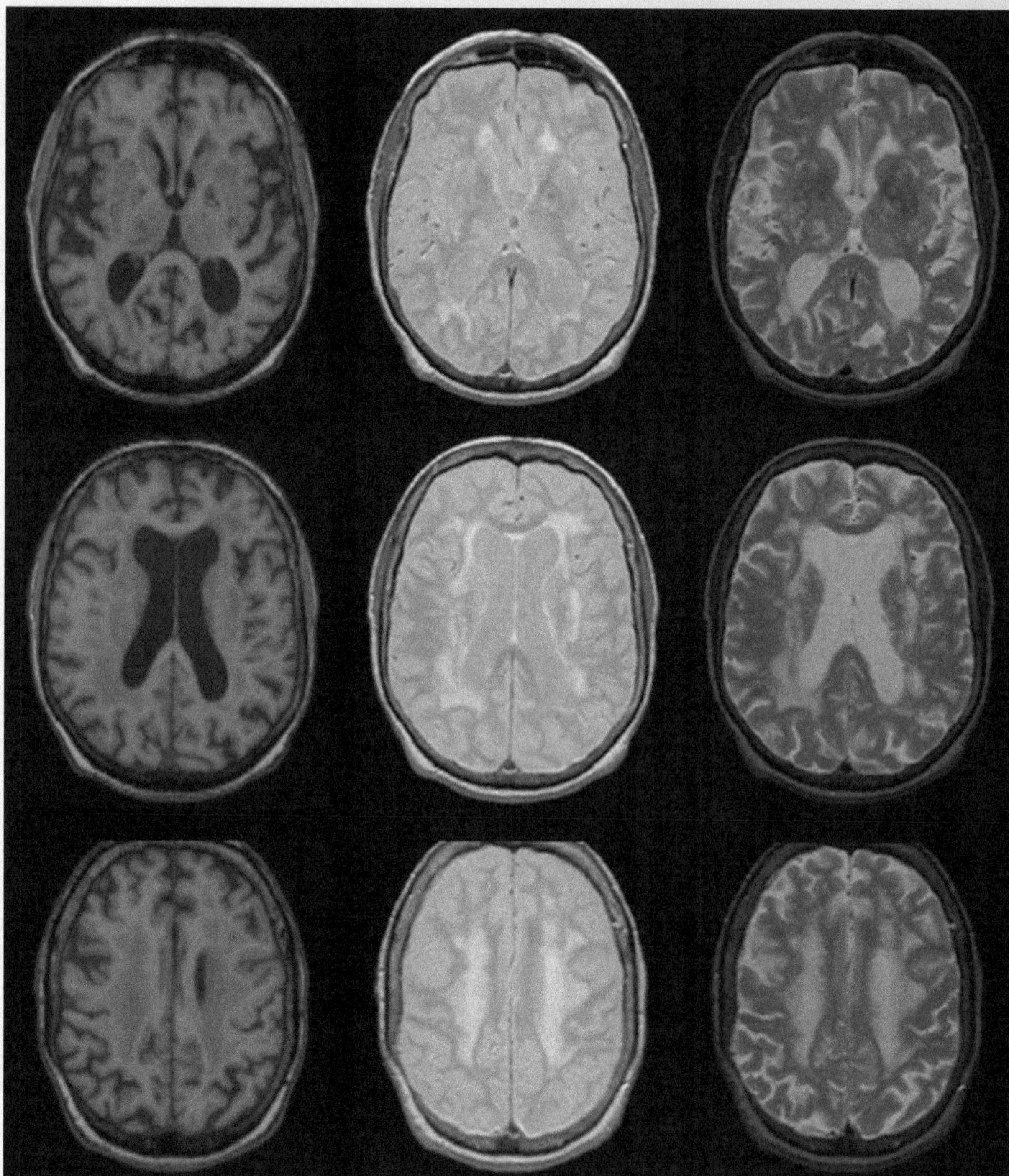

Figure 4.5 Case 3: MRI (T1, PD, and T2 weighted) shows severe confluent deep white matter changes (grade 7–8), SBI in the right lateral thalamus, and mineralization of the globus pallidi.

Neurofibrillary tangles and neuritic plaques were found in the hippocampus, but not neocortex (Braak and Braak stage IV, CERAD sparse). Acute infarcts were found in both cortex and white matter. In addition, there were multiple cortical microinfarcts and diffuse white matter demyelination (better explained by arteriolosclerosis than CAA or Wallerian degeneration). Final pathologic diagnosis is MCI due to mixed SVD and early AD.

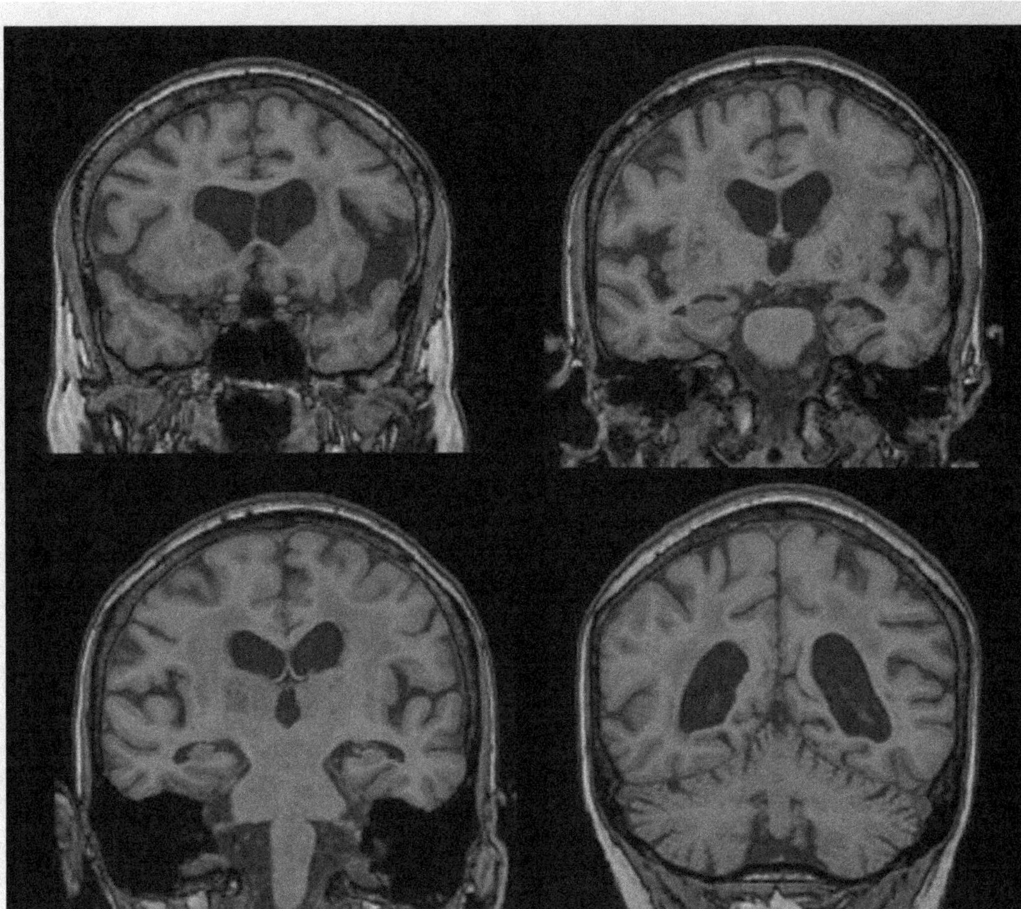

Figure 4.6 Case 3: coronal T1-weighted MRI shows 3+ atrophy by Scheltens' scale [110] of both hippocampi and moderate cerebral atrophy.

Clinical subtypes of VCI

VCI has been categorized in many ways including heritability (e.g., CADASIL), location (e.g., SVD, strategic), clinical presentation (poststroke dementia (PSD); Binswanger's syndrome), or MRI findings (e.g., SBI). We review several common nonmutually exclusive syndromes.

PSD

In hospital- and community-based series, it has been shown that stroke doubles the risk of dementia. The incidence of dementia within 6–12 months' poststroke is about 20%, and the risk of delayed dementia, including AD, is also doubled after stroke [13] (Figure 4.7). In Olmsted County, Minnesota, prevalent dementia was 30% immediately after stroke; incident dementia was 7% 1 year poststroke and rose to 48% 25 years after stroke [48]. Compared to normal controls, history of stroke doubles the risk of dementia over 10 years [14].

Risk factors for dementia at the time of stroke include fewer years of education, older age, diabetes mellitus, atrial fibrillation, and recurrent stroke [49]. Stroke locations associated with higher likelihood of cognitive impairment include left hemisphere, anterior and posterior cerebral artery distribution, multiple infarcts, and strategic infarcts (see following text) [13]. Neuroimaging variables associated with PSD include SBI, WMH, and global and medial temporal atrophy [13].

Concomitant AD is also a major risk factor for PSD. About 15–30% of persons with PSD have a history of dementia before stroke [50, 51], and approximately one-third have significant MTA [52]. Case 2 is an example in which severe MTA was shown on MRI (Figure 4.4), and a diagnosis of mixed AD and CVD was confirmed at autopsy.

Strategic infarct dementia

A dementia syndrome might result from a single infarct placed in a strategic location. The left angular gyrus, inferomesial temporal, and mesial frontal lobe are considered strategic locations perfused by large arteries. Frontal-subcortical loops are strategic networks for executive function. These networks include the prefrontal cortex, head of the caudate, anterior and dorsomedial

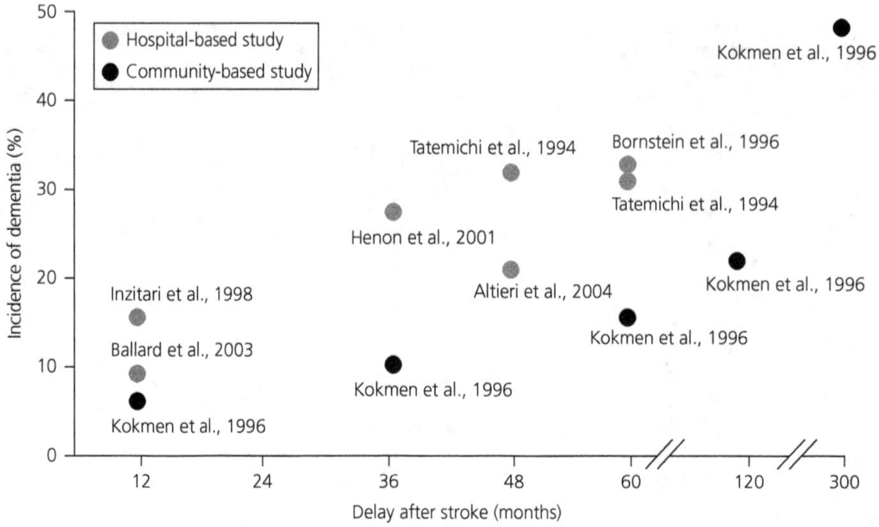

Figure 4.7 Incidence of poststroke dementia at different time intervals after stroke onset in hospital-based studies (gray) and community-based studies (black). When the reference appears several times, data provided correspond to different assessments at different time intervals in the same cohort of patients. Source: Leys et al. [13]. Reproduced with permission from Elsevier.

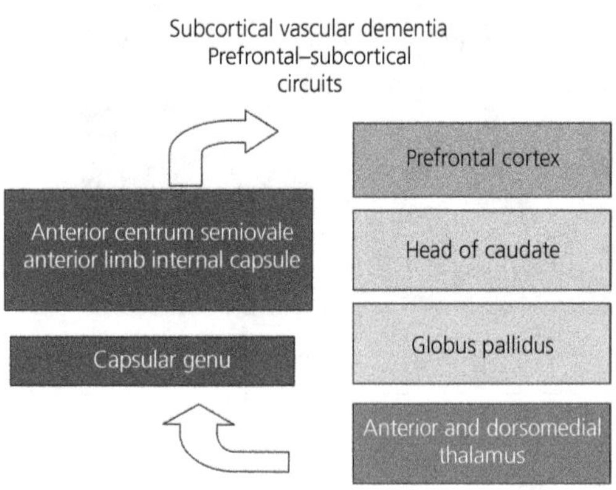

Figure 4.8 Prefrontal-subcortical circuits important for executive function.

thalamic nuclei, capsular genu, and anterior limb of the internal capsule [53, 54] (Figure 4.8). The dementia syndrome associated with thalamic infarcts is characterized by marked apathy, impaired attention and mental control, and anterograde and retrograde amnesia [45, 55, 56]. In case 1, lesions in the right anterior thalamic nucleus and the genu of the left internal capsule demonstrate strategic infarcts.

SVD is defined by VBI confined mainly to subcortical white and gray matter. Small vessel infarcts account for 25% of subjects hospitalized for strokes and make up nearly 60% of asymptomatic strokes in community-based studies [26]. In addition to PSD and strategic infarct dementia due to small vessel disease, lacunar state and Binswanger's syndrome all fall under the umbrella of SVD.

Lacunar state (etat lacunaire) is an extreme phenotype of SVD, characterized by multiple lacunar infarcts in the basal ganglia, thalamus, and white matter. Clinical features included sudden-onset hemiparesis, lack of volition, akinetic mutism, dysarthria, pseudobulbar palsy and affect, small-stepped gait, and urinary incontinence [57]. Prior to MRI, the distribution of lacunes in subcortical gray matter and white matter, especially of the frontal lobe, was documented by autopsy [57, 58].

The pathological hallmark of Binswanger's syndrome is prominent demyelination of the deep white matter, ascribed to stenosis of the deep penetrating medullary arteries [59, 60]. A triad of slowly progressive dementia, gait apraxia, and urinary incontinence might be confused clinically with normal pressure hydrocephalus (NPH). Neuroimaging, however, shows severe cerebral atrophy and widening of the sulci in Binswanger's syndrome, indicating a secondary ex vacuo type of ventriculomegaly.

CADASIL

CADASIL (see Chapter 12) offers a prototypic example of "pure" SVD without concomitant AD. Extracellular domains of NOTCH3 protein accumulate in the smooth muscle walls of small arterioles [61, 62]. CADASIL is associated with migraine, depression, and seizures beginning in early adulthood, followed by recurrent ischemic events and progressive cognitive decline [63, 64]. Prominent slowing and impairment in executive function, with relative preservation of recall and receptive language, are noted on neuropsychological testing [65]. Severity of cognitive impairment correlates better with lacunar infarcts rather than WMH or microbleeds [66, 67].

Subclinical VBI

Symptomatic stroke is the tip of the iceberg of VBI. In the Rotterdam study, the prevalence of SBI was five times greater than symptomatic stroke [26]. SBI should be differentiated from CSF-filled perivascular spaces (PVS) [68], which are sometimes

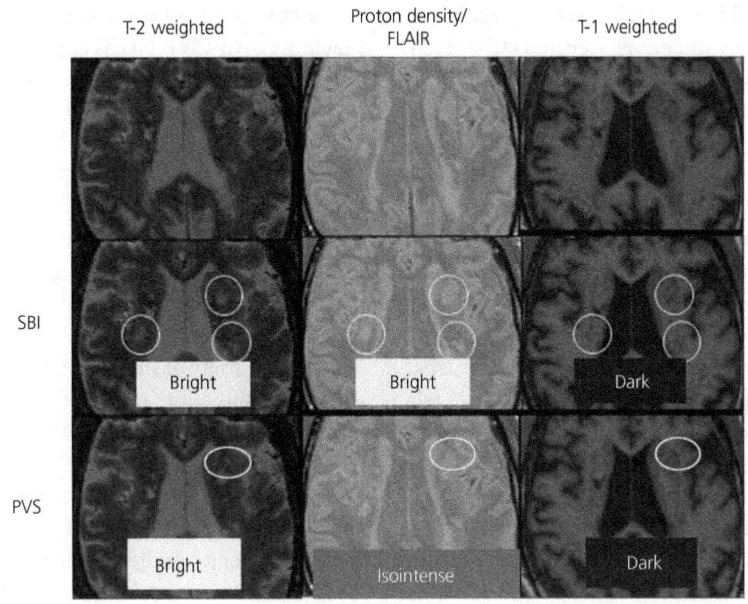

Figure 4.9 Both SBI and perivascular spaces (PVS) are bright on T2-weighted sequences. On proton density or fluid-attenuated inversion recovery (FLAIR) sequences, however, SBI are hyperintense (bright), whereas perivascular spaces (PVS) are isointense, compared to cerebrospinal fluid (CSF). On T1-weighted sequences, both SBI and PVS are hypointense or dark.

especially prominent in the putamen and infraputaminal regions, as well as near the anterior commissure [69] (Figure 4.9). Rarefaction of the periventricular and deep white matter can be seen as leukoaraiosis (LA) on CT scan [70] and as WMH on FLAIR or T2-weighted MRI [71]. Semiquantitative white matter intensity scales are useful to communicate the severity of WMH in clinical practice. In cross-sectional studies, WMH ratings are associated with mild impairment on the Modified Mini-Mental State (3MS) exam [72]. In longitudinal MRI studies, incident SBI and worsening WMH correlate with cognitive decline, especially information processing speed [73–75], supporting the relevance of SBI and WMH as presymptomatic targets for risk reduction. CMBs are small, round, or ovoid hypointensities, of <10 mm in diameter, evident on T2* gradient-recall echo (T2*GRE) and susceptibility-weighted (SWI) MRI sequences [30]. The presence of CMBs, which are considered a marker of small vessel pathology due to either hypertensive vasculopathy or CAA, may be an independent contributor to cognitive impairment. Location of CMBs suggests underlying pathology. Deep and lobar CMBs have been associated with hypertensive vasculopathy versus strictly lobar CMBs with CAA. The sensitivity and specificity of these associations has not yet been studied. Cognitive deficits may vary depending on the location of CMBs, mostly affecting executive function, speed of processing, and other nonmemory cognitive domains [76, 77]. Recently, in a Japanese cohort of subjects with vascular risk factors ($n = 729$), the presence of ≥2 CMBs or mixed lobar and deep CMBs was associated with increased risk of all-cause dementia, independent of other risk factors (age, sex, education, and *APOE* ε4 status) [78].

Evaluation and diagnosis

Clinical evaluation

The clinical evaluation for VCI follows the established approach to the evaluation of cognitive impairment: a thorough history (from both the patient and a reliable informant); physical examination, including screening mental state examination, with emphasis on complete neurologic (focal neurological signs, gait disturbance) and cardiovascular components (funduscopic examination of retinal vessels, carotid bruit, cardiac arrhythmia); laboratory testing (left ventricular hypertrophy, renal insufficiency); and neuroimaging (brain CT or MRI). At the present time, structural MRI provides the most sensitive and specific measure of VBI [79]. Emphasis is placed on identification by history of vascular risk factors (hypertension, hyperlipidemia, diabetes, heart disease) for risk reduction and on the pattern of cognitive and affective disturbance and functional decline for symptomatic treatment, management, and support.

Neuropsychological testing

There is no single characteristic behavioral profile for VCI. Memory impairment in VCI is variable, tends to be of the dysexecutive rather than amnestic type, and responds better to cueing or recognition formats. WMH and SBI are often associated with decreased processing speed and executive function. In contrast to AD in which semantic fluency usually is more affected than phonemic fluency, in VCI, they generally are equally affected [80]. Microinfarcts have been associated with lower perceptual speed and semantic and episodic memory deficits independent of macroscopic infarcts or AD pathology [6].

Inclusion of Trails B, verbal fluency, clock drawing, digit symbol substitution, episodic memory (including free and cued recall), language, and visuospatial domains has been recommended by a 2005 North American workshop [81].

Clinical diagnosis

A diagnosis of VCI is typically made using one of several diagnostic criteria (Table 4.3). In comparing diagnostic criteria, it is useful to consider (i) evidence of cognitive impairment/dementia, (ii) evidence of VBI, and (iii) likelihood that VBI is causing VCI. The Hachinski Ischemic Score [38] assigns 1 or 2 points to a list of risk factors, signs, and symptoms associated with stroke. DSM-IV [39] and ICD-10 [42] leave assessment of causal relationship between VBI and VCI to the judgment of the clinician. For a diagnosis of probable VaD, the California ADDTC criteria [41] allow either a temporal relationship between VBI and VCI or evidence of two or more infarcts on a neuroimaging study. Temporal relationship is required for a diagnosis of probable VaD by NINDS-AIREN criteria [40], thereby increasing the stringency of these criteria.

More recent clinical criteria were published for the diagnosis of VCI by the AHA/ASA in 2011 [43]. These rely on evidence of VBI present by structural neuroimaging and establish causality based on temporal relationship and correlation between type of VBI and cognitive deficits. In addition, the International Society for Vascular Behavioral and Cognitive Disorders (VASCOG) has recently proposed a new set of criteria [82]. Updated DSM-5 criteria have been released [44] and propose a change in terminology from VaD or VCI to major or minor neurocognitive impairment due to CVD.

With the advent of in vivo biomarkers for the detection of amyloid accumulation in the brain, new diagnostic criteria for specific types of VCI are being proposed, that is, the Seoul criteria for Pittsburgh imaging compound B [PiB]-negative SVD based on clinical and MRI variables [83]. These criteria are based on the exclusion of coexistent AD pathology by amyloid PET scan and demonstration of VBI on MRI in patients that present with VCI. In their small cohort of patients ($n=77$), this criteria had 49% sensitivity and 100% specificity. This needs confirmation and further validation in large clinicopathological cohorts.

Criteria for the SVD subtype of VCI emphasize slowing of cognition, executive dysfunction (impairment in selective attention, abstract reasoning, and mental flexibility), depression, extrapyramidal signs, and gait disturbance [84]. In an autopsy-confirmed study, a "low executive" profile was 67% sensitive and 86% specific in distinguishing SVD from AD (positive likelihood ratio = 4.7) [85]. Although the sample size was small, the reference groups were defined by neuropathology, thereby avoiding the circularity that often occurs when comparison groups are defined clinically. The study suggests modest clinical utility of the executive dysfunction profile for SVD.

The neurobehavioral approach is illustrated for the three case presentations above and utilizes structure–function correlations in interpreting neuropsychological and neuroimaging studies (Table 4.4). An advantage is allowance for the dependent assessment of likelihood of VCI and AD and thus the diagnosis of mixed VCI/AD. The approach is applicable for MCI/CIND as well as dementia syndromes, although validation is needed.

CSF biomarkers

Further studies to determine markers that reflect the health and reactivity of intracerebral blood vessels and blood–brain barrier (BBB) integrity are needed. To date, no validated CSF biomarkers have been established to support the diagnosis of VCI, although a variety of substances have been proposed as measure of BBB dysfunction in CVD, including albumin index and matrix metalloproteinase-9 (MMP-9) [86].

Neuropathologic contributions to diagnosis and understanding

Neuropathologic studies determine the type and severity of CVD and severity and distribution of AD pathology. In contrast to AD, there is no gold standard for the neuropathologic diagnosis of VCI. Typically, the reference standard is based on evidence of infarcts in neocortex, without considering the causal relationship between VBI and VCI. With these caveats, the clinical criteria for VaD show high specificity and moderate sensitivity [87]. Several longitudinal cohort studies with high autopsy rates (Religious Orders Study, Honolulu-Asia Aging Study, Baltimore Longitudinal Study of Aging) underscore (i) the high prevalence of mixed vascular and neurodegenerative pathologies in late life and (ii) the additive risk of cerebral infarcts and AD pathology for cognitive impairment [9–11]. They also disclose the importance of microinfarcts [6] and hippocampal sclerosis [88] for cognitive impairment and memory loss and remind us that these lesions often go undetected or unsuspected until autopsy.

Treatment

Primary prevention: Identification and reduction of stroke risk factors

The type of underlying CVD (e.g., arteriosclerosis or CAA) should be considered. It is likely that reduction of vascular risk factors for arteriosclerosis can significantly reduce vascular contributions to pure vascular and mixed dementia. The beneficial effects of treating hypertension, diabetes mellitus, and dyslipidemia vis-à-vis risk of stroke are well established by randomized clinical trials. Evidence-based official guidelines have been disseminated [89], but all too often fall short in implementation. Primary or secondary prevention trials that include cognitive outcome measures are still limited (Table 4.5), often begin too late in life, and do not include sensitive cognitive outcome measures. In a meta-analysis of several placebo-controlled trials (SHEP, Sys-Eur, HYVET, and PROGRESS), treatment of hypertension was associated with reduction in the combined

Table 4.5 Primary and secondary prevention: clinical trials that include a cognition outcome measure.

	Antihypertensive	Duration of follow-up (years)	Main results for dementia	Significance
Primary prevention				
SHEP (1991) *N*=4736	Diuretic (chlorthalidone) and/or beta blocker (atenolol) or reserpine	4.5	16% reduction in dementia	n.s.
Syst-Eur (1998) *N*=2418	Ca channel blocker (dihydropyridine) with or without beta blocker (enalapril maleate) and/or diuretic (hydrochlorothiazide)	2.0	50% (0 to 76%) reduction in dementia	*P*=0.05
SCOPE (2003) *N*=4937	ARB (candesartan cilexetil) and/or diuretics	3.7	7% increased risk in active arm (but only 3.2/1.6 mmHg reduction in BP in treatment vs. control arm)	*P*>0.20
HYVET (2008) *N*=3336	Diuretic (indapamide) with or without ACEI (perindopril)	2.2	14% (−9 to 23%) reduction in dementia Trial stopped early because of significant reduction in stroke and mortality)	*P*=0.2
Secondary prevention				
PROGRESS (2003) *N*=6104	ACEI (perindopril) with or without diuretic (indapamide)	4.0	12% (−8 to 28%) reduction in dementia	*P*=0.2
PRoFESS (2008) *N*=20332	ARB (telmisartan)	2.4	No reduction of the risk of dementia	*P*=0.48

risk ratio (HR 0.87, 0.76–1.00, $p=0.045$) [90]. The Syst-Eur trial [91, 92] suggested that treatment of 1000 patients for 5 years could prevent 20 cases of dementia (95% CI, 7–33). In PROGRESS, a secondary prevention trial among persons with previous stroke or TIA [93], treatment with perindopril plus or minus indapamide showed a 19% relative risk reduction in cognitive decline and WMH progression over 4 years compared to placebo [94]. The Memory in Diabetes (MIND) substudy of the ACCORD trial will determine whether interventions for type 2 diabetes reduce cognitive decline and structural brain changes [95]. In the PROSPER study, no difference in cognitive decline was found among subjects treated with pravastatin compared to placebo after a mean follow-up period of 42 months [96]. In the Women's Antioxidant Cardiovascular Study, antioxidant supplementation did not slow cognitive change among women with preexisting cardiovascular disease or risk factors [97]. There are several promising prospective cohort studies, but currently, no clinical trials of omega-3 fatty acids [98] or exercise [99, 100] in the prevention of VCI. Two large trials for primary prevention of VCI are ongoing. The ASPREE trial [101] is a clinical trial evaluating (every 6 months) the prevention of cardiovascular disease and VaD with low-dose aspirin in the elderly (subjects ≥65 years); the study is expected to be completed in 2017. The Systolic Blood Pressure Intervention Trial: Memory and Cognition in Decreased Hypertension (SPRINT-MIND) [102] looks to see if tighter blood pressure control parameters over an average of about 5 years reduces the risk of incident dementia, reduces the rate of cognitive decline, and in a subset further decreases the volume of small vessel ischemic vascular disease.

For secondary prevention, a recent paper evaluating outcomes of a large community-based stroke registry from London, United Kingdom, found that "appropriate vascular risk management," defined as clinically indicated use of antihypertensives, antithrombotic agents, and lipid-lowering drugs, was associated with reduced long-term risk of cognitive impairment assessed by the Mini-Mental State Examination in patients with ischemic strokes without history of atrial fibrillation [103]. Independent effects were seen with antihypertensives, a combination of aspirin and dipyridamole, and statins. No effects on cognition were seen in patients with history of atrial fibrillation or hemorrhagic stroke.

From a population perspective, based on comprehensive reviews of the literature, and assuming a causal relation and intervention at the correct age for prevention of 10% per decade in the prevalence of each of seven risk factors (diabetes, midlife hypertension, midlife obesity, smoking, depression, cognitive inactivity or low educational attainment, and physical inactivity), it has been estimated that the prevalence of AD could be reduced by 8.3% worldwide by 2050 [104]. This would translate to 1.1–3.0 million AD cases worldwide and 184,000–492,000 cases in the United States [105]. Five of these risks are vascular risk factors (i.e., midlife hypertension, diabetes mellitus, midlife hyperlipidemia, smoking, sedentary lifestyle, as well as depression and low educational attainment). Arguably, the epidemiological diagnosis of AD may well include cases with subclinical VBI or mixed AD/VBI, in which case the projected risk reduction in dementia cases may predominantly reflect reduction in VBI contributions to dementia.

Treatment of cognitive symptoms

Positive effects of cholinesterase inhibitors and memantine have been reported in randomized, double-blind, placebo-controlled trials of VaD. A meta-analysis showed favorable effects of cholinesterase inhibitors on cognitive outcomes, but not for global

	Drug		Placebo		Weight (%)	WMD (fixed) (95% CI)
	n	Mean (SD)	*n*	Mean (SD)		
Donepezil 5 mg vs placebo						
307	196	−0.96 (5.49)	194	0.72 (5.64)	21.09	−1.68 (−2.78 to −0.58)
308	199	−1.75 (4.70)	180	−0.10 (5.36)	24.76	−0.65 (−2.67 to −0.63)
319	648	−0.71 (5.18)	326	0.00 (5.18)	54.16	−0.71 (−1.40 to −0.02)
Subtotal	1043		700		100.00	−1.15 (−1.65 to −0.64)
Test for heterogeneity: $\chi^2 = 3.37$; df2 ($p = 0.19$); $I^2 = 40.70\%$						
Test for overall effect: $p<0.00001$						
Donepezil 10 mg vs placebo						
307	195	−1.52 (5.74)	194	0.72 (5.64)	52.11	−2.24 (−3.37 to −1.11)
308	194	−2.19 (6.27)	180	−0.10 (5.36)	47.89	−2.09 (−3.27 to −0.91)
Subtotal	389		374		100.00	−2.17 (−2.98 to −1.35)
Test for heterogeneity: $\chi^2 = 0.03$; df1 ($p = 0.86$); $I^2 = 0\%$						
Test for overall effect: $p<0.00001$						
Galantamine 24 mg vs placebo						
GAL-INT-6	149	−2.00 (6.10)	77	0.00 (6.76)	19.42	−2.00 (−3.80 to −0.20)
GAL-INT-26	367	−1.80 (5.94)	373	−0.30 (6.32)	80.58	−1.50 (−2.38 to −0.62)
Subtotal	516		450		100.00	−1.60 (−2.39 to −0.80)
Test for heterogeneity: $\chi^2 = 0.24$; df1 ($p = 0.63$); $I^2 = 0\%$						
Test for overall effect: $p<0.0001$						
Rivastigmine 12 mg vs placebo						
Vantag E	360	−0.70 (7.21)	338	0.40 (6.99)	100.00	−1.10 (−2.15 to −0.05)
Test for overall effect: $p=0.04$					100.00	−1.10 (−2.15 to −0.05)
Memantine 20 mg vs placebo						
MMM300	147	−0.40 (5.70)	141	1.60 (6.10)	45.77	−2.00 (−3.36 to −0.64)
MMM500	277	0.53 (7.02)	261	2.28 (7.77)	54.23	−1.75 (−3.00 to −0.50)
Subtotal	424		402		100.00	−1.86 (−2.79 to −0.94)
Test for heterogeneity: $\chi^2 = 0.07$; df1 ($p = 0.79$); $I^2 = 0\%$						
Test for overall effect: $p<0.0001$						

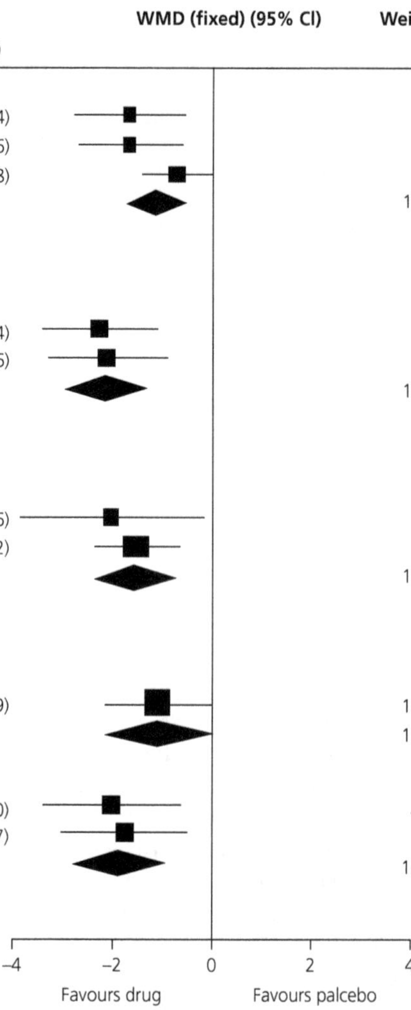

Figure 4.10 Meta-analysis of double-blind placebo-controlled trials of cholinesterase inhibitors and memantine for vascular dementia. Cognitive outcomes on the ADAS-Cog subscale (change from baseline) in vascular dementia patients in cholinesterase inhibitors and memantine trials by drug and dose (last observation carried forward sample); WMD, weighted mean difference. Source: Kavirajan and Schneider [106]. Reproduced with permission from Elsevier.

impressions of change [106] (Figure 4.10). Despite a more rigorous implementation of diagnostic criteria, it remains difficult to parse contributions of mixed AD. Unlike AD, loss of cholinergic neurons in the basal forebrain is not characteristic of VaD. Disruption of cholinergic pathways by severe WMH in Binswanger's syndrome [107] and CADASIL [108, 109], however, has been demonstrated. In CADASIL, treatment with donepezil was associated with improvement in a secondary measure of executive function [110]. Cholinesterase inhibitors were generally well tolerated, although associated with an increase in gastrointestinal side effects; they should be avoided in patients with heart block. Cholinesterase inhibitors and memantine have been approved for the treatment of VaD in some countries, but not in the United States. At this time, guidelines for VCI should follow guidelines for the prevention and treatment of stroke.

Summary

CVD is the second leading cause of cognitive impairment in late life. The manifestations of VCI are widely heterogeneous in severity, pathophysiology, and neurobehavioral phenotype depending upon site, size, and sum of VBI. MRI might show preclinical evidence of VBI (e.g., SBI and WMH), which is associated with impairment in executive function. One-third of patients experience PSD and if not initially affected are at twice the risk of developing subsequent cognitive impairment over the ensuing 10 years. Neuropathology studies show that AD and VBI often occur together and exert additive adverse effects on cognition. CADASIL represents the prototype for pure small vessel type of VCI and has greatly advanced our understanding of underlying pathophysiology and brain–behavior correlations. Many risk factors for sporadic VBI (e.g., hypertension, diabetes mellitus, dyslipidemia) are modifiable, although double-blind placebo-controlled trials are often inconclusive because they are started too late, are too short in duration, or lack sufficiently sensitive cognitive outcome measures. Cholinesterase inhibitors and memantine show mild benefits for cognitive, but not global endpoints in trials. They are not currently approved by the US Food and Drug Administration for the symptomatic treatment of VCI, but are approved in some other countries. By and large, the means for early detection and prevention of VCI are known. The major challenge remains one of diligent clinical practice and public health implementation. It has been projected that a 10% reduction in seven risk factors (including five vascular risk factors) for 10 years could result in an 8% reduction in incident dementia cases.

References

1 Tomlinson BE, Blessed G, Roth M. Observations on the brains of demented old people. *J Neurol Sci.* 1970;**11**(3):205–42.

2 Vermeer SE, Hollander M, van Dijk EJ, Hofman A, Koudstaal PJ, Breteler MM. Silent brain infarcts and white matter lesions increase stroke risk in the general population: the Rotterdam Scan Study. *Stroke.* 2003;**34**(5):1126–9.

3 Iadecola C. The pathobiology of vascular dementia. *Neuron.* 2013;**80**(4):844–66.

4 Grinberg LT, Thal DR. Vascular pathology in the aged human brain. *Acta Neuropathol.* 2010;**119**(3):277–90.

5 Schneider JA, Arvanitakis Z, Bang W, Bennett DA. Mixed brain pathologies account for most dementia cases in community-dwelling older persons. *Neurology.* 2007;**69**(24):2197–204.

6 Arvanitakis Z, Leurgans SE, Barnes LL, Bennett DA, Schneider JA. Microinfarct pathology, dementia, and cognitive systems. *Stroke.* 2011;**42**(3):722–7.

7 Soontornniyomkij V, Lynch MD, Mermash S, Pomakian J, Badkoobehi H, Clare R, et al. Cerebral microinfarcts associated with severe cerebral beta-amyloid angiopathy. *Brain Pathol.* 2010;**20**(2): 459–67.

8 Snowdon DA, Greiner LH, Mortimer JA, Riley KP, Greiner PA, Markesbery WR. Brain infarction and the clinical expression of Alzheimer disease. The nun study *JAMA.* 1997;**277**(10):813–7.

9 Schneider JA, Wilson RS, Bienias JL, Evans DA, Bennett DA. Cerebral infarctions and the likelihood of dementia from Alzheimer disease pathology. *Neurology.* 2004;**62**(7):1148–55.

10 White L. Brain lesions at autopsy in older Japanese-American men as related to cognitive impairment and dementia in the final years of life: a summary report from the Honolulu-Asia aging study. *J Alzheimers Dis.* 2009;**18**(3):713–25.

11 Troncoso JC, Zonderman AB, Resnick SM, Crain B, Pletnikova O, O'Brien RJ. Effect of infarcts on dementia in the Baltimore longitudinal study of aging. *Ann Neurol.* 2008;**64**(2):168–76.

12 Toledo JB, Arnold SE, Raible K, Brettschneider J, Xie SX, Grossman M, et al. Contribution of cerebrovascular disease in autopsy confirmed neurodegenerative disease cases in the National Alzheimer's Coordinating Centre. *Brain.* 2013;**136**(Pt 9):2697–706.

13 Leys D, Henon H, Mackowiak-Cordoliani MA, Pasquier F. Poststroke dementia. *Lancet Neurol.* 2005;**4**(11):752–9.

14 Ivan CS, Seshadri S, Beiser A, Au R, Kase CS, Kelly-Hayes M, et al. Dementia after stroke: the Framingham Study. *Stroke.* 2004;**35**(6): 1264–8.

15 Rocca WA, Kokmen E. Frequency and distribution of vascular dementia. *Alzheimer Dis Assoc Disord.* 1999;**13**(Suppl 3):S9–14.

16 Knopman DS, Rocca WA, Cha RH, Edland SD, Kokmen E. Incidence of vascular dementia in Rochester, Minn, 1985–1989. *Arch Neurol.* 2002;**59**(10):1605–10.

17 Ravaglia G, Forti P, Maioli F, Martelli M, Servadei L, Brunetti N, et al. Incidence and etiology of dementia in a large elderly Italian population. *Neurology.* 2005;**64**(9):1525–30.

18 Jin YP, Di Legge S, Ostbye T, Feightner JW, Hachinski V. The reciprocal risks of stroke and cognitive impairment in an elderly population. *Alzheimers Dement.* 2006;**2**(3):171–8.

19 Peila R, White LR, Petrovich H, Masaki K, Ross GW, Havlik RJ, et al. Joint effect of the APOE gene and midlife systolic blood pressure on late-life cognitive impairment: the Honolulu-Asia aging study. *Stroke.* 2001;**32**(12):2882–9.

20 Peila R, Rodriguez BL, Launer LJ. Type 2 diabetes, APOE gene, and the risk for dementia and related pathologies: the Honolulu-Asia aging Study. *Diabetes.* 2002;**51**(4):1256–62.

21 Elias MF, Elias PK, Sullivan LM, Wolf PA, D'Agostino RB. Obesity, diabetes and cognitive deficit: the Framingham Heart Study. *Neurobiol Aging.* 2005;**26** (Suppl 1):11–6.

22 Solomon A, Kivipelto M, Wolozin B, Zhou J, Whitmer RA. Midlife serum cholesterol and increased risk of Alzheimer's and vascular dementia three decades later. *Dement Geriatr Cogn Disord.* 2009; **28**(1):75–80.

23 Solomon A, Kareholt I, Ngandu T, Wolozin B, Macdonald SW, Winblad B, et al. Serum total cholesterol, statins and cognition in non-demented elderly. *Neurobiol Aging.* 2009;**30**(6):1006–9.

24 Longstreth WT, Jr., Bernick C, Manolio TA, Bryan N, Jungreis CA, Price TR. Lacunar infarcts defined by magnetic resonance imaging of 3660 elderly people: the Cardiovascular Health Study. *Arch Neurol.* 1998;**55**(9):1217–25.

25 Longstreth WT, Jr., Manolio TA, Arnold A, Burke GL, Bryan N, Jungreis CA, et al. Clinical correlates of white matter findings on cranial magnetic resonance imaging of 3301 elderly people. The cardiovascular health study. *Stroke* 1996;**27**(8):1274–82.

26 Vermeer SE, Koudstaal PJ, Oudkerk M, Hofman A, Breteler MM. Prevalence and risk factors of silent brain infarcts in the population-based Rotterdam Scan Study. *Stroke.* 2002;**33**(1):21–5.

27 Vermeer SE, Den Heijer T, Koudstaal PJ, Oudkerk M, Hofman A, Breteler MM. Incidence and risk factors of silent brain infarcts in the population-based Rotterdam Scan Study. *Stroke.* 2003;**34**(2):392–6.

28 Vermeer SE, Prins ND, den Heijer T, Hofman A, Koudstaal PJ, Breteler MM. Silent brain infarcts and the risk of dementia and cognitive decline. *N Engl J Med.* 2003;**348**(13):1215–22.

29 Debette S, Beiser A, DeCarli C, Au R, Himali JJ, Kelly-Hayes M, et al. Association of MRI markers of vascular brain injury with incident stroke, mild cognitive impairment, dementia, and mortality: the Framingham Offspring Study. *Stroke.* 2010;**41**(4):600–6.

30 Yates PA, Villemagne VL, Ellis KA, Desmond PM, Masters CL, Rowe CC. Cerebral microbleeds: a review of clinical, genetic, and neuroimaging associations. *Front Neurol.* 2014;**4**:205.

31 Tournier-Lasserve E, Joutel A, Melki J, Weissenbach J, Lathrop GM, Chabriat H, et al. Cerebral autosomal dominant arteriopathy with subcortical infarcts and leukoencephalopathy maps to chromosome 19q12. *Nat Genet.* 1993;**3**(3):256–9.

32 Joutel A, Corpechot C, Ducros A, Vahedi K, Chabriat H, Mouton P, et al. Notch3 mutations in CADASIL, a hereditary adult-onset condition causing stroke and dementia. *Nature*. 1996;**383**(6602):707–10.

33 Hara K, Shiga A, Fukutake T, Nozaki H, Miyashita A, Yokoseki A, et al. Association of HTRA1 mutations and familial ischemic cerebral small-vessel disease. *N Engl J Med*. 2009;**360**(17):1729–39.

34 Revesz T, Holton JL, Lashley T, Plant G, Frangione B, Rostagno A, et al. Genetics and molecular pathogenesis of sporadic and hereditary cerebral amyloid angiopathies. *Acta Neuropathol*. 2009;**118**(1):115–30.

35 Greenberg SM, Rebeck GW, Vonsattel JP, Gomez-Isla T, Hyman BT. Apolipoprotein E epsilon 4 and cerebral hemorrhage associated with amyloid angiopathy. *Ann Neurol*. 1995;**38**(2):254–9.

36 Scheltens P, Leys D, Barkhof F, Huglo D, Weinstein HC, Vermersch P, et al. Atrophy of medial temporal lobes on MRI in "probable" Alzheimer's disease and normal ageing: diagnostic value and neuropsychological correlates. *J Neurol Neurosurg Psychiatry*. 1992; **55**(10):967–72.

37 D'Agostino RB, Wolf PA, Belanger AJ, Kannel WB. Stroke risk profile: adjustment for antihypertensive medication. The Framingham Study. *Stroke*. 1994;**25**(1):40–3.

38 Hachinski VC, Lassen NA, Marshall J. Multi-infarct dementia. A cause of mental deterioration in the elderly. *Lancet*. 1974;**2**(7874): 207–10.

39 American Psychiatric Association. *Task Force on DSM-IV. Diagnostic and statistical manual of mental disorders: DSM-IV*. 4th ed. Washington, DC: American Psychiatric Association; 1994.

40 Roman GC, Tatemichi TK, Erkinjuntti T, Cummings JL, Masdeu JC, Garcia JH, et al. Vascular dementia: diagnostic criteria for research studies. Report of the NINDS-AIREN International Workshop. *Neurology*. 1993;**43**(2):250–60.

41 Chui HC, Victoroff JI, Margolin D, Jagust W, Shankle R, Katzman R. Criteria for the diagnosis of ischemic vascular dementia proposed by the State of California Alzheimer's disease diagnostic and treatment centers. *Neurology*. 1992;**42**(3 Pt 1):473–80.

42 World Health Organization., ebrary Inc. *The ICD-10 classification of mental and behavioural disorders diagnostic criteria for research*. Geneva: World Health Organization, 1993:xiii, 248 p. 24 cm.

43 Gorelick PB, Scuteri A, Black SE, Decarli C, Greenberg SM, Iadecola C, et al. Vascular contributions to cognitive impairment and dementia: a statement for healthcare professionals from the american heart association/american stroke association. *Stroke*. 2011;**42**(9):2672–713.

44 American Psychiatric Association. *Diagnostic and Statistical Manual of Mental Disorders*. 5th ed. Arlington, VA: APA; 2013.

45 Bogousslavsky J, Regli F, Uske A. Thalamic infarcts: clinical syndromes, etiology, and prognosis. *Neurology*. 1988;**38**(6):837–48.

46 Tatemichi TK, Desmond DW, Prohovnik I, Cross DT, Gropen TI, Mohr JP, et al. Confusion and memory loss from capsular genu infarction: a thalamocortical disconnection syndrome? *Neurology*. 1992;**42**(10):1966–79.

47 Petersen RC, Smith GE, Waring SC, Ivnik RJ, Tangalos EG, Kokmen E. Mild cognitive impairment: clinical characterization and outcome. *Arch Neurol*. 1999;**56**(3):303–8.

48 Kokmen E, Whisnant JP, O'Fallon WM, Chu CP, Beard CM. Dementia after ischemic stroke: a population-based study in Rochester, Minnesota (1960–1984). *Neurology*. 1996;**46**(1):154–9.

49 Srikanth VK, Quinn SJ, Donnan GA, Saling MM, Thrift AG. Long-term cognitive transitions, rates of cognitive change, and predictors of incident dementia in a population-based first-ever stroke cohort. *Stroke*. 2006;**37**(10):2479–83.

50 Pohjasvaara T, Mantyla R, Aronen HJ, Leskela M, Salonen O, Kaste M, et al. Clinical and radiological determinants of prestroke cognitive decline in a stroke cohort. *J Neurol Neurosurg Psychiatry*. 1999;**67**(6):742–8.

51 Cordoliani-Mackowiak MA, Henon H, Pruvo JP, Pasquier F, Leys D. Poststroke dementia: influence of hippocampal atrophy. *Arch Neurol*. 2003;**60**(4):585–90.

52 Bastos-Leite AJ, van der Flier WM, van Straaten EC, Staekenborg SS, Scheltens P, Barkhof F. The contribution of medial temporal lobe atrophy and vascular pathology to cognitive impairment in vascular dementia. *Stroke*. 2007;**38**(12):3182–5.

53 Cummings JL. Frontal-subcortical circuits and human behavior. *Arch Neurol*. 1993;**50**(8):873–80.

54 Tatemichi TK, Desmond DW, Prohovnik I. Strategic infarcts in vascular dementia. A clinical and brain imaging experience. *Arzneimittelforschung*. 1995;**45**(3A):371–85.

55 Katz DI, Alexander MP, Mandell AM. Dementia following strokes in the mesencephalon and diencephalon. *Arch Neurol*. 1987;**44**(11): 1127–33.

56 Stuss DT, Guberman A, Nelson R, Larochelle S. The neuropsychology of paramedian thalamic infarction. *Brain Cogn*. 1988;**8**(3):348–78.

57 Ishii N, Nishihara Y, Imamura T. Why do frontal lobe symptoms predominate in vascular dementia with lacunes? *Neurology*. 1986;**36**(3):340–5.

58 Dozono K, Ishii N, Nishihara Y, Horie A. An autopsy study of the incidence of lacunes in relation to age, hypertension, and arteriosclerosis. *Stroke*. 1991;**22**(8):993–6.

59 Roman GC. Senile dementia of the Binswanger type. A vascular form of dementia in the elderly. *JAMA*. 1987;**258**(13):1782–8.

60 Bennett DA, Wilson RS, Gilley DW, Fox JH. Clinical diagnosis of Binswanger's disease. *J Neurol Neurosurg Psychiatry*. 1990;**53**(11):961–5.

61 Okeda R, Arima K, Kawai M. Arterial changes in cerebral autosomal dominant arteriopathy with subcortical infarcts and leukoencephalopathy (CADASIL) in relation to pathogenesis of diffuse myelin loss of cerebral white matter: examination of cerebral medullary arteries by reconstruction of serial sections of an autopsy case. *Stroke*. 2002;**33**(11):2565–9.

62 Miao Q, Paloneva T, Tuisku S, Roine S, Poyhonen M, Viitanen M, et al. Arterioles of the lenticular nucleus in CADASIL. *Stroke*. 2006;**37**(9):2242–7.

63 Dichgans M, Mayer M, Uttner I, Bruning R, Muller-Hocker J, Rungger G, et al. The phenotypic spectrum of CADASIL: clinical findings in 102 cases. *Ann Neurol*. 1998;**44**(5):731–9.

64 Desmond DW, Moroney JT, Lynch T, Chan S, Chin SS, Mohr JP. The natural history of CADASIL: a pooled analysis of previously published cases. *Stroke*. 1999;**30**(6):1230–3.

65 Peters N, Opherk C, Danek A, Ballard C, Herzog J, Dichgans M. The pattern of cognitive performance in CADASIL: a monogenic condition leading to subcortical ischemic vascular dementia. *Am J Psychiatry*. 2005;**162**(11):2078–85.

66 Liem MK, van der Grond J, Haan J, van den Boom R, Ferrari MD, Knaap YM, et al. Lacunar infarcts are the main correlate with cognitive dysfunction in CADASIL. *Stroke*. 2007;**38**(3):923–8.

67 Viswanathan A, Gschwendtner A, Guichard JP, Buffon F, Cumurciuc R, O'Sullivan M, et al. Lacunar lesions are independently associated with disability and cognitive impairment in CADASIL. *Neurology*. 2007;**69**(2):172–9.

68 van Swieten JC, van den Hout JH, van Ketel BA, Hijdra A, Wokke JH, van Gijn J. Periventricular lesions in the white matter on magnetic resonance imaging in the elderly. A morphometric correlation with arteriolosclerosis and dilated perivascular spaces. *Brain.* 1991;**114** (Pt 2):761–74.

69 Pullicino PM, Miller LL, Alexandrov AV, Ostrow PT. Infraputaminal "lacunes". Clinical and pathological correlations. *Stroke.* 1995;**26**(9): 1598–602.

70 Hachinski VC, Potter P, Merskey H. Leukoaraiosis. *Arch Neurol.* 1987;**44**(1):21–3.

71 Fazekas F, Schmidt R, Scheltens P. Pathophysiologic mechanisms in the development of age-related white matter changes of the brain. *Dement Geriatr Cogn Disord.* 1998;**9**(Suppl 1):2–5.

72 van Straaten EC, Fazekas F, Rostrup E, Scheltens P, Schmidt R, Pantoni L, et al. Impact of white matter hyperintensities scoring method on correlations with clinical data: the LADIS study. *Stroke.* 2006;**37**(3):836–40.

73 Longstreth WT, Jr., Arnold AM, Beauchamp NJ, Jr., Manolio TA, Lefkowitz D, Jungreis C, et al. Incidence, manifestations, and predictors of worsening white matter on serial cranial magnetic resonance imaging in the elderly: the Cardiovascular Health Study. *Stroke.* 2005;**36**(1):56–61.

74 van Dijk EJ, Prins ND, Vrooman HA, Hofman A, Koudstaal PJ, Breteler MM. Progression of cerebral small vessel disease in relation to risk factors and cognitive consequences: Rotterdam Scan study. *Stroke.* 2008;**39**(10):2712–9.

75 Carey CL, Kramer JH, Josephson SA, Mungas D, Reed BR, Schuff N, et al. Subcortical lacunes are associated with executive dysfunction in cognitively normal elderly. *Stroke.* 2008;**39**(2):397–402.

76 Martinez-Ramirez S, Greenberg SM, Viswanathan A. Cerebral microbleeds: overview and implications in cognitive impairment. *Alzheimers Res Ther.* 2014;**6**(3):33.

77 Charidimou A, Werring DJ. Cerebral microbleeds and cognition in cerebrovascular disease: an update. *J Neurol Sci.* 2012;**322**(1–2): 50–5.

78 Miwa K, Tanaka M, Okazaki S, Yagita Y, Sakaguchi M, Mochizuki H, et al. Multiple or mixed cerebral microbleeds and dementia in patients with vascular risk factors. *Neurology.* 2014;**83**(7):646–53.

79 Jagust WJ, Zheng L, Harvey DJ, Mack WJ, Vinters HV, Weiner MW, et al. Neuropathological basis of magnetic resonance images in aging and dementia. *Ann Neurol.* 2008;**63**(1):72–80.

80 Tierney MC, Black SE, Szalai JP, Snow WG, Fisher RH, Nadon G, et al. Recognition memory and verbal fluency differentiate probable Alzheimer disease from subcortical ischemic vascular dementia. *Arch Neurol.* 2001;**58**(10):1654–9.

81 Hachinski V, Iadecola C, Petersen RC, Breteler MM, Nyenhuis DL, Black SE, et al. National institute of neurological disorders and stroke-canadian stroke network vascular cognitive impairment harmonization standards. *Stroke.* 2006;**37**(9):2220–41.

82 Sachdev P, Kalaria R, O'Brien J, Skoog I, Alladi S, Black SE, et al. Diagnostic criteria for vascular cognitive disorders: a VASCOG statement. *Alzheimer Dis Assoc Disord.* 2014;**28**(3):206–18.

83 Kim GH, Lee JH, Seo SW, Ye BS, Cho H, Kim HJ, et al. Seoul criteria for PiB(-) subcortical vascular dementia based on clinical and MRI variables. *Neurology.* 2014;**82**(17):1529–35.

84 Erkinjuntti T, Inzitari D, Pantoni L, Wallin A, Scheltens P, Rockwood K, et al. Research criteria for subcortical vascular dementia in clinical trials. *J Neural Transm Suppl* 2000;**59**:23–30.

85 Reed BR, Mungas DM, Kramer JH, Ellis W, Vinters HV, Zarow C, et al. Profiles of neuropsychological impairment in autopsy-defined Alzheimer's disease and cerebrovascular disease. *Brain.* 2007;**130** (Pt 3):731–9.

86 Rosenberg GA, Bjerke M, Wallin A. Multimodal markers of inflammation in the subcortical ischemic vascular disease type of vascular cognitive impairment. *Stroke.* 2014;**45**(5):1531–8.

87 Gold G, Bouras C, Canuto A, Bergallo MF, Herrmann FR, Hof PR, et al. Clinicopathological validation study of four sets of clinical criteria for vascular dementia. *Am J Psychiatry.* 2002; **159**(1):82–7.

88 Zarow C, Sitzer TE, Chui HC. Understanding hippocampal sclerosis in the elderly: epidemiology, characterization, and diagnostic issues. *Curr Neurol Neurosci Rep.* 2008;**8**(5):363–70.

89 Goldstein LB, *A primer on stroke prevention and treatment: an overview based on AHA/ASA guidelines.* Chichester, UK/Hoboken, NJ: Wiley-Blackwell; 2009.

90 Peters R, Beckett N, Forette F, Tuomilehto J, Clarke R, Ritchie C, et al. Incident dementia and blood pressure lowering in the hypertension in the very elderly trial cognitive function assessment (HYVET-COG): a double-blind, placebo controlled trial. *Lancet Neurol.* 2008;**7**(8):683–9.

91 Forette F, Seux ML, Staessen JA, Thijs L, Birkenhager WH, Babarskiene MR, et al. Prevention of dementia in randomised double-blind placebo-controlled systolic hypertension in Europe (Syst-Eur) trial. *Lancet.* 1998;**352**(9137):1347–51.

92 Forette F, Seux ML, Staessen JA, Thijs L, Babarskiene MR, Babeanu S, et al. The prevention of dementia with antihypertensive treatment: new evidence from the systolic hypertension in Europe (Syst-Eur) study. *Arch Intern Med.* 2002;**162**(18):2046–52.

93 Tzourio C, Anderson C, Chapman N, Woodward M, Neal B, MacMahon S, et al. Effects of blood pressure lowering with perindopril and indapamide therapy on dementia and cognitive decline in patients with cerebrovascular disease. *Arch Intern Med.* 2003;**163**(9): 1069–75.

94 Dufouil C, Chalmers J, Coskun O, Besancon V, Bousser MG, Guillon P, et al. Effects of blood pressure lowering on cerebral white matter hyperintensities in patients with stroke: the PROGRESS (Perindopril Protection Against Recurrent Stroke Study) magnetic resonance imaging substudy. *Circulation.* 2005;**112**(11):1644–50.

95 Cukierman-Yaffe T, Gerstein HC, Williamson JD, Lazar RM, Lovato L, Miller ME, et al. Relationship between baseline glycemic control and cognitive function in individuals with type 2 diabetes and other cardiovascular risk factors: the action to control cardiovascular risk in diabetes-memory in diabetes (ACCORD-MIND) trial. *Diabetes Care.* 2009;**32**(2):221–6.

96 Trompet S, van Vliet P, de Craen AJ, Jolles J, Buckley BM, Murphy MB, et al. Pravastatin and cognitive function in the elderly. Results of the PROSPER study. *J Neurol.* 2010;**257**(1):85–90.

97 Kang JH, Cook NR, Manson JE, Buring JE, Albert CM, Grodstein F. Vitamin E, vitamin C, beta carotene, and cognitive function among women with or at risk of cardiovascular disease: the women's antioxidant and cardiovascular study. *Circulation.* 2009;**119**(21): 2772–80.

98 Beydoun MA, Kaufman JS, Satia JA, Rosamond W, Folsom AR. Plasma n-3 fatty acids and the risk of cognitive decline in older adults: the atherosclerosis risk in communities study. *Am J Clin Nutr.* 2007;**85**(4):1103–11.

99 Sturman MT, Morris MC, Mendes de Leon CF, Bienias JL, Wilson RS, Evans DA. Physical activity, cognitive activity, and cognitive decline in a biracial community population. *Arch Neurol.* 2005;**62**(11):1750–4.

100 Ravaglia G, Forti P, Lucicesare A, Pisacane N, Rietti E, Bianchin M, et al. Physical activity and dementia risk in the elderly: findings from a prospective Italian study. *Neurology.* 2008;**70**(19 Pt 2):1786–94.

101 Nelson MR, Reid CM, Ames DA, Beilin LJ, Donnan GA, Gibbs P, et al. Feasibility of conducting a primary prevention trial of low-dose aspirin for major adverse cardiovascular events in older people in Australia: results from the ASPirin in reducing events in the elderly (ASPREE) pilot study. *Med J Aust.* 2008;**189**(2):105–9.

102 SPRINT. 2014; [online] https://www.sprinttrial.org (accessed September 5, 2014).

103 Douiri A, McKevitt C, Emmett ES, Rudd AG, Wolfe CD. Long-term effects of secondary prevention on cognitive function in stroke patients. *Circulation.* 2013;**128**(12):1341–8.

104 Norton S, Matthews FE, Barnes DE, Yaffe K, Brayne C. Potential for primary prevention of Alzheimer's disease: an analysis of population-based data. *Lancet Neurol.* 2014;**13**(8):788–94.

105 Barnes DE, Yaffe K. The projected effect of risk factor reduction on Alzheimer's disease prevalence. *Lancet Neurol.* 2011;**10**(9):819–28.

106 Kavirajan H, Schneider LS. Efficacy and adverse effects of cholinesterase inhibitors and memantine in vascular dementia: a meta-analysis of randomised controlled trials. *Lancet Neurol.* 2007;**6**(9):782–92.

107 Tomimoto H, Ohtani R, Shibata M, Nakamura N, Ihara M. Loss of cholinergic pathways in vascular dementia of the Binswanger type. *Dement Geriatr Cogn Disord.* 2005;**19**(5–6):282–8.

108 Mesulam M, Siddique T, Cohen B. Cholinergic denervation in a pure multi-infarct state: observations on CADASIL. *Neurology.* 2003;**60**(7):1183–5.

109 Keverne JS, Low WC, Ziabreva I, Court JA, Oakley AE, Kalaria RN. Cholinergic neuronal deficits in CADASIL. *Stroke.* 2007;**38**(1):188–91.

110 Dichgans M, Markus HS, Salloway S, Verkkoniemi A, Moline M, Wang Q, et al. Donepezil in patients with subcortical vascular cognitive impairment: a randomised double-blind trial in CADASIL. *Lancet Neurol.* 2008;**7**(4):310–8.

111 Scheltens P, Launer LJ, Barkhof F, Weinstein HC, van Gool WA. Visual assessment of medial temporal lobe atrophy on magnetic resonance imaging: interobserver reliability. *J Neurol.* 1995;**242**(9):557–60.

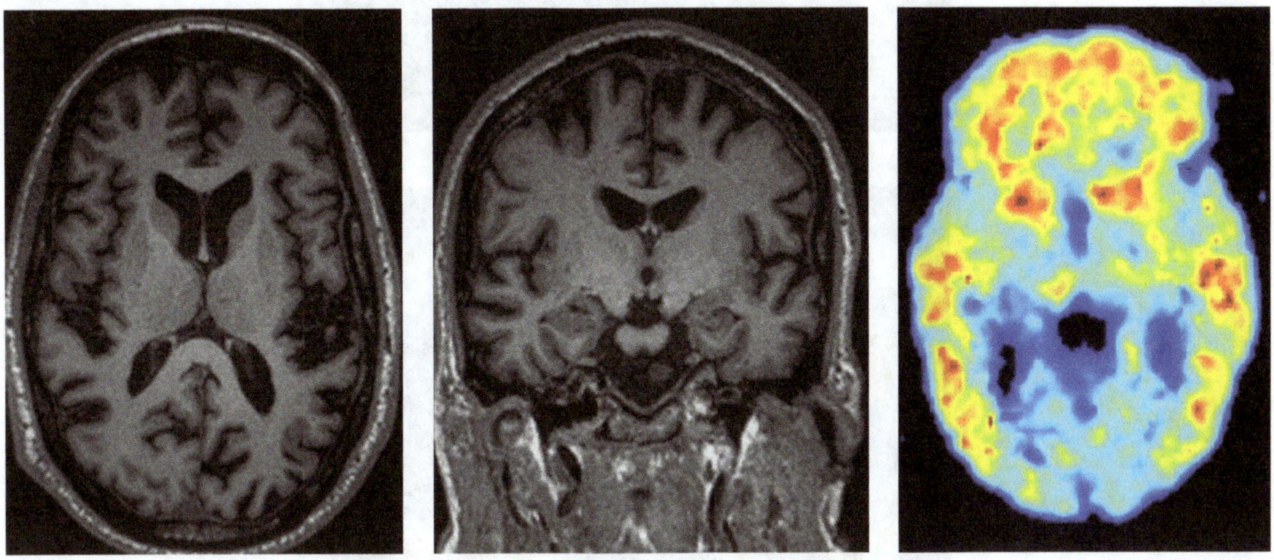

Figure 3.2 (**a**) Axial T1-weighted MRI of case 2 showing left parietal atrophy. (**b**) Coronal T1-weighted MRI showing normal hippocampal size. (**c**) PIB-PET showing cortical PIB binding (yellow to red indicate increasing spectrum of PIB binding). Orientation of MRIs is radiologic (left is right). Orientation of PET scan is neurological (right is right).

Non-Alzheimer's and Atypical Dementia, First Edition. Edited by Michael D. Geschwind and Caroline Racine Belkoura.
© 2016 John Wiley & Sons, Ltd. Published 2016 by John Wiley & Sons, Ltd.

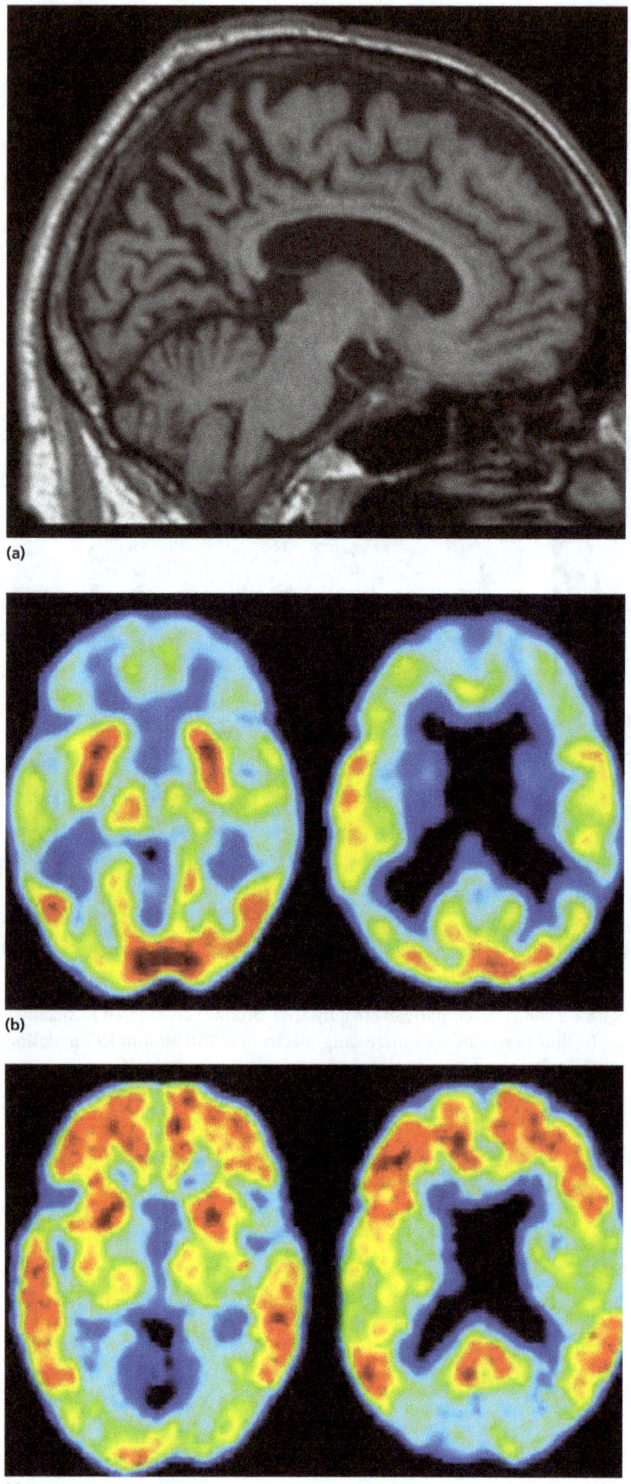

Figure 3.4 (**a**) Sagittal T1-weighted MRI showing parietal and occipital atrophy. (**b**) FDG-PET showing hypometabolism in frontal and parietal cortices. (**c**) PIB-PET showing diffuse cortical binding. Orientation is neurological.

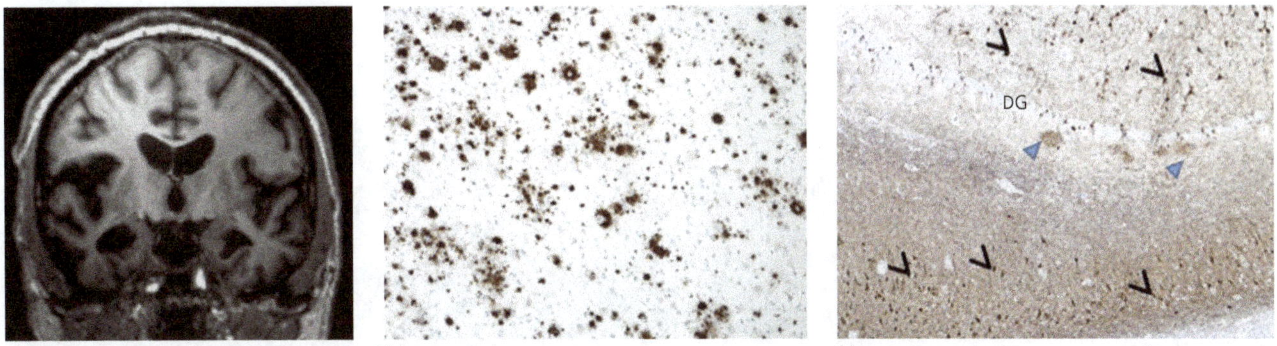

(a) (b) (c)

Figure 3.5 (**a**) Coronal T1-weighted MRI showing bilateral (right > left) temporal and right parietal (not shown) atrophy; orientation is radiological. (**b**) His pathology showed AD characteristic amyloid-beta-positive plaques (brown) in the middle frontal gyrus (4G8 (anti-amyloid-beta) immunohistochemistry; 100x). (**c**) AD characteristic tau-positive inclusions in the hippocampus. Neurofibrillary tangles (arrows), neuritic plaques (arrow heads), and neuropil threads (brown background) are present (CP13 (anti-phosphorylated tau) immunohistochemistry; 40x). DG, dentate gyrus.

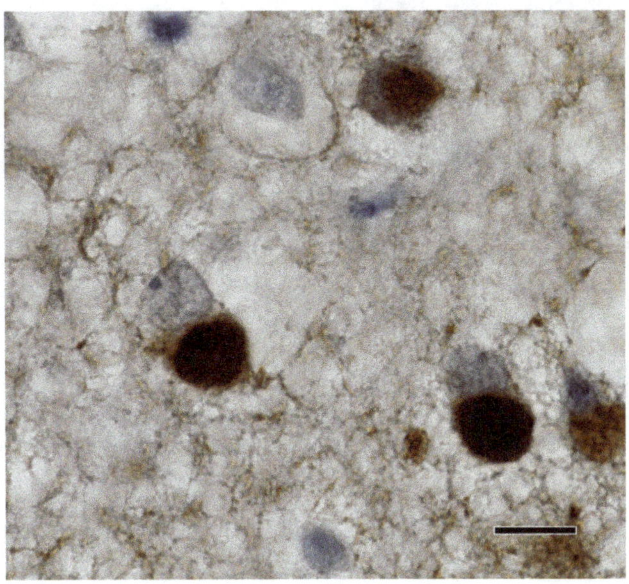

Figure 5.4 Pick bodies in the left midinsula in a 74-year-old woman with nonfluent variant PPA due to Pick's disease. Immunohistochemistry for 3-repeat tau, hematoxylin counterstain. Reproduced with permission of W.W. Seeley.

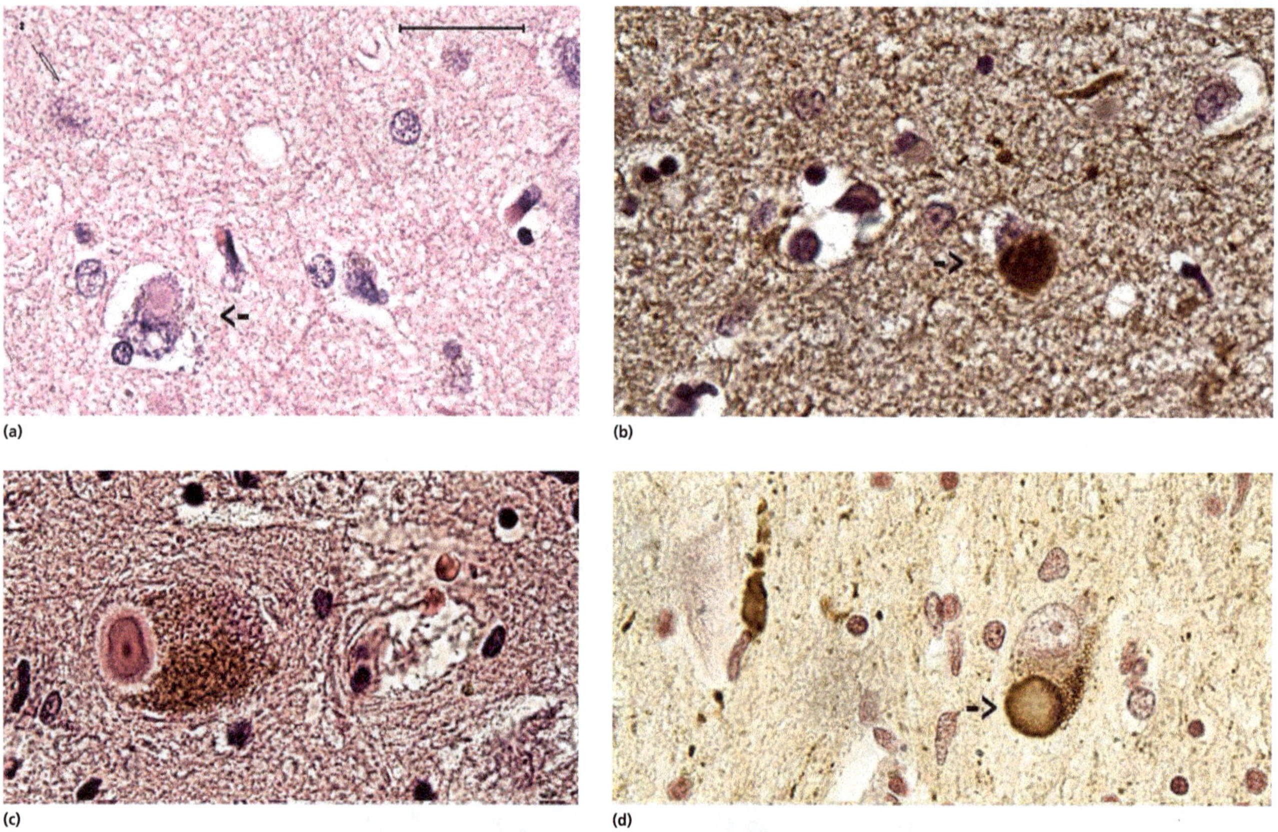

(a) (b) (c) (d)

Figure 6.2 High magnification neuropathology from a DLB case. Cortical (**a**) and nigral (**c**) LBs after staining with hematoxylin and eosin. Note that cortical LBs are smaller and lack the halo that typifies LBs within the substantia nigra. Images (**b**) and (**d**) are taken after immunostaining DLB tissue with antibodies against alpha-synuclein. Cortical (**b**) and nigral LBs (**d**) both stand out. The entire inclusion stains in the cortex, but only the halo in the substantia nigra contains alpha-synuclein. Arrows point to the LBs in all images. All images at 60× magnification. Scale bar is 30 μm.

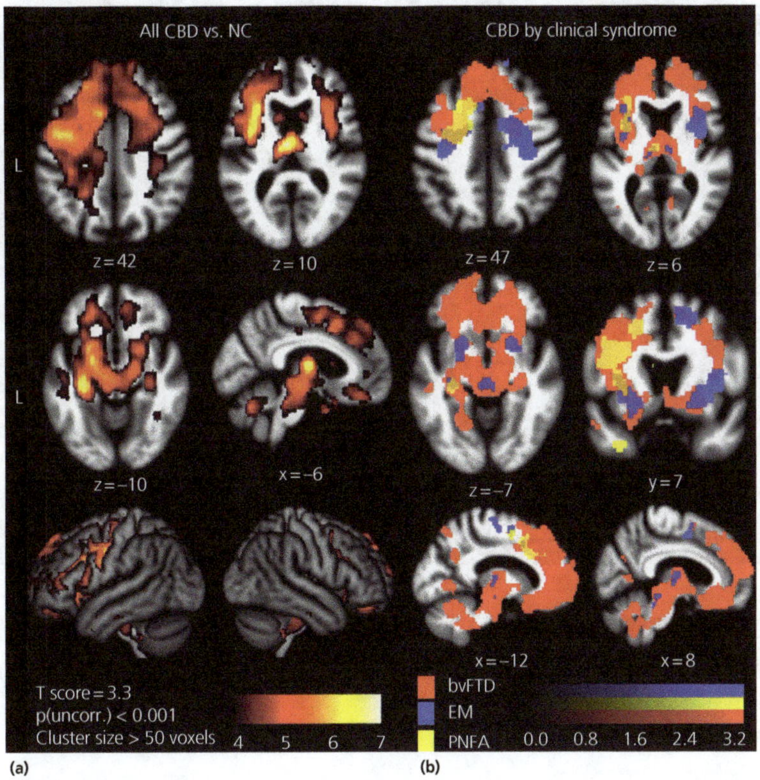

Figure 7.5 Statistical parametric mapping version 5 (SPM5) voxel-based morphometry (VBM) MRI analysis contrasting gray and white matter volume in **(a)** a cohort of patients with corticobasal degeneration (CBD) (N= 13) with healthy older controls (NC, N=44) who had VBM-compatible 1.5T structural T1 scans and **(b)** the three main clinical syndromes seen in CBD compared to NC viewed on a DARTEL-derived template based on 48 healthy controls (voxel resolution: 1 mm). Patients with VBM-compatible scans in the three CBD clinical syndromes included nfvPPA (N=4), EM-CBD (N=5), and bvFTD-CBD (N=3). Source: Lee et al. [8]. Reproduced with permission of Wiley.

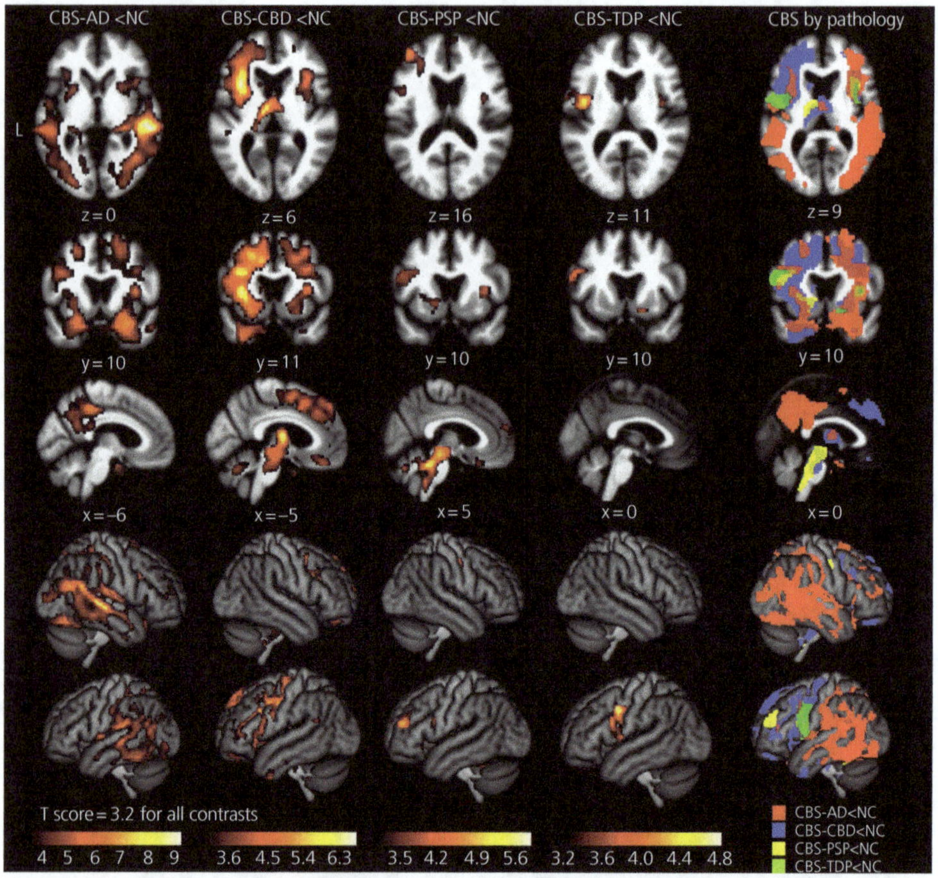

(a) (b)

Figure 7.6 SPM5 VBM analysis showing the patterns of gray and white matter volume loss in **(a)** left panel: each CBS subgroup, all with autopsy studies (CBS-AD (N=7), CBS-CBD (N=11), CBS-PSP (N=4), and CBS-TDP (N=3)) relative to healthy controls (NC, N=44) and **(b)** right panel: all three CBS subgroups combined relative to NC viewed on a DARTEL-derived template based on 48 healthy controls (voxel resolution: 1 mm). Source: Lee et al. [8]. Reproduced with permission of Wiley.

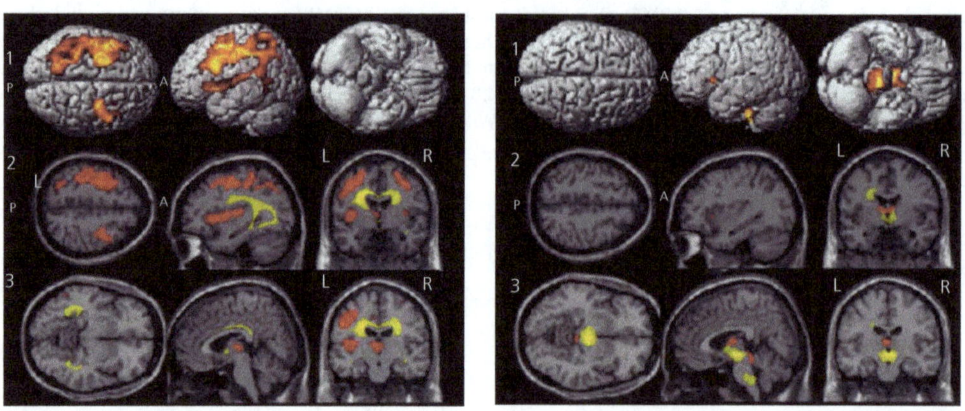

Figure 7.7 Regions of brain atrophy in patients with corticobasal syndrome (CBS) and progressive supranuclear palsy syndrome (PSP-S) relative to controls. VBM-identified regions of decreased gray and white matter volume in 14 CBS and 15 PSP-S patients relative to 80 age-matched control subjects are displayed on a normal adult brain template (P<0.05, corrected). **(a)** CBS patients versus controls. **(b)** PSP patients versus controls. Row 1 shows the regions of significant gray matter loss rendered on a healthy subject's brain. Row 2 shows regions of significant gray (displayed in red) and white (displayed in yellow) matter loss relative to controls at the following Montreal Neurological Institute (MNI) coordinates: x=−33, y=−4, and z=49. Row 3 shows regions of significant gray (displayed in red) and white (displayed in yellow) matter loss relative to controls at the following MNI coordinates: x=5, y=−15, and z=−8. A indicates anterior; P, posterior. Source: Boxer et al. [82]. Reproduced with permission of the American Medical Association.

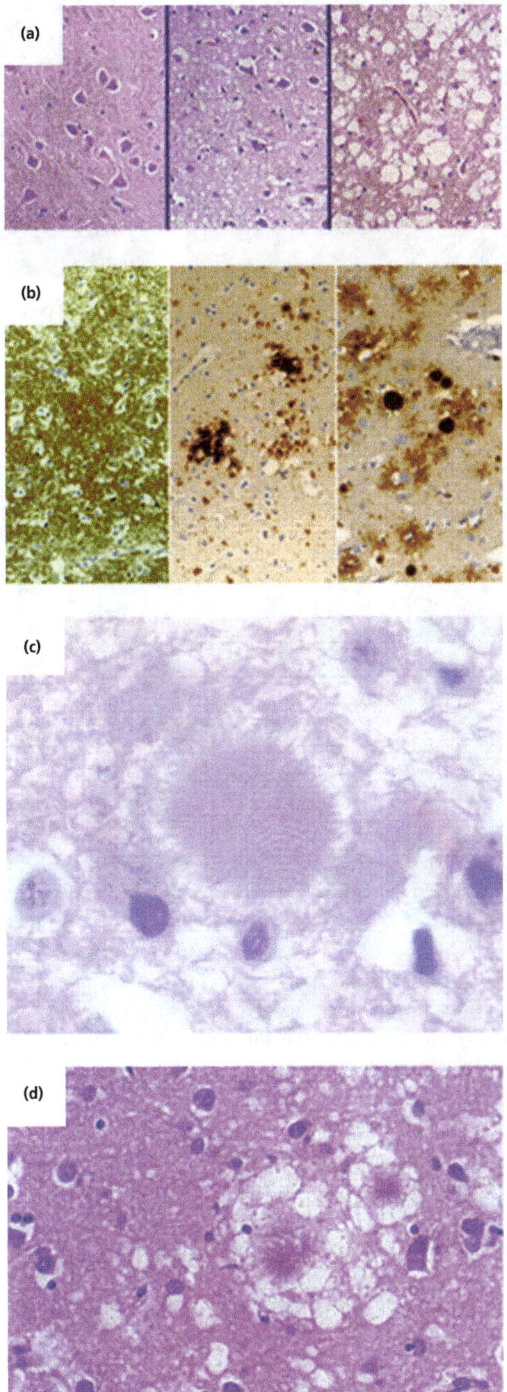

Figure 9.3 Neuropathological findings in prion diseases. **(a)** In sporadic CJD, some brain areas may have no (hippocampal end plate, left), mild (subiculum, middle), or severe (temporal cortex, right) spongiform change. Hematoxylin and eosin (H&E) stain. **(b)** Cortical sections immunostained for PrP^{Sc} in sporadic CJD: synaptic (left), patchy/perivacuolar (middle), or plaque type (right) patterns of PrP^{Sc} deposition. **(c)** Large kuru-type plaque, H&E stain. **(d)** Typical "florid" plaques in vCJD, H&E stain. Source: Adapted from Budka [98]. Reproduced with permission of Oxford University Press.

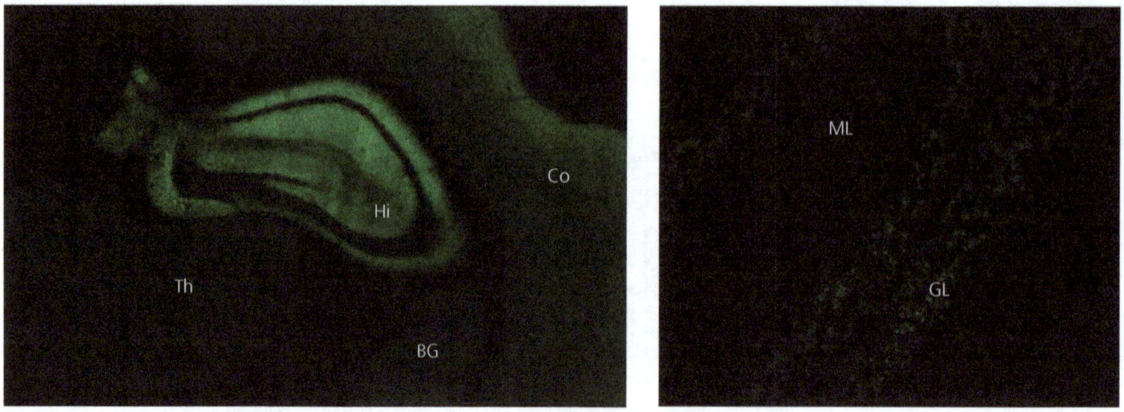

Figure 10.2 NMDAR antibody (relevant to Case 2). Indirect immunofluorescence staining pattern of patient's serum on a composite of mouse neural tissue, provided courtesy of Dr. Vanda A. Lennon, Neuroimmunology Laboratory, Mayo Clinic, Rochester, MN. Hippocampus (Hi) stains brighter than cerebral cortex (Co), basal ganglia (BG), and thalamus (Th). Granular layer (GL) of cerebellum also stains brightly, typical for NMDAR antibody; molecular layer (ML) is negative.

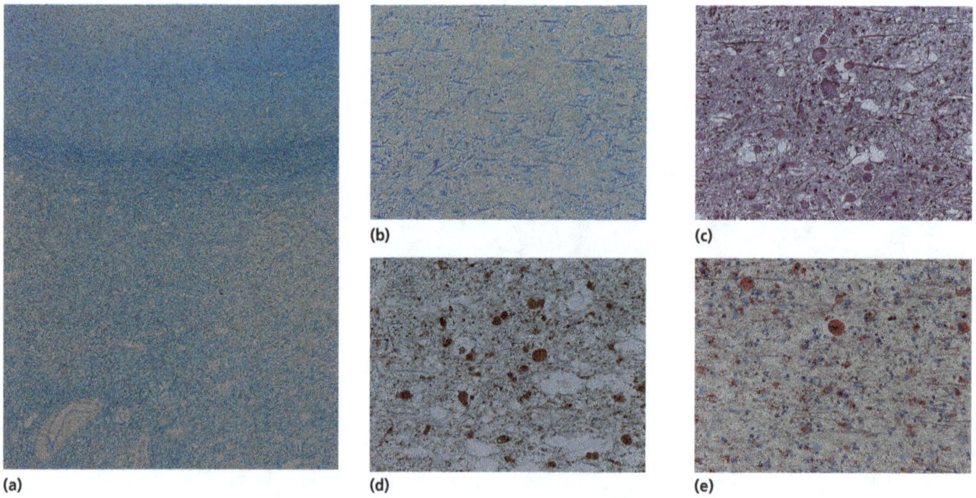

Figure 12.5 White matter lesions of the motor cortex from an ALSP/HDLS case. **(a)** Marked myelin loss of the subcortical white matter with spared U-fiber, KB staining. **(b–d)** Numerous axonal spheroids in the white matter lesion: **(b)** KB staining, **(c)** Bodian staining, and **(d)** immunohistochemistry for ubiquitin. **(e)** Abundant sudanophilic macrophages (*arrowhead*) in the white matter, Sudan III (*KB* Klüver–Barrera). *Bar* **(a)** 400 μm, **(b–e)** 90 μm. Source: Itoh et al. [24]. Reproduced with permission of Springer.

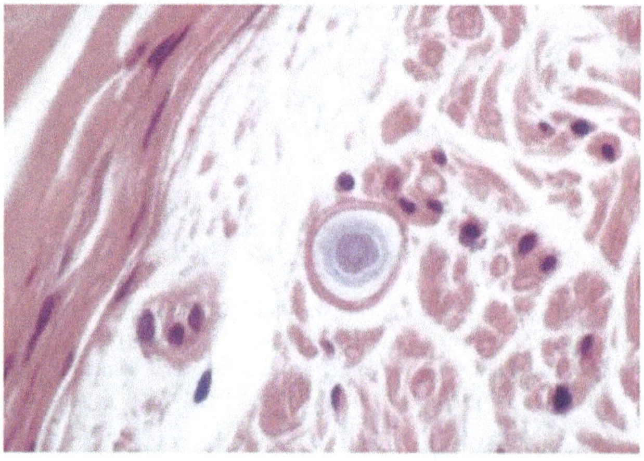

Figure 12.7 Sural nerve biopsy in APBD showing intra-axonal basophilic inclusions (polyglucosan bodies) in several nerve fascicles (light microscopy, H&E stain). Further investigations showed that the storage material is not membrane bound, is diastase resistant, and is PAS positive (not shown).

CHAPTER 5
Frontotemporal dementia

David C. Perry and Howard J. Rosen
University of California, San Francisco, San Francisco, CA, USA

Introduction and definition of terms

Arnold Pick first described a patient with progressive behavior and language deterioration and left temporal lobe atrophy in 1892. Based upon subsequent cases described by Pick and pathological findings described by Alois Alzheimer, the entity of Pick's disease was recognized [1, 2]. Although the terminology has changed over time and the term frontotemporal dementia (FTD) has gained favor, the hallmark features of these disorders remain a progressive deterioration in personality and behavior and/or language impairment. Rather than being one homogeneous disorder, FTD is now understood as including multiple distinct clinical subtypes that can be caused by several pathological processes.

The nomenclature in the field has been inconsistent and confusing. In this chapter, the term FTD will be used to refer to any of the three core clinical syndromes of FTD. These include the behavioral variant of FTD (bvFTD), which presents primarily with changes in personality and socioemotional function, and two variants of primary progressive aphasia (PPA), including the semantic variant PPA (svPPA) and the nonfluent/agrammatic variant PPA (nfv-PPA). The term frontotemporal lobar degeneration (FTLD) will be used to describe the associated pathological entities. This chapter focuses on the clinical features of the FTD syndromes and on FTLD as a whole and its diverse clinical, pathological, and genetic features as well as current treatment approaches. Research in FTD has also identified links between FTD and other neurological syndromes, including corticobasal syndrome (CBS), progressive supranuclear palsy (PSP) and motor neuron disease (MND), which are associated with FTLD pathology and are often considered as part of the FTLD spectrum. PSP and CBS are discussed in detail in other chapters of this volume, but the disorders will be reviewed here in order to highlight their relationships with FTD.

Epidemiology

Although FTD was previously felt to be a rare entity, current data indicates that it is the third most common neurodegenerative cause of dementia, behind Alzheimer's disease (AD) and Lewy body dementias [3, 4]. Prevalence estimates have varied, but in one study in the Netherlands, it was estimated at 2.7/100 000 [5]. A study conducted in Rochester, Minnesota, indicated that in patients whose dementia begins prior to age 60, FTD is as common as AD [6]. Onset is most commonly in the sixth decade but has been described as early as the third decade and as late as the ninth [5].

Survival from disease onset in FTLD is shorter than in AD. The longest survival is in svPPA at 11.9 years from onset, and the shortest is in patients with FTD and coexisting MND (approximately 2 years). Disease durations in bvFTD and nfv-PPA are intermediate, at 8.7 years and 9.4 years, respectively [7].

Core FTD clinical syndromes

Case 1

A 55 year-old woman was noted at work to be keeping an inaccurate tally of inventory and 4 years before presentation was fired after making inappropriate comments and gestures about her boss to one of his friends at work. Two years before presentation, her personality gradually changed, and she began to swear more frequently, would burp in public, and would talk to strangers about her sex life. She became less engaged in group activities and was thought to be depressed. She watched more television and when she was unable to figure out the remote control would sit and stare at the blank screen. She seemed indifferent to her family members' feelings and called her daughter "ugly." Over time, she started to develop new habits, including collecting artificial flowers and insisting that the clocks in the house be synchronized down to the second. She began craving sweet foods and eating whole bags of cookies in a sitting and gained 30 pounds.

On presentation to the clinic, she was asked why she was visiting the clinic, and said, "I have some problems," but could not elaborate. She recognized that she had lost her job but said it was because of unreasonable demands from her boss. On examination, she had increased speech output and would use the same phrases repetitively, but her speech was fluent and sensible, and she followed complex commands accurately. She would not persist in following commands, for instance, she would close her eyes when asked by the examiner but repeatedly opened them immediately before the examiner asked her to (motor impersistence). She would stare at the examiner for long periods of time and repeatedly interrupted the examination to tell jokes. The rest of the physical neurological exam was unremarkable.

Non-Alzheimer's and Atypical Dementia, First Edition. Edited by Michael D. Geschwind and Caroline Racine Belkoura.
© 2016 John Wiley & Sons, Ltd. Published 2016 by John Wiley & Sons, Ltd.

On neuropsychological testing, she scored 27/30 on the Mini-Mental State Examination (MMSE), had a flat learning curve on a test of verbal memory, and had particular difficulty with tasks of executive function, such as the Stroop interference task (i.e., words for colors printed in different colored ink, and patient must state the color of the ink; if the word blue is written in green ink, they must say "green") and verbal fluency, particularly phonemic fluency as she named only 4 words beginning with the letter D in 1 min with perseveration on one of the words. Her MRI scan showed right greater than left frontotemporal atrophy with particular orbitofrontal and caudate atrophy (Figure 5.1).

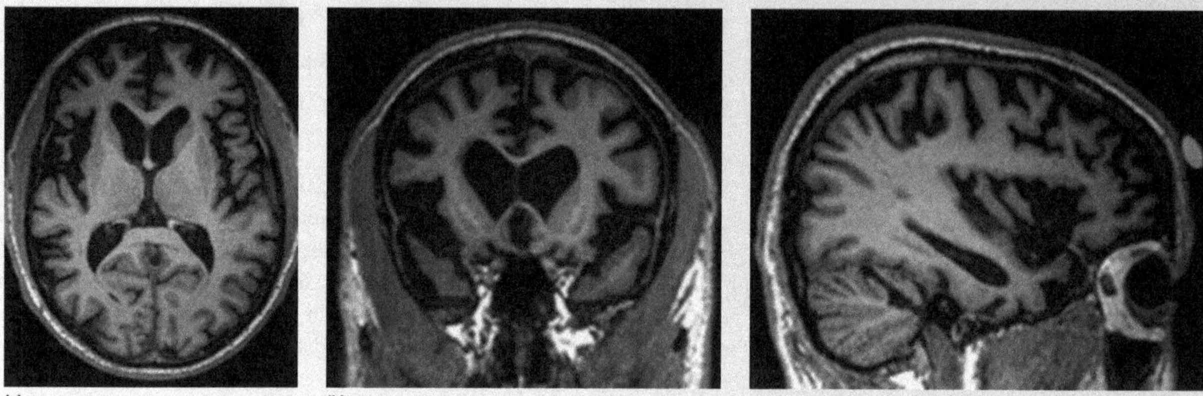

(a) (b) (c)

Figure 5.1 MRI axial (**a**), coronal (**b**), and sagittal (**c**) T1 showing bifrontal atrophy associated with behavioral variant FTD (bvFTD), greater on the right than left.

bvFTD

Symptoms in bvFTD

Sometimes referred to as frontal variant or simply as FTD, bvFTD is the most common presentation of FTD, comprising about 50% of cases, with svPPA and nfv-PPA making up the other 50% [8]. The symptoms begin with insidious changes in behavior and personality. Frequently, these are felt to be either psychiatric in nature or to represent a "midlife crisis" [9]. Typical early symptoms include disinhibition, apathy, loss of empathy, changes in eating behaviors, and compulsive behaviors. A lack of insight into their symptoms is typical in bvFTD. A distinction between a disinhibited subtype and an apathetic subtype has been proposed [10], though these features tend to be coexistent. The disinhibited acts often include socially inappropriate behaviors such as touching strangers, lack of manners or appropriate response to social cues, or impulsive or antisocial actions such as stealing. Apathy in bvFTD includes a loss of interest or motivation as well as decreased initiation of behavior. Affected patients are often described as cold, unfeeling, and indifferent to the emotions of others. This lack of empathy can be illustrated by dramatic examples such as telling jokes at funerals. Typical eating behaviors include both overeating and a change in food preference, with more consumption of sweet or high-carbohydrate foods, and sometimes development of food fads, such as insisting on foods from certain establishments or foods of a certain color. Repetitive motor behaviors are common, including simple stereotypic behaviors such as tapping or rubbing, or compulsive behaviors such as hoarding, checking, cleaning, and arranging.

Curiously, a subset of patients who meet clinical criteria for bvFTD do not progress over time or progress very slowly [11]. Imaging and neuropsychological performance in this group are normal. This group has been referred to as FTD phenocopy, implying that the etiology in these cases is not FTLD, though this has yet to be established, and the etiology of clinical symptoms and reason for lack of progression are not known.

Imaging

Both structural and functional brain imaging reveal abnormalities that can help support a diagnosis of bvFTD. Structural imaging with CT or MRI typically shows a pattern of atrophy that is generally most prominent in the frontal and/or anterior temporal lobes. If there is asymmetry, the right hemisphere is often more affected [12]. The earliest structures affected include the anterior insula, anterior cingulate, and orbitofrontal cortices [13], which are much less severely affected in AD [14]. The reason for the selective vulnerability of these regions in FTD is not known, but it has been noted that these regions are the only location of large bipolar projection cells called von Economo neurons [15]. These neurons are found only in humans, great apes, certain whales, dolphins, and elephants and are particularly targeted in bvFTD. It has been suggested that the introduction of these phylogenetically new cells into these brain regions might have induced some vulnerability [16]. The significant involvement of these paralimbic structures that are known to be involved in emotional processing [17, 18] explains the prominence of socioemotional dysfunction in bvFTD, as specific symptoms have been correlated with structural atrophy in particular portions of this network, particularly the medial prefrontal and anterior cingulate with apathy and right anterior temporal and right medial frontal atrophy with loss of empathy [19, 20]. The eating behavior changes have been correlated with orbitofrontal, right insular, striatal, and most recently hypothalamic atrophy [21–23]. For repetitive behaviors, simple stereotypies correlate with striatal atrophy[24], and complex compulsions have been variably associated with the orbitofrontal, caudate, and temporal lobe, particularly asymmetric temporal lobe atrophy [25, 26].

Whereas structural imaging usually demonstrates specific patterns of regional atrophy in bvFTD, functional brain imaging such as positron emission tomography using fluorodeoxyglucose (FDG-PET) and single-photon emission computed tomography using Tc-hexamethylpropyleneamine oxime (HMPAO-SPECT), which images cerebral perfusion, has also been frequently used to demonstrate corresponding frontotemporal abnormalities in bvFTD [27, 28].

Neuropsychological testing

Early in the course of bvFTD, patients typically perform well on traditional neuropsychological measures [29], because most of these tasks assess executive functions mediated by the dorsolateral prefrontal cortex, an area spared in early bvFTD, rather than behaviors reliant on the medial and orbital frontal lobe that are affected early in the disease [30]. Degeneration of the regions affected in bvFTD results in deficits in social cognition. Accordingly, studies have demonstrated that bvFTD patients are impaired at recognition of emotion [31], recognition of sarcasm [32], and ability to appreciate another's point of view (theory of mind) [33]. Efforts are currently underway to develop assessment tools that examine these abilities and can be used in the clinical setting, with appropriate normative data. As bvFTD progresses to involve the more dorsal frontal regions, patients develop deficits in traditional tests of executive functions, such as the Trails B task, which assesses the ability to flexibly switch between two different types of responses [34]; the Stroop interference task, which assesses the ability to inhibit automatic or "prepotent" responses [34]; and phonemic fluency, which assesses the ability to continually generate novel responses [35]. Whereas everyday memory is often relatively spared in bvFTD, performance on tests of verbal and visual memory is variable [36, 37]. Similarly, visuospatial function is relatively spared, though performance on tasks might be affected by poor planning or organization [38].

Diagnosis

Criteria published in 1994 [39] and 1998 [40] were used most commonly for diagnosis, and the 1998 Neary criteria are shown in Table 5.1. These criteria proved difficult to use in clinical practice because not all patients meet the major criteria and many of the minor criteria occur too inconsistently to be clinically useful [41]. New, simpler criteria that were proposed by an international consensus panel have shown good reliability and improved sensitivity (Table 5.2) [42, 43]. The new criteria make use of current knowledge about biomarkers to increase the

Table 5.1 1998 Neary consensus criteria for behavioral variant frontotemporal dementia.

Core diagnostic features (all needed for diagnosis)
Insidious onset and gradual progression
Early decline in social interpersonal conduct
Early impairment in regulation of personal conduct
Early emotional blunting
Early loss of insight
Supportive behavioral diagnostic features
Decline in personal hygiene and grooming
Mental rigidity and inflexibility
Distractibility and impersistence
Hyperorality and dietary changes
Perseverative and stereotyped behavior
Utilization behavior
Supportive speech and language diagnostic features
Altered speech output with economic, aspontaneous or pressed speech
Stereotypy of speech
Echolalia
Perseveration
Mutism
Supportive physical diagnostic features
Primitive reflexes
Incontinence
Akinesia, rigidity, and tremor
Low or labile blood pressure
Investigations
Neuropsychology: impairment on frontal tests in the absence of severe amnesia, aphasia, or perceptual disorder
Brain imaging: predominant frontal or anterior temporal abnormality
EEG: normal

Table 5.2 Proposed international consensus criteria for bvFTD.

I. Required criterion—progressive deterioration of behavior and/or cognition by observation or history

II. Possible bvFTD—3 of 6 required

- A. Early behavioral disinhibition—socially inappropriate behavior, loss of manners or decorum, or impulsive actions
- B. Early apathy or inertia
- C. Early loss of sympathy or empathy
- D. Early perseverative, stereotyped, or compulsive/ritualistic behavior
- E. Hyperorality and dietary changes
- F. Neuropsychological profile: executive/generation deficits with relative sparing of memory and visuospatial functions

III. Probable bvFTD (all of the following required)

- A. Meets criteria for possible bvFTD
- B. Significant functional decline
- C. Imaging results consistent with bvFTD (frontal and/or anterior temporal atrophy on CT or MRI or frontal hypoperfusion or hypometabolism on SPECT or PET)

IV. bvFTD with definite FTLD pathology (1 and either 2 or 3 required)

- A. Meets criteria for possible or probable bvFTD
- B. Histopathological evidence of FTLD on biopsy or at postmortem
- C. Presence of a known pathogenic mutation

V. Exclusion criteria for bvFTD—criteria A and B must both be answered negatively; criterion C can be positive for possible bvFTD but must be negative for probable bvFTD

- A. Pattern of deficits is better accounted for by other nervous system or medical disorders
- B. Behavioral disturbance is better accounted for by a psychiatric diagnosis
- C. Biomarkers strongly indicative of Alzheimer's disease or other neurodegenerative processes

certainty of diagnosis. Thus, although clinical features can be used to make a diagnosis of possible bvFTD, imaging findings consistent with bvFTD, such as PET hypometabolism or frontal lobe atrophy, or mutations associated with bvFTD are necessary to increase the certainty to probable. The use of imaging is supported by studies showing that imaging enhances the diagnostic accuracy [28].

PPA

PPA refers to progressive disorders in which language deterioration is the most prominent symptom and the primary cause of a patient's impairment for the initial period of the illness [44]. There are three syndromes within this category: svPPA (previously referred to as semantic dementia), nfv-PPA (also referred to as progressive nonfluent aphasia), and logopenic variant primary progressive aphasia (lvPPA). Whereas svPPA and nfv-PPA are usually associated with FTLD pathology, lvPPA is usually associated with underlying AD pathology, and because of this relationship, it will be discussed in more detail in the chapter on atypical AD. Logopenic aphasia, as seen in lvPPA, is characterized by hesitant speech and profound difficulty with word finding but relatively preserved word comprehension, and brain imaging usually shows left posterior temporal and parietal abnormalities.

svPPA

Symptoms in svPPA

svPPA is characterized by progressive deterioration in knowledge about words and objects. It begins with word finding and sometimes subtle word recognition difficulties and progresses to involve loss of knowledge about objects. Patients have fluent, empty speech without motor impairment or agrammatism. The disease usually appears to begin in the left temporal pole although patients with right greater than left temporal atrophy are not uncommon, and such patients present with more behavioral symptoms typical of bvFTD in the early phases and more subtle semantic loss [45]. As the disease progresses and involves the left temporal lobe more, typical semantic loss develops. When the

Case 2

A 61-year-old right-handed man presented with symptoms beginning one and a half years ago with trouble remembering the names of people he had known for 15 years. He then began having difficulty coming up with words. He would ask his wife what various words mean, including "what is an éclair?" and "what are immunizations?" When his wife asked him to get a mallet from the garage, he returned with a variety of items, none of which were a mallet. A neighbor came over to borrow an oil filter wrench, and he sent the neighbor to look in his tools because he was not able to identify it himself. More recently, he developed trouble planning and multitasking. He developed a rigid routine regarding eating the exact same breakfast daily and a fixation on somatic complaints including neck pain and lightheadedness.

Neurologic examination was notable for semantic paraphasias with fluent, tangential speech. Neuropsychological testing was notable for impaired naming, scoring 2/15 on the Boston Naming Test, and he only identified another two pictures with cues and multiple choice. There are some of the objects he was able to describe vaguely, such as a seahorse, which was "an animal in the water somewhere." On the Peabody Picture Vocabulary Test, which asks patients to point to pictures that match words read by the examiner (i.e., banister), he scored below expectations at 7/16. MRI showed prominent left temporal atrophy (see Figure 5.2). This patient's history is most consistent with svPPA.

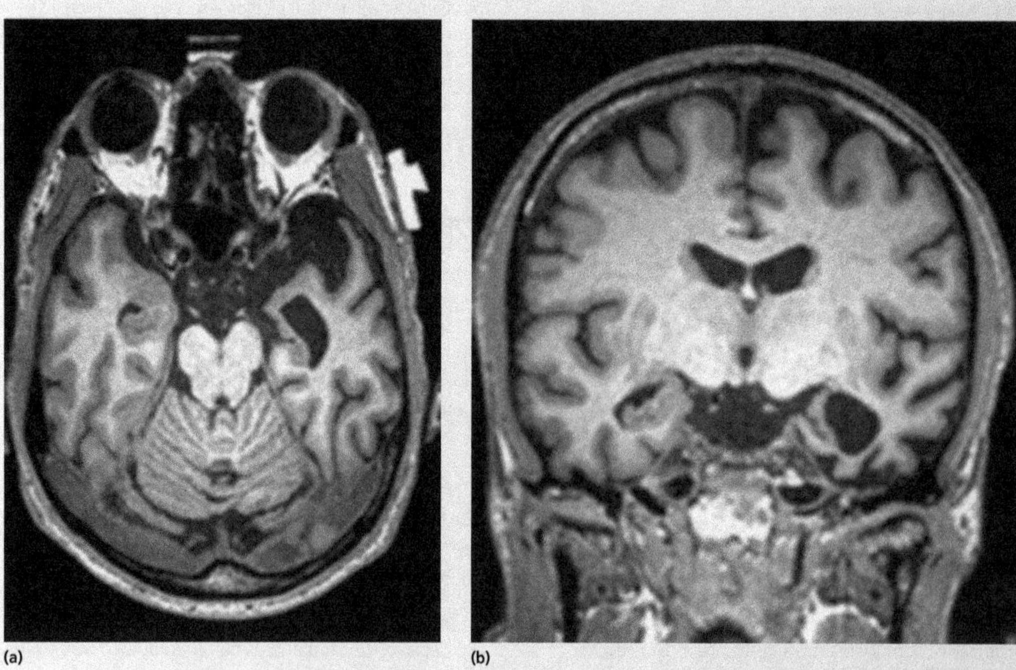

(a) (b)

Figure 5.2 Axial (**a**) and coronal (**b**) T1 MRI showing left anterior temporal lobe atrophy associated with semantic variant PPA (svPPA).

disease begins on the right, knowledge about faces also is often an early deficit, for instance, not recognizing very famous faces of politicians or entertainers [46]. Left-sided predominance is more common than right-sided predominance by a 3:1 margin [45]. Whether the disease begins on the right or left, svPPA patients usually develop behavioral symptoms typical of bvFTD within 3 or 4 years of onset, presumably because of the spread of the disease from temporal to frontal structures [47].

Imaging

Dramatic anterior temporal atrophy can easily be appreciated on MRI [47], and it is usually remarkably asymmetric, although bilateral [48]. Frontal atrophy may be found at later stages.

Neuropsychological testing

Patients with svPPA will perform poorly on tests of confrontational naming, single-word comprehension (word to picture matching), and category fluency. They often display surface dyslexia, an inability to correctly pronounce irregular written words (such as knight, yacht, etc.). Those with right temporal involvement might also have difficulty on tasks of recognizing famous faces. Verbal memory is typically impaired above and beyond the language deficits secondary to mesial temporal lobe involvement and in many cases concomitant hippocampal sclerosis. Visuospatial and executive functions tend to be relatively preserved [49].

nfv-PPA

Symptoms in nfv-PPA

nfv-PPA is characterized by slow, effortful speech, apraxia of speech and agrammatism (decreased use of grammatical function words). Nonfluency refers to a reduced rate of speech. Apraxia of speech involves problems with the motor speech production and involves sound distortions. For example, pronunciation of a complicated phonological word such as "catastrophe" by someone with speech apraxia would result in the word sounding different with each attempt, whereas with a cerebellar dysarthria the sound errors would be the same or similar each time the word is spoken. Phonological errors with variable substitutions of syllables with each attempt at pronunciation of a word are heard. Comprehension is generally spared. Motor signs (typically parkinsonism) are often found on examination, particularly if the underlying pathology is corticobasal

Case 3

A 74-year-old gentleman began to notice difficulty enunciating beginning about 2 years prior to presentation. He says he knows the words he wants to say, but can't get them out. He stumbles over words, mispronounces them, and must slow his speech down in order to pronounce things better and to find the words he wants to say. Being under stress, such as public speaking, is particularly likely to worsen his difficulties. His wife says sometimes he will use the wrong tense of a verb or will say the wrong word, such as saying "hose" instead of "nose." He notes no trouble with comprehension. Neither he nor his wife has noted any other areas of thinking difficulty. He is still doing crossword puzzles and paying their bills.

On examination, he was alert and attentive and followed commands quickly and accurately. His speech was slow and effortful, with frequent pauses in between and even within words. He had trouble pronouncing phonemically complex words, making many attempts with varying results. For instance, when asked to pronounce the word anachronistic, he said "acrononistic...ananochronoristic...acronistic...." The remainder of his neurological exam was unremarkable except for slightly decreased arm swing on the right during walking. He scored poorly on verbal fluency but did well on most other cognitive tasks. MRI showed atrophy in the left insular/perisylvian region (Figure 5.3). Based on his clinical history, exam, and MRI, his diagnosis is most consistent nfv-PPA.

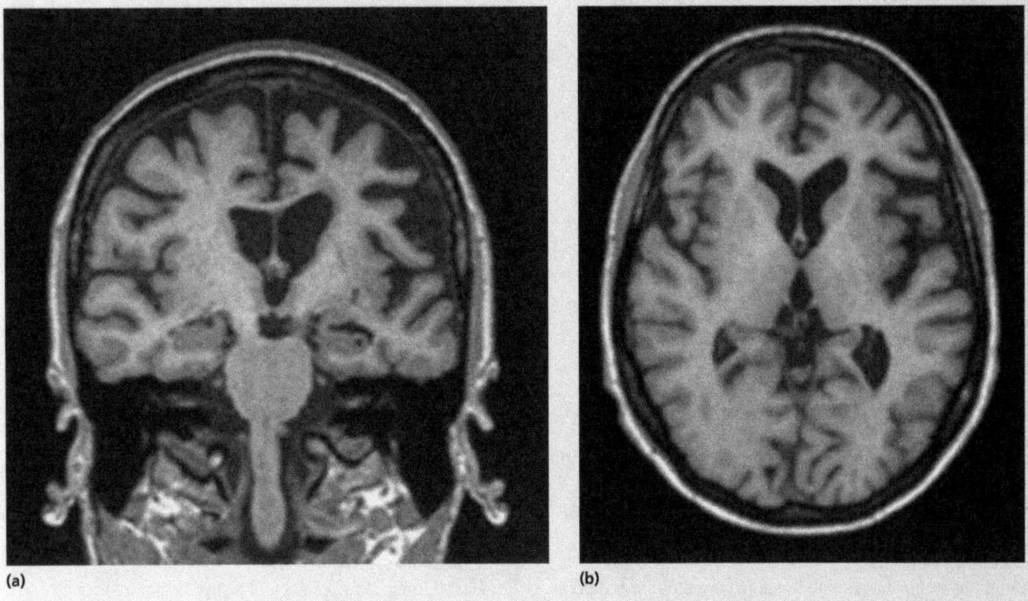

(a) (b)

Figure 5.3 Coronal (**a**) and axial (**b**) T1 MRI showing left perisylvian atrophy associated with nfv-PPA.

degeneration (CBD) or PSP. Depression is common. Although behavioral and personality changes can develop over time in nfv-PPA, they have less of the dramatic socioemotional dysfunction seen in bvFTD and svPPA [50].

Imaging

Asymmetric atrophy and hypometabolism of the left inferior frontal/perisylvian area is the characteristic imaging finding [51, 52].

Neuropsychological testing

Nonfluent speech with apraxia of speech and impaired grammar are found. Frequently, there are substitutions of incorrect sounds in a word, called phonemic paraphasias. Verbal fluency is typically reduced, and naming may also be impaired. Executive dysfunction is often subtle early in the disease but typically becomes more apparent with progression due to extensive involvement of the left lateral prefrontal cortex. Visuospatial skills and memory abilities are relatively spared early in the course of the disease [51].

Table 5.3 1998 Neary consensus criteria for semantic variant.

Core diagnostic features
Insidious onset and gradual progression
Language disorder characterized by:
1. Progressive, fluent, empty spontaneous speech
2. Loss of word meaning, manifest by impaired naming and comprehension
3. Semantic paraphasias

Perceptual disorder characterized by:
1. Prosopagnosia: impaired recognition of identity of familiar faces and/or
2. Associative agnosia: impaired recognition of object identity

Preserved perceptual matching and drawing reproduction
Preserved single-word repetition
Preserved ability to read aloud and write to dictation orthographically regular words

Supportive speech and language diagnostic features
Press of speech
Idiosyncratic word usage
Absence of phonemic paraphasias
Surface dyslexia and dysgraphia
Preserved calculation

Supportive behavior features
Loss of sympathy and empathy
Narrowed preoccupations
Parsimony

Supportive physical signs
Absent or late primitive reflexes
Akinesia, rigidity, and tremor

Investigations
Neuropsychology
1. Profound semantic loss, manifest in failure of word comprehension and naming and/or face and object recognition
2. Preserved phonology and syntax, elementary perceptual processing, spatial skills, and day-to-day memorizing

Electroencephalography: normal
Brain imaging (structural and/or functional): predominant anterior temporal abnormality (symmetric or asymmetric)

PPA diagnosis

Diagnostic criteria from 1998 have been used until recently for these aphasic syndromes [40] (Tables 5.3 and 5.5). New knowledge about the clinical and imaging features and of PPA has led to new criteria for these disorders (see Tables 5.4 and 5.6) [53].

Table 5.4 Diagnostic criteria for semantic variant PPA.

Core diagnostic features
Insidious onset and gradual progression
Nonfluent spontaneous speech with at least one of the following: agrammatism, phonemic paraphasias, anomia

Supportive speech and language features
Stuttering or oral apraxia
Impaired repetition
Alexia, agraphia
Early preservation of word meaning
Late mutism

Supportive behavior features
Early preservation of social skills
Late behavioral changes similar to FTD

Supportive physical signs
Late contralateral primitive reflexes, akinesia, rigidity, and tremor

Investigations
Neuropsychology: nonfluent aphasia in the absence of severe amnesia or perceptuospatial disorder
Electroencephalography: normal or minor asymmetric slowing
Brain imaging (structural and/or functional): asymmetric abnormality predominantly affecting dominant (usually left) hemisphere

Table 5.5 1998 Neary consensus criteria for progressive nonfluent aphasia.

Patients must meet criteria for primary progressive aphasia (modified from Mesulam)
Both of the following **core features** must be present:
1. Poor confrontation naming
2. Impaired single-word comprehension

At least three of the following other features must be present:
- Poor object knowledge
- Surface dyslexia and/or dysgraphia
- Spared repetition
- Spared motor speech and grammar

Imaging-supported SV-PPA diagnosis
Both of the following criteria must be present:
- Clinical diagnosis of SV-PPA
- Imaging must show one or more of the following results:
  - Predominant anterior temporal lobe atrophy on MRI
  - Predominant anterior temporal hypoperfusion or hypometabolism on SPECT or PET

SV-PPA with definite pathology
Clinical diagnosis (criterion 1 below) and either criterion 2 or 3 must be present:
- Clinical diagnosis of SV-PPA
- Histopathological evidence of a specific pathology

Presence of a known pathogenic mutation

Table 5.6 Diagnostic criteria for nonfluent PPA.

Patients must meet criteria for primary progressive aphasia (modified from Mesulam)
At least one of the following core features must be present:
1. Agrammatism in language production
2. Effortful, halting speech with inconsistent sound errors and distortions (apraxia of speech)

At least two of three of the following other features must be present:
1. Impaired comprehension of syntactically complex sentences
2. Spared single-word comprehension
3. Spared object knowledge

Imaging-supported nfv-PPA diagnosis
Both of the following criteria must be present:
1. Clinical diagnosis of nfv-PPA
2. Imaging must show one or more of the following results:
   - Predominant left posterior fronto-insular atrophy on MRI
   - Predominant left posterior fronto-insular hypoperfusion or hypometabolism on SPECT or PET

nfv-PPA with definite pathology
Clinical diagnosis (criterion 1 below) and either criterion 2 or 3 must be present:
1. Clinical diagnosis of nfv-PPA
2. Histopathological evidence of a specific pathology (e.g., FTLD-tau, FTLD-TDP, AD)
3. Presence of a known pathogenic mutation

Other clinical syndromes associated with FTD

Although bvFTD, svPPA, and nfv-PPA are the core FTD clinical syndromes, several other neurodegenerative syndromes are associated with FTLD pathology at autopsy and have overlapping clinical features. These syndromes are now often included in discussions of FTD as "FTD spectrum" or "FTLD spectrum" and include features of MND and parkinsonism.

Frontotemporal dementia with motor neuron disease

About 10 to 15% of patients with FTD also develop MND similar to amyotrophic lateral sclerosis (ALS, also known as Lou Gehrig's disease) [54], and this combination is associated with the most rapid progression of FTD subtypes and shortest survival [7]. MND is most likely to occur with bvFTD, although it occurs with any of the three core FTD syndromes. MND is characterized by muscular weakness, atrophy, and fasciculations due to degeneration of spinal cord anterior horn cells, as well as pyramidal signs such as spastic tone and hyperreflexia due to degeneration of neurons in the primary motor cortex. Symptoms more frequently involve the bulbar muscles (tongue, face, those associated with swallowing), when MND is associated with FTD. Either cognitive or motor symptoms present first. When FTD is associated with MND, patients sometimes have strong, uncontrollable bursts of laughing or crying, referred to as pseudobulbar affect (PBA) [55], and PBA in the setting of FTD should prompt investigations for MND. The behavioral symptoms in frontotemporal dementia with motor neuron disease (FTD-MND) are similar to those occurring in FTD without MND, although psychotic symptoms are more common in FTD-MND [56]. Imaging in FTD-MND sometimes is less dramatic than in FTD without MND but can include atrophy around premotor areas extending to the precentral gyrus [57]. Although ALS was traditionally thought to be very rarely associated with dementia, the occurrence of MND in the setting of FTD prompted research to more closely examine the cognition of ALS patients. These studies revealed that approximately 20% of patients presenting to neuromuscular clinics with only motor complaints actually have substantial cognitive and behavioral problems consistent with a diagnosis FTD [58] and up to 50% of ALS patients have more subtle cognitive deficits detectable using psychometric or quantitative assessment—findings which further cemented the link between FTD and ALS [58, 59].

PSP and CBS

PSP and CBS have traditionally been included in neurological texts as atypical forms of parkinsonism. These are discussed in detail in Chapter 7, so will only be briefly mentioned here. Many PSP patients develop cognitive difficulties suggesting frontal lobe dysfunction, and they frequently develop behavioral and/or language symptoms seen in bvFTD and nfv-PPA. Some PSP patients initially suffer from these cognitive or behavioral symptoms, with minimal or very subtle motor difficulties, and later develop the typical motor features of PSP. This symptomatic overlap and association with the pathological features of FTLD has led to its inclusion with FTD-spectrum disorders.

CBS is also a disorder where the true spectrum of clinical presentation is in flux. Traditionally, CBS (often referred to by the pathological term CBD) was described as a cognitive and motor disorder with markedly asymmetric movement difficulties including tremor and myoclonus, rigidity and dystonia, alien limb (tendency for the limb to move on its own and sometimes interfere with movements of other limbs), and asymmetric sensory problems suggesting somatosensory cortex dysfunction. Studies have also described language difficulties similar to nfv-PPA or less commonly lvPPA and profound visuospatial disturbances and neglect of the left side of space [60, 61]. Recent studies have suggested that many CBS patients, even with asymmetric motor symptoms, have AD pathology [62, 63] and those with AD pathology have more temporoparietal atrophy [64]. When CBD is found pathologically, patients can present with the asymmetrical motor symptoms and cognitive and behavioral deficits typical of frontal lobe dysfunction similar to those seen in bvFTD, and they may not have significant motor deficits [65].

Neuropathology

One of the challenges facing clinicians who see patients with neurodegenerative disorders is translating a patient's presenting clinical syndrome into a prediction of the underlying molecular and histopathology. These correlations will be more relevant as treatments are developed that target the molecular basis of disease. Unfortunately, this prediction is made more complicated by the fact that the clinical syndromes that comprise FTD are associated with varied underlying pathologies.

All subtypes of FTLD pathology show gross frontal and temporal lobe atrophy as well as neuronal loss, variable gliosis, and microvacuolation [66]. The different subtypes are differentiated from each other by the types of neuronal inclusions and other morphological features. The earliest reports of FTLD described Pick bodies [2], which were later recognized to contain hyperphosphorylated tau proteins. Subsequently, many cases of FTLD were described with tau inclusions, but not necessarily Pick bodies; however, this only accounted for about half of cases of FTLD. The pathological descriptions for the other half have evolved over time, having been described for many years as dementia lacking distinctive histopathology (DLDH) [67]. Subsequently, new staining techniques demonstrated that many patients that would have been called DLDH actually show tau-negative ubiquitinated inclusions, termed FTLD-U. In 2006, it was discovered that the ubiquitinated protein in most of these cases is the 43 kDa TAR DNA-binding protein (TDP-43) [68]. Now, it is recognized that these two pathologies, tau inclusions or TDP-43 inclusions, are approximately found in equal frequencies in bvFTD and account for the majority of cases [69]. Recently, it was discovered that patients showing inclusions with the fused in sarcoma (FUS) protein now explain most of rest of the FTLD-U cases [70].

Tau

The tau protein, which is also called microtubule-associated protein tau (MAPT), is coded on chromosome 17 and is important for stabilizing microtubules and thus supports molecular transport within neurons [71]. Tau exists in two forms created by alternative splicing, which leads to a 3-amino-acid sequence repeat form (3R) and a 4 repeat form (4R). Both forms are present in normal cells, but some pathologies are associated predominantly with one form or the other. Pick bodies, the classic histopathology in FTLD, contain the 3R form of tau (seen in Figure 5.4). Achromatic ballooned neurons, or Pick cells, are seen in association with Pick bodies, and many patients have Pick cells without Pick bodies. Other pathological settings with predominant tau pathology include FTDP-17, a genetic form associated with mutations in the *MAPT* gene, and this is a mixture of 3R and 4R tau. The rarer tangle-dominant dementia (TDD) and the Guam ALS parkinsonism–dementia complex are also 3R + 4R mixtures. CBD and PSP are both 4R tau forms. CBD is associated with tau immunoreactive astrocytic plaques and glial threads and coils. PSP is characterized by globose neurofibrillary tangles and tufted astrocytes [72]. Argyrophilic grain disease (AGD) and multiple system tauopathy with dementia are rarer 4R tau pathologies [72].

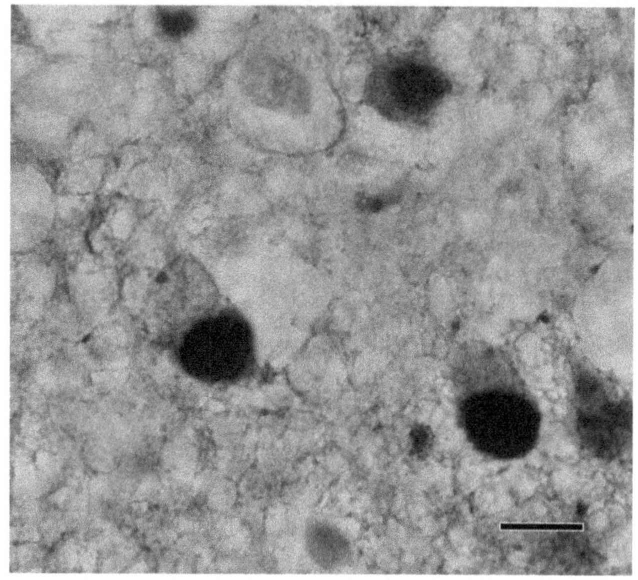

Figure 5.4 Pick bodies in the left midinsula in a 74-year-old woman with nonfluent variant PPA due to Pick's disease. Immunohistochemistry for 3-repeat tau, hematoxylin counterstain. Reproduced with permission of W.W. Seeley. (*See insert for color representation of the figure.*)

TDP-43

The functions of the TDP-43 protein are not completely understood, but it is a normal constituent of neurons. In these circumstances, staining is limited to the nuclei, which is consistent with data indicating that TDP-43 is a regulator of DNA transcription [73]. In FTLD, TDP-43 inclusions are found in the cytoplasm, and various patterns of staining have been recognized based on whether the TDP-43 appears to be collecting mostly in cytoplasmic inclusions, neurites, or both. This classification is important because certain pathological subtypes are associated with specific clinical presentations (discussed in the next section). A harmonized classification [74] of the two prior systems [75, 76] recognizes four types of TDP-43 pathology. Type A has frequent small dystrophic neurites and neuronal cytoplasmic inclusions and might have neuronal intranuclear inclusions. Type B has numerous neuronal cytoplasmic inclusions in superficial and deep cortical layers with infrequent neurites, and Type C includes long dystrophic neurites in superficial layers and few neuronal cytoplasmic inclusions. Type D is relatively rare and includes dystrophic neurites and intranuclear inclusions. At the time that the link between TDP-43 and FTLD was discovered, TDP-43 was also found to be present in the majority of patients with ALS, which provides a pathological basis for the clinical links between ALS and FTD noted earlier [68, 77].

FUS

FUS pathology was initially discovered in patients with familial ALS and soon thereafter in patients with FTD [78]. Basophilic inclusion body disease (BIBD) [79], neuronal intermediate filament inclusion disease (NIFID) [80], and atypical FTLD-U (aFTLD-U) are rare pathologies in the FTLD spectrum that are now attributed to FUS pathology as well.

Other

There still remain some cases without inclusions in the DLDH category, as well as cases termed FTD-3 that will be discussed later with the corresponding genetic mutation.

Clinicopathological correlation

Overall, the relationship between the specific clinical presentation and the molecular and histopathology is far from a one-to-one correlation (see Figure 5.5), but some clinical presentations are fairly predictive of specific pathologies.

svPPA usually is caused by TDP-43 pathology, specifically type C [74, 81], though it can also be caused by AD and very rarely by tau pathology [82]. nfv-PPA is often caused by tau pathology, usually PSP or CBD [52], though it can be the result of other pathologies as well [83]. FTD-MND is caused by TDP-43 type B pathology. Type A pathology is seen in patients with familial FTD associated with progranulin mutations (see following text) and can cause multiple other sporadic FTD syndromes. Type D pathology is also associated with familial cases of FTD, inclusion body myositis, and Paget's disease of bone due to mutations in valosin-containing protein (VCP) [74, 81].

Clinically, patients with FUS pathology have a young age of onset and often have a psychiatric presentation [70]. Their imaging is associated with more caudate atrophy than is seen in other FTLD pathologies [84].

Whereas svPPA and nfv-PPA are strongly associated with specific pathologies, bvFTD is associated about equally with tau or TDP-43 pathology, and no clinical features are currently recognized as predicting the subtype. Some patients with bvFTD have AD pathology at autopsy [85]. In some cases, this is seen in addition to FTLD pathology, but in many of these cases, AD pathology appears to be the only cause (i.e., frontal variant of AD).

When the supranuclear gaze difficulties characteristic of PSP are present, PSP pathology is highly likely [86]. As noted earlier, the clinical features of CBS can be associated with various pathologies, including AD, and the features predicting CBD pathology are still being resolved.

The development of additional biomarkers to identify the molecular subtype in each case of FTD is currently of great interest. For those patients with clinical features of FTD but underlying AD pathology, CSF levels of tau and Aβ42 have shown promise for discriminating between FTLD and AD [87]. PET ligands are also available for detecting amyloid plaques in vivo, providing another approach for making this distinction [88], particularly in patients with atypical presentations who are considered diagnostic dilemmas [89]. Recent work has suggested that it might be possible to distinguish FTLD-tau from FTLD-TDP based on assaying multiple specific CSF analytes [90, 91]. Low progranulin levels measured in serum, plasma, and CSF have been found in patients with progranulin mutations [92–94]. One study suggested that elevated serum TDP-43 levels might be useful [95]. Neurofilament light chains have also been found to be elevated in FTD and to correlate with disease severity [96]. All of these tests, however, must still be considered preliminary.

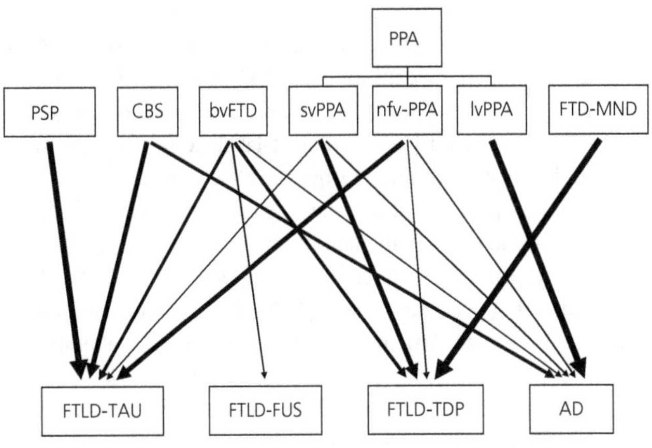

Figure 5.5 Clinical and pathologic correlates between FTD-spectrum syndromes and FTLD pathologies. PSP = progressive supranuclear palsy; CBS = corticobasal syndrome; bvFTD = behavioral variant frontotemporal dementia; PPA = primary progressive aphasia; svPPA = semantic variant primary progressive aphasia; nfv-PPA = nonfluent variant primary progressive aphasia; lvPPA = logopenic variant primary progressive aphasia; FTD-MND = frontotemporal dementia with motor neuron disease; FTLD-tau = frontotemporal lobar degeneration with tau pathology; FTLD-TDP = FTLD with TAR DNA-binding protein 43 (TDP-43) pathology; FTLD-FUS = FTLD with fused in sarcoma (FUS) pathology; AD = Alzheimer's disease.

Genetics

The majority of cases of FTD are sporadic and there is no clear pattern of inheritance. About 10% are associated with an autosomal dominant inheritance pattern. Forty percent of patients have a family history of dementia or psychiatric conditions but do not necessarily have a clear inheritance pattern [97]. There are two haplotypes of tau, H1 and H2, and the H1/H1 genotype has been associated with an increased risk of developing 4R tau disorders, PSP or CBD [98, 99].

MAPT

There are more than 40 different currently recognized disease-causing mutations of the *MAPT* gene, which is found on chromosome 17. Carriers of this gene develop symptoms at a younger age than sporadic or other genetic cases (52 years old compared to 62 years old for *PGRN* mutations in one series [100]), and imaging reveals a more symmetric pattern of atrophy with more temporal lobe atrophy than other genetic cases [101]. There is also some suggestion that different mutations are associated with different patterns of atrophy [102].

PGRN

Mutations in the progranulin gene (also on chromosome 17) cause a wide variety of clinical presentations, including not only symptoms of bvFTD but also parkinsonism, memory impairment, hallucinations or delusions, and a nonfluent aphasia (often without apraxia of speech). The atrophy pattern on MRI tends to be more asymmetric and more posterior than other forms of FTLD [103]. The mechanism by which *PGRN* mutations lead to TDP-43 pathology is currently unclear, though multiple pathways have been implicated, including neuroinflammation and impaired lysosomal function [104]. PGRN mutations have been found in patients with AD copathology, suggesting that these mutations may also be an AD risk factor [105]. As opposed to *MAPT*, mutations in *PGRN* lead to haploinsufficiency, rather than a toxic gain of function [106].

C9ORF72

A recently discovered hexanucleotide repeat expansion on chromosome 9 (*C9ORF72*) has been found to be the most common cause of both familial FTD and familial ALS [107, 108]. This expansion may be found in 11–29% of familial FTD, 24% of familial ALS, and 2–4% of sporadic FTD or ALS [107, 109]. The clinical syndrome in these patients is most commonly bvFTD, ALS, or FTD-MND [110], but PPA subtypes have also been described [111, 112]. Psychosis has been described as a more common feature with *C9ORF72* than in nonmutation carriers [111]. Some cases of slowly progressive bvFTD, thought to have been FTD phenocopies, have also been found to carry *C9ORF72* mutations [113]. Mutation carriers have been found to have FTLD-TDP pathology (types A or B), and TDP-negative p62-positive inclusions in the cerebellum are a specific pathologic feature [112, 114, 115]. Formation and intracellular accumulation of RNA foci have been proposed as a putative disease mechanism [107]. Dipeptide repeat proteins translated from the hexanucleotide repeat have also been found [116], though it is not clear if these are pathogenic as they do not colocalize with neurodegenerative findings, with other TDP-43 pathology, or correspond with the clinical phenotype in these cases [117].

CHMP-2B

The gene *CHMP-2B* (charged multivesicular body protein 2B, also referred to as chromatin-modifying protein 2B) is found on chromosome 3, encodes a component of the endosomal sorting complex required for transport III, and causes the type of FTLD known as FTD-3. It is not associated with tau, TDP-43, or FUS pathology. It is extremely rare and only described in a few families, one Danish [118] and another Belgian.

VCP

Mutations of the VCP on chromosome 9 are associated most commonly with inclusion body myositis and in some affected individuals also with Paget's disease of bone and FTD. *VCP* mutations have also been associated with familial ALS [119].

Other

Several studies have looked for additional genes or epigenetic risk factors that might confer risk for development of FTD. Whereas variants in several genes have been found to increase risk in single studies [120, 121], these results have not yet been replicated. Recent genome-wide association studies (GWAS) in clinical [122] and pathologically confirmed cases [123] of FTD have suggested other genes that confer risk of developing the disease and point to cellular pathways that may be involved in its development. Epigenetic factors, such as methylation or histone modification, may also be relevant and lead to therapeutic targets in FTD [124]. Mutations in the *TARDBP* and *FUS* genes have been found and linked mostly to familial ALS, with rare associations with an FTD presentation.

Treatment

There are no US FDA-approved medications for the treatment of FTD. There is limited evidence regarding symptomatic treatment. Treatments directed at specific molecular targets are currently being developed.

Symptomatic

Nonpharmacologic methods of dealing with behavioral symptoms are important, particularly given the lack of proven pharmacologic treatments. Caregiver education is important and can help caregivers to realize that rational debate or argument often is not helpful in modifying the patient's behavior. (See Chapter 15 regarding patient management.)

The pharmacologic agents used in AD are not necessarily useful in FTD, which affects different neural networks. FTD is not associated with a cholinergic deficit, and there is no strong evidence for the use of cholinesterase inhibitors in FTD. Donepezil showed no beneficial cognitive effect in one open-label trial and resulted in worsening of behavior [125]. An open-label study of rivastigmine showed improvement in neuropsychiatric symptoms but not cognition [126], and another study of galantamine showed a nonsignificant trend toward language improvement in a cohort of PPA patients that might have included some with lvPPA (who likely had underlying AD pathology) [127]. There is no compelling evidence for the use of memantine. Though two open-label studies showed that the medication is well tolerated [128, 129], a double-blind placebo-controlled trial in France showed no improvement with memantine after 1 year [130], and a subsequent study in the United States confirmed a lack of benefit [131].

Behavioral symptoms can be treated with antidepressants, particularly serotonergic agents. Open-label studies of fluoxetine, fluvoxamine, sertraline, and paroxetine have shown efficacy in controlling behaviors [132, 133]. Paroxetine was effective in a placebo-controlled study [134], though a separate, very brief randomized study of this drug showed no effect [135]. Trazodone has also been shown effective in one study [136]. There is no evidence for the use of mood-stabilizing agents. Antipsychotic medications should be used with caution given the unfavorable side effect profile and US FDA black box warning. Quetiapine has less D2 receptor antagonism, making it a more appealing choice for avoiding extrapyramidal side effects. Some data show benefit for olanzapine [137] (one open-label study), aripiprazole [138], and risperidone (single case reports) [139].

Disease-modifying

The ultimate goal of treatment is not only to ameliorate symptoms but also to cure disease. Current efforts are underway to develop medications to target tau and TDP-43 pathology. Tau-active drugs in development include those that prevent tau kinase activity to block phosphorylation, those that clear tau aggregates, microtubule stabilizers, and aggregation inhibitors. The neuroactive peptide davunetide had shown a benefit on microtubule stabilization and decreased tau phosphorylation in preclinical studies, but it was recently shown to be ineffective in PSP [140], although it is not clear that the drug had adequate brain penetration in this study. Progranulin mutations result in their deleterious effect through haploinsufficiency, so treatments aimed at this molecular pathology are intended to increase progranulin levels. Many other treatment trials for FTD and related disorders are underway (see www.clinicaltrials.gov).

Conclusions

The term FTD encompasses multiple distinct clinical phenotypes with personality, behavior, and language changes, as well as extrapyramidal syndromes and MND. It is caused by multiple distinct pathologies and in some cases genetic mutations. Treatments are currently symptomatic, but molecular-based treatments are currently in development.

References

1 Pick A. Uber die Beziehungen der senilen Hirnatrophie zur Aphasie. *Prager Medizinische Wochenschrift* 1892;**17**:165–167.

2 Alzheimer A. Uber eigenartige Krankheitsfalle des sparteren Alters. *Psychiatr Nervenkr Z Gesamte Neurol Psychiatr* 1911;**4**:356–385.

3 Ratnavalli E, Brayne C, Dawson K, Hodges JR. The prevalence of frontotemporal dementia. *Neurology* 2002 Jun 11;**58**(11):1615–1621.

4 Brunnstrom H, Gustafson L, Passant U, Englund E. Prevalence of dementia subtypes: a 30-year retrospective survey of neuropathological reports. *Arch Gerontol Geriatr* 2009 Jul–Aug;**49**(1):146–149.

5 Rosso SM, Donker Kaat L, Baks T, Joosse M, de Koning I, Pijnenburg Y, et al. Frontotemporal dementia in the Netherlands: patient characteristics and prevalence estimates from a population-based study. *Brain* 2003 Sep;**126**(Pt 9):2016–2022.

6 Knopman DS, Petersen RC, Edland SD, Cha RH, Rocca WA. The incidence of frontotemporal lobar degeneration in Rochester, Minnesota, 1990 through 1994. *Neurology* 2004 Feb 10;**62**(3):506–508.

7 Roberson ED, Hesse JH, Rose KD, Slama H, Johnson JK, Yaffe K, et al. Frontotemporal dementia progresses to death faster than Alzheimer disease. *Neurology* 2005 Sep 13;**65**(5):719–725.

8 Johnson JK, Diehl J, Mendez MF, Neuhaus J, Shapira JS, Forman M, et al. Frontotemporal lobar degeneration: demographic characteristics of 353 patients. *Arch Neurol* 2005 June 1;**62**(6):925–930.

9 Woolley JD, Khan BK, Murthy NK, Miller BL, Rankin KP. The diagnostic challenge of psychiatric symptoms in neurodegenerative disease: rates of and risk factors for prior psychiatric diagnosis in patients with early neurodegenerative disease. *J Clin Psychiatry* 2011 Feb;**72**(2):126–133.

10 Neary D, Snowden JS, Northen B, Goulding P. Dementia of frontal lobe type. *J Neurol Neurosurg Psychiatry* 1988 Mar;**51**(3):353–361.

11 Kipps CM, Nestor PJ, Fryer TD, Hodges JR. Behavioral variant frontotemporal dementia: not all it seems? *Neurocase* 2007 Aug;**13**(4):237–247.

12 Fukui T, Kertesz A. Volumetric study of lobar atrophy in Pick complex and Alzheimer's disease. *J Neurol Sci* 2000 Mar 15;**174**(2): 111–121.

13 Seeley WW, Crawford R, Rascovsky K, Kramer JH, Weiner M, Miller BL, et al. Frontal paralimbic network atrophy in very mild behavioral variant frontotemporal dementia. *Arch Neurol* 2008; **65**(2):249.

14 Liu W, Miller BL, Kramer JH, Rankin K, Wyss-Coray C, Gearhart R, et al. Behavioral disorders in the frontal and temporal variants of frontotemporal dementia. *Neurology* 2004 Mar 9;**62**(5):742–748.

15 Seeley WW, Carlin DA, Allman JM, Macedo MN, Bush C, Miller BL, et al. Early frontotemporal dementia targets neurons unique to apes and humans. *Ann Neurol* 2006 Dec;**60**(6):660–667.

16 Seeley WW. Selective functional, regional, and neuronal vulnerability in frontotemporal dementia. *Curr Opin Neurol* 2008 Dec;**21**(6):701–707.

17 Lane RD, Reiman EM, Axelrod B, Yun LS, Holmes A, Schwartz GE. Neural correlates of levels of emotional awareness. Evidence of an interaction between emotion and attention in the anterior cingulate cortex. *J Cogn Neurosci* 1998 Jul;**10**(4):525–535.

18 Craig AD. Interoception: the sense of the physiological condition of the body. *Curr Opin Neurobiol* 2003 Aug;**13**(4):500–505.

19 Rosen HJ, Allison SC, Schauer GF, Gorno-Tempini ML, Weiner MW, Miller BL. Neuroanatomical correlates of behavioral disorders in dementia. *Brain* 2005 Nov;**128**(Pt 11):2612–2625.

20 Rankin KP, Gorno-Tempini ML, Allison SC, Stanley CM, Glenn S, Weiner MW, et al. Structural anatomy of empathy in neurodegenerative disease. *Brain* 2006 Nov;**129**(Pt 11):2945–2956.

21 Woolley JD, Gorno-Tempini ML, Seeley WW, Rankin K, Lee SS, Matthews BR, et al. Binge eating is associated with right orbitofrontal-insular-striatal atrophy in frontotemporal dementia. *Neurology* 2007 Oct 2;**69**(14):1424–1433.

22 Whitwell JL, Sampson EL, Loy CT, Warren JE, Rossor MN, Fox NC, et al. VBM signatures of abnormal eating behaviors in frontotemporal lobar degeneration. *Neuroimage* 2007 Mar;**35**(1):207–213.

23 Piguet O, Petersen A, Yin Ka Lam B, Gabery S, Murphy K, Hodges JR, et al. Eating and hypothalamus changes in behavioral-variant frontotemporal dementia. *Ann Neurol* 2011;**69**(2):312–319.

24 Josephs KA, Whitwell JL, Jack CR, Jr. Anatomic correlates of stereotypies in frontotemporal lobar degeneration. *Neurobiol Aging* 2008 Dec;**29**(12):1859–1863.

25 Rosso SM, Roks G, Stevens M, de Koning I, Tanghe HLJ, Kamphorst W, et al. Complex compulsive behavior in the temporal variant of frontotemporal dementia. *J Neurol* 2001 Nov;**248**(11):965–970.

26 Ames D, Cummings JL, Wirshing WC, Quinn B, Mahler M. Repetitive and compulsive behavior in frontal lobe degenerations. *J Neuropsychiatry Clin Neurosci* 1994 Spring;**6**(2):100–113.

27 Ishii K, Sakamoto S, Sasaki M, Kitagaki H, Yamaji S, Hashimoto M, et al. Cerebral glucose metabolism in patients with frontotemporal dementia. *J Nucl Med* 1998 Nov;**39**(11):1875–1878.

28 Foster NL, Heidebrink JL, Clark CM, Jagust WJ, Arnold SE, Barbas NR, et al. FDG-PET improves accuracy in distinguishing frontotemporal dementia and Alzheimer's disease. *Brain* 2007 October 01; **130**(10):2616–2635.

29 Gregory CA, Serra-Mestres J, Hodges JR. Early diagnosis of the frontal variant of frontotemporal dementia: how sensitive are standard neuroimaging and neuropsychologic tests? *Neuropsychiatry Neuropsychol Behav Neurol* 1999 Apr;**12**(2):128–135.

30 Krueger CE, Laluz V, Rosen HJ, Neuhaus JM, Miller BL, Kramer JH. Double dissociation in the anatomy of socioemotional disinhibition and executive functioning in dementia. *Neuropsychology* 2011 Mar;**25**(2):249–259.

31 Lough S, Kipps CM, Treise C, Watson P, Blair JR, Hodges JR. Social reasoning, emotion and empathy in frontotemporal dementia. *Neuropsychologia* 2006;**44**(6):950–958.

32 Kosmidis MH, Aretouli E, Bozikas VP, Giannakou M, Ioannidis P. Studying social cognition in patients with schizophrenia and patients with frontotemporal dementia: theory of mind and the perception of sarcasm. *Behav Neurol* 2008;**19**(1–2):65–69.

33 Gregory C, Lough S, Stone V, Erzinclioglu S, Martin L, Baron-Cohen S, et al. Theory of mind in patients with frontal variant frontotemporal dementia and Alzheimer's disease: theoretical and practical implications. *Brain* 2002 Apr;**125**(Pt 4):752–764.

34 Strauss E, Sherman EMS, Spreen O. *A compendium of neuropsychological tests: administration, norms, and commentary*. 3rd ed. New York: Oxford University Press; 2006.

35 Henry JD, Crawford JR. A meta-analytic review of verbal fluency performance following focal cortical lesions. *Neuropsychology* 2004 Apr;**18**(2):284–295.

36 Hornberger M, Piguet O, Graham AJ, Nestor PJ, Hodges JR. How preserved is episodic memory in behavioral variant frontotemporal dementia? *Neurology* 2010 Feb 9;**74**(6):472–479.

37 Pasquier F, Grymonprez L, Lebert F, Van der Linden M. Memory impairment differs in frontotemporal dementia and Alzheimer's disease. *Neurocase* 2001;**7**(2):161–171.

38 Kramer JH, Jurik J, Sha SJ, Rankin KP, Rosen HJ, Johnson JK, et al. Distinctive neuropsychological patterns in frontotemporal dementia, semantic dementia, and Alzheimer disease. *Cogn Behav Neurol* 2003 Dec;**16**(4):211–218.

39 Clinical and neuropathological criteria for frontotemporal dementia. The Lund and Manchester Groups. *J Neurol Neurosurg Psychiatry* 1994 Apr;**57**(4):416–418.

40 Neary D, Snowden JS, Gustafson L, Passant U, Stuss D, Black S, et al. Frontotemporal lobar degeneration: a consensus on clinical diagnostic criteria. *Neurology* 1998 Dec;**51**(6):1546–1554.

41 Rascovsky K, Hodges JR, Kipps CM, Johnson JK, Seeley WW, Mendez MF, et al. Diagnostic criteria for the behavioral variant of frontotemporal dementia (bvFTD): current limitations and future directions. *Alzheimer Dis Assoc Disord* 2007 Oct-Dec;**21**(4):S14–8.

42 Rascovsky K, Hodges JR, Knopman D, Mendez MF, Kramer JH, Neuhaus J, et al. Sensitivity of revised diagnostic criteria for the behavioral variant of frontotemporal dementia. *Brain* 2011 Aug 2; **134**(9):2456–2477.

43 Lamarre AK, Rascovsky K, Bostrom A, Toofanian P, Wilkins S, Sha SJ, et al. Interrater reliability of the new criteria for behavioral variant frontotemporal dementia. *Neurology* 2013 May 21;**80**(21): 1973–1977.

44 Mesulam MM. Primary progressive aphasia. *Ann Neurol* 2001 Apr;**49**(4):425–432.

45 Thompson SA, Patterson K, Hodges JR. Left/right asymmetry of atrophy in semantic dementia: behavioral-cognitive implications. *Neurology* 2003 Nov 11;**61**(9):1196–1203.

46 Snowden JS, Thompson JC, Neary D. Knowledge of famous faces and names in semantic dementia. *Brain* 2004 Apr 1;**127**(4):860–872.

47 Seeley WW, Bauer AM, Miller BL, Gorno-Tempini ML, Kramer JH, Weiner M, et al. The natural history of temporal variant frontotemporal dementia. *Neurology* 2005 Apr 26;**64**(8):1384–1390.

48 Rosen HJ, Gorno-Tempini ML, Goldman WP, Perry RJ, Schuff N, Weiner M, et al. Patterns of brain atrophy in frontotemporal dementia and semantic dementia. *Neurology* 2002 Jan 22;**58**(2):198–208.

49 Hodges JR, Patterson K, Ward R, Garrard P, Bak T, Perry R, et al. The differentiation of semantic dementia and frontal lobe dementia (temporal and frontal variants of frontotemporal dementia) from early Alzheimer's disease: a comparative neuropsychological study. *Neuropsychology* 1999 Jan;**13**(1):31–40.

50 Rosen HJ, Allison SC, Ogar JM, Amici S, Rose K, Dronkers N, et al. Behavioral features in semantic dementia vs other forms of progressive aphasias. *Neurology* 2006 Nov 28;**67**(10):1752–1756.

51 Gorno-Tempini ML, Dronkers NF, Rankin KP, Ogar JM, Phengrasamy L, Rosen HJ, et al. Cognition and anatomy in three variants of primary progressive aphasia. *Ann Neurol* 2004 Mar;**55**(3): 335–346.

52 Josephs KA, Duffy JR, Strand EA, Whitwell JL, Layton KF, Parisi JE, et al. Clinicopathological and imaging correlates of progressive aphasia and apraxia of speech. *Brain* 2006 Jun;**129**(Pt 6):1385–1398.

53 Gorno-Tempini ML, Hillis AE, Weintraub S, Kertesz A, Mendez M, Cappa SF, et al. Classification of primary progressive aphasia and its variants. *Neurology* 2011 Mar 15;**76**(11):1006–1014.

54 Lomen-Hoerth C, Anderson T, Miller B. The overlap of amyotrophic lateral sclerosis and frontotemporal dementia. *Neurology* 2002 Oct 8;**59**(7):1077–1079.

55 Chang JL, Lomen-Hoerth C, Murphy J, Henry RG, Kramer JH, Miller BL, et al. A voxel-based morphometry study of patterns of brain atrophy in ALS and ALS/FTLD. *Neurology* 2005 Jul 12;**65**(1):75–80.

56 Lillo P, Garcin B, Hornberger M, Bak TH, Hodges JR. Neurobehavioral features in frontotemporal dementia with amyotrophic lateral sclerosis. *Arch Neurol* 2010 Jul;**67**(7):826–830.

57 Whitwell JL, Jack CR, Jr, Senjem ML, Josephs KA. Patterns of atrophy in pathologically confirmed FTLD with and without motor neuron degeneration. *Neurology* 2006 Jan 10;**66**(1):102–104.

58 Murphy JM, Henry RG, Langmore S, Kramer JH, Miller BL, Lomen-Hoerth C. Continuum of frontal lobe impairment in amyotrophic lateral sclerosis. *Arch Neurol* 2007 April 1;**64**(4):530–534.

59 Lomen-Hoerth C, Murphy J, Langmore S, Kramer JH, Olney RK, Miller B. Are amyotrophic lateral sclerosis patients cognitively normal? *Neurology* 2003 Apr 8;**60**(7):1094–1097.

60 Rebeiz JJ, Kolodny EH, Richardson EP, Jr. Corticodentatonigral degeneration with neuronal achromasia. *Arch Neurol* 1968 Jan 1; **18**(1):20–33.

61 Gorno-Tempini ML, Murray RC, Rankin KP, Weiner MW, Miller BL. Clinical, cognitive and anatomical evolution from nonfluent progressive aphasia to corticobasal syndrome: a case report. *Neurocase* 2004 Dec;**10**(6):426–436.

62 Boeve BF, Maraganore DM, Parisi JE, Ahlskog JE, Graff-Radford N, Caselli RJ, et al. Pathologic heterogeneity in clinically diagnosed corticobasal degeneration. *Neurology* 1999 Sep 11;**53**(4):795–800.

63 Hu WT, Rippon GW, Boeve BF, Knopman DS, Petersen RC, Parisi JE, et al. Alzheimer's disease and corticobasal degeneration presenting as corticobasal syndrome. *Mov Disord* 2009 Jul 15;**24**(9):1375–1379.

64 Whitwell JL, Jack CR, Jr, Boeve BF, Parisi JE, Ahlskog JE, Drubach DA, et al. Imaging correlates of pathology in corticobasal syndrome. *Neurology* 2010 Nov 23;**75**(21):1879–1887.

65 Lee SE, Rabinovici GD, Mayo MC, Wilson SM, Seeley WW, DeArmond SJ, et al. Clinicopathological correlations in corticobasal degeneration. *Ann Neurol* 2011 Aug;**70**(2):327–40.

66 Brun A. Frontal lobe degeneration of non-Alzheimer type. I. *Neuropathol Arch Gerontol Geriatr* 1987 Sep;**6**(3):193–208.

67 Knopman DS, Mastri AR, Frey WH, 2nd, Sung JH, Rustan T. Dementia lacking distinctive histologic features: a common non-Alzheimer degenerative dementia. *Neurology* 1990 Feb;**40**(2):251–256.

68 Neumann M, Sampathu DM, Kwong LK, Truax AC, Micsenyi MC, Chou TT, et al. Ubiquitinated TDP-43 in frontotemporal lobar degeneration and amyotrophic lateral sclerosis. *Science* 2006 Oct 6;**314**(5796):130–133.

69 Snowden J, Neary D, Mann D. Frontotemporal lobar degeneration: clinical and pathological relationships. *Acta Neuropathol* 2007 Jul;**114**(1):31–38.

70 Urwin H, Josephs KA, Rohrer JD, Mackenzie IR, Neumann M, Authier A, et al. FUS pathology defines the majority of tau- and TDP-43-negative frontotemporal lobar degeneration. *Acta Neuropathol* 2010 Jul;**120**(1):33–41.

71 Weingarten MD, Lockwood AH, Hwo SY, Kirschner MW. A protein factor essential for microtubule assembly. *Proc Natl Acad Sci U S A* 1975 May;**72**(5):1858–1862.

72 Cairns NJ, Bigio EH, Mackenzie IR, Neumann M, Lee VM, Hatanpaa KJ, et al. Neuropathologic diagnostic and nosologic criteria for frontotemporal lobar degeneration: consensus of the consortium for frontotemporal lobar degeneration. *Acta Neuropathol* 2007 Jul;**114**(1):5–22.

73 Buratti E, Baralle FE. Multiple roles of TDP-43 in gene expression, splicing regulation, and human disease. *Front Biosci* 2008 Jan 1;**13**: 867–878.

74 Mackenzie IR, Neumann M, Baborie A, Sampathu DM, Du Plessis D, Jaros E, et al. A harmonized classification system for FTLD-TDP pathology. *Acta Neuropathol* 2011 Jul;**122**(1):111–113.

75 Sampathu DM, Neumann M, Kwong LK, Chou TT, Micsenyi M, Truax A, et al. Pathological heterogeneity of frontotemporal lobar degeneration with ubiquitin-positive inclusions delineated by ubiquitin immunohistochemistry and novel monoclonal antibodies. *Am J Pathol* 2006 Oct;**169**(4):1343–1352.

76 Mackenzie IR, Baborie A, Pickering-Brown S, Du Plessis D, Jaros E, Perry RH, et al. Heterogeneity of ubiquitin pathology in frontotemporal lobar degeneration: classification and relation to clinical phenotype. *Acta Neuropathol* 2006 Nov;**112**(5):539–549.

77 Mackenzie IRA, Bigio EH, Ince PG, Geser F, Neumann M, Cairns NJ, et al. Pathological TDP-43 distinguishes sporadic amyotrophic lateral sclerosis from amyotrophic lateral sclerosis with SOD1 mutations. *Ann Neurol* 2007;**61**(5):427–434.

78 Neumann M, Rademakers R, Roeber S, Baker M, Kretzschmar HA, Mackenzie IR. A new subtype of frontotemporal lobar degeneration with FUS pathology. *Brain* 2009 Nov;**132**(Pt 11):2922–2931.

79 Munoz DG, Neumann M, Kusaka H, Yokota O, Ishihara K, Terada S, et al. FUS pathology in basophilic inclusion body disease. *Acta Neuropathol* 2009 Nov;**118**(5):617–627.

80 Neumann M, Roeber S, Kretzschmar HA, Rademakers R, Baker M, Mackenzie IR. Abundant FUS-immunoreactive pathology in neuronal intermediate filament inclusion disease. *Acta Neuropathol* 2009 Nov;**118**(5):605–616.

81 Rohrer JD, Geser F, Zhou J, Gennatas ED, Sidhu M, Trojanowski JQ, et al. TDP-43 subtypes are associated with distinct atrophy patterns in frontotemporal dementia. *Neurology* 2010 Dec 14;**75**(24):2204–2211.

82 Davies RR, Hodges JR, Kril JJ, Patterson K, Halliday GM, Xuereb JH. The pathological basis of semantic dementia. *Brain* 2005 Sep;**128** (Pt 9):1984–1995.

83 Kertesz A, McMonagle P, Blair M, Davidson W, Munoz DG. The evolution and pathology of frontotemporal dementia. *Brain* 2005 Sep;**128**(Pt 9):1996–2005.

84 Josephs KA, Whitwell JL, Parisi JE, Petersen RC, Boeve BF, Jack CR, Jr, et al. Caudate atrophy on MRI is a characteristic feature of FTLD-FUS. *Eur J Neurol* 2010 Jul;**17**(7):969–975.

85 Forman MS, Farmer J, Johnson JK, Clark CM, Arnold SE, Coslett HB, et al. Frontotemporal dementia: clinicopathological correlations. *Ann Neurol* 2006;**59**(6):952–962.

86 Litvan I, Agid Y, Calne D, Campbell G, Dubois B, Duvoisin RC, et al. Clinical research criteria for the diagnosis of progressive supranuclear palsy (Steele-Richardson-Olszewski syndrome): report of the NINDS-SPSP international workshop. *Neurology* 1996 Jul;**47**(1):1–9.

87 Irwin DJ, Trojanowski JQ, Grossman M. Cerebrospinal fluid biomarkers for differentiation of frontotemporal lobar degeneration from Alzheimer's disease. *Front Aging Neurosci* 2013 Feb 21;**5**:6.

88 Rabinovici GD, Furst AJ, O'Neil JP, Racine CA, Mormino EC, Baker SL, et al. 11C-PIB PET imaging in Alzheimer disease and frontotemporal lobar degeneration. *Neurology* 2007 Apr 10; **68**(15):1205–1212.

89 Sanchez-Juan P, Ghosh PM, Hagen J, Gesierich B, Henry M, Grinberg LT, et al. Practical utility of amyloid and FDG-PET in an academic dementia center. *Neurology* 2014 Jan 21;**82**(3):230–238.

90 Hu WT, Chen-Plotkin A, Grossman M, Arnold SE, Clark CM, Shaw LM, et al. Novel CSF biomarkers for frontotemporal lobar degenerations. *Neurology* 2010 Dec 7;**75**(23):2079–2086.

91 Hu WT, Watts K, Grossman M, Glass J, Lah JJ, Hales C, et al. Reduced CSF p-Tau181 to Tau ratio is a biomarker for FTLD-TDP. *Neurology* 2013 Nov 26;**81**(22):1945–1952.

92 Coppola G, Karydas A, Rademakers R, Wang Q, Baker M, Hutton M, et al. Gene expression study on peripheral blood identifies progranulin mutations. *Ann Neurol* 2008 Jul;**64**(1):92–96.

93 Sleegers K, Brouwers N, Van Damme P, Engelborghs S, Gijselinck I, van der Zee J, et al. Serum biomarker for progranulin-associated frontotemporal lobar degeneration. *Ann Neurol* 2009 May;**65**(5): 603–609.

94 Ghidoni R, Benussi L, Glionna M, Franzoni M, Binetti G. Low plasma progranulin levels predict progranulin mutations in frontotemporal lobar degeneration. *Neurology* 2008 Oct 14; **71**(16):1235–1239.

95 Foulds P, McAuley E, Gibbons L, Davidson Y, Pickering-Brown SM, Neary D, et al. TDP-43 protein in plasma may index TDP-43 brain pathology in Alzheimer's disease and frontotemporal lobar degeneration. *Acta Neuropathol* 2008 Aug;**116**(2):141–146.

96 Scherling CS, Hall T, Berisha F, Klepac K, Karydas A, Coppola G, et al. Cerebrospinal fluid neurofilament concentration reflects disease severity in frontotemporal degeneration. *Ann Neurol* 2014 Jan;**75**(1):116–126.
97 Goldman JS, Farmer JM, Wood EM, Johnson JK, Boxer A, Neuhaus J, et al. Comparison of family histories in FTLD subtypes and related tauopathies. *Neurology* 2005 Dec 13;**65**(11):1817–1819.
98 Baker M, Litvan I, Houlden H, Adamson J, Dickson D, Perez-Tur J, et al. Association of an extended haplotype in the tau gene with progressive supranuclear palsy. *Hum Mol Genet* 1999 Apr;**8**(4): 711–715.
99 Houlden H, Baker M, Morris HR, MacDonald N, Pickering-Brown S, Adamson J, et al. Corticobasal degeneration and progressive supranuclear palsy share a common tau haplotype. *Neurology* 2001 Jun 26;**56**(12):1702–1706.
100 Seelaar H, Kamphorst W, Rosso SM, Azmani A, Masdjedi R, de Koning I, et al. Distinct genetic forms of frontotemporal dementia. *Neurology* 2008 Oct 14;**71**(16):1220–1226.
101 Whitwell JL, Jack CR, Jr, Boeve BF, Senjem ML, Baker M, Rademakers R, et al. Voxel-based morphometry patterns of atrophy in FTLD with mutations in MAPT or PGRN. *Neurology* 2009 Mar 3;**72**(9):813–820.
102 Whitwell JL, Jack CR, Jr, Boeve BF, Senjem ML, Baker M, Ivnik RJ, et al. Atrophy patterns in IVS10+16, IVS10+3, N279K, S305N, P301L, and V337M MAPT mutations. *Neurology* 2009 Sep 29;**73**(13):1058–1065.
103 Beck J, Rohrer JD, Campbell T, Isaacs A, Morrison KE, Goodall EF, et al. A distinct clinical, neuropsychological and radiological phenotype is associated with progranulin gene mutations in a large UK series. *Brain* 2008 March 01;**131**(3):706–720.
104 Ward ME, Miller BL. Potential mechanisms of progranulin-deficient FTLD. *J Mol Neurosci* 2011 Nov;**45**(3):574–582.
105 Perry DC, Lehmann M, Yokoyama JS, Karydas A, Lee JJ, Coppola G, et al. Progranulin mutations as risk factors for Alzheimer disease. *JAMA Neurol* 2013 Jun;**70**(6):774–778.
106 Gass J, Cannon A, Mackenzie IR, Boeve B, Baker M, Adamson J, et al. Mutations in progranulin are a major cause of ubiquitin-positive frontotemporal lobar degeneration. *Hum Mol Genet* 2006 Oct 15;**15**(20):2988–3001.
107 DeJesus-Hernandez M, Mackenzie I, Boeve B, Boxer A, Baker M, Rutherford N, et al. Expanded GGGGCC hexanucleotide repeat in noncoding region of C9ORF72 causes chromosome 9p-linked FTD and ALS. *Neuron* 2011 Oct 20;**72**(2):245–256.
108 Renton A, Majounie E, Waite A, Simón-Sánchez J, Rollinson S, Gibbs J, et al. A hexanucleotide repeat expansion in C9ORF72 is the cause of chromosome 9p21-linked ALS-FTD. *Neuron* 2011 Oct 20;**72**(2):257–268.
109 Simon-Sanchez J, Dopper EG, Cohn-Hokke PE, Hukema RK, Nicolaou N, Seelaar H, et al. The clinical and pathological phenotype of C9ORF72 hexanucleotide repeat expansions. *Brain* 2012 Mar;**135**(Pt 3):723–735.
110 Sha SJ, Takada LT, Rankin KP, Yokoyama JS, Rutherford NJ, Fong JC, et al. Frontotemporal dementia due to C9ORF72 mutations: clinical and imaging features. *Neurology* 2012 Sep 4;**79**(10): 1002–1011.
111 Snowden JS, Rollinson S, Thompson JC, Harris JM, Stopford CL, Richardson AM, et al. Distinct clinical and pathological characteristics of frontotemporal dementia associated with C9ORF72 mutations. *Brain* 2012 Mar;**135**(Pt 3):693–708.
112 Hsiung GY, Dejesus-Hernandez M, Feldman HH, Sengdy P, Bouchard-Kerr P, Dwosh E, et al. Clinical and pathological features of familial frontotemporal dementia caused by C9ORF72 mutation on chromosome 9p. *Brain* 2012 Mar;**135**(Pt 3):709–722.
113 Khan BK, Yokoyama JS, Takada LT, Sha SJ, Rutherford NJ, Fong JC, et al. Atypical, slowly progressive behavioral variant frontotemporal dementia associated with C9ORF72 hexanucleotide expansion. *J Neurol Neurosurg Psychiatry* 2012 Apr;**83**(4):358–364.
114 Al-Sarraj S, King A, Troakes C, Smith B, Maekawa S, Bodi I, et al. p62 positive, TDP-43 negative, neuronal cytoplasmic and intranuclear inclusions in the cerebellum and hippocampus define the pathology of C9orf72-linked FTLD and MND/ALS. *Acta Neuropathol* 2011 Dec;**122**(6):691–702.
115 Murray ME, DeJesus-Hernandez M, Rutherford NJ, Baker M, Duara R, Graff-Radford NR, et al. Clinical and neuropathologic heterogeneity of c9FTD/ALS associated with hexanucleotide repeat expansion in C9ORF72. *Acta Neuropathol* 2011 Dec;**122** (6):673–690.
116 Mori K, Weng SM, Arzberger T, May S, Rentzsch K, Kremmer E, et al. The C9orf72 GGGGCC repeat is translated into aggregating dipeptide-repeat proteins in FTLD/ALS. *Science* 2013 Mar 15;**339** (6125):1335–1338.
117 Mackenzie IR, Arzberger T, Kremmer E, Troost D, Lorenzl S, Mori K, et al. Dipeptide repeat protein pathology in C9ORF72 mutation cases: clinico-pathological correlations. *Acta Neuropathol* 2013 Dec;**126**(6):859–879.
118 Gydesen S, Brown JM, Brun A, Chakrabarti L, Gade A, Johannsen P, et al. Chromosome 3 linked frontotemporal dementia (FTD-3). *Neurology* 2002 Nov 26;**59**(10):1585–1594.
119 Johnson JO, Mandrioli J, Benatar M, Abramzon Y, Van Deerlin VM, Trojanowski JQ, et al. Exome sequencing reveals VCP mutations as a cause of familial ALS. *Neuron* 2010 Dec 9;**68** (5):857–864.
120 Borroni B, Ghezzi S, Agosti C, Archetti S, Fenoglio C, Galimberti D, et al. Preliminary evidence that VEGF genetic variability confers susceptibility to frontotemporal lobar degeneration. *Rejuvenation Res* 2008 Aug;**11**(4):773–780.
121 Rademakers R, Eriksen JL, Baker M, Robinson T, Ahmed Z, Lincoln SJ, et al. Common variation in the miR-659 binding-site of GRN is a major risk factor for TDP43-positive frontotemporal dementia. *Hum Mol Genet* 2008 Dec 1;**17**(23):3631–3642.
122 Ferrari R, Hernandez DG, Nalls MA, Rohrer JD, Ramasamy A, Kwok JB, et al. Frontotemporal dementia and its subtypes: a genome-wide association study. *Lancet Neurol* 2014 Jul;**13**(7): 686–699.
123 Van Deerlin VM, Sleiman PM, Martinez-Lage M, Chen-Plotkin A, Wang LS, Graff-Radford NR, et al. Common variants at 7p21 are associated with frontotemporal lobar degeneration with TDP-43 inclusions. *Nat Genet* 2010 Mar;**42**(3):234–239.
124 Veerappan CS, Sleiman S, Coppola G. Epigenetics of Alzheimer's disease and frontotemporal dementia. *Neurotherapeutics* 2013 Oct;**10**(4):709–721.
125 Mendez MF, Shapira JS, McMurtray A, Licht E. Preliminary findings: behavioral worsening on donepezil in patients with frontotemporal dementia. *Am J Geriatr Psychiatry* 2007 Jan; **15**(1):84–87.
126 Moretti R, Torre P, Antonello RM, Cattaruzza T, Cazzato G, Bava A. Rivastigmine in frontotemporal dementia: an open-label study. *Drugs Aging* 2004;**21**(14):931–937.

127 Kertesz A, Morlog D, Light M, Blair M, Davidson W, Jesso S, et al. Galantamine in frontotemporal dementia and primary progressive aphasia. *Dement Geriatr Cogn Disord* 2008;**25**(2):178–185.

128 Diehl-Schmid J, Forstl H, Perneczky R, Pohl C, Kurz A. A 6-month, open-label study of memantine in patients with frontotemporal dementia. *Int J Geriatr Psychiatry* 2008 Jul;**23**(7):754–759.

129 Boxer AL, Lipton AM, Womack K, Merrilees J, Neuhaus J, Pavlic D, et al. An open-label study of memantine treatment in 3 subtypes of frontotemporal lobar degeneration. *Alzheimer Dis Assoc Disord* 2009 Jul–Sep;**23**(3):211–217.

130 Vercelletto M, Boutoleau-Bretonniere C, Volteau C, Puel M, Auriacombe S, Sarazin M, et al. Memantine in behavioral variant frontotemporal dementia: negative results. *J Alzheimers Dis* 2011 Jan 1;**23**(4):749–759.

131 Boxer AL, Knopman DS, Kaufer DI, Grossman M, Onyike C, Graf-Radford N, et al. Memantine in patients with frontotemporal lobar degeneration: a multicentre, randomised, double-blind, placebo-controlled trial. *Lancet Neurol* 2013 Feb;**12**(2):149–156.

132 Swartz JR, Miller BL, Lesser IM, Darby AL. Frontotemporal dementia: treatment response to serotonin selective reuptake inhibitors. *J Clin Psychiatry* 1997 May;**58**(5):212–216.

133 Ikeda M, Shigenobu K, Fukuhara R, Hokoishi K, Maki N, Nebu A, et al. Efficacy of fluvoxamine as a treatment for behavioral symptoms in frontotemporal lobar degeneration patients. *Dement Geriatr Cogn Disord* 2004;**17**(3):117–121.

134 Moretti R, Torre P, Antonello RM, Cazzato G, Bava A. Frontotemporal dementia: paroxetine as a possible treatment of behavior symptoms. A randomized, controlled, open 14-month study. *Eur Neurol* 2003;**49**(1):13–19.

135 Deakin JB, Rahman S, Nestor PJ, Hodges JR, Sahakian BJ. Paroxetine does not improve symptoms and impairs cognition in frontotemporal dementia: a double-blind randomized controlled trial. *Psychopharmacology (Berl)* 2004 Apr;**172**(4):400–408.

136 Lebert F, Stekke W, Hasenbroekx C, Pasquier F. Frontotemporal dementia: a randomised, controlled trial with trazodone. *Dement Geriatr Cogn Disord* 2004;**17**(4):355–359.

137 Moretti R, Torre P, Antonello RM, Cazzato G, Griggio S, Bava A. Olanzapine as a treatment of neuropsychiatric disorders of Alzheimer's disease and other dementias: a 24-month follow-up of 68 patients. *Am J Alzheimers Dis Other Demen* 2003 Jul–Aug;**18**(4): 205–214.

138 Fellgiebel A, Muller MJ, Hiemke C, Bartenstein P, Schreckenberger M. Clinical improvement in a case of frontotemporal dementia under aripiprazole treatment corresponds to partial recovery of disturbed frontal glucose metabolism. *World J Biol Psychiatry* 2007;**8**(2):123–126.

139 Curtis RC, Resch DS. Case of pick's central lobar atrophy with apparent stabilization of cognitive decline after treatment with risperidone. *J Clin Psychopharmacol* 2000 Jun;**20**(3): 384–385.

140 Boxer AL, Lang AE, Grossman M, Knopman DS, Miller BL, Schneider LS, et al. Davunetide in patients with progressive supranuclear palsy: a randomised, double-blind, placebo-controlled phase 2/3 trial. *Lancet Neurol* 2014;**13**(7):676–685.

CHAPTER 6

Lewy body dementias (DLB/PDD)

Carol F. Lippa[1] and Katherine L. Possin[2]

[1] Drexel University College of Medicine, Philadelphia, PA, USA
[2] University of California, San Francisco, San Francisco, CA, USA

Introduction

Dementia is characterized by cognitive impairment severe enough to interfere with daily functioning [1]. Alzheimer's disease (AD) is the most common dementia subtype, accounting for more than half of all dementia cases. In AD, memory loss is the most significant aspect of cognitive impairment [2]. Dementia with Lewy bodies (DLB) is probably the second most common dementia, affecting nearly one-quarter of dementia subjects. In contrast to AD, core diagnostic criteria of DLB include visual hallucinations, parkinsonism, and fluctuations of attention and alertness (see Table 6.1). These symptoms are rare in cognitively normal elderly individuals and early AD patients [4]. Other features in DLB include rapid eye movement (REM) sleep behavior disorder (RBD), other sleep dysfunctions, syncope, transient impairment in consciousness, delusions, depression, and early incontinence [5–7]. The diagnosis of DLB is important to make because treatment specifics differ from those used in other dementias. For example, DLB patients are more susceptible to neuroleptic hypersensitivity than AD patients [8].

Patients with Parkinson's disease (PD) often develop cognitive decline and up to 80% will progress to dementia (Parkinson's disease with dementia (PDD), [4]). PDD differs from DLB in the temporal sequence of initial symptoms, but with progression, the syndromes and pathology become similar. Both involve progressive cognitive decline involving visuospatial, attentional, and executive functions. Psychiatric disturbances include visual hallucinations, anxiety, apathy, and depression. The motor symptoms are similar in PDD and DLB, and both have more axial symptoms, postural instability, and gait difficulty than nondemented PD [9]. Both are characterized pathologically by intracytoplasmic inclusions containing ubiquitin and alpha-synuclein called Lewy bodies (LBs). PDD and DLB brains have a loss of the neurotransmitters acetylcholine and dopamine [10].

Nosology

Historical issues/nomenclature

PD was first profiled in 1817 by James Parkinson in "An Essay on the Shaking Palsy." He described the classic motor symptoms of PD but reported "the senses and intellects being uninjured" [11]. It is now increasingly recognized, however, that many patients newly diagnosed with PD have cognitive impairment associated with their disease and that many of these patients will go on to develop a dementia syndrome.

The initial autopsy descriptions of patients with DLB were written by Dr. Okazaki [12]. They described patients with progressive dementia but without the motor symptoms of PD whose brains had cortical LBs. This was followed by detailed clinicopathologic descriptions of DLB cases by Kenji Kosaka [13] who reviewed all available literature cases and noted a characteristic clinical syndrome. Since the original descriptions, immunohistochemistry with antibodies to components of LBs (antiubiquitin and anti-alpha-synuclein antibodies) has made diagnosis easier, and we now realize that DLB is a common disorder. In 1996, McKeith et al. established the first consensus criteria for DLB and formalized the term "dementia with Lewy bodies."

The discoveries of α-synuclein mutations in families with autosomal dominant PD [14] and of α-synuclein as the main component of LBs [15] linked PDD and DLB from a biologic standpoint. The DLB/PDD Working Group recommended the use of a single term and model "Lewy body disorders" (LBD), encompassing these two syndromes and nondemented PD, to study disease pathogenesis, new treatments, and biomarkers [16].

Multiple system atrophy (MSA) is a rare neurodegenerative disorder that, as with DLB and PDD, is related to a disturbance of alpha-synuclein, although, in MSA, inclusions are within glial

Non-Alzheimer's and Atypical Dementia, First Edition. Edited by Michael D. Geschwind and Caroline Racine Belkoura.
© 2016 John Wiley & Sons, Ltd. Published 2016 by John Wiley & Sons, Ltd.

Table 6.1 Comparison of DLB and PDD.

DLB	PDD
Central feature Dementia: progressive cognitive decline that interferes with social or occupational function. Prominent or persistent memory impairment may not be an early feature but is usually evident with progression. Prominent deficits on tests of attention, executive function, and visuospatial ability **Core features** (two sufficient for probable, one for possible) Fluctuating cognition with variations in attention and alertness Recurrent visual hallucinations Spontaneous parkinsonism	**Core features** (both must be present for probable diagnosis) 1. Diagnosis of PD according to Queen Square Brain Bank criteria 2. Dementia Insidious onset and slow progression, developing after established PD Impairment in more than one cognitive domain Decline from the premorbid level Deficits severe enough to impair daily life independent of impairment ascribable to the motor or autonomic symptoms of PD
Suggestive features (one or more + in presence of one or more core features sufficient for probable; one or more but without any core features sufficient for possible) REM sleep behavior disorder Severe neuroleptic sensitivity Low dopamine transporter uptake in the basal ganglia (SPECT and PET imaging) **Supportive features (commonly present, but no diagnostic specificity)** Repeated falls and syncope Transient loss of consciousness Severe autonomic dysfunction Hallucinations in other modalities Systematized delusions Depression Relative preservation of medial temporal lobe volume on CT/MRI Generalized low uptake on SPECT/PET perfusion scan with reduced occipital activity Abnormal (low uptake) MIBG myocardial scintigraphy Prominent slow-wave activity on EEG with temporal lobe transient sharp waves	**Associated clinical features** 1. Cognitive features: Attention: impairment in spontaneous and focused attention, performance may fluctuate Executive functions: impairment in tasks requiring initiation, planning, concept formation, rule-finding, set shifting, or set maintenance; impaired mental speed (bradyphrenia) Visuospatial function: impairment in tasks requiring visuospatial orientation, perception, or construction Memory: impairment in free recall of recent events or in tasks requiring learning; memory usually improves with cueing; recognition is usually better than free recall Language: core functions preserved 2. Behavioral features: Apathy Changes in personality and mood Hallucinations: mostly visual, formed visions of people and animals Delusions: usually paranoid or phantom boarder Excessive daytime sleepiness
Less likely if Cerebrovascular disease (focal neurologic signs or on brain imaging) Other physical illnesses or brain disorders sufficient to account for part or total of the clinical picture Parkinsonism appears only in severe dementia	**Less likely if (don't exclude but diagnosis uncertain)** Coexistence of any other abnormalities which may cause cognitive impairment, but judged not to be the cause of dementia, for example, presence of relevant vascular disease in imaging Time interval between the development of motor and cognitive symptoms is not known **Features suggesting other conditions (impossible to reliably diagnose PDD)** Cognitive and behavioral symptoms appearing solely in the context of other conditions including systemic diseases or drug intoxication or major depression Features compatible with "probable vascular dementia" criteria according to NINDS-AIREN criteria

Adapted from McKeith [3] and Emre [4].

cells, rather than neurons. An in-depth description of MSA is outside the scope of this chapter; however, the syndrome is characterized by a combination of autonomic, parkinsonian, and cerebellar features. When parkinsonian features predominate, the term MSA-P is used; when cerebellar features predominate, the term MSA-C is used. Dementia is infrequent and in fact is listed as a nonsupportive feature in current consensus criteria [17]. Less severe cognitive impairment is common in MSA, however, and might be intermediate in severity to that of DLB and PD patients of similar disease duration [18].

Epidemiology

Approximately 1% of the population over 60 years old suffers from PD, increasing to 4% in older age groups, with slightly higher prevalence in men than women [19, 20]. Approximately 30% of PD patients are estimated to have dementia, which is four to six times higher than controls [21]. Longitudinal PD cohort studies suggest up to 80% of PD patients exhibit dementia before death [22]. About 15–20% of dementia cases involve DLB, whereas approximately 6% are due to PDD [23]. Monogenetic forms of LB disorders represent less than 10% of LBD cases; the majority of cases result from interactions among susceptibility genes and environmental risk factors [24]. A recent case–control study looking at 19 risk factors in 147 DLB subjects compared with cognitively normal controls, as well as an AD cohort, found that compared to controls, DLB subjects were more liked to have depression, history of anxiety, and a family history of PD and to carry ApoE4 alleles, but were less likely to have cancer or use caffeine. Compared to AD subjects, DLB subjects were more likely to be male, about 2 years younger (72.5 vs. 74.9), highly educated, have a family history of PD, have no ApoE4 alleles, and have had an oophorectomy before age 45 [25].

Case study

A 74-year-old gentleman without significant past medical history was referred for neurological consultation for a 2-year history of difficulties concentrating. He lost track of conversations, had trouble reading, and had problems getting lost. His general intellect was intact; he reported no memory loss and had no difficulties with specific activities but felt he was less productive. Irritability was his only behavioral symptom. He was on no medications. Family history was notable only for a brother with PD who had a L-DOPA-responsive tremor.

General physical examination was normal. Neurological examination disclosed an alert, pleasant patient. His Mini-Mental State Examination [26] (MMSE) score was 25/30, losing 1 point for recall, 3 points for spelling WORLD backward, and 1 point for copying the pentagons. Language skills and comprehension were intact, but he had problems with attentional tasks. Cranial nerve, motor, and gait examination was normal, with the exception of an abnormal glabellar response. Head CT and blood work for reversible causes of dementia was normal. An atypical presentation of early stage of AD was suspected, and an annual follow-up was recommended.

One year later, he had decreased activities of daily living, sometimes requiring help in cutting his food, needing his clothes laid out for him, occasionally putting on a garment backward or inside out, and often shaving incompletely. He was occasionally visually disoriented at home and had more difficulty with routine tasks such as shoveling snow and piling it in illogical places. Once, he walked the dog but returned home without him. He slept more and took daytime naps. Behaviorally, he was mildly depressed, was quieter, and was having well-formed, usually visual and occasionally threatening hallucinations typically involving people from his past. He imagined that his (deceased) brother was living with them and insisted on making plans for him to have a bedroom. He stumbled and his gait was slower. He was alert but looked "a little lost." Vital signs, including orthostatics, and general physical examination remained normal. Neurologically, he was pleasant and cooperative but hypophonic. His MMSE was 15/30, losing 5 points on orientation—1 for registration, 1 for delayed recall, 5 for spelling the WORLD backward, 1 for a 3-step command, 1 for copying the pentagons, and 1 for repetition. Most language skills and comprehension were intact. Cranial nerve examination was remarkable only for a mild restriction in upgaze. Motor examination revealed normal strength, bulk but increased muscle tone with mild cogwheel rigidity, and symmetrically brisk reflexes. There was no resting tremor, but a slight postural tremor. Gait testing revealed a mildly stooped posture, shuffling, and reduced stride length. Plantar responses were flexor, but marked frontal release signs developed including a suck, snout, and palmomental responses as well as bilateral grasp reflexes. Sensory examination was intact to primary and cortical sensory modalities. He was diagnosed with an extrapyramidal dementia of unclear etiology.

He progressed gradually and died 2 years later, 5 years after onset. His brain weight was normal (1330 grams) and showed no focal atrophy with normal ventricle size. The substantia nigra and locus ceruleus were depigmented. LBs were frequent including the amygdala and the adjacent entorhinal cortex/parahippocampal gyrus and were also present in the cingulate gyrus and lower layers of the frontal, temporal, and parietal lobe cortex. The substantia nigra and locus ceruleus showed neuronal loss and LBs in some remaining neurons. There were no neurofibrillary tangles (NFTs), but numerous diffuse amyloid plaques were scattered in the cerebral cortex, and moderate amyloid angiopathy was seen. Although there was some Alzheimer's pathology, as he did not have NFTs, he did not meet NIA-Reagan or CERAD criteria for AD [27]. His final pathological diagnosis was DLB.

DLB/PDD clinical features

Diagnostic criteria

Diagnostic criteria specific for dementia associated with PD (PDD) were proposed in 2007 by the Movement Disorder Society Task Force [4]. Diagnosis of PDD requires a dementia syndrome with insidious onset and slow progression, developing with the context of established PD (Table 6.1). The dementia must involve a decline in multiple cognitive domains severe enough to impair daily life. A probable diagnosis requires impairment in at least two of the following: attention, executive functions, visuospatial functions, or memory retrieval. Behavioral features including apathy, changes in personality and mood including depression or anxiety, hallucinations, delusions, or excessive daytime sleepiness support the diagnosis.

Diagnostic criteria for DLB were proposed in 1996 [28] and refined in 2005 [3] by the DLB Consortium (Table 6.2).

Table 6.2 Bedside tests to evaluate cognitive features in PDD/DLB.

Attention: serial 7 s, months, or days backward
Memory: learning a word list with delayed free recall, recall versus recognition
Executive functions: verbal fluency, trail making, clock drawing
Visuospatial functions: copying intersecting pentagons or a three-dimensional cube
Language: confrontation naming, understanding complex sentences

According to the original criteria, probable DLB is characterized by dementia associated with any two of the following three core features: (i) fluctuating cognition or level of consciousness, (ii) visual hallucinations, and (iii) spontaneous parkinsonian motor signs. The refined criteria include suggestive features: RBD, neuroleptic sensitivity, and low dopamine transporter uptake in the basal ganglia demonstrated by SPECT or PET imaging. Probable DLB can also be diagnosed if one or more of these suggestive features are present along with one or more core features. The new recommendations contain provisions for a probabilistic basis for the pathologic diagnosis of DLB based on the predominance of cortical and limbic LBs relative to the density of neurofibrillary tangles. Cases with LBs in the setting of extensive AD-type pathology are classified as having a "low likelihood" of DLB.

Neurological exam and motor features

Motor signs in DLB and PDD include the classic triad of akinesia, rigidity, and tremor, which might be responsive to dopamine replacement, and axial symptoms, which are considered less responsive [4]. Extrapyramidal motor symptoms are present in about half of DLB patients at presentation, and they eventually occur in most of the remaining patients [29]. In comparison to PD, in DLB, there usually is more axial rigidity and postural instability. Gait is disrupted earlier in DLB than PD, and falls are not uncommon. Although resting tremor is a common presenting symptom in PD, DLB patients more typically have an intention or position tremor, if present at all. Their rigidity might lack the classical cogwheel quality that is the hallmark of PD. The gait of DLB patients is similar to PD/PDD and includes postural instability, a stooped posture, and festination [9]. Deep tendon reflexes are generally symmetrical in DLB, and frontal release signs might include palmomental responses and a glabellar response.

In PDD, patients often present with asymmetrical resting tremor and other classical features of PD including cogwheel rigidity. Postural instability and gait disorder is associated with accelerated cognitive decline and subsequent dementia, whereas patients with tremor less commonly develop early dementia [30].

Clinical assessment of motor dysfunction is difficult when dementia is severe; however, a subscale of the Unified PD Rating Scale [31] contains five items (resting tremor, action tremor, bradykinesia, loss of facial expression, and rigidity) that can be reliably assessed independent of dementia severity.

Cognitive features

The neuropsychological phenotype of both DLB and PDD is characterized by impairments in visuospatial and executive functions and also by fluctuations in attention and arousal, with core language functions relatively preserved [32–34]. When matched for dementia severity, the cognitive profiles of PDD and DLB are similar or indistinguishable [35, 36], although some studies suggest greater attentional impairment in DLB [37]. In comparison to AD, LB dementia patients show worse visuospatial, attentional, and executive impairments, whereas AD patients show more severe memory impairment [38]. An absence of visuospatial impairment early in the course of dementia is unusual in LBD and suggests a different etiology [39]. Figure 6.1 presents an example of figure copy performance in DLB that illustrates visuospatial impairment.

PD patients do not evidence dementia at onset; there is, however, increasing recognition that milder cognitive impairment is

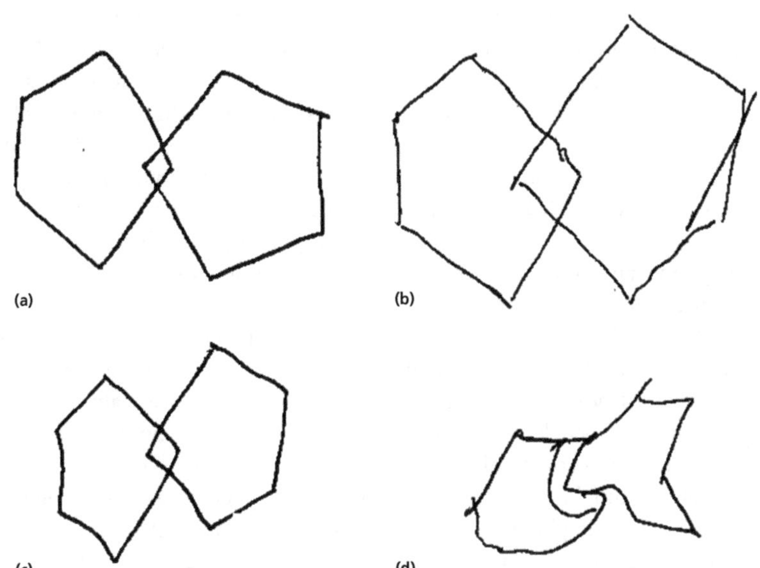

Figure 6.1 Patients were asked to copy the image exactly. Image **(a)** is the original figure that patients were asked to copy. Image **(b)** is the reproduced image from an 80-year-old patient with Alzheimer's disease. Note that the patient struggles with reproducing one of the pentagons but the spatial aspects of the figure are easily identifiable. Image **(c)** is from a cognitively intact 82-year-old elderly individual. Image **(d)** shows an attempt by an 80-year-old patient with probable DLB; although cognitive symptoms were mild, he is unable to reproduce the spatial aspects of the figures.

common [40]. Working memory, selective attention, inhibitory processing, cognitive flexibility, and learning are often impacted early and attributed primarily to nigrostriatal dopamine loss causing disruption of frontal-striatal circuitry function [41], although depletion in noradrenergic and cholinergic neurotransmitter systems have also been implicated [42, 43]. The emergence of impairment on tasks with a more posterior cortical basis (figure copy or semantic fluency) might signal the transition of the disease from the brainstem to the neocortex and indicate that progression to dementia is likely [44].

Bedside cognitive testing is useful to gauge the severity of cognitive impairment and its response to cholinesterase inhibitors, to diagnose cognitive impairment in PD, and to differentiate DLB from other diseases. The MMSE [26] is not sensitive to LBD because it emphasizes language and memory over executive function and visuospatial skills [45]. The Montreal Cognitive Assessment (MoCA; www.mocatest.org) is more sensitive to LBD; the recommended cutoff for dementia in PD is 20/30 [46]. Suggested methods for brief assessment are listed in Table 6.2. Patients exhibiting cognitive impairment on a brief exam might require more detailed neurocognitive testing.

Neuropsychiatric features

Neuropsychiatric disturbances are common in LBD and contribute to reduced quality of life [47], caregiver distress [48], and increased risk for nursing home admission [49]. In a study of 537 patients with PDD using the Neuropsychiatric Inventory (NPI), the most common symptoms were depression (58%), apathy (54%), anxiety (49%), and hallucinations (44%).

Depression is more common in LB dementias than in AD [50] and equally common in PD, PDD, and DLB [5]. Depression is listed as a supportive feature in DLB criteria [3]. Anxiety often predates PD by many years [51]. Panic disorder, generalized anxiety disorder, and social phobia are prevalent, and depression is often comorbid [52]. Apathy is common in PD and DLB and is associated with cognitive decline [53, 54]. The pathophysiology of depression, anxiety, and apathy in LB dementia might involve reductions in dopamine, noradrenaline, and serotonin [55–58], and depression has been associated with LBs in the amygdala [59].

Although depression, anxiety, and apathy are frequent in other dementias, visual hallucinations are more specific to LBD [60]. Hallucinations occur in 45–65% of PD and 60–80% of DLB patients, with much lower rates in early AD (4–8%) [4]. In patients with PDD or DLB and hallucinations, most experienced daily complex hallucinations (i.e., people or animals) [61]. Auditory and tactile hallucinations less commonly occur. Hallucinations in DLB are associated with LBs in the temporal cortex [62] and with hypoperfusion on single-photon emission tomography in the left ventral occipital gyrus and bilateral parietal areas [63]. Hallucinations are associated with cholinergic deficits [64] and often respond to cholinesterase inhibitors.

Delusions are also common in LB dementia. Capgras syndrome, for example, is characterized by the delusional belief that a person, usually someone who is closely related, has been replaced by an imposter. For example, a patient might say "she looks like my wife, but she is not my wife." When occurring early, Capgras syndrome is suggestive of LB dementia; however, it also occurs in late-stage AD. In a study of 47 patients with Capgras syndrome, 38 were clinically diagnosed with a neurodegenerative disease, and of those, 26 had LBD, whereas only 7 had AD (only two subjects were pathology proven, however) [65].

Preclinical symptoms

Recognition of premotor and predementia phases of LBD, which might span 20 years or more, is guiding the search for predictive biomarkers as well as risk factors. RBD is a common early feature of synucleinopathies and has been estimated to precede PD and DLB by a decade on average [66–68], with some patients showing clear RBD up to 50 years before LBD has clinically manifested [69]. Infrequent bowel movements were associated with the development of PD, with a mean 10-year latency [70], and in a large aging cohort without PD or dementia, infrequent bowel movements were associated with a fourfold risk of incidental LBs at autopsy [71]. Psychiatric symptoms (especially anxiety) might also predate PD [51, 72, 73]. High scores on the composite neuroticism scale of the Minnesota Multiphasic Personality Inventory also predict PD even when administered at ages 20–39 years [73].

Comorbidities

Parasomnias help to distinguish DLB/PDD from nonsynucleinopathies. The most striking is RBD, in which patients act out dreams during REM sleep. Loss of muscle atonia during REM sleep leads to violent vocalizations and thrashing. Individuals diagnosed with RBD have been estimated to have a 41% risk of developing a neurodegenerative disease in 10 years [68], and the presence of RBD in a patient with suspected neurodegenerative disease supports the diagnosis of a synucleinopathy [66]. Considering its specificity for LBD, physicians should be encouraged to ask about RBD during the initial history taking in any dementia patient [74]. Diagnosis can be confirmed by polysomnography [75]. Other sleep disorders in DLB, PDD, and PD include insomnia, sleep apnea, excessive daytime fatigue, and restless legs syndrome [76]. Treating these disorders can improve quality of life. Clonazepam or melatonin at bedtime is often used as first-line treatment [77].

Another supportive feature of DLB that is uncommon in other dementias is neuroleptic hypersensitivity, which involves an acute worsening of rigidity, psychosis, confusion, and impaired consciousness, following neuroleptic use [8, 78]. This occurs in DLB and PDD and might be life threatening.

Other comorbidities suggestive of DLB/PDD include autonomic symptoms such as orthostatic hypotension, constipation, incontinence, and impotence, which are less common in early AD. Falls, syncope, and transient losses of consciousness also occur.

Atypical presentations

When patients present with classical features of LBD, diagnostic specificity is high. Unfortunately, atypical presentations are common [79, 80]. Concurrent pathology (especially neurofibrillary tangles) impacts the symptoms and signs, leading to an amnestic/Alzheimer-like phenotype. The more plentiful the tau pathology in DLB, the more clinical features mimic AD [81]. The issue of overlap pathology is challenging but needs to be dealt with as over 75% of DLB patients have concurrent pathology. Vascular pathology is common in LBD and might contribute to cognitive decline and the severity of motor symptoms [82, 83]. Lastly, in advanced disease, the clinical (cognitive and motor) features of all dementias merge, and diagnosis is almost impossible based on physical examination [84].

Differential diagnosis

Differentiation of DLB from PDD is made on temporal information alone (i.e., cognitive decline within 1 year of motor symptoms is called DLB, otherwise PDD); however, no biologically defined differences reliably differentiate these conditions, and treatment is similar.

When cognitive symptoms predominate, differentiation from AD is important. Early memory loss is milder early in the course of DLB and PDD. Attention and alertness fluctuate frequently in DLB, and family members might note that the patient's cognition fluctuates significantly both within and across days, often irrespective of medications or environment, while in AD, cognitive impairment tends to be more chronic and exacerbated under conditions of increased cognitive demand. Daytime drowsiness, excessive daytime naps, prolonged staring into space, and disorganized speech are also more suggestive of DLB than AD [85].

Employment of standardized criteria for DLB, PDD, and other degenerative conditions will help the physician exclude other dementia diagnoses (Tables 6.1 and 6.3), including progressive supranuclear palsy, MSA, Creutzfeldt–Jakob disease, and corticobasal syndrome (CBS). Patients with cerebrovascular disease often have extrapyramidal features when ischemic changes involve subcortical regions. Medication effects, tumors, and normal pressure hydrocephalus also might mimic LBD. When the diagnosis remains unclear, functional imaging or cerebrospinal fluid (CSF) studies (for beta-amyloid and tau for AD diagnosis) might be of benefit.

Table 6.3 Differential diagnosis of DLB/PDD.

Etiology	Distinguishing features
Degenerative	
Progressive supranuclear palsy	Gait disorder with postural instability; often presents with falls; supranuclear gaze palsy (vertical), poor bulbar control
Corticobasal syndrome	Alien limb phenomenon, limb apraxia, complex tremor, cortical sensory loss, dystonic features, myoclonus, aphasia
Multiple system atrophy	Early autonomic dysfunction; ataxia; cerebellar signs; early speech changes and falls; usually minimal to response to levodopa, and if there is response, it is not sustained
Frontotemporal dementia with parkinsonism	Often early onset; sometimes autosomal dominant inheritance; cognitive profile might show progressive aphasia and deterioration of demeanor in addition to attentional and executive losses
Prion diseases	Rapid progression with dementia and ataxia; DWI/ADC brain MRI with cortical ribboning and/or hyperintense deep nuclei
Secondary parkinsonian syndromes	
Vascular parkinsonism	Abrupt onset, stepwise progression (but don't often occur); vascular risk factors; subcortical infarcts or white matter lesions on MRI, particularly in the brainstem
Normal pressure hydrocephalus	Classically triad of cognitive impairment, gait apraxia, and urinary incontinence; subacute onset; should have risk factors for hydrocephalus (e.g., prior head trauma, CNS infection or bleed); CT or MRI show enlarged ventricles (out of proportion to cortical tissue loss), transependymal CSF flow
Drug/medication induced	Relevant drug exposure (e.g., dopamine receptor blockers, reserpine, lithium, tetrabenazine, MPTP, carbon monoxide, manganese, mercury, others); often symmetrical, may improve when exposure is eliminated
Infectious	Postencephalitic parkinsonism, neurocysticercosis, syphilis, HIV encephalitis, Whipple's disease
Structural brain lesions (tumor, trauma)	Focal symptoms and signs; abnormal neuroimaging studies

Neuroimaging findings

Structural neuroimaging can rule out other diagnoses, but gross structural brain changes in DLB, PD and PDD are nonspecific, so they are of limited diagnostic use [86]. Greater atrophy in the medial temporal lobe occurs in AD [87], whereas putaminal atrophy is sometimes useful to support DLB versus AD [88].

Presynaptic dopaminergic terminal loss is present in LBD, so functional dopamine transporter imaging often helps distinguish DLB from dementias where the nigrostriatal system remains intact [89]; however, it cannot distinguish DLB from vascular dementia, MSA, and progressive supranuclear palsy because the nigrostriatal tracts might be disrupted.

Laboratory findings

At present, there is no blood, CSF, or urine test that can establish the diagnosis of DLB or PDD. Routine blood work to assess the patient for B12 deficiency, neurosyphilis, vasculitis, endocrine dysfunction, vitamin deficiency, and organ failure should be done on all patients to rule out medical conditions that cause problems with movement or cognition. Vascular risk factors should be reviewed, and effort should be made to maximize medical management of all vascular risks. CSF studies for beta-amyloid and tau might help establish a diagnosis of AD and predict cognitive decline in patients with PD [90], but CSF alpha-synuclein assessments are not currently commercially available.

Pathophysiology and pathology

Neuropathology

The pathological inclusion diagnostic of DLB and PDD is the LB (see Figure 6.2). LBs are round, cytoplasmic inclusions. Nigral LBs, present in all LB disorders, have a distinctive clear halo. Cortical LBs are present in limbic and/or neocortical regions in DLB and are often observed in smaller numbers in PD and PDD. They might compress the nuclei; however, they lack the halo of nigral LBs, and so diagnosis requires a keen, experienced eye. Immunohistochemical stains to ubiquitin and alpha-synuclein facilitate diagnosis.

Both nigral and cortical LBs are composed of filamentous forms of alpha-synuclein and ubiquitin fibers. In the substantia nigra, the halo consists of alpha-synuclein, and the core is composed of other neurofilaments. Cortical LBs stain diffusely for alpha-synuclein and ubiquitin. In addition, thinner, elongate alpha-synuclein aggregates occur in presynaptic terminals (Lewy neurites). Lewy neurites are coupled with the loss of the corresponding (postsynaptic dendritic) spines [91]. The composition of alpha-synuclein epitopes in LBs and Lewy neurites are indistinguishable in DLB and PDD [92].

The regional distribution of LBs differs between PDD and DLB with greater nigral neuronal loss in PDD than DLB and more alpha-synuclein pathology in the striatum and cortex in DLB [93]. Although LB burden is only a weak correlate of disease severity [94, 95], the regional distribution of pathology might influence neurological features.

Beta-amyloid plaques are evident in most DLB patients [96, 97]. In PDD, neocortical plaques are less common and most

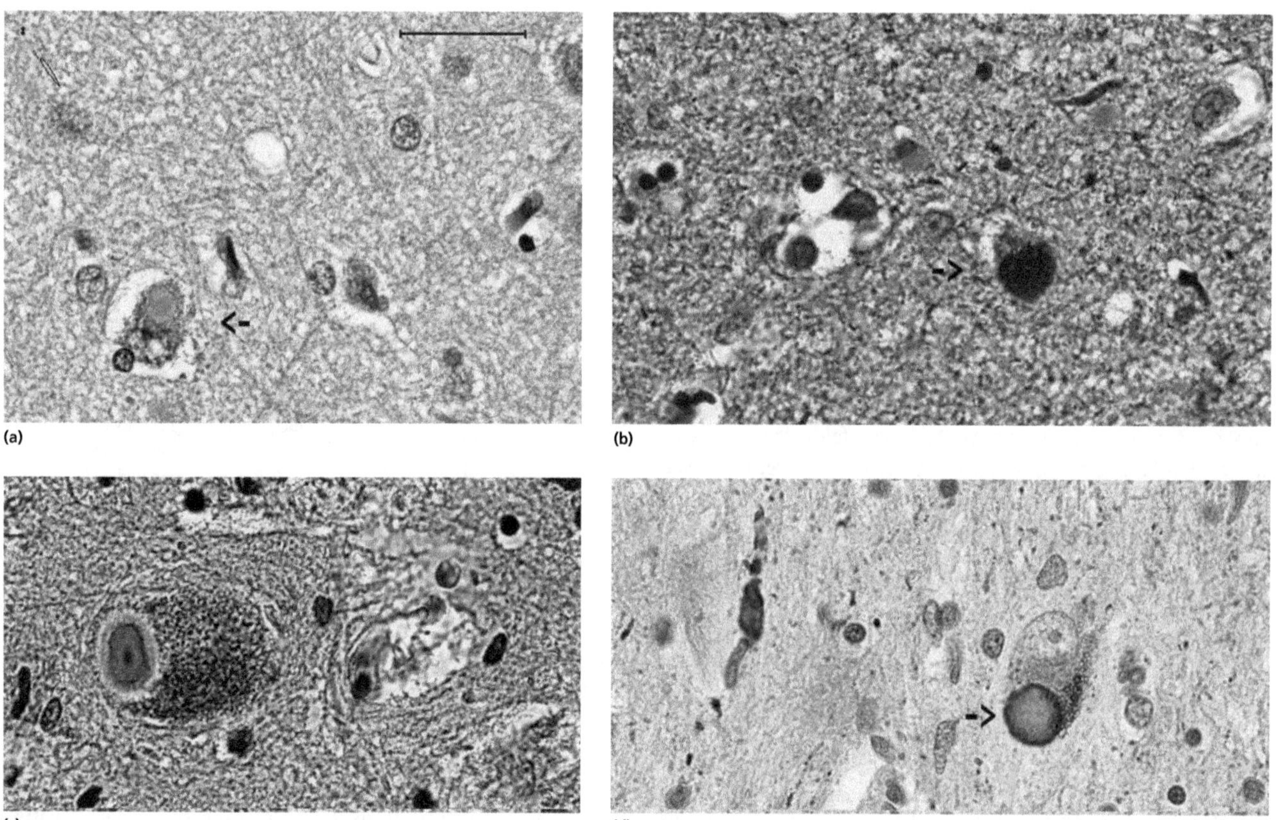

Figure 6.2 High magnification neuropathology from a DLB case. Cortical **(a)** and nigral **(c)** LBs after staining with hematoxylin and eosin. Note that cortical LBs are smaller and lack the halo that typifies LBs within the substantia nigra. Images **(b)** and **(d)** are taken after immunostaining DLB tissue with antibodies against alpha-synuclein. Cortical **(b)** and nigral LBs **(d)** both stand out. The entire inclusion stains in the cortex, but only the halo in the substantia nigra contains alpha-synuclein. Arrows point to the LBs in all images. All images at 60× magnification. Scale bar is 30 μm. (*See insert for color representation of the figure.*)

often seen in those with early dementia [95]. The greater the neuritic pathology, the more the DLB patient resembles AD clinically [81]. Additionally, beta-amyloid plaques and tau aggregates are associated with LB formation in the amygdala [98].

Pathology of case 1

The pathology of case 1 demonstrates some of the points described earlier. Case 1 had pure DLB and a normal brain size with no atrophy of the hippocampus, parahippocampal gyrus, amygdala, or cortex. Brain size and medial temporal lobe structures might be normal in DLB. The more severe the AD pathology, the smaller the volume of the hippocampal complex [99]. Although the number of LBs correlates poorly with the degree of dementia [100], the occurrence of widespread LBs differentiates LBD from the other dementia subtypes. Those with nigral, limbic, or neocortical LBs are more likely to have symptoms referable to motor, behavioral/psychiatric, or cognitive issues, respectively. Case 1 had symptoms related to all three spheres and had LBs in neocortical, limbic, and nigral areas. Cortical LBs account for his disorganization and executive dysfunction (frontal) and visuospatial impairment (temporo- and parieto-occipital). The visual hallucinations correspond to his LBs in lateral/posterior temporal lobe and parieto-occipital areas. His mood changes and psychotic symptoms are consistent with his limbic LBs. The substantia nigra was depigmented (with neuronal dropout), and it showed neuronal loss with classical LBs in remaining neurons, explaining his parkinsonism. The absence of tau aggregates and vascular pathology correlates with his typical DLB phenotype.

Genetic issues and risks

Although PD and its associated dementias are usually sporadic in origin, 5–10% of the patients have monogenic forms of the disease. These cases are more typically early onset and are associated with LRRK2, SNCA, or GBA genes [101]. Tau and progranulin mutations (chromosome 17) cause frontotemporal dementia but sometimes have clinical features that overlap with DLB or PDD [102]. The majority of patients with early-onset autosomal dominant forms of AD and half of the elderly individuals with trisomy 21 (Down's syndrome) have LBs and might show extrapyramidal features [103, 104].

The basic pathogenic mechanism underlying LB formation seems to be similar in cases with sporadic and genetic etiologies. The situation is complicated, however, because some patients meeting clinical criteria for DLB do not have LBs or abnormalities of alpha-synuclein. For example, LRRK2 abnormalities are sometimes associated with LBs, but other times they are associated with tau or ubiquitin pathology [105].

Biochemistry

Alpha-synuclein is the hallmark pathological protein in the LB disorders. Ubiquitin is also present in LBs, but it also is seen in other pathological inclusions. Normally, alpha-synuclein is expressed widely in the CNS and in presynaptic nerve terminals. In LBs, alpha-synuclein aggregates into insoluble fibrils. Epitope mapping studies of alpha-synuclein in PD and DLB synucleinopathies show comparable profiles [106].

Over the past few years, it has become increasingly recognized that alpha-synuclein can act in a prion-like manner, spreading from cell to cell in vitro and in vivo, which might help explain the spread of neurodegeneration in the brains of patients with synucleinopathies [107–110]. Some of the earliest indications of the potential spread of alpha-synuclein were discovered in some patients with PD whom had undergone therapeutic fetal tissue transplants; at autopsy, 11–16 years after the transplant, the fetal neurons had alpha-synuclein deposits, suggesting that β-sheet-rich alpha-synuclein prions propagated from the host neurons into the transplanted fetal cells and induced a change in the structure of α-synuclein and the formation of LBs [111–113]. This led to an explosion of research investigating the potential spread of alpha-synuclein. In one paper, the Trojanowski and Lee laboratories showed that pathological alpha-synuclein derived from animals or entirely synthetic alpha-synuclein preformed fibrils (PFFs) when injected into mice overexpressing alpha-synuclein greatly accelerated the formation and propagation of pathological inclusions throughout the mouse nervous system that were highly reminiscent of LBs and Lewy neurites [114]. In a follow-up paper, they showed that a single injection of synthetic alpha-synuclein fibrils into the striatum of wild-type nontransgenic mice caused cell-to-cell transmission of pathological alpha-synuclein and Parkinson's-like Lewy pathology in regions connected anatomically, leading to a disease reminiscent of PD [115]. Thus, there is now a growing body of evidence suggesting that pathological alpha-synuclein can act in a prion-like manner, spreading from cell-to-cell and inducing the formation of normal alpha-synuclein into a misfolded, pathologic form [116]. This helps explain the mechanism of spread of pathological alpha-synuclein in the brain of PD, PDD, and DLB described by Heiko Braak and colleagues more than a decade ago [117].

Biomarkers

Effective diagnostic biomarkers for DLB/PDD do not currently exist, but are needed to improve differential diagnosis when symptoms are atypical (Table 6.3). Biomarkers are also needed to prognosticate, follow progression, and monitor response an individual's response to treatment.

In addition to traditional PET scans, which might help to distinguish AD from DLB (greater occipital hypoperfusion in DLB), imaging with Pittsburgh compound B (PIB) might help determine beta-amyloid burden in PDD and DLB [118, 119]. Beta-amyloid occurs commonly in both conditions, but the burden is greater in DLB [97]. Cortical cholinergic deficits are more severe in DLB and PDD than other dementias, and thus PET tracers specific for cholinergic function might prove to be useful biomarkers [120, 121]. Dopamine transporter imaging (of striatal nerve terminals) can also discriminate PDD and DLB from AD, but not always from vascular dementia [122].

CSF biomarkers are commercially available for AD, but there is need for specific alpha-synuclein (LB) biomarkers. Serum alpha-synuclein oligomer assays are under investigation [123]. A SPECT or PET ligand for aggregated alpha-synuclein would also be beneficial for diagnosis.

Treatment and management

Treatment and management of LB dementia includes early diagnosis and treatment or management of cognitive impairment, psychiatric symptoms, and motor symptoms and monitoring and management of autonomic dysfunction and sleep disorders. LB dementia patients can decompensate quickly when faced with infection, metabolic stress, or changes in the environment; these risks should be closely monitored. To avoid adverse reactions, physicians should carefully monitor medications, introduce new medications one at a time, and prescribe minimal doses. Medications with anticholinergic effects should be avoided because they can worsen the psychiatric and cognitive syndrome. Nonpharmacological interventions, including physical and occupational therapy, community resources, and home care, are discussed in Chapter 15 and should be tried prior to medications when feasible. For example, psychotic symptoms can often be managed more effectively and safely by changes in the patient's environment.

Cholinesterase inhibitors are the first-line treatment for cognitive impairment in LB dementias. DLB and PDD are associated with reduced acetylcholine, which contributes to the attentional and psychiatric symptoms and functional deficits [124, 125]. Several treatment studies have shown positive effects of cholinesterase inhibitors on cognitive impairment (especially attention and cognitive fluctuations), neuropsychiatric symptoms (especially visual hallucinations, apathy, and anxiety), sleep disturbances, and functional domains [126–131]. DLB patients probably are the most responsive to cholinesterase inhibitors of any of the dementias. Gastrointestinal symptoms and/or vivid dreams sometimes occur. Treated patients should be monitored closely for orthostatic hypotension. Due to potential cardiac conduction blocks occurring or worsening with cholinesterase inhibitors, a baseline EKG prior to starting treatment is recommended. Rivastigmine was approved by the US Food and Drug Administration for treating PDD in 2006. Memantine, an NMDA antagonist, is well tolerated, but its efficacy for cognitive impairment in PDD and DLB is not clear [132, 133].

Dopaminergic therapy is the mainstay for extrapyramidal symptom treatment in LBD. Clinicians should aim for the lowest acceptable dose of levodopa monotherapy to avoid exacerbating psychiatric symptoms and causing delirium [129]; in our experience, DLB patients often respond to carbidopa/levodopa doses in the range of 25/100 mg three times per day or less. Levodopa responsiveness in DLB and PDD has not been extensively studied, but the improvement of symptoms is generally considered to be less than that seen in uncomplicated PD possibly due to greater intrinsic striatal degeneration [93] and motor symptoms without dopaminergic origin.

Depression and anxiety are common in LBD and can be treated with SSRIs or SNRIs. Tricyclics are also effective but can cause orthostatic hypotension, sedation, and cognitive impairment. If treatment is required for RBD, clonazepam, melatonin, or low-dose quetiapine can be tried. For psychotic symptoms, atypical antipsychotic medications must be used cautiously due to the risk of motor and cognitive side effects [78]; consider using atypicals, such as quetiapine, with less extrapyramidal side effects. Traditional neuroleptics should be avoided due to the high rates of neuroleptic hypersensitivity reactions in these patients [8].

For a nice review on pharmacological and nonpharmacological management of DLB, see the article by Boot et al. [134]. The melatonin agonist ramelteon, used to treat sleep disturbances, has been found in a small DLB case series to reduce visual hallucinations, excessive daytime sleepiness, and even RBD [135].

The symptomatic treatments available do not modify the disease course. The current search for disease-modifying drugs is focused primarily on preventing alpha-synuclein misfolding and fibril formation and aggregation [16, 136].

Summary

DLB and PDD are particularly challenging disorders to diagnose and treat because of the complexity of cognitive, behavioral, and motor features involved and because of the frequent presence of overlapping pathology complicating the presentation. Diagnostic criteria identify LB dementia patients when presentations are typical. Better biomarkers are needed to clarify the primary diagnosis when symptoms are not clear-cut. Several symptomatic treatments are available. There is need for disease-modifying agents. Agents that impact the aggregation of alpha-synuclein hold particular promise as future agents for early intervention.

References

1 American Psychiatric Association. *Diagnostic and statistical manual of mental disorders*. Vol. Revised 4th ed. 2000, Washington, DC: American Psychiatric Association.

2 Petersen, R.C., et al., Alzheimer's disease neuroimaging initiative (ADNI): clinical characterization. *Neurology*, 2010. **74**(3): pp. 201–9.

3 McKeith, I.G., et al., Diagnosis and management of dementia with Lewy bodies: third report of the DLB consortium. *Neurology*, 2005. **65**(12): pp. 1863–72.

4 Emre, M., et al., Clinical diagnostic criteria for dementia associated with Parkinson's disease. *Mov Disord*, 2007. **22**(12): pp. 1689–707; quiz 1837.

5 Aarsland, D., et al., A comparative study of psychiatric symptoms in dementia with Lewy bodies and Parkinson's disease with and without dementia. *Int J Geriatr Psychiatry*, 2001. **16**(5): pp. 528–36.

6 Ballard, C., et al., Attention and fluctuating attention in patients with dementia with Lewy bodies and Alzheimer disease. *Arch Neurol*, 2001. **58**(6): pp. 977–82.
7 Horimoto, Y., et al., Autonomic dysfunctions in dementia with Lewy bodies. *J Neurol*, 2003. **250**(5): pp. 530–3.
8 McKeith, I., et al., Neuroleptic sensitivity in patients with senile dementia of Lewy body type. *BMJ*, 1992. **305**(6855): pp. 673–8.
9 Burn, D.J., et al., Extrapyramidal features in Parkinson's disease with and without dementia and dementia with Lewy bodies: a cross-sectional comparative study. *Mov Disord*, 2003. **18**(8): pp. 884–9.
10 Klein, J.C., et al., Neurotransmitter changes in dementia with Lewy bodies and Parkinson disease dementia in vivo. *Neurology*. **74**(11): pp. 885–92.
11 Parkinson, J., An essay on the shaking palsy. 1817. *J Neuropsychiatry Clin Neurosci*, 2002. **14**(2): pp. 223–36; discussion 222.
12 Okazaki, H., L.E. Lipkin, and S.M. Aronson, Diffuse intracytoplasmic ganglionic inclusions (Lewy type) associated with progressive dementia and quadriparesis in flexion. *J Neuropathol Exp Neurol*, 1961. **20**: pp. 237–44.
13 Kosaka, K., et al., Diffuse type of Lewy body disease: progressive dementia with abundant cortical Lewy bodies and senile changes of varying degree—a new disease? *Clin Neuropathol*, 1984. **3**(5): pp. 185–92.
14 Polymeropoulos, M.H., et al., Mutation in the alpha-synuclein gene identified in families with Parkinson's disease. *Science*, 1997. **276**(5321): pp. 2045–7.
15 Spillantini, M.G., et al., Alpha-synuclein in Lewy bodies. *Nature*, 1997. **388**(6645): pp. 839–40.
16 Lippa, C.F., et al., DLB and PDD boundary issues: diagnosis, treatment, molecular pathology, and biomarkers. *Neurology*, 2007. **68**(11): pp. 812–9.
17 Gilman, S., et al., Second consensus statement on the diagnosis of multiple system atrophy. *Neurology*, 2008. **71**(9): pp. 670–6.
18 Kao, A.W., et al., Cognitive and neuropsychiatric profile of the synucleinopathies: Parkinson disease, dementia with Lewy bodies, and multiple system atrophy. *Alzheimer Dis Assoc Disord*, 2009. **23**(4): pp. 365–70.
19 Elbaz, A., et al., Risk tables for parkinsonism and Parkinson's disease. *J Clin Epidemiol*, 2002. **55**(1): pp. 25–31.
20 de Lau, L.M. and M.M. Breteler, Epidemiology of Parkinson's disease. *Lancet Neurol*, 2006. **5**(6): pp. 525–35.
21 Aarsland, D. and M.W. Kurz, The epidemiology of dementia associated with Parkinson's disease. *Brain Pathol*, 2010. **20**(3): pp. 633–9.
22 Hely, M.A., et al., The Sydney multicenter study of Parkinson's disease: the inevitability of dementia at 20 years. *Mov Disord*, 2008. **23**(6): pp. 837–44.
23 Aarsland, D., et al., Frequency and case identification of dementia with Lewy bodies using the revised consensus criteria. *Dement Geriatr Cogn Disord*, 2008. **26**(5): pp. 445–52.
24 Lesage, S. and A. Brice, Parkinson's disease: from monogenic forms to genetic susceptibility factors. *Hum Mol Genet*, 2009. **18**(R1): pp. R48–59.
25 Boot, B.P., et al., Risk factors for dementia with Lewy bodies: a case-control study. *Neurology*, 2013. **81**(9): pp. 833–40.
26 Folstein, M.F., S.E. Folstein, and P.R. McHugh, "Mini-mental state." A practical method for grading the cognitive state of patients for the clinician. *J Psychiatr Res*, 1975. **12**(3): pp. 189–98.
27 Gearing, M., et al., The consortium to establish a registry for Alzheimer's disease (CERAD). Part X. Neuropathology confirmation of the clinical diagnosis of Alzheimer's disease. *Neurology*, 1995. **45**(3 Pt 1): pp. 461–6.
28 McKeith, I.G., et al., Consensus guidelines for the clinical and pathologic diagnosis of dementia with Lewy bodies (DLB): report of the consortium on DLB international workshop. *Neurology*, 1996. **47**(5): pp. 1113–24.
29 Aarsland, D., et al., Comparison of extrapyramidal signs in dementia with Lewy bodies and Parkinson's disease. *J Neuropsychiatry Clin Neurosci*, 2001. **13**(3): pp. 374–9.
30 Alves, G., et al., Changes in motor subtype and risk for incident dementia in Parkinson's disease. *Mov Disord*, 2006. **21**(8): pp. 1123–30.
31 Fahn, S. and R. Elton, Unified Parkinson's disease rating scale, in *Recent developments in Parkinson's disease*, S. Fahn, D. Marsden, and D. Calne, Editors. 1987, Macmillan: London. pp. 153–63.
32 Collerton, D., et al., Systematic review and meta-analysis show that dementia with Lewy bodies is a visual-perceptual and attentional-executive dementia. *Dement Geriatr Cogn Disord*, 2003. **16**(4): pp. 229–37.
33 Mosimann, U.P., et al., Visual perception in Parkinson disease dementia and dementia with Lewy bodies. *Neurology*, 2004. **63**(11): pp. 2091–6.
34 Troster, A.I., Neuropsychological characteristics of dementia with Lewy bodies and Parkinson's disease with dementia: differentiation, early detection, and implications for "mild cognitive impairment" and biomarkers. *Neuropsychol Rev*, 2008. **18**(1): pp. 103–19.
35 Ballard, C.G., et al., Fluctuations in attention: PD dementia vs DLB with parkinsonism. *Neurology*, 2002. **59**(11): pp. 1714–20.
36 Janvin, C.C., et al., Cognitive profiles of individual patients with Parkinson's disease and dementia: comparison with dementia with Lewy bodies and Alzheimer's disease. *Mov Disord*, 2006. **21**(3): pp. 337–42.
37 Perriol, M.P., et al., Disturbance of sensory filtering in dementia with Lewy bodies: comparison with Parkinson's disease dementia and Alzheimer's disease. *J Neurol Neurosurg Psychiatry*, 2005. **76**(1): pp. 106–8.
38 Calderon, J., et al., Perception, attention, and working memory are disproportionately impaired in dementia with Lewy bodies compared with Alzheimer's disease. *J Neurol Neurosurg Psychiatry*, 2001. **70**(2): pp. 157–64.
39 Tiraboschi, P., et al., What best differentiates Lewy body from Alzheimer's disease in early-stage dementia? *Brain*, 2006. **129**(Pt 3): pp. 729–35.
40 Aarsland, D., et al., Cognitive impairment in incident, untreated Parkinson disease: the Norwegian ParkWest study. *Neurology*, 2009. **72**(13): pp. 1121–6.
41 Cools, R., Dopaminergic modulation of cognitive function-implications for L-DOPA treatment in Parkinson's disease. *Neurosci Biobehav Rev*, 2006. **30**(1): pp. 1–23.
42 Mattila, P.M., et al., Choline acetytransferase activity and striatal dopamine receptors in Parkinson's disease in relation to cognitive impairment. *Acta Neuropathol*, 2001. **102**(2): pp. 160–6.
43 Kehagia, A.A., R.A. Barker, and T.W. Robbins, Neuropsychological and clinical heterogeneity of cognitive impairment and dementia in patients with Parkinson's disease. *Lancet Neurol*, 2007. **9**(12): pp. 1200–1213.
44 Williams-Gray, C.H., et al., Evolution of cognitive dysfunction in an incident Parkinson's disease cohort. *Brain*, 2007. **130**(Pt 7): pp. 1787–98.

45 Hoops, S., et al., Validity of the MoCA and MMSE in the detection of MCI and dementia in Parkinson disease. *Neurology*, 2009. **73**(21): pp. 1738–45.

46 Dalrymple-Alford, J.C., et al., The MoCA: well-suited screen for cognitive impairment in Parkinson disease. *Neurology*, **75**(19): pp. 1717–25.

47 Bostrom, F., et al., Patients with dementia with Lewy bodies have more impaired quality of life than patients with Alzheimer disease. *Alzheimer Dis Assoc Disord*, 2007. **21**(2): pp. 150–4.

48 Aarsland, D., et al., Mental symptoms in Parkinson's disease are important contributors to caregiver distress. *Int J Geriatr Psychiatry*, 1999. **14**(10): pp. 866–74.

49 Aarsland, D., et al., Predictors of nursing home placement in Parkinson's disease: a population-based, prospective study. *J Am Geriatr Soc*, 2000. **48**(8): pp. 938–42.

50 Fritze, F., et al., Depression in mild dementia: associations with diagnosis, APOE genotype and clinical features. *Int J Geriatr Psychiatry*, 2011. **26**(10): pp. 1054–61.

51 Shiba, M., et al., Anxiety disorders and depressive disorders preceding Parkinson's disease: a case-control study. *Mov Disord*, 2000. **15**(4): pp. 669–77.

52 Dissanayaka, N.N., et al., Anxiety disorders in Parkinson's disease: prevalence and risk factors. *Mov Disord*, 2010. **25**(7): pp. 838–45.

53 Pedersen, K.F., et al., Occurrence and risk factors for apathy in Parkinson disease: a 4-year prospective longitudinal study. *J Neurol Neurosurg Psychiatry*, 2009. **80**(11): pp. 1279–82.

54 Ricci, M., et al., Clinical findings, functional abilities and caregiver distress in the early stage of dementia with Lewy bodies (DLB) and Alzheimer's disease (AD). *Arch Gerontol Geriatr*, 2009. **49**(2): pp. e101–4.

55 Barone, P., Neurotransmission in Parkinson's disease: beyond dopamine. *Eur J Neurol*, 2010. **17**(3): pp. 364–76.

56 Cummings, J.L. and D.L. Masterman, Depression in patients with Parkinson's disease. *Int J Geriatr Psychiatry*, 1999. **14**(9): pp. 711–8.

57 Temel, Y., et al., Parkinson's disease, DBS and suicide: a role for serotonin? *Brain*, 2009. **132**(Pt 10): pp. e126; author reply e127.

58 Remy, P., et al., Depression in Parkinson's disease: loss of dopamine and noradrenaline innervation in the limbic system. *Brain*, 2005. **128**(Pt 6): pp. 1314–22.

59 Lopez, O.L., et al., Lewy bodies in the amygdala increase risk for major depression in subjects with Alzheimer disease. *Neurology*, 2006. **67**(4): pp. 660–5.

60 Engelborghs, S., et al., Neuropsychiatric symptoms of dementia: cross-sectional analysis from a prospective, longitudinal Belgian study. *Int J Geriatr Psychiatry*, 2005. **20**(11): pp. 1028–37.

61 Mosimann, U.P., et al., Characteristics of visual hallucinations in Parkinson disease dementia and dementia with Lewy bodies. *Am J Geriatr Psychiatry*, 2006. **14**(2): pp. 153–60.

62 Harding, A.J., G.A. Broe, and G.M. Halliday, Visual hallucinations in Lewy body disease relate to Lewy bodies in the temporal lobe. *Brain*, 2002. **125**(Pt 2): pp. 391–403.

63 Nagahama, Y., et al., Neural correlates of psychotic symptoms in dementia with Lewy bodies. *Brain*, 2010. **133**(Pt 2): pp. 557–67.

64 Ballard, C., et al., Delusions associated with elevated muscarinic binding in dementia with Lewy bodies. *Ann Neurol*, 2000. **48**(6): pp. 868–76.

65 Josephs, K.A., Capgras syndrome and its relationship to neurodegenerative disease. *Arch Neurol*, 2007. **64**(12): pp. 1762–6.

66 Boeve, B.F., et al., Synucleinopathy pathology and REM sleep behavior disorder plus dementia or parkinsonism. *Neurology*, 2003. **61**(1): pp. 40–5.

67 Schenck, C.H., S.R. Bundlie, and M.W. Mahowald, Delayed emergence of a parkinsonian disorder in 38% of 29 older men initially diagnosed with idiopathic rapid eye movement sleep behaviour disorder. *Neurology*, 1996. **46**(2): pp. 388–93.

68 Postuma, R.B., et al., Quantifying the risk of neurodegenerative disease in idiopathic REM sleep behavior disorder. *Neurology*, 2009. **72**(15): pp. 1296–300.

69 Claassen, D.O., et al., REM sleep behavior disorder preceding other aspects of synucleinopathies by up to half a century. *Neurology*. **75**(6): pp. 494–9.

70 Abbott, R.D., et al., Frequency of bowel movements and the future risk of Parkinson's disease. *Neurology*, 2001. **57**(3): pp. 456–62.

71 Abbott, R.D., et al., Bowel movement frequency in late-life and incidental Lewy bodies. *Mov Disord*, 2007. **22**(11): pp. 1581–6.

72 Ishihara-Paul, L., et al., Prospective association between emotional health and clinical evidence of Parkinson's disease. *Eur J Neurol*, 2008. **15**(11): pp. 1148–54.

73 Bower, J.H., et al., Anxious personality predicts an increased risk of Parkinson's disease. *Mov Disord*. **25**(13): pp. 2105–13.

74 Boeve, B.F. and C.B. Saper, REM sleep behavior disorder: a possible early marker for synucleinopathies. *Neurology*, 2006. **66**(6): pp. 796–7.

75 Fantini, M.L., L. Ferini-Strambi, and J. Montplaisir, Idiopathic REM sleep behavior disorder: toward a better nosologic definition. *Neurology*, 2005. **64**(5): pp. 780–6.

76 Menza, M., et al., Sleep disturbances in Parkinson's disease. *Mov Disord*. **25** Suppl 1: pp. S117–22.

77 Boeve, B.F., M.H. Silber, and T.J. Ferman, Melatonin for treatment of REM sleep behavior disorder in neurologic disorders: results in 14 patients. *Sleep Med*, 2003. **4**(4): pp. 281–4.

78 Aarsland, D., et al., Neuroleptic sensitivity in Parkinson's disease and parkinsonian dementias. *J Clin Psychiatry*, 2005. **66**(5): pp. 633–7.

79 Litvan, I., et al., Clinical features differentiating patients with postmortem confirmed progressive supranuclear palsy and corticobasal degeneration. *J Neurol*, 1999. **246** Suppl 2: pp. II1–5.

80 Lopez, O.L., et al., Accuracy of four clinical diagnostic criteria for the diagnosis of neurodegenerative dementias. *Neurology*, 1999. **53**(6): pp. 1292–9.

81 Merdes, A.R., et al., Influence of Alzheimer pathology on clinical diagnostic accuracy in dementia with Lewy bodies. *Neurology*, 2003. **60**(10): pp. 1586–90.

82 Isojima, D., et al., Vascular complications in dementia with Lewy bodies: a postmortem study. *Neuropathology*, 2006. **26**(4): pp. 293–7.

83 Lee, S.J., et al., Influence of white matter hyperintensities on the cognition of patients with Parkinson disease. *Alzheimer Dis Assoc Disord*, 2010. **24**(3): pp. 227–33.

84 Nelson, P.T., et al., Low sensitivity in clinical diagnoses of dementia with Lewy bodies. *J Neurol* **257**(3): pp. 359–66.

85 Ferman, T.J., et al., DLB fluctuations: specific features that reliably differentiate DLB from AD and normal aging. *Neurology*, 2004. **62**(2): pp. 181–7.

86 Burton, E.J., et al., Cerebral atrophy in Parkinson's disease with and without dementia: a comparison with Alzheimer's disease, dementia with Lewy bodies and controls. *Brain*, 2004. **127**(Pt 4): pp. 791–800.

87 Whitwell, J.L., et al., Focal atrophy in dementia with Lewy bodies on MRI: a distinct pattern from Alzheimer's disease. *Brain*, 2007. **130**(Pt 3): pp. 708–19.

88 Cousins, D.A., et al., Atrophy of the putamen in dementia with Lewy bodies but not Alzheimer's disease: an MRI study. *Neurology*, 2003. **61**(9): pp. 1191–5.

89 McKeith, I., et al., Sensitivity and specificity of dopamine transporter imaging with 123I-FP-CIT SPECT in dementia with Lewy bodies: a phase III, multicentre study. *Lancet Neurol*, 2007. **6**(4): pp. 305–13.

90 Siderowf, A., et al., CSF amyloid {beta} 1-42 predicts cognitive decline in Parkinson disease. *Neurology*, 2010. **75**(12): pp. 1055–61.

91 Kramer, M.L. and W.J. Schulz-Schaeffer, Presynaptic alpha-synuclein aggregates, not Lewy bodies, cause neurodegeneration in dementia with Lewy bodies. *J Neurosci*, 2007. **27**(6): pp. 1405–10.

92 Baba, M., et al., Aggregation of alpha-synuclein in Lewy bodies of sporadic Parkinson's disease and dementia with Lewy bodies. *Am J Pathol*, 1998. **152**(4): pp. 879–84.

93 Duda, J.E., et al., Novel antibodies to synuclein show abundant striatal pathology in Lewy body diseases. *Ann Neurol*, 2002. **52**(2): pp. 205–10.

94 Samuel, W., et al., Neocortical lewy body counts correlate with dementia in the Lewy body variant of Alzheimer's disease. *J Neuropathol Exp Neurol*, 1996. **55**(1): pp. 44–52.

95 Selikhova, M., et al., A clinico-pathological study of subtypes in Parkinson's disease. *Brain*, 2009. **132**(Pt 11): pp. 2947–57.

96 Edison, P., et al., Amyloid load in Parkinson's disease dementia and Lewy body dementia measured with [11C]PIB positron emission tomography. *J Neurol Neurosurg Psychiatry*, 2008. **79**(12): pp. 1331–8.

97 Gomperts, S.N., et al., Imaging amyloid deposition in Lewy body diseases. *Neurology*, 2008. **71**(12): pp. 903–10.

98 Lippa, S.M., C.F. Lippa, and H. Mori, Alpha-Synuclein aggregation in pathological aging and Alzheimer's disease: the impact of beta-amyloid plaque level. *Am J Alzheimers Dis Other Demen*, 2005. **20**(5): pp. 315–8.

99 Lippa, C.F., R. Johnson, and T.W. Smith, The medial temporal lobe in dementia with Lewy bodies: a comparative study with Alzheimer's disease. *Ann Neurol*, 1998. **43**(1): pp. 102–6.

100 Harding, A.J. and G.M. Halliday, Cortical Lewy body pathology in the diagnosis of dementia. *Acta Neuropathol*, 2001. **102**(4): pp. 355–63.

101 Alcalay, R.N., et al., Frequency of known mutations in early-onset Parkinson disease: implication for genetic counseling: the consortium on risk for early onset Parkinson disease study. *Arch Neurol*. **67**(9): pp. 1116–22.

102 Wider, C. and Z.K. Wszolek, Etiology and pathophysiology of frontotemporal dementia, Parkinson disease and Alzheimer disease: lessons from genetic studies. *Neurodegener Dis*, 2008. **5**(3–4): pp. 122–5.

103 Lippa, C.F., et al., Lewy bodies contain altered alpha-synuclein in brains of many familial Alzheimer's disease patients with mutations in presenilin and amyloid precursor protein genes. *Am J Pathol*, 1998. **153**(5): pp. 1365–70.

104 Lippa, C.F., et al., Antibodies to alpha-synuclein detect Lewy bodies in many Down's syndrome brains with Alzheimer's disease. *Ann Neurol*, 1999. **45**(3): pp. 353–7.

105 Zimprich, A., et al., Mutations in LRRK2 cause autosomal-dominant parkinsonism with pleomorphic pathology. *Neuron*, 2004. **44**(4): pp. 601–7.

106 Lippa, C.F., et al., Alpha-synuclein in familial Alzheimer disease: epitope mapping parallels dementia with Lewy bodies and Parkinson disease. *Arch Neurol*, 2001. **58**(11): pp. 1817–20.

107 Frost, B. and M.I. Diamond, The expanding realm of prion phenomena in neurodegenerative disease. *Prion*, 2009. **3**(2): pp. 74–7.

108 Frost, B. and M.I. Diamond, Prion-like mechanisms in neurodegenerative diseases. *Nat Rev Neurosci*, 2010. **11**(3): pp. 155–9.

109 Yonetani, M., et al., Conversion of wild-type alpha-synuclein into mutant-type fibrils and its propagation in the presence of A30P mutant. *J Biol Chem*, 2009. **284**(12): pp. 7940–50.

110 Polymenidou, M. and D.W. Cleveland, Prion-like spread of protein aggregates in neurodegeneration. *J Exp Med*, 2012. **209**(5): pp. 889–93.

111 Kordower, J.H., et al., Lewy body-like pathology in long-term embryonic nigral transplants in Parkinson's disease. *Nat Med*, 2008. **14**(5): pp. 504–6.

112 Kordower, J.H., et al., Transplanted dopaminergic neurons develop PD pathologic changes: a second case report. *Mov Disord*, 2008. **23**(16): pp. 2303–6.

113 Li, J.Y., et al., Lewy bodies in grafted neurons in subjects with Parkinson's disease suggest host-to-graft disease propagation. *Nat Med*, 2008. **14**(5): pp. 501–3.

114 Luk, K.C., et al., Intracerebral inoculation of pathological alpha-synuclein initiates a rapidly progressive neurodegenerative alpha-synucleinopathy in mice. *J Exp Med*, 2012. **209**(5): pp. 975–86.

115 Luk, K.C., et al., Pathological alpha-synuclein transmission initiates Parkinson-like neurodegeneration in nontransgenic mice. *Science*, 2012. **338**(6109): pp. 949–53.

116 Prusiner, S.B., Biology and genetics of prions causing neurodegeneration. *Annu Rev Genet*, 2013. **47**: pp. 601–23.

117 Braak, H., et al., Staging of brain pathology related to sporadic Parkinson's disease. *Neurobiol Aging*, 2003. **24**(2): pp. 197–211.

118 Burack, M.A., et al., In vivo amyloid imaging in autopsy-confirmed Parkinson disease with dementia. *Neurology*. **74**(1): pp. 77–84.

119 Burn, D.J. and J.T. O'Brien, Use of functional imaging in Parkinsonism and dementia. *Mov Disord*, 2003. **18** Suppl 6: pp. S88–95.

120 Bohnen, N.I., et al., Cortical cholinergic function is more severely affected in parkinsonian dementia than in Alzheimer disease: an in vivo positron emission tomographic study. *Arch Neurol*, 2003. **60**(12): pp. 1745–8.

121 Lippa, C.F., T.W. Smith, and E. Perry, Dementia with Lewy bodies: choline acetyltransferase parallels nucleus basalis pathology. *J Neural Transm*, 1999. **106**(5–6): pp. 525–35.

122 Brooks, D.J. and P. Piccini, Imaging in Parkinson's disease: the role of monoamines in behavior. *Biol Psychiatry*, 2006. **59**(10): pp. 908–18.

123 El-Agnaf, O.M., et al., Detection of oligomeric forms of alpha-synuclein protein in human plasma as a potential biomarker for Parkinson's disease. *Faseb J*, 2006. **20**(3): pp. 419–25.

124 Shimada, H., et al., Mapping of brain acetylcholinesterase alterations in Lewy body disease by PET. *Neurology*, 2009. **73**(4): pp. 273–8.

125 Bohnen, N.I., et al., Cognitive correlates of cortical cholinergic denervation in Parkinson's disease and parkinsonian dementia. *J Neurol*, 2006. **253**(2): pp. 242–7.

126 Olin, J.T., D. Aarsland, and X. Meng, Rivastigmine in the treatment of dementia associated with Parkinson's disease: effects on activities of daily living. *Dement Geriatr Cogn Disord.* **29**(6): pp. 510–5.

127 Wesnes, K.A., et al., Benefits of rivastigmine on attention in dementia associated with Parkinson disease. *Neurology*, 2005. **65**(10): pp. 1654–6.

128 Emre, M., et al., Rivastigmine for dementia associated with Parkinson's disease. *N Engl J Med*, 2004. **351**(24): pp. 2509–18.

129 McKeith, I., et al., Dementia with Lewy bodies. *Lancet Neurol*, 2004. **3**(1): pp. 19–28.

130 Samuel, W., et al., Better cognitive and psychopathologic response to donepezil in patients prospectively diagnosed as dementia with Lewy bodies: a preliminary study. *Int J Geriatr Psychiatry*, 2000. **15**(9): pp. 794–802.

131 Burn, D., et al., Effects of rivastigmine in patients with and without visual hallucinations in dementia associated with Parkinson's disease. *Mov Disord*, 2006. **21**(11): pp. 1899–907.

132 Leroi, I., et al., Randomized controlled trial of memantine in dementia associated with Parkinson's disease. *Mov Disord*, 2009. **24**(8): pp. 1217–21.

133 Aarsland, D., et al., Memantine in patients with Parkinson's disease dementia or dementia with Lewy bodies: a double-blind, placebo-controlled, multicentre trial. *Lancet Neurol*, 2009. **8**(7): pp. 613–8.

134 Boot, B.P., et al., Treatment of dementia with Lewy bodies. *Curr Treat Options Neurol*, 2013. **15**(6): pp. 738–64.

135 Kasanuki, K., et al., Effectiveness of ramelteon for treatment of visual hallucinations in dementia with Lewy bodies: a report of 4 cases. *J Clin Psychopharmacol*, 2013. **33**(4): pp. 581–3.

136 Amer, D.A., G.B. Irvine, and O.M. El-Agnaf, Inhibitors of alpha-synuclein oligomerization and toxicity: a future therapeutic strategy for Parkinson's disease and related disorders. *Exp Brain Res*, 2006. **173**(2): pp. 223–33.

CHAPTER 7

Corticobasal degeneration and progressive supranuclear palsy

Suzee E. Lee and Bruce L. Miller
University of California, San Francisco, San Francisco, CA, USA

History and nomenclature

Corticobasal degeneration

In 1968, Rebeiz and colleagues first described three patients with a progressive movement disorder and swollen neurons with poorly staining inclusions found at autopsy, a condition they named "corticodentatonigral degeneration with neuronal achromasia" [1]. Although the authors noted neuropathological overlap with Pick's disease, they believed that the clinical features of these patients were inconsistent with Pick's. Subsequent groups emphasized motor features of the disease, including focal reflex myoclonus, alien limb phenomena, apraxia, rigidity and akinesia, postural–action tremor, limb dystonia, hyperreflexia, and postural instability [2, 3]. Other researchers classified these patients as a subtype of Pick's disease, emphasizing behavioral and cognitive symptoms in addition to extrapyramidal features of the condition [4]. Over time, this disorder came to be known as corticobasal degeneration. Neuronal aggregates in CBD were shown to consist of the microtubule-associated protein tau (MAPT) [5], drawing links to other tau-associated disorders, including PSP, progressive aphasia [6], and Pick's disease [7].

Progressive supranuclear palsy

In 1964, Richardson, Olszewski, and Steele observed a syndrome of postural instability, supranuclear gaze palsy with prominent downgaze difficulty, spastic facies, axial rigidity, and dementia with personality changes [9]. Neuropathological studies revealed "cell loss, gliosis, neurofibrillary tangles, granulovacuolar degeneration and demyelination in various regions of the basal ganglia, brainstem and cerebellum"; these pathological changes bore a striking resemblance to postencephalitic parkinsonism and the parkinsonism–dementia complex of Guam [9]. Subsequent studies confirmed the consistency of clinical findings [10, 11], and clinical consensus criteria for PSP were established in 1996 (Table 7.1) [12]. Neuronal aggregates found in PSP consist of tau protein [13], linking PSP to other tau disorders.

Autopsy series highlight the clinical heterogeneity of CBD and PSP. Thus, the terms corticobasal syndrome [14] and progressive supranuclear palsy syndrome distinguish the clinically defined syndrome from the pathological entities, CBD and PSP. For the remainder of this chapter, we will use the terms CBD and PSP to refer to pathologically defined diseases and CBS and PSP syndrome to refer to the clinically defined syndromes.

Epidemiology

Typically, symptoms in pathologically proven CBD emerge between the sixth and eighth decades of life [15]. To our knowledge, the youngest patient with pathologically confirmed CBD had symptom onset at age 45 [15]. Both women and men are affected with some studies citing higher rates in women [16]. To date, there have been no population-based studies of CBD, and CBD is regarded as a rare neurodegenerative disorder, although studies have estimated of 4.9 cases per 100 000 people in the United States [17] and 1.7 per 100 000 in Japan [18a]. Mean age at onset in a series of 267 patients with CBD was 64 years with a disease duration of 6.6 years [18b].

A study from the United Kingdom found that an age-adjusted prevalence of PSP is approximately 5 per 100 000 [19, 20]. Men appear to have a slightly higher incidence of PSP. A study in the United States showed an average annual incidence rate of

Non-Alzheimer's and Atypical Dementia, First Edition. Edited by Michael D. Geschwind and Caroline Racine Belkoura.
© 2016 John Wiley & Sons, Ltd. Published 2016 by John Wiley & Sons, Ltd.

Table 7.1 NINDS–SPSP clinical criteria for PSP (1996).

I. Mandatory inclusion criteria
  A. PSP possible
    1. Gradually progressive disorder
    2. Onset at age 40 or later
    3. Either vertical (upward or downward gaze) supranuclear palsy **or** both slowing of vertical saccades and prominent postural instability with falls in the first year of disease onset
    4. No evidence of other diseases that could explain the foregoing features, as indicated by mandatory exclusion criteria
  B. PSP probable
    1. Gradually progressive disorder
    2. Onset at age 40 or later
    3. Vertical (upward or downward gaze) supranuclear palsy and prominent postural instability with falls in the first year of disease onset
    4. No evidence of other diseases that could explain the foregoing features, as indicated by mandatory exclusion criteria
  C. Definite
    1. Clinically probable or possible PSP and histopathologic evidence of typical PSP

II. Mandatory exclusion criteria
  A. Recent history of encephalitis
  B. Alien limb syndrome, cortical sensory deficits, focal frontal, or temporoparietal atrophy
  C. Hallucinations or delusions unrelated to dopaminergic therapy
  D. Cortical dementia of Alzheimer's type (severe amnesia and aphasia or agnosia, according to NINCDS-ADRA criteria)
  E. Prominent, early cerebellar symptoms or prominent, early unexplained dysautonomia (marked hypotension and urinary disturbances)
  F. Severe, asymmetric parkinsonian signs (i.e., bradykinesia)
  G. Neuroradiologic evidence of relevant structural abnormality (i.e., basal ganglia or brainstem infarcts, lobar atrophy)
  H. Whipple's disease, confirmed by polymerase chain reaction, if indicated

III. Supportive criteria
  A. Symmetric akinesia or rigidity, proximal more than distal
  B. Abnormal neck posture, especially retrocollis
  C. Poor or absent response of parkinsonism to levodopa therapy
  D. Early dysphagia and dysarthria
  E. Early onset of cognitive impairment including at least two of the following: apathy, impairment in abstract thought, decreased verbal fluency, utilization or imitation behavior, or frontal release signs

5.3 per 100 000 person-years, and incidence was higher in men than women [21]. Most patients with PSP are affected in the sixth decade of life, with ages of presentation ranging from the 50s to the 60s [22, 23].

Studies of the MAPT gene (*MAPT*) reveal overrepresentation of the H1 MAPT haplotype in both CBD and PSP [24, 25]. Association between the H1/H1 genotypes also occurs with FTD [26, 27] and primary progressive aphasia [28]. H1/H1 is the common genotype found with near 100% prevalence in Japanese and approximately 70% in Caucasians [29, 30]. In one cohort of 64 Caucasian patients with PSP, the prevalence of the H1 haplotype was greater than 90%, with 87.5% H1/H1 and 12.5% H1/H2 [24].

Clinical features of corticobasal syndrome

In the 1980s, clinicians in the movement disorder community suggested that CBD was a progressive neurodegenerative condition characterized by asymmetric parkinsonism, apraxia, myoclonus, dystonia, and alien limb syndrome [1–3]. Clinicopathological studies eventually demonstrated that the CBS clinical syndrome poorly predicts CBD pathology [14]. Despite CBD's initial characterization as a movement disorder, CBD also manifests frontal lobe degeneration presenting with cognitive and behavioral symptoms [8, 31], with motor symptoms sometimes emerging only during advanced disease stages [8, 32–35]. Thus, the absence of early motor findings does not exclude CBD from the picture. Moreover, features of bvFTD, nfvPPA, and CBS may overlap or evolve within individual patients throughout the disease course [33, 36]. The three main clinical presentations of CBD include a motor syndrome with prominent, early executive dysfunction, nfvPPA, and bvFTD [8]. Case studies are presented below as examples.

Case 1 Executive–motor syndrome

A 68-year-old right-handed woman started having difficulty with balance 4 years prior to presentation. Initially, she tripped on uneven ground, usually with her right foot, although her leg was not weak. Three years before presentation, she noted trouble with organizing and multitasking; memory seemed intact. She noted progressive difficulty controlling her right leg. Once, she tried to step over her grandchild's toy on the ground, but her right leg remained in the air, and she could not put it down. When seated, she noticed difficulty crossing her right leg over her left. She gradually lost dexterity of her right hand, and her handwriting deteriorated. About 1 year ago, her right forearm moved suddenly and uncontrollably, knocking over a vase of flowers. Her gait slowed. Six months before presentation, she developed increasing apathy and social withdrawal, slowing losing interest in her grandchildren and ending most of her social relationships.

On exam, affect was sad and facies were masked. On primary gaze, there were no square wave jerks. Saccadic eye movement testing showed increased latency to initiating saccadic eye movements in all directions, with normal velocity and full excursion of extraocular movements. There was moderate cogwheel rigidity in the upper extremities, more prominent on the right, and hypertonia in the right lower extremity. Mild axial rigidity was present. Strength was full. A mild, high-frequency bilateral postural hand tremor was present, more prominent on the right. There was no rest tremor. Deep tendon reflexes were symmetric and 2+; plantar response was flexor bilaterally. Sensory exam was intact. Gait revealed diminished arm swing, worse on the right, with mild shuffling and difficulty with turns. She intermittently held her right arm in a flexed posture.

Neuropsychological testing revealed significant deficits in executive function, particularly with verbal fluencies and set-shifting. Mild deficits in naming and episodic memory were noted. Visuospatial skills were intact. A brain MRI revealed focal atrophy in dorsomedial frontal cortex and insula and bilateral primary motor cortices (see Figure 7.1).

In subsequent evaluations, her gait grew progressively worse, and her memory deteriorated. She developed retrocollis, and severe appendicular rigidity ensued. She had trouble with swallowing and began to choke, particularly when drinking liquids. She grew nonverbal but remained cooperative on examination. She died 5 years after symptom onset. Autopsy showed CBD.

As described in the case above, the executive–motor syndrome presents with extrapyramidal syndromes including axial or appendicular rigidity, dystonia, and progressive loss of limb function, findings classically associated with CBS. Poor performance on executive function measures occurs early during the disease course. Perirolandic, supplementary motor area, striatal and insular atrophy are associated with the executive–motor syndrome [8].

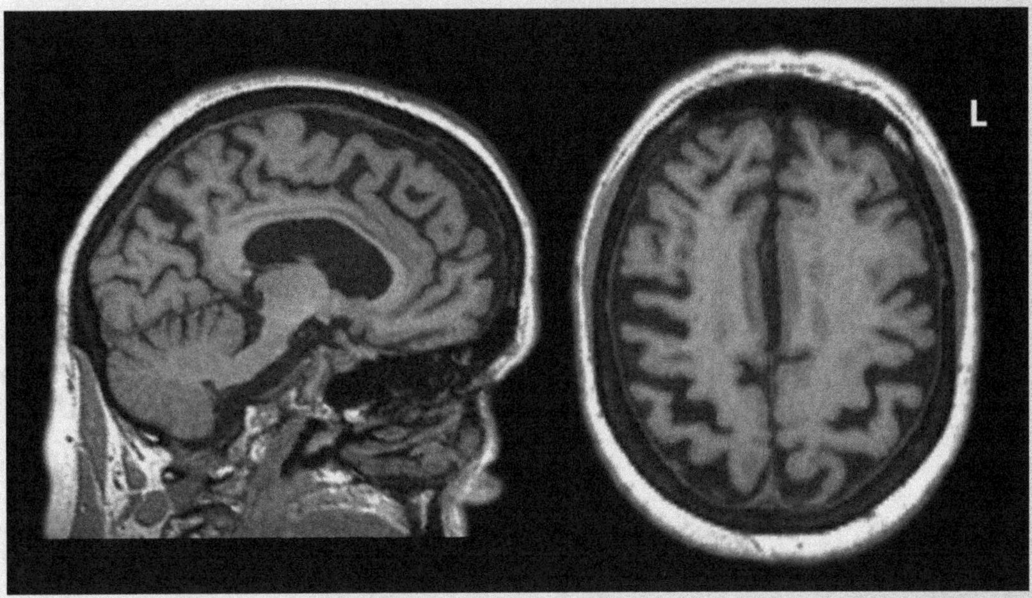

Figure 7.1 Brain MRI in executive–motor CBD. T1-weighted brain MRI of a 68-year-old right-handed woman with pathological-proven CBD with an executive–motor syndrome. Sagittal MRI (left) shows dorsolateral frontal atrophy, and axial MRI (right) shows bilateral parietal atrophy, particularly in the primary motor cortex. Orientation is radiological (left is right).

Case 2 Nonfluent variant primary progressive aphasia

A 54-year-old right-handed woman first noted difficulty with speaking 3 years prior to evaluation. Initially, she had trouble finding words in conversation, and pauses in her speech evolved into stuttering. Even though she knew what she wanted to say, her speech grew slow and effortful. Her speech was slurred; she made frequent phonemic paraphasic errors, and she occasionally stressed the wrong syllable in pronouncing words. Her speech grew agrammatical and she tended to omit articles and conjunctions. She had no difficulty with comprehension, reading, or spelling. About 1 year prior to evaluation, behavioral symptoms emerged. She compulsively arranged the books on her coffee table with the edges aligned. She also took food from her family members' plates without permission. Six months prior, she developed difficulty using her right hand and began to use her left hand to pick up objects. Her right arm appeared stiff, and she frequently held it fixed at her side.

On exam, she was cooperative. Speech was effortful, dysarthric, and agrammatical. Apraxia of speech and orobuccal apraxia were noted, but limb apraxia was absent. There were no square wave jerks and saccadic eye movements were normal. There was mild cogwheel rigidity in the right upper extremity, but no axial rigidity. Strength was full. A mild, high-frequency postural right-hand tremor was present. Deep tendon reflexes were symmetric and 2+; plantar response was flexor bilaterally. Sensory exam was normal. Gait revealed diminished arm swing on the right with normal stride and turns.

Neuropsychological testing revealed significant deficits in language testing, including naming and repetition. Verbal memory and executive function were impaired, but the prominence of her language impairments rendered the interpretation of other cognitive testing less clear. Visuospatial skills were intact. A brain MRI revealed severe focal left insular and left inferior frontal gyrus atrophy with mild atrophy in bilateral orbitofrontal cortex and medial frontal regions (see Figure 7.2).

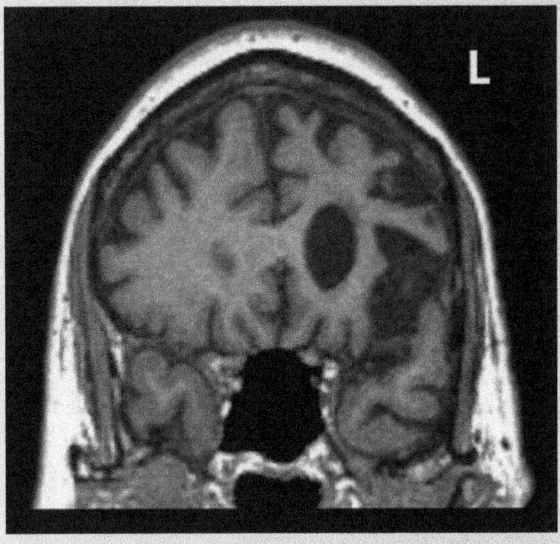

Figure 7.2 Brain MRI in nonfluent variant primary progressive aphasia secondary to CBD. Coronal T1-weighted brain MRI of a 54-year-old right-handed woman showing severe focal left insular and left inferior frontal gyrus atrophy with mild atrophy in bilateral orbitofrontal cortex and medial frontal regions. Orientation is radiological.

Over the next few years, she developed severe right-sided rigidity and grew mute. She had involuntary movements in her right hand and foot, which also intermittently assumed dystonic postures, and eventually had trouble using utensils in her left hand. On exam, her eye movements were extremely limited, and she had right-sided visual neglect. She died 7 years after symptom onset; at autopsy, she was diagnosed with CBD.

Features of nfvPPA include agrammatism with effortful, halting speech and impaired comprehension of syntactically complicated sentences, with spared single-word comprehension and object knowledge [37]. Left frontoinsular atrophy on MRI or hypometabolism on PET might be observed. Some studies suggest that nfvPPA correlates most strongly with FTLD-tau within the FTLD spectrum [8, 38–40] although FTLD-TDP pathology [8, 41] has also been found underlying nfvPPA.

Case 3 Behavioral variant frontotemporal dementia

A 64-year-old gentleman began to develop personality changes 7 years prior to evaluation. He developed a newfound interest in painting, and began to wear bizarre, brightly colored outfits. Over the next several years, his obsession with painting burgeoned, and he created hundreds of pieces of art. He also became less risk-averse. Previously conservative with money, he developed an interest in gambling, both winning and losing large amounts of money in casinos. He became a "born-again" Christian 5 years prior to evaluation and began praying several times a day. He was evaluated by a psychiatrist who diagnosed him with depression and started an SSRI, which did not significantly alleviate his symptoms.

Four years after his personality changes began, he developed short-term memory difficulty. Word-finding difficulties emerged and he spoke less. He grew emotionally blunted and withdrawn. In the few months prior to evaluation, his family noted that his gait grew slower and that he had a hand tremor.

On exam, he remained quiet and had a flat affect. Speech was clear and grammatical, but he spoke only in short phrases. Cranial nerve, motor, reflex, and sensory examination appeared normal. Gait exam revealed diminished right arm swing with normal stride and turns.

Neuropsychological testing revealed significant deficits in memory, language, and executive function. Visuospatial skills were intact. A brain MRI revealed bilateral frontoinsular and dorsomedial frontal and dorsolateral prefrontal atrophy, more prominent on the right (see Figure 7.3).

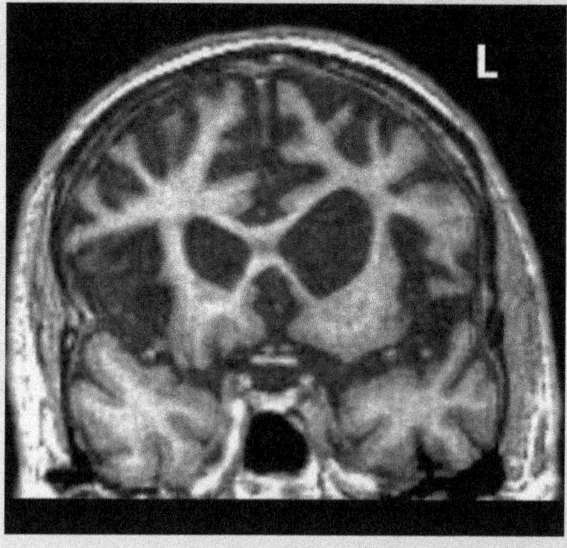

Figure 7.3 Brain MRI in behavioral variant frontotemporal dementia secondary to CBD. Coronal T1-weighted brain MRI in a 64-year-old gentleman showing bilateral frontoinsular, dorsomedial frontal, and dorsolateral prefrontal atrophy. Orientation is radiological.

In follow-up evaluations, his postural hand tremor worsened. When walking, he developed dystonic posturing of his right arm. He stopped initiating conversations and needed to be monitored and encouraged to perform basic activities of daily living, such as toileting and grooming. His speech grew sparser and he answered questions with single words. He died 12 years after his initial symptoms of personality changes. Autopsy revealed CBD.

The earliest and more salient features of behavioral variant frontotemporal dementia (bvFTD) include changes in behavior and personality [42]. bvFTD clinical criteria include early behavioral disinhibition, apathy or inertia, and loss of sympathy or empathy, compulsive behaviors ranging from simple repetitive movements to complex, ritualistic behaviors, and hyperorality or dietary changes, such as altered food preferences, binge eating or drinking alcohol, and placing inedible objects in the mouth. Often, behavioral changes are misdiagnosed as psychiatric disease early in the disease course. Typically, visuospatial skills and memory are spared early in bvFTD. Frontal and temporal brain atrophy on MRI brain or hypometabolism on PET scans emerges.

Correlation between CBS and CBD

Clinicopathological correlation studies attest to the significant challenges of diagnosing CBD. Autopsy studies demonstrate that the sensitivities of CBS for CBD are poor ranging from 31 to 56% [8, 32, 34, 43]. The pathologies underlying CBS are protean and include CBD, tauopathies other than CBD (including PSP, Pick's disease, frontotemporal dementia, and parkinsonism linked to tau mutations on chromosome 17 (FTDP-17)), frontotemporal lobar degeneration with TAR DNA-binding protein-43 (TDP-43) immunoreactive inclusions (FTLD-TDP), Alzheimer's disease (AD), dementia with Lewy bodies (DLB), and Creutzfeldt–Jakob disease [38–40, 43–46]. Recent autopsy series have shown that underlying CBD pathology is found in only 35–55% of all patients who present with CBS during life [8, 38, 40, 44, 47, 48]. PSP pathology commonly manifests as CBS with one study citing nearly 50% of 21 CBS patients with PSP at autopsy [40].

Conversely, many patients with autopsy-confirmed CBD are not suspected of having the disease during life [38, 44, 47, 49, 50]. As described previously, the clinical presentations of CBD are heterogeneous and include bvFTD, nfvPPA, PSP syndrome, Parkinson's disease (PD), AD, and occasionally posterior cortical atrophy (PCA) [8, 40, 49, 51, 52], rendering diagnosis challenging. Based on 267 pathologically confirmed CBD cases, new criteria for possible and probable CBD have been established [18b]. These 2013 criteria for possible CBD include insidious onset and gradual progression, with symptoms lasting at least 1 year, with one of four clinical syndromes (possible corticobasal syndrome, frontal behavioral–spatial syndrome or nonfluent/agrammatic primary progressive aphasia, PSP syndrome) with an additional feature of CBS. The more stringent criteria for probable CBD include those for possible but also require age at onset to be greater than 50 years and no family history of similar conditions or known tau mutations [18b]. Future studies are necessary to determine the sensitivity and specificity of the new CBD criteria.

Despite attempts to characterize symptoms and signs predictive of CBD pathology, the overlap of these symptoms and signs with other neurodegenerative diseases makes pathological prediction at the bedside extremely challenging. Although cortical symptoms and signs for CBD have historically included visuospatial deficits, limb apraxia, and cortical sensory loss, these parietal lobe-associated features are not specific for CBD pathology and are common in AD [8]. Although memory and visuospatial deficits in CBS may suggest underlying AD in group studies, it remains unclear how such deficits improve diagnosis at individual patient level [8]. Motor symptoms in CBD may be absent up to 8 years after symptom onset, and motor symptoms classically associated with CBS are not exclusive to CBD pathology, presenting in similar rates in patients with CBS with underlying AD, PSP, FTLD-TDP, or mixed pathologies [8]. Quantitative eye movement studies of CBS suggested that saccadic eye movement latency is increased with relatively preserved velocity in CBD [53–57, 57a], although an eye movement study of autopsy-proven CBD suggests similar saccadic latency and velocity compared with controls, but impairments on an antisaccade task [57b]. This contrasts with the saccadic eye movement changes in PSP, in which the velocity of movements are slowed with relatively preserved latency [53, 54, 57b].

Neuropsychological testing in patients with CBS shows impairments in attention, executive function, and/or language impairments, with memory relatively less affected [8, 32, 34, 50, 58–60]. Although some studies have demonstrated that poorer performance on visual and verbal memory measures suggests underlying AD pathology in CBS [8, 46], the utility of neuropsychological testing in predicting CBD pathology remains unproven for individual patients.

Although the symptoms, signs, and neuropsychological profile described previously have been associated with CBD, they are variably present in individual patients. In patients with CBS, the presence or absence of any specific clinical sign or symptom does not reliably predict CBD pathology [8]. Furthermore, although asymmetry has been stressed as a core feature of CBD, several studies have revealed that CBD can emerge with symmetric parkinsonism and with symmetric brain degeneration [8, 61–63].

Clinical features of progressive supranuclear palsy syndrome

Progressive supranuclear palsy was first defined as a neurodegenerative syndrome consisting of supranuclear vertical gaze palsy, axial dystonia with a hypererect posture, bradykinesia, rigidity, and early falls [9]. In 1996, clinical consensus criteria for PSP syndrome defined core features as a progressive course of impairment beginning after the age of 40, with supranuclear gaze palsy, slowing of vertical saccadic eye movements, and postural instability with falls in the first year of onset (Table 7.1) [12].

Case study: A 63-year-old man developed problems with concentration 5 years prior to evaluation. Previously excellent with multitasking, he described significant difficulty keeping track of more than one activity simultaneously. He described his thinking as slowed, although memory remained intact. He grew more outspoken, started telling his coworkers exactly what he thought of them, and became less aware of putting himself and others in uncomfortable situations. Three years prior to evaluation, he fell when attempting to stand up from a reclining chair. His speech grew softer and slurred, particularly when he was tired. Two years prior to evaluation, he walked more slowly and he developed a shuffling gait. He fell frequently, usually when arising from sitting to standing. One fall resulted in a fractured elbow. Despite awareness of his worsening balance, he could not comply with his family's pleas to be more cautious when walking. He described difficulty looking downward and seeing objects on the ground. Mild emotional triggers caused him to laugh and cry easily and grew more disinhibited in social situations. Previously outgoing, he became quieter and more passive. He developed urinary frequency at night with occasional urinary incontinence. A trial of levodopa/carbidopa resulted in no improvement in his symptoms.

On exam, he was cooperative. Certain topics, such as his favorite sports team and his dog, invariably provoked uncontrollable laughter, even when the topics were not amusing to him. Speech was mildly dysarthric and aprosodic. He had masked facies and the procerus sign was present. There were square wave jerks in primary gaze. Vertical saccadic velocity was reduced, with downgaze more affected than upgaze; horizontal saccades appeared normal. Downgaze excursion was limited by about 50%. Severe axial rigidity and mild symmetric rigidity appeared in all limbs. Tremor and dysmetria were absent. Repetitive finger, hand, and foot movements were diminutive. Deep tendon reflexes were 2+ in the extremities, and plantar responses were flexor. Sensory exam appeared normal. Gait examination showed diminished left arm swing; a rigid, hypererect posture; and mild retropulsive instability. Neuropsychological testing revealed deficits only in executive function and indicated that his responses were error prone and impulsive. Memory, language, and visuospatial skills were intact. An MRI brain revealed mild midbrain atrophy (see Figure 7.4). He was given a clinical diagnosis of PSP.

In subsequent evaluations, his falls became increasingly frequent, occurring up to several times per day, despite his family's efforts to prevent falls. Eventually, he became wheelchair bound. He grew more apathetic and rarely initiated conversations or engaged with others. Downgaze became completely absent, and he could not see food on his plate. He developed severe dysarthria and dysphagia, which required a modified diet to prevent aspiration. He died of pneumonia 5 years after his first symptom. Autopsy confirmed PSP.

The classical PSP syndrome features severe gait and balance impairment with bradykinesia leading to frequent falls, dysarthria and dysphagia, and gaze palsy. In addition to motor and oculomotor abnormalities, patients with PSP syndrome often harbor behavioral changes and executive function deficits showing clinical overlap with bvFTD [64–66]. A subset of patients with PSP syndrome manifest a predominant behavioral presentation that precedes motor symptoms; in such cases, early falls might not be present [65, 67, 68]. Prominent behavioral changes often emerge, with apathy and disinhibition being the most common [67]. In contrast to bvFTD, neuropsychiatric symptoms such as hyperorality and repetitive motor behaviors occur less commonly. Psychotic symptoms are uncommon in PSP syndrome [69]. Memory difficulties in PSP syndrome are usually mild and usually involve retrieval rather than recognition deficits [59].

Downward gaze palsy is a strong predictor of autopsy-proven PSP [70], and horizontal square wave jerks on primary gaze may emerge. Oculomotor abnormalities are present in CBS, AD, and FTD spectrum disorders; however, abnormalities in vertical greater than horizontal saccadic velocity and gaze excursion are more typical of PSP [57b]. Although patients with PSP, CBS, and AD have abnormalities in saccadic gain (maintaining accuracy of saccadic eye movements by adjusting saccadic amplitude relative to the target distance) and range of eye movement excursion, patients with PSP have the most prominent decrements in saccadic gain [53–56]. With supranuclear gaze palsy, the oculocephalic reflex is intact early in the disease course but disappears in later disease stages. Other ocular abnormalities often include square wave jerks, blepharospasm, eyelid opening apraxia, and reduced blink rate [71].

Supportive diagnostic features include symmetric akinesia or rigidity that is proximal more than distal, dysphagia and dysarthria, abnormal neck posture (retrocollis), urinary incontinence, and cognitive impairment. The procerus sign, caused by contraction of the corrugator and orbicularis oculi muscles leading to wrinkles in the glabellar region and the bridge of the nose, may give a furrowed-brow appearance [72, 73]. In contrast to PD, tremor is often absent and rigidity is axial rather than appendicular. Postural instability typically is an early symptom, causing frequent falls. Early in the disease course, falls might be provoked by uneven surfaces. As motor symptoms progress, however, falls can be unpredictable, with no known provocation. The etiology of the falls is multifactorial; impaired downgaze, poor postural reflexes and instability, and impulsivity all contribute to fall risk.

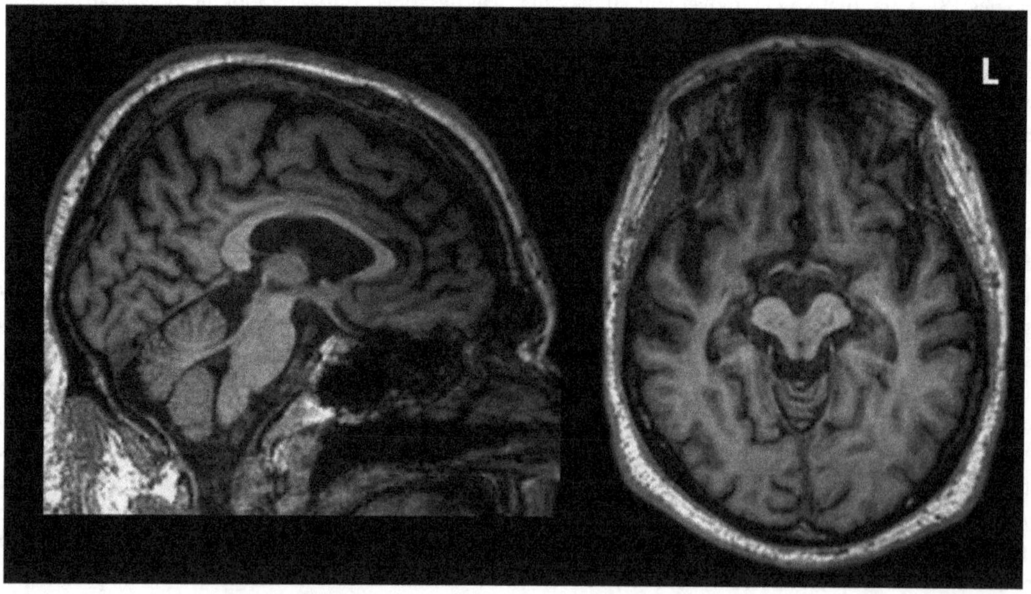

Figure 7.4 Brain MRI in progressive supranuclear palsy syndrome secondary to CBD. T1-weighted brain MRI in a 63-year-old gentleman showing mild midbrain atrophy in sagittal (left) and axial (right) planes.

Correlation between PSP syndrome and PSP

About one-half to two-thirds of those diagnosed with PSP at autopsy were suspected to have PSP at presentation [44, 68, 70, 74–77]. Other clinical syndromes associated with PSP include PD, CBS, and MSA [43, 75]. In some series, about half of patients with CBS showed PSP pathology [40, 48]. About 80% of patients diagnosed with PSP syndrome during life show PSP at autopsy [68, 74]. Other autopsy diagnoses of those with PSP syndrome include DLB, AD, MSA, CBD, Pick's disease, and FTDP-17 [76]. There is substantial clinical overlap between PSP and CBD.

Diagnostic studies

Laboratory tests

Currently, there are no laboratory tests for CBD or PSP, and diagnosis is based on clinical evaluation. In diagnostic evaluation of patients with cognitive impairment, laboratory tests should be done to rule out medical causes of cognitive decline, including vitamin B12 deficiency, thyroid dysfunction, syphilis, and HIV, if risk factors are suspected in patients. Cerebrospinal fluid (CSF) diagnostic biomarkers are currently being explored, although none has yet been approved for clinical use (see Pathophysiology and Pathology, "Biomarkers").

Neuroimaging

Quantitative brain imaging studies reveal distinct atrophy patterns arising in CBD and PSP, and studies have assessed atrophy patterns in CBS and PSP syndrome in attempts to determine underlying predictors of pathology. Major sites of degeneration in pathologically proven CBD include the frontal lobes, basal ganglia, and brainstem (Figure 7.5) [8, 78]. Although historically CBD was described as a frontoparietal disease [63], voxel-based morphometry (VBM) studies demonstrate that frontal and striatal degeneration, rather than parietal atrophy, dominates [8, 78]. One study showed that although heterogeneous clinical syndromes such as nfvPPA, bvFTD, and an executive–motor phenotype result from CBD, common regions of atrophy across all three syndromes include bilateral dorsomedial prefrontal cortex, supplementary motor area, perirolandic cortex, and striatum, suggesting that these are the core regions affected by CBD [8].

VBM studies demonstrate that dorsomedial frontal cortex, perirolandic cortex, and dorsal insula atrophy arise in all

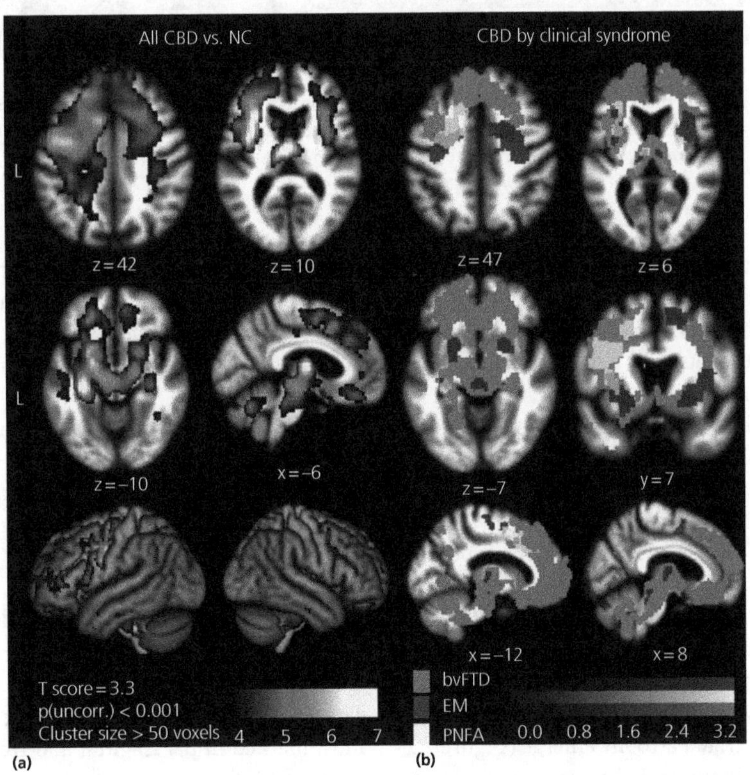

Figure 7.5 Statistical parametric mapping version 5 (SPM5) voxel-based morphometry (VBM) MRI analysis contrasting gray and white matter volume in **(a)** a cohort of patients with corticobasal degeneration (CBD) ($N=13$) with healthy older controls (NC, $N=44$) who had VBM-compatible 1.5T structural T1 scans and **(b)** the three main clinical syndromes seen in CBD compared to NC viewed on a DARTEL-derived template based on 48 healthy controls (voxel resolution: 1 mm). Patients with VBM-compatible scans in the three CBD clinical syndromes included nfvPPA ($N=4$), EM-CBD ($N=5$), and bvFTD-CBD ($N=3$). Source: Lee et al. [8]. Reproduced with permission of Wiley. (*See insert for color representation of the figure.*)

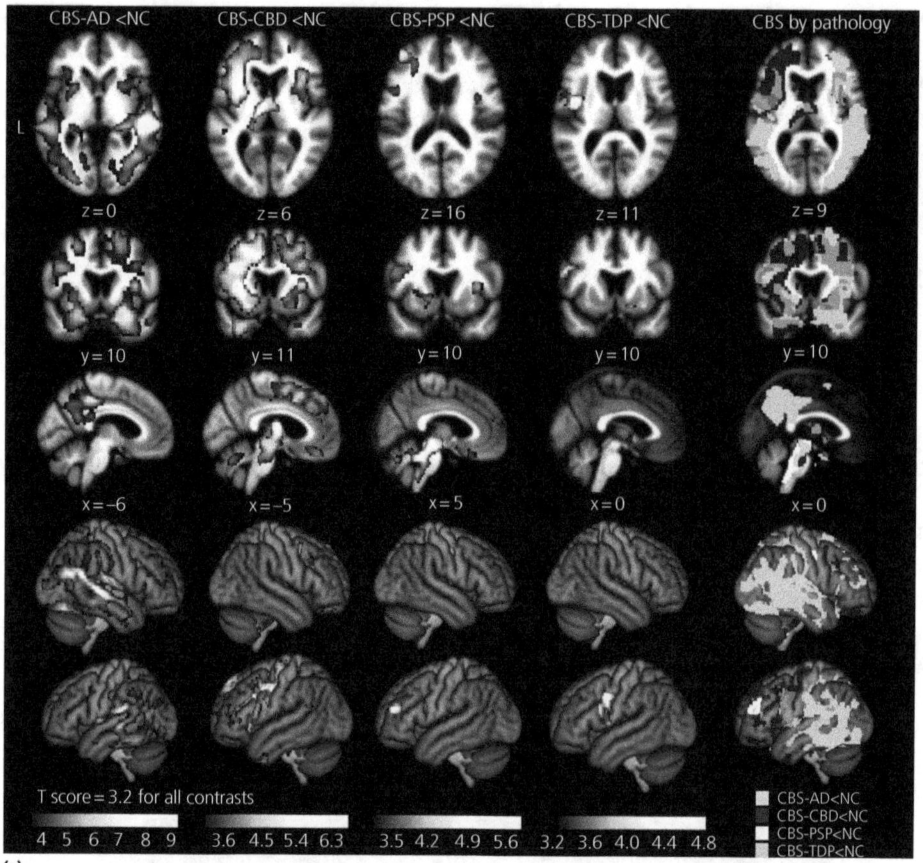

Figure 7.6 SPM5 VBM analysis showing the patterns of gray and white matter volume loss in **(a)** left panel: each CBS subgroup, all with autopsy studies (CBS-AD ($N=7$), CBS-CBD ($N=11$), CBS-PSP ($N=4$), and CBS-TDP ($N=3$)) relative to healthy controls (NC, $N=44$) and **(b)** right panel: all three CBS subgroups combined relative to NC viewed on a DARTEL-derived template based on 48 healthy controls (voxel resolution: 1 mm). Source: Lee et al. [8]. Reproduced with permission of Wiley. (*See insert for color representation of the figure.*)

patients with CBS regardless of underlying pathology (Figure 7.6) [8, 78]. Underlying FTLD histopathology was associated with atrophy extending into frontal cortex and brainstem, whereas extension into precuneus and temporoparietal cortex correlates with underlying AD.

In PSP, dilation of the third ventricle and prominent dorsal midbrain atrophy, with a diminished anteroposterior diameter, appear, although visual inspection of these structures fails to discriminate PSP from other disorders such as CBD, PD, or multiple system atrophy. Studies quantifying the midbrain anteroposterior diameter reveal mixed results, with some showing complete differentiation between PSP, PD, and MSA [79], while others show overlap between groups [80].

Most imaging studies have examined patients with clinically defined PSP. On VBM analysis in PSP syndrome, frontal [81], pons, thalamus, and striatal atrophy emerge (Figure 7.7) [82]. Atrophy in the midbrain and cerebral peduncles on VBM distinguishes PSP syndrome from clinical PD [83]. A VBM study of 13 patients with autopsy-proven PSP showed subcortical and brainstem atrophy, consistent with previous studies, but also atrophy in premotor cortex and supplementary motor area [63]. Similarly, all imaging studies with diffusion-weighted imaging and DTI and magnetic resonance spectroscopy have been performed in PSP syndrome, and the clinical diagnostic utility of such imaging modalities remains uncertain [84a].

Amyloid PET imaging was recently FDA approved by the FDA for clinical use and can help identify AD pathology in patients with CBS. Pilot studies of tau PET ligands in order to detect tau pathology in vivo are underway [84b].

Pathology and pathophysiology

CBD

The gross pathology of CBD reveals narrow cortical gyri, most marked in parasagittal and frequently perirolandic cortices, and inferior frontal and temporal cortices; atrophy can be asymmetric [85]. The substantia nigra appears pale. According to a working group supported by the Office of Rare Diseases of the National Institutes of Health (ORD NIH), the minimal pathological features for CBD include cortical and

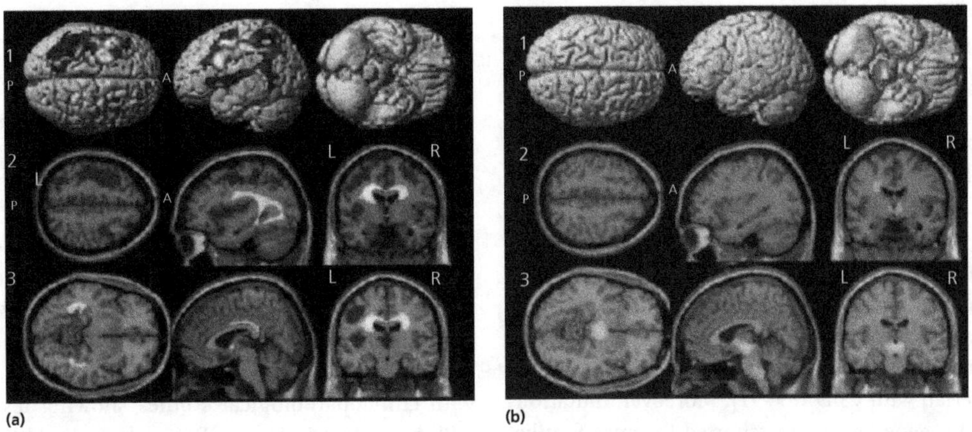

Figure 7.7 Regions of brain atrophy in patients with corticobasal syndrome (CBS) and progressive supranuclear palsy syndrome (PSP-S) relative to controls. VBM-identified regions of decreased gray and white matter volume in 14 CBS and 15 PSP-S patients relative to 80 age-matched control subjects are displayed on a normal adult brain template ($P<0.05$, corrected). **(a)** CBS patients versus controls. **(b)** PSP patients versus controls. Row 1 shows the regions of significant gray matter loss rendered on a healthy subject's brain. Row 2 shows regions of significant gray (displayed in red) and white (displayed in yellow) matter loss relative to controls at the following Montreal Neurological Institute (MNI) coordinates: $x=-33$, $y=-4$, and $z=49$. Row 3 shows regions of significant gray (displayed in red) and white (displayed in yellow) matter loss relative to controls at the following MNI coordinates: $x=5$, $y=-15$, and $z=-8$. A indicates anterior; P, posterior. Source: Boxer et al. [82]. Reproduced with permission of the American Medical Association. *(See insert for color representation of the figure.)*

striatal tau-positive neuronal and glial lesions, with astrocytic plaques and threadlike lesions present both in gray and white matter and neuronal loss in cortical regions and the substantia nigra [2, 86]. Swollen (i.e., achromatic or ballooned) cortical neurons often are present in CBD, but as they are absent in some cases, they were not considered essential for the ORD NIH criteria [86–88]. Coiled bodies, which are tau-positive oligodendroglial inclusions, are found in CBD and PSP, but at a lower density than astrocytic inclusions [85].

Tau protein has six isoforms which harbor either 3 or 4 tubulin-binding repeats, referred to as 3R and 4R isoforms, respectively. Tau inclusions in CBD and PSP are hyperphosphorylated and consist of the 4R tau protein. Tau protein assists in microtubule assembly and stability and is highly expressed in axons. Hyperphosphorylation of tau alters its binding affinity for microtubules and increases its aggregation into multimers [89b, c].

PSP

The gross pathology of PSP reveals mild frontal atrophy but prominent midbrain atrophy, with loss of dopaminergic neurons in the substantia nigra and subthalamic nucleus. The cerebellar dentate nucleus and superior cerebellar peduncle show neuronal loss [95]. On microscopy, characteristics of PSP include neuronal loss, gliosis, and flame-shaped and globose neurofibrillary tangles in the basal ganglia and brainstem. Mild neuronal loss and gliosis occur in the thalamus and striatum and the nucleus basalis of Meynert [96].

Neurofibrillary tangles are composed of paired helical filaments and straight filaments of tau protein [97]. The tangles are similar to those seen in AD; however, they consist nearly entirely of the 4R isoform of the tau protein [13]. Although both CBD and PSP are 4R tauopathies, the biochemical profiles of the tau proteins of each disease have different tau protein cleavage fragments [98, 99]. Gallyas stain and tau immunohistochemistry reveal NFTs in neurons but also argyrophilic, tau-positive inclusions in astrocytes and oligodendrocytes. Tufted astrocytes represent a hallmark of PSP pathology and emerge in the motor cortex and striatum [100, 101]. In oligodendrocytes, tau-positive, argyrophilic, perinuclear fibers appear as coiled bodies [102].

Quantitative studies of tau burden have been performed in PSP to determine whether clinical PSP variants are associated with variations in pathological features [103–105]. Across all subtypes, the subthalamic nucleus, substantia nigra, and globus pallidus are most severely affected by tau pathology [103, 104, 106].

Biomarkers

Because CBD and PSP pathologies are characterized by tau inclusions, several studies have explored CSF total tau and phosphorylated tau levels. Nearly all of these studies were performed with clinically diagnosed patients without autopsy studies, limiting the scope and power of these analyses.

Studies in CBS are mixed, with studies reporting higher CSF total tau levels in CBS than PSP syndrome and controls [111, 112] and others finding no difference between CBS, PSP syndrome, and controls [113, 114]. For PSP syndrome, two studies reported CSF total tau levels within normal range [111, 115].

Other CSF analytes in CBS and PSP syndrome have been studied. Two studies showed no differences in CSF Abeta42 levels in CBS or PSP syndrome compared with controls

[116, 117], although a subsequent study found that levels are reduced in PSP syndrome and CBS [114]. In one blinded study of 70 patients (21 with PSP syndrome), levels of CSF neurofilament heavy chain, a measure of axonal damage, were significantly higher in PSP syndrome compared with PD and controls [118a].

Genetics

The etiology and pathophysiology of CBD and PSP remain unknown. Although CBD is considered a sporadic disease with most patients reporting no family history, patients with *MAPT* mutations may present with CBS and also demonstrate pathological overlap with CBD [89–91]. Moreover, mutations in the progranulin gene have been reported to cause familial CBS [92–94]. Studies of the *MAPT* gene have demonstrated overrepresentation of the H1/H1 *MAPT* haplotype in both CBD and PSP [24, 25].

For PSP, most cases are sporadic, although familial and genetic factors influencing the development of the disease occur in a subset of patients. One study reported that 33% of patients with PSP have a first-degree relative with parkinsonism or dementia [107], and there are strong associations with genetic variants in *MAPT* [24, 108, 109] and chromosome 1q31 [110]. A genome-wide association study for PSP described several new susceptibility genes associated with PSP, but the functional relevance of these genetic loci to PSP pathology remains to be determined [118b].

Treatments

At present, there are no FDA-approved treatments for CBD or PSP. Anti-tau agents are under investigation in clinical trials. In CBS, if the suspected underlying pathology is AD, a trial of an acetylcholinesterase inhibitor may be indicated.

Patients with CBD and PSP are typically unresponsive to dopaminergic medications, such as carbidopa/levodopa, although some report mild benefit, even at low doses, that is often transient [119]. Thus, a trial of levodopa is warranted. Neuroleptic medications should be avoided when possible due to their extrapyramidal side effects and the risk of death. Depression occurs frequently; thus, antidepressant medications are indicated [120]. Many patients benefit from serotonin reuptake inhibitors, perhaps because of an underlying dysfunction in the serotonergic system in PSP and related disorders.

Supportive care measures include speech pathology and dysphagia evaluations to prevent aspiration risk. Dystonia and blepharospasm often are ameliorated with botulinum toxin injections [119]. Physical therapy and exercise aid in maintaining mobility and range of motion; stationary recumbent bicycling might be useful for those with significant fall risk. Occupational therapy and home safety evaluations can help minimize fall risk.

Summary

Corticobasal degeneration and progressive supranuclear palsy are 4R tauopathies with heterogeneous presentations and considerable clinical and pathological overlap. Though historically CBD was initially defined as a movement disorder and motor symptoms eventually emerge at some point during the CBD disease course, clinicopathological series reveal that CBD predominantly involves frontal degeneration with the most common syndromes showing executive dysfunction, nonfluent aphasia, and behavioral presentations. Neuropathologies presenting as CBS range widely, with clinicopathological studies showing less than 40% of CBS having underlying CBD pathology. Although PSP syndrome usually predicts PSP, early diagnosis remains a challenge. As with CBD, early behavioral and cognitive features in PSP are likely underreported. The advent of serological, CSF, and imaging biomarkers such as amyloid and tau PET will be crucial to the diagnosis and monitoring of future treatments.

References

1 Rebeiz, J.J., E.H. Kolodny, and E.P. Richardson, Jr., Corticodentatonigral degeneration with neuronal achromasia. *Arch Neurol*, 1968. **18**(1): p. 20–33.

2 Gibb, W.R., P.J. Luthert, and C.D. Marsden, Corticobasal degeneration. *Brain*, 1989. **112** (Pt 5): p. 1171–92.

3 Riley, D.E., Lane A.E., Lewis A., et al., Cortical-basal ganglionic degeneration. *Neurology*, 1990. **40**(8): p. 1203–12.

4 Constantinidis, J., J. Richard, and R. Tissot, Pick's disease. Histological and clinical correlations. *Eur Neurol*, 1974. **11**(4): p. 208–17.

5 Wakabayashi, K., Oyanagi K., Makifuchi T, et al., Corticobasal degeneration: etiopathological significance of the cytoskeletal alterations. *Acta Neuropathol*, 1994. **87**(6): p. 545–53.

6 Arima, K., Uesugi H., Fujita I., et al., Corticonigral degeneration with neuronal achromasia presenting with primary progressive aphasia: ultrastructural and immunocytochemical studies. *J Neurol Sci*, 1994. **127**(2): p. 186–97.

7 Buee Scherrer, V., Hof P.R., Buee L., et al., Hyperphosphorylated tau proteins differentiate corticobasal degeneration and Pick's disease. *Acta Neuropathol*, 1996. **91**(4): p. 351–9.

8 Lee S.E., Rabinovici G.D., Mayo M.C., et al., Clinicopathological correlations in corticobasal degeneration. *Ann Neurol*, 2011. **70**(2): p. 327–40.

9 Steele, J.C., J.C. Richardson, and J. Olszewski, Progressive supranuclear palsy. A heterogeneous degeneration involving the brain stem, basal ganglia and cerebellum with vertical gaze and pseudobulbar palsy, Nuchal Dystonia and Dementia. *Arch Neurol*, 1964. **10**: p. 333–59.

10 David, N.J., E.A. Mackey, and J.L. Smith, Further observations in progressive supranuclear palsy. *Neurology*, 1968. **18**(4): p. 349–56.

11 Steele, J.C., Progressive supranuclear palsy. *Brain*, 1972. **95**(4): p. 693–704.

12 Litvan, I., Agid Y., Calne D., et al., Clinical research criteria for the diagnosis of progressive supranuclear palsy (Steele-Richardson-Olszewski syndrome): report of the NINDS-SPSP international workshop. *Neurology*, 1996. **47**(1): p. 1–9.
13 Chambers, C.B., Lee J.M., Troncoso J.C., et al., Overexpression of four-repeat tau mRNA isoforms in progressive supranuclear palsy but not in Alzheimer's disease. *Ann Neurol*, 1999. **46**(3): p. 325–32.
14 Boeve, B.F., A.E. Lang, and I. Litvan, Corticobasal degeneration and its relationship to progressive supranuclear palsy and frontotemporal dementia. *Ann Neurol*, 2003. **54** Suppl 5: p. S15–9.
15 Wenning, G.K., Litvan I., Jankovic J., et al., Natural history and survival of 14 patients with corticobasal degeneration confirmed at postmortem examination. *J Neurol Neurosurg Psychiatry*, 1998. **64**(2): p. 184–9.
16 Mahapatra, R.K., Edwards M.J., Schott J.M., et al., Corticobasal degeneration. *Lancet Neurol*, 2004. **3**(12): p. 736–43.
17 Togasaki, D.M. and C.M. Tanner, Epidemiologic aspects. *Adv Neurol*, 2000. **82**: p. 53–9.
18 (a) Morimatsu, M. and K. Negoro, [Provisional diagnostic criteria of corticobasal degeneration (CBD) and the survey of patients with CBD in Japan]. *Rinsho Shinkeigaku*, 2002. **42**(11): p. 1150–3; (b) Armstrong, M.J., Litvan, I., Lang, A.E., et al., Criteria for the diagnosis of corticobasal degeneration. *Neurology*, 2013. **80**(5): p. 496–503.
19 Nath, U., Ben-Shlomo Y., Thomson R.G., et al., The prevalence of progressive supranuclear palsy (Steele-Richardson-Olszewski syndrome) in the UK. *Brain*, 2001. **124**(Pt 7): p. 1438–49.
20 Schrag, A., Y. Ben-Shlomo, and N.P. Quinn, Prevalence of progressive supranuclear palsy and multiple system atrophy: a cross-sectional study. *Lancet*, 1999. **354**(9192): p. 1771–5.
21 Bower, J.H., Maraganore D.M., McDonnell S.K., et al., Incidence of progressive supranuclear palsy and multiple system atrophy in Olmsted County, Minnesota, 1976 to 1990. *Neurology*, 1997. **49**(5): p. 1284–8.
22 Maher, E.R. and A.J. Lees, The clinical features and natural history of the Steele-Richardson-Olszewski syndrome (progressive supranuclear palsy). *Neurology*, 1986. **36**(7): p. 1005–8.
23 Golbe, L.I., Davis P.H., Schoenberg B.S., et al., Prevalence and natural history of progressive supranuclear palsy. *Neurology*, 1988. **38**(7): p. 1031–4.
24 Baker, M., Litvan I., Houlden H., et al., Association of an extended haplotype in the tau gene with progressive supranuclear palsy. *Hum Mol Genet*, 1999. **8**(4): p. 711–5.
25 Houlden, H., Baker M., Morris HR, et al., Corticobasal degeneration and progressive supranuclear palsy share a common tau haplotype. *Neurology*, 2001. **56**(12): p. 1702–6.
26 Verpillat, P., Camuzat A., Hannequin D., et al., Association between the extended tau haplotype and frontotemporal dementia. *Arch Neurol*, 2002. **59**(6): p. 935–9.
27 Hughes, A., D. Mann, and S. Pickering-Brown, Tau haplotype frequency in frontotemporal lobar degeneration and amyotrophic lateral sclerosis. *Exp Neurol*, 2003. **181**(1): p. 12–6.
28 Sobrido, M.J., Abu-Khalil A., Weintraub S., et al., Possible association of the tau H1/H1 genotype with primary progressive aphasia. *Neurology*, 2003. **60**(5): p. 862–4.
29 Conrad, C., Amano N., Andreadis A., et al., Differences in a dinucleotide repeat polymorphism in the tau gene between Caucasian and Japanese populations: implication for progressive supranuclear palsy. *Neurosci Lett*, 1998. **250**(2): p. 135–7.
30 Evans, W., Fung H.C., Steele J., et al., The tau H2 haplotype is almost exclusively Caucasian in origin. *Neurosci Lett*, 2004. **369**(3): p. 183–5.
31 Vanvoorst, W.A., Greenaway M.C., Boeve B.F., et al., Neuropsychological findings in clinically atypical autopsy confirmed corticobasal degeneration and progressive supranuclear palsy. *Parkinsonism Relat Disord*, 2008. **14**(4): p. 376–8.
32 Grimes, D.A., A.E. Lang, and C.B. Bergeron, Dementia as the most common presentation of cortical-basal ganglionic degeneration. *Neurology*, 1999. **53**(9): p. 1969–74.
33 Kertesz, A., McMongale P., Blair M., et al., The evolution and pathology of frontotemporal dementia. *Brain*, 2005. **128**(Pt 9): p. 1996–2005.
34 Murray, R., Neumann M., Forman M.S., et al., Cognitive and motor assessment in autopsy-proven corticobasal degeneration. *Neurology*, 2007. **68**(16): p. 1274–83.
35 Geda, Y.E., Beove B.F., Negash S., et al., Neuropsychiatric features in 36 pathologically confirmed cases of corticobasal degeneration. *J Neuropsychiatry Clin Neurosci*, 2007. **19**(1): p. 77–80.
36 Kertesz, A., Davidson W., McCabe P., et al., Primary progressive aphasia: diagnosis, varieties, evolution. *J Int Neuropsychol Soc*, 2003. **9**(5): p. 710–9.
37 Gorno-Tempini, M.L., Hillis A.E., Weintraub S., et al., Classification of primary progressive aphasia and its variants. *Neurology*, 2011. **76**(11): p. 1006–14.
38 Boeve, B.F., Maraganore D.M., Parisi J.E., et al. Pathologic heterogeneity in clinically diagnosed corticobasal degeneration. *Neurology*, 1999. **53**(4): p. 795–800.
39 Josephs, K.A. and D.W. Dickson, Diagnostic accuracy of progressive supranuclear palsy in the society for progressive supranuclear palsy brain bank. *Mov Disord*, 2003. **18**(9): p. 1018–26.
40 Josephs, K.A., Petersen R.C., Knopman D.S., et al., Clinicopathologic analysis of frontotemporal and corticobasal degenerations and PSP. *Neurology*, 2006. **66**(1): p. 41–8.
41 Rohrer, J.D., Geser F., Zhou J., et al., TDP-43 subtypes are associated with distinct atrophy patterns in frontotemporal dementia. *Neurology*. 2010. **75**(24): p. 2204–11.
42 Rascovsky, K., Hodges J.R., Knopman D., et al., Sensitivity of revised diagnostic criteria for the behavioral variant of frontotemporal dementia. *Brain*. 2011;**134**(Pt 9): p. 2456–77.
43 Ling, H., O'Sullivan S.S., Holton J.L., et al., Does corticobasal degeneration exist? A clinicopathological re-evaluation. *Brain*, 2010. **133**(Pt 7): p. 2045–57.
44 Litvan, I., Agid Y., Goetz C., et al., Accuracy of the clinical diagnosis of corticobasal degeneration: a clinicopathologic study. *Neurology*, 1997. **48**(1): p. 119–25.
45 Hu, W.T., Rippon G.W., Boeve B.F., et al., Alzheimer's disease and corticobasal degeneration presenting as corticobasal syndrome. *Mov Disord*, 2009. **24**(9): p. 1375–9.
46 Shelley, B.P., Hodges J.R., Kipps C.M., et al., Is the pathology of corticobasal syndrome predictable in life? *Mov Disord*, 2009. **24**(11): p. 1593–9.
47 Mackenzie, I.R., Neumann M., Bigio E.H., et al., Nomenclature and nosology for neuropathologic subtypes of frontotemporal lobar degeneration: an update. *Acta Neuropathol*, 2010. **119**(1): p. 1–4.
48 Wadia, P.M. and A.E. Lang, The many faces of corticobasal degeneration. *Parkinsonism Relat Disord*, 2007. **13** Suppl 3: p. S336–40.

49 Josephs, K.A., Duffy J.R., Strand E.A., et al., Clinicopathological and imaging correlates of progressive aphasia and apraxia of speech. *Brain*, 2006. **129**(Pt 6): p. 1385–98.

50 Kertesz, A., Martinez-Lage P., Davidson W., et al., The corticobasal degeneration syndrome overlaps progressive aphasia and frontotemporal dementia. *Neurology*, 2000. **55**(9): p. 1368–75.

51 Schneider, J.A., Watts R.L., Gearing M., et al., Corticobasal degeneration: neuropathologic and clinical heterogeneity. *Neurology*, 1997. **48**(4): p. 959–69.

52 Alladi, S., Xuereb J., Bak T., et al., Focal cortical presentations of Alzheimer's disease. *Brain*, 2007. **130**(Pt 10): p. 2636–45.

53 Rivaud-Pechoux, S., Vidailhet M., Gallouedec G., et al., Longitudinal ocular motor study in corticobasal degeneration and progressive supranuclear palsy. *Neurology*, 2000. **54**(5): p. 1029–32.

54 Garbutt, S., Matlin A., Hellmuth J., et al., Oculomotor function in frontotemporal lobar degeneration, related disorders and Alzheimer's disease. *Brain*, 2008. **131**(Pt 5): p. 1268–81.

55 Vidailhet, M., Rivaud S., Gouider-Khouja N., et al., Eye movements in parkinsonian syndromes. *Ann Neurol*, 1994. **35**(4): p. 420–6.

56 Rottach, K.G., Riley D.E., DiScenna A.O., et al., Dynamic properties of horizontal and vertical eye movements in parkinsonian syndromes. *Ann Neurol*, 1996. **39**(3): p. 368–77.

57 (a) Rivaud-Pechoux, S., Vaidailhet M., Brandel J.P., et al., Mixing pro- and antisaccades in patients with parkinsonian syndromes. *Brain*, 2007. **130**(Pt 1): p. 256–64; (b) Boxer, A.L., Garbutt, S., Seeley, W.W., et al., Saccade abnormalities in autopsy-confirmed frontotemporal lobar degeneration and Alzheimer disease. *Arch Neurol*, (2012). **69**(4): p. 509–517.

58 Graham, N.L., T.H. Bak, and J.R. Hodges, Corticobasal degeneration as a cognitive disorder. *Mov Disord*, 2003. **18**(11): p. 1224–32.

59 Pillon, B., Blin J, Vidailhet M, et al., The neuropsychological pattern of corticobasal degeneration: comparison with progressive supranuclear palsy and Alzheimer's disease. *Neurology*, 1995. **45**(8): p. 1477–83.

60 Belfor, N., Amici S., Boxer A.L., et al., Clinical and neuropsychological features of corticobasal degeneration. *Mech Ageing Dev*, 2006. **127**(2): p. 203–7.

61 Groschel, K., Hauser T.K., Luft A., et al., Magnetic resonance imaging-based volumetry differentiates progressive supranuclear palsy from corticobasal degeneration. *Neuroimage*, 2004. **21**(2): p. 714–24.

62 Hassan, A., Whitwell J.l., Boeve B.F., et al., Symmetric corticobasal degeneration (S-CBD). *Parkinsonism Relat Disord*, 2010. **16**(3): p. 208–214.

63 Josephs, K.A., Whitwell J.L., Dickson D.W., et al., Voxel-based morphometry in autopsy proven PSP and CBD. *Neurobiol Aging*, 2008. **29**(2): p. 280–9.

64 Nath, U., Ben-Shlomo Y., Thomson R.G., et al., Clinical features and natural history of progressive supranuclear palsy: a clinical cohort study. *Neurology*, 2003. **60**(6): p. 910–6.

65 Donker Kaat, L., Boon A.J., Kamphorst W., et al., Frontal presentation in progressive supranuclear palsy. *Neurology*, 2007. **69**(8): p. 723–9.

66 Kertesz, A. and P. McMonagle, Behavior and cognition in corticobasal degeneration and progressive supranuclear palsy. *J Neurol Sci*, 2010. **289**(1–2): p. 138–43.

67 Litvan, I., Mega M.S., Cumming J.L., et al., Neuropsychiatric aspects of progressive supranuclear palsy. *Neurology*, 1996. **47**(5): p. 1184–9.

68 Osaki, Y., Ben-Shlomo Y., Lees A.J., et al., Accuracy of clinical diagnosis of progressive supranuclear palsy. *Mov Disord*, 2004. **19**(2): p. 181–9.

69 Bak, T.H., Caine D., Hearn V.C., et al., Visuospatial functions in atypical parkinsonian syndromes. *J Neurol Neurosurg Psychiatry*, 2006. **77**(4): p. 454–6.

70 Litvan, I., Agid Y., Jankovic J., et al., Accuracy of clinical criteria for the diagnosis of progressive supranuclear palsy (Steele-Richardson-Olszewski syndrome). *Neurology*, 1996. **46**(4): p. 922–30.

71 Golbe, L.I., P.H. Davis, and F.E. Lepore, Eyelid movement abnormalities in progressive supranuclear palsy. *Mov Disord*, 1989. **4**(4): p. 297–302.

72 Batla, A., R. Nehru, and T. Vijay, Vertical wrinkling of the forehead or procerus sign in progressive supranuclear palsy. *J Neurol Sci* **298**(1–2): p. 148–9.

73 Romano, S. and C. Colosimo, Procerus sign in progressive supranuclear palsy. *Neurology*, 2001. **57**(10): p. 1928.

74 Hughes, A.J., Daniel S.E., Ben-Shlomo Y., et al., The accuracy of diagnosis of parkinsonian syndromes in a specialist movement disorder service. *Brain*, 2002. **125**(Pt 4): p. 861–70.

75 Morris, H.R., Gibb G., Katzenschlager R., et al., Pathological, clinical and genetic heterogeneity in progressive supranuclear palsy. *Brain*, 2002. **125**(Pt 5): p. 969–75.

76 Daniel, S.E., V.M. de Bruin, and A.J. Lees, The clinical and pathological spectrum of Steele-Richardson-Olszewski syndrome (progressive supranuclear palsy): a reappraisal. *Brain*, 1995. **118** (Pt 3): p. 759–70.

77 Litvan, I., Grimes D.A., Lang A.E., et al., Clinical features differentiating patients with postmortem confirmed progressive supranuclear palsy and corticobasal degeneration. *J Neurol*, 1999. **246** Suppl 2: p. II1–5.

78 Whitwell, J.L., Jack C.R. Jr, Boeve B.F., et al., Imaging correlates of pathology in corticobasal syndrome. *Neurology*, 2010. **75**(21): p. 1879–87.

79 Oba, H., Yagashita A., Terada H., et al., New and reliable MRI diagnosis for progressive supranuclear palsy. *Neurology*, 2005. **64**(12): p. 2050–5.

80 Quattrone, A., Nicoletti G., Messina D., et al., MR imaging index for differentiation of progressive supranuclear palsy from Parkinson disease and the Parkinson variant of multiple system atrophy. *Radiology*, 2008. **246**(1): p. 214–21.

81 Brenneis, C., Seppi K., Schocke M., et al., Voxel based morphometry reveals a distinct pattern of frontal atrophy in progressive supranuclear palsy. *J Neurol Neurosurg Psychiatry*, 2004. **75**(2): p. 246–9.

82 Boxer, A.L., Geschwind M.D., Belfor N., et al., Patterns of brain atrophy that differentiate corticobasal degeneration syndrome from progressive supranuclear palsy. *Arch Neurol*, 2006. **63**(1): p. 81–6.

83 Price, S., Paviour D., Scahill R., et al., Voxel-based morphometry detects patterns of atrophy that help differentiate progressive supranuclear palsy and Parkinson's disease. *Neuroimage*, 2004. **23**(2): p. 663–9.

84 (a) Stamelou, M., Knake S., Oertel W.H., et al., Magnetic resonance imaging in progressive supranuclear palsy. *J Neurol.* 2011. **258**(4): p. 549–58; (b) Okamura N., Furumoto S., Fodero-Tavoletti M.T., et al. Non-invasive assessment of Alzheimer's disease neurofibrillary pathology using 18F-THK5105 PET. *Brain.* 2014;**137**(Pt 6): p. 1762–71.

85 Cairns, N.J., Bigio E., Mackenzie I.R., et al., Neuropathologic diagnostic and nosologic criteria for frontotemporal lobar degeneration: consensus of the consortium for frontotemporal lobar degeneration. *Acta Neuropathol*, 2007. **114**(1): p. 5–22.

86 Dickson, D.W., Bergeron C., Chin S.S., et al., Office of rare diseases neuropathologic criteria for corticobasal degeneration. *J Neuropathol Exp Neurol*, 2002. **61**(11): p. 935–46.

87 Komori, T., Arai N., Oda M., et al., Astrocytic plaques and tufts of abnormal fibers do not coexist in corticobasal degeneration and progressive supranuclear palsy. *Acta Neuropathol*, 1998. **96**(4): p. 401–8.

88 Feany, M.B. and D.W. Dickson, Widespread cytoskeletal pathology characterizes corticobasal degeneration. *Am J Pathol*, 1995. **146**(6): p. 1388–96.

89 (a) Bugiani, O., Murrell J.R., Giaccone G., et al., Frontotemporal dementia and corticobasal degeneration in a family with a P301S mutation in tau. *J Neuropathol Exp Neurol*, 1999. **58**(6): p. 667–77; (b) Grundke-Iqbal, I., Iqbal, K., Quinlan, M., et al., Microtubule-associated protein tau. A component of Alzheimer paired helical filaments. *J Biol Chem*, 1986. **261**(13), 6084–6089.; (c) Witman, G.B., Cleveland, D.W., Weingarten, M.D., et al., Tubulin requires tau for growth onto microtubule initiating sites. *Proc Natl Acad Sci*, 1976. **73**(11), 4070–4074.

90 Spillantini, M.G., Yoshida H., Rizzini C., et al., A novel tau mutation (N296N) in familial dementia with swollen achromatic neurons and corticobasal inclusion bodies. *Ann Neurol*, 2000. **48**(6): p. 939–43.

91 Rossi, G., Marelli C., Farina L., et al., The G389R mutation in the MAPT gene presenting as sporadic corticobasal syndrome. *Mov Disord*, 2008. **23**(6): p. 892–5.

92 Yu, C.E., Bird T.D., Bekris L.M., et al., The spectrum of mutations in progranulin: a collaborative study screening 545 cases of neurodegeneration. *Arch Neurol*, 2010 **67**(2): p. 161–70.

93 Rohrer, J.D., Beck J., Warren J.D., et al., Corticobasal syndrome associated with a novel 1048_1049insG progranulin mutation. *J Neurol Neurosurg Psychiatry*, 2009. **80**(11): p. 1297–8.

94 Masellis, M., Momeni P., Meschino W., et al., Novel splicing mutation in the progranulin gene causing familial corticobasal syndrome. *Brain*, 2006. **129**(Pt 11): p. 3115–23.

95 Dickson, D.W., Ahmed Z., Algom A.A., et al., Neuropathology of variants of progressive supranuclear palsy. *Curr Opin Neurol*, 2010. **23**(4): p. 394–400.

96 Tagliavini, F., Pilleri G., Bouras C., et al., The basal nucleus of Meynert in patients with progressive supranuclear palsy. *Neurosci Lett*, 1984. **44**(1): p. 37–42.

97 Hauw, J.J., Daniel S.E., Dickson D., et al., Preliminary NINDS neuropathologic criteria for Steele-Richardson-Olszewski syndrome (progressive supranuclear palsy). *Neurology*, 1994. **44**(11): p. 2015–9.

98 Arai, T., Ikeda K, Akiyama H, et al., Identification of amino-terminally cleaved tau fragments that distinguish progressive supranuclear palsy from corticobasal degeneration. *Ann Neurol*, 2004. **55**(1): p. 72–9.

99 Arai, T., Ikeda K., Akiyama H., et al., Intracellular processing of aggregated tau differs between corticobasal degeneration and progressive supranuclear palsy. *Neuroreport*, 2001. **12**(5): p. 935–8.

100 Nishimura, M., Namba Y., Ikeda K., et al., Glial fibrillary tangles with straight tubules in the brains of patients with progressive supranuclear palsy. *Neurosci Lett*, 1992. **143**(1–2): p. 35–8.

101 Matsusaka, H., Ikeda K., Akiyama H., et al., Astrocytic pathology in progressive supranuclear palsy: significance for neuropathological diagnosis. *Acta Neuropathol*, 1998. **96**(3): p. 248–52.

102 Arima, K., Nakamura M., Sunohara N., et al., Ultrastructural characterization of the tau-immunoreactive tubules in the oligodendroglial perikarya and their inner loop processes in progressive supranuclear palsy. *Acta Neuropathol*, 1997. **93**(6): p. 558–66.

103 Williams, D.R., de Silva R., Paviour D.C., et al., Characteristics of two distinct clinical phenotypes in pathologically proven progressive supranuclear palsy: Richardson's syndrome and PSP-parkinsonism. *Brain*, 2005. **128**(Pt 6): p. 1247–58.

104 Williams, D.R., Holton J.L., Strand C., et al., Pathological tau burden and distribution distinguishes progressive supranuclear palsy-parkinsonism from Richardson's syndrome. *Brain*, 2007. **130**(Pt 6): p. 1566–76.

105 Wakabayashi, K. and H. Takahashi, Pathological heterogeneity in progressive supranuclear palsy and corticobasal degeneration. *Neuropathology*, 2004. **24**(1): p. 79–86.

106 Williams, D.R., Holton J.L., Strand K., et al., Pure akinesia with gait freezing: a third clinical phenotype of progressive supranuclear palsy. *Mov Disord*, 2007. **22**(15): p. 2235–41.

107 Donker Kaat, L., Boon A.J., Azmani A., et al., Familial aggregation of parkinsonism in progressive supranuclear palsy. *Neurology*, 2009. **73**(2): p. 98–105.

108 Pittman, A.M., Myers A.J., Abou-Sleiman P., et al., Linkage disequilibrium fine mapping and haplotype association analysis of the tau gene in progressive supranuclear palsy and corticobasal degeneration. *J Med Genet*, 2005. **42**(11): p. 837–46.

109 Rademakers, R., Melquist S., Cruts M., et al., High-density SNP haplotyping suggests altered regulation of tau gene expression in progressive supranuclear palsy. *Hum Mol Genet*, 2005. **14**(21): p. 3281–92.

110 Dickson, D.W., R. Rademakers, and M.L. Hutton, Progressive supranuclear palsy: pathology and genetics. *Brain Pathol*, 2007. **17**(1): p. 74–82.

111 Urakami, K., Wada K., Sasaki H., et al., Diagnostic significance of tau protein in cerebrospinal fluid from patients with corticobasal degeneration or progressive supranuclear palsy. *J Neurol Sci*, 2001. **183**(1): p. 95–8.

112 Mitani, K., Furiya Y., Uchihara T., et al., Increased CSF tau protein in corticobasal degeneration. *J Neurol*, 1998. **245**(1): p. 44–6.

113 Arai, H., Morikawa Y., Higuchi M., et al., Cerebrospinal fluid tau levels in neurodegenerative diseases with distinct tau-related pathology. *Biochem Biophys Res Commun*, 1997. **236**(2): p. 262–4.

114 Noguchi, M., Yoshita M., Matsumoto Y., et al., Decreased beta-amyloid peptide42 in cerebrospinal fluid of patients with progressive supranuclear palsy and corticobasal degeneration. *J Neurol Sci*, 2005. **237**(1–2): p. 61–5.

115 Borroni, B., Malinverno M., Gardoni F., et al., Tau forms in CSF as a reliable biomarker for progressive supranuclear palsy. *Neurology*, 2008. **71**(22): p. 1796–803.

116 Verbeek, M.M., Abdo W.F., De Jong D., et al., Cerebrospinal fluid Abeta42 levels in multiple system atrophy. *Mov Disord*, 2004. **19**(2): p. 238–40; author reply 240–1.

117 Holmberg, B., Johnels B., Blennow K., et al., Cerebrospinal fluid Abeta42 is reduced in multiple system atrophy but normal in Parkinson's disease and progressive supranuclear palsy. *Mov Disord*, 2003. **18**(2): p. 186–90.

118 (a) Brettschneider, J., Petzold A., Sussmuth S.D., et al., Neurofilament heavy-chain NfH(SMI35) in cerebrospinal fluid supports the differential diagnosis of Parkinsonian syndromes. *Mov Disord*, 2006. **21**(12): p. 2224–7; (b) Höglinger, G.U., Melhem, N.M., Dickson, D.W., Sleiman, P.M.A., Wang, L.-S., Klei, L., et al., Identification of common variants influencing risk of the tauopathy progressive supranuclear palsy. *Nat Genet*, 2011. **43**(7), 699–705.

119 Kompoliti, K., Goetz C.G., Litvan I., et al., Pharmacological therapy in progressive supranuclear palsy. *Arch Neurol*, 1998. **55**(8): p. 1099–102.

120 Stamelou, M., de Silva R., Arias-Carrion O., et al., Rational therapeutic approaches to progressive supranuclear palsy. 2010. *Brain*. **133**(Pt 6): p. 1578–90.

CHAPTER 8

Repeat expansion diseases and dementia

Praveen Dayalu[1], Roger L. Albin[1,2] and Henry Paulson[1]
[1] University of Michigan, Ann Arbor, MI, USA
[2] VAAAHS GRECC, Ann Arbor, MI, USA

Introduction

More than 20 neurological disorders are caused by DNA repeat expansions, many of which are associated with neurodegeneration. Relatively few of these disorders, however, will be considered in the patient undergoing evaluation for atypical dementia. The principal reason why these diseases are not high on the differential diagnosis of dementia is that most heritable repeat expansion disorders do not include prominent cortical or subcortical loss as a primary site of degeneration. The most notable exception to this is Huntington's disease (HD), in which progressive cognitive impairment is a hallmark feature. HD is the most common among the nine diseases known to be caused by polyglutamine-encoding CAG repeat expansions. The other eight polyglutamine diseases include six dominantly inherited spinocerebellar ataxias (SCAs 1,2,3,6, 7, and 17), dentatorubral-pallidoluysian atrophy (DRPLA), and the motor neuron disorder, spinobulbar muscular atrophy (SMA). Of the non-HD polyglutamine disorders, only SCA17 typically manifests with progressive cognitive impairment that culminates in dementia, although about a third of SCA2 patients develop dementia as well [1–4]. Whereas most patients with SCA17 also have significant ataxia and cerebellar atrophy, the cognitive symptoms often begin early and sometimes dominate the clinical picture before cerebellar or basal ganglionic signs surface. Other SCAs including SCA1, SCA2, SCA3, and SCA8 can also have cognitive deficits, albeit milder than SCA17, but will not be discussed in this chapter. The other relatively common repeat expansion disease associated with age-related dementia is fragile X-associated tremor/ataxia syndrome (FXTAS), which is caused by a modest noncoding CGG expansion.

We begin with a detailed overview of HD because it is an important and readily diagnosed form of atypical dementia associated with basal ganglionic signs and symptoms. In discussing the differential diagnosis of HD, we touch on other disorders involving the basal ganglia in which cognitive impairment can be prominent, including the much rarer Huntington's disease-like 2 (HDL2) disorder, which is caused by a repeat expansion in a different gene (junctophilin-3). We then briefly discuss SCA17 as the primary SCA in which dementia is a very common, and sometimes presenting, feature. Finally, we discuss FXTAS, which displays broad heterogeneity in phenotype, with progressive movement disorder, ataxia, and cognitive impairment being the most common manifestations. When discussing FXTAS, we remind the reader that among sporadic forms of progressive ataxia associated with cognitive impairment, multiple system atrophy (MSA) is perhaps the most common disorder.

HD

Nosology

History/nomenclature

In 1872, physician George Huntington reported a familial chorea on Long Island, noted previously by his father and grandfather, also physicians [5]. More than a century later, Huntington's vivid writings are a remarkably complete description of the disease that now bears his name. He described chorea as "dancing propensities" in which there "seems to exist some hidden power, something that is playing tricks, as it were, upon the will." At first, this inherited disease began "as an ordinary chorea might begin, by the irregular and spasmodic action of certain muscles as of the face, arms, etc. These movements gradually increase when muscles hitherto unaffected take on the spasmodic action...." He noted that the disease was "confined to ... a few families ... hardly ever manifesting itself until adult or middle life, and then coming on gradually but surely, increasing by degrees, and often occupying years in its development, until the hapless sufferer is but a quivering wreck of his former self." Huntington also commented on the mind, which "becomes more or less impaired, in many amounting to insanity while in others, mind and body both gradually fail until death relieves them of their sufferings."

Non-Alzheimer's and Atypical Dementia, First Edition. Edited by Michael D. Geschwind and Caroline Racine Belkoura.
© 2016 John Wiley & Sons, Ltd. Published 2016 by John Wiley & Sons, Ltd.

Regarding the inheritance pattern, he noted: "When either or both parents have shown manifestations … one or more of the offspring almost invariably suffer from the disease … but if by any chance these children go through a life without it, the thread is broken…." Finally, he noted the relentless, fatal course: "I have never known a recovery … it seems at least to be one of the incurables."

Epidemiology

HD is the most common polyglutamine neurodegenerative disease. In the United States and Canada, approximately 30 000 people carry the diagnosis, and an estimated 150 000 more are at risk. HD is most prevalent in those of European descent, approximately 10–15/100 000 [6, 7]. Pockets of particularly high prevalence, probably due to founder effects, include the Lake Maracaibo region of Venezuela and regions of Scotland and Tasmania [8–10]. Prevalence rates are much lower in populations of non-European ancestry [11]. Males and females are equally at risk. Median age of diagnosis approximates 40, with a wide range in age of onset. Onset before age 20 or after age 65 is relatively rare. Death generally occurs 15–20 years after diagnosis [12]. The combination of typical midlife onset and dominant inheritance pulls entire families down the social scale and devastates the lives of patients, mutation carriers, and unaffected family members alike.

Genetic epidemiology

HD is an autosomal dominant disorder. In the general population, there are on average 17–20 CAG repeats in the HTT gene [13]. With a CAG repeat of 40 or more, a person will develop HD with 100% certainty, but with repeats of 36–39, there is incomplete penetrance. CAG repeat lengths of 6–26 do not cause disease and are thus considered "normal." The intermediate range, from 27 to 35 repeats, does not cause HD with a few reported exceptions [14]. Notably, all alleles of 27 repeats and higher are unstable and prone to expand in future generations, particularly when transmitted by a male parent. Whereas the great majority of HD patients have an affected parent, up to 10% of cases result from new expansions into the disease range [15, 16]. In European populations, there are specific HTT haplotypes, involving polymorphisms in other regions of the gene, that might promote CAG repeat instability [17]. The appearance of earlier and more severe symptoms in successive generations, known as "anticipation," reflects CAG instability with further expansions from one generation to the next.

Case presentation

Sonia H, a waitress aged 42, started drinking whiskey every evening. At first, her husband and sons thought this was related to arguments with her coworkers. A year later, her family noted that she often "flew off the handle" at minor issues. Her boss noted a new tendency to drop platters and break dishes. Others suspected her of illegal substance abuse because of her mildly slurred speech and increasing fidgetiness. At age 44, after she struggled to plan her traditional Thanksgiving dinner, her family brought her to a neurologist.

Sonia's parents were alive and healthy in their 70s. Her older brother was also well. She knew of no more distant family members with a movement disorder, dementia, or prominent psychiatric problems. Her only medications were citalopram for "moods" and omeprazole. She did not smoke. Other than intermittently heavy alcohol, she denied substance abuse.

In the office, she was irritable toward her family, offering curt denials of their reports. When her son described her new compulsion to count cash at home, she snapped, "It isn't your money, so what do you care!" Her speech was irregular in volume and emphasis. She denied involuntary movements, but her family thought she looked "restless." Throughout the interview, there were occasional brief random movements: pursing of her lips, raising of her eyebrows, tilting of her head, extending or flexing a finger or wrist, and inverting a foot.

On the Montreal Cognitive Assessment (MoCA), she scored 23/30. She lost 1 point each for trails test, serial 7s, digits backward, delayed recall, and sentence repetition. She lost 2 points for concrete responses on abstraction. She could not complete the Luria maneuver unless cued verbally: "fist, edge, palm." On motor examination, her involuntary movements were brought out when she counted backward with hands outstretched; in particular, there were "piano-playing" finger movements. She blinked and moved her head when initiating saccades. She could not keep her tongue protruded for a full 10 s; it flicked briefly back into her mouth at 8 s. Finger tapping was slightly slowed on the left. Hand pronation–supination was clumsy bilaterally. Heel–knee–shin was slightly irregular bilaterally. Her gait was stable and narrow based but with occasional random shoulder, trunk, and hand movements creating a vaguely puppetlike appearance. She sidestepped twice in a 10-step tandem walk. On pullback testing, she took 3 steps to maintain her balance.

The neurologist concluded that Sonia had chorea, mild ataxia, and cognitive deficits typical of executive dysfunction. Given her change in personality and behavior, he was most concerned about HD. The lack of a family history, however, was puzzling. His differential diagnosis also included other heredodegenerative diseases (Wilson's disease, neuroacanthocytosis, DRPLA, SCA17), inflammatory disorders (SLE, antiphospholipid antibody syndrome, demyelinating disease, CNS angiitis), unrecognized substance abuse with complications, thyroid disease, or chronic CNS infection (e.g., HIV).

Vitamin B12 level, TSH, and a comprehensive metabolic panel had been unremarkable. The neurologist advised the patient and her family that HD was the most common cause of adult-onset chronic chorea. He informed them that if HD testing was clearly negative, he would initiate a broader workup including brain MRI. The patient and her family were referred to a genetic counselor to discuss the implications of testing for the HD gene.

Testing revealed 44 CAG repeats in one HTT allele and 17 in the other. Sonia received the diagnosis of HD at a subsequent visit, with her family present. Her teenage sons were informed that they, too, were at risk for HD, though they were asymptomatic. The neurologist informed them that after reaching age 18, they could receive predictive testing if they so chose. As to why both of Sonia's elderly parents were unaffected, the neurologist explained that one of them might carry an unstable CAG repeat expansion of less than 40 that was not fully penetrant. Other explanations could include nonpaternity.

Sonia's citalopram was increased to 40 mg per day to help with irritability, anxiety, and obsessions. She was referred to occupational therapy to help her compensate for her decline in coordination. Her husband asked for treatment of her "restlessness"; however, the neurologist noted that Sonia herself was not aware of or disabled by her mild chorea, so he persuaded the family that antichorea therapy was not necessary at this time. He informed the family of support and advocacy resources in HD, as well as research opportunities at the nearby academic medical center.

Clinical features

Overview and natural history

The classic clinical triad in HD is (i) a progressive motor disorder, notably with chorea but also with varying degrees of dystonia, bradykinesia, rigidity, ataxia, dysphagia, and loss of postural reflexes; (ii) progressive cognitive disturbance culminating in dementia; and (iii) various behavioral disturbances including depression, anxiety, apathy, obsessive–compulsive behaviors, outbursts, and occasionally delusions or psychosis. A cognitive or behavioral syndrome is often the first manifestation, a fact that is often clearer in retrospect. Weight loss is another common symptom [18].

Motor disorder

Though chorea is only a small part of motor dysfunction in HD, it remains its most recognizable feature. Chorea often begins as fleeting, suppressible random "fidgety" movements, seen best in the distal extremities. With time, chorea becomes insuppressible and more overt, involving larger and more proximal muscles. Chorea might incorporate fragments of complex purposeful movements such as straightening one's hair. Motor impersistence is often seen in chorea. The "flycatcher's tongue," for example, describes a difficulty in keeping the tongue protruded beyond the lips. Most patients with chorea are not aware of the extent of their involuntary movements; some deny it altogether. Others report that the movements are embarrassing, exhausting, or injurious. In many patients, worsening chorea develops the sinuous, writhing quality known as athetosis. The combination of athetosis and the more rapid movements of chorea is termed choreoathetosis. Severe chorea–choreoathetosis exhibits violent flinging of the limbs or trunk and can be accompanied by traumatic injuries.

Saccadic eye movement abnormalities occur early and persist throughout the disease. Saccades are slow to initiate, often requiring a head movement or a blink to break fixation. Saccadic velocities often become slow as the disease progresses [19]. Patients usually do not complain of associated visual problems.

Ataxia, manifested by dysmetria and dysrhythmia, is common in HD, especially as disease advances. Ataxia might be apparent in speech, finger–nose, and heel–knee–shin testing and a broader-based gait with impaired tandem walking. Dystonia, a more sustained posturing or twisting, is common in HD. Bradykinesia refers to slower and reduced amplitude of movement: for example, diminished facial expression, reduced spontaneous gesturing, reduced finger tap speed and size, reduced arm swing, and small steps. Well before HD manifests, gene-positive individuals show increased variability of voluntary motor measures such as finger tap and tongue protrusion force [20].

There is considerable motor heterogeneity from patient to patient. In general, younger-onset patients are more likely to present with bradykinesia, rigidity, and dystonia; juvenile HD patients may lack chorea altogether and look more like they have Parkinson's disease (PD) (known as the "Westphal variant" of HD). These individuals have a relatively high prevalence of epilepsy [21]. Even within a given HD patient's disease course, the motor abnormalities evolve across a continuum: chorea early in the disease often progresses to superimposed dystonia as the disease advances [22], culminating often in striking bradykinesia, rigidity, and poor postural reflexes in late stages. Progressive motor failure is a major cause of life-ending complications; falls and serious injuries become increasingly common. Weight loss in HD occurs even early in the disease, independent of chorea, and might represent a metabolic or homeostatic alteration due to the disease [23]; dysphagia in late HD only exacerbates this problem.

Cognitive disorder

Dementia is sometimes an underappreciated facet of HD and especially serious because it strikes in the prime of life. Unlike elderly demented adults, HD patients often lack adult children who can assist with planning and care. Marriages and families are disrupted, and children lose an effective parent. With increasing difficulty at work, years of income are lost.

A recent large-scale prospective observational analysis of premanifest persons [24] showed declines in several measures, including working memory, attention, and verbal fluency, consistent with prior studies. These deficits were worse for subjects approaching their expected motor onset. Prediagnosis cognitive impairment, as measured via neuropsychological testing, may serve as an important outcome measure in future clinical trials of potential preventive agents.

By the time of diagnosis, most subjects with HD have cognitive impairment clearly evident on neuropsychological testing. Patients typically have difficulty with multitasking, focus, short-term memory, and learning new skills, although these problems are often first noted by family members. Early in the disease, these difficulties are usually not sufficient to impede most activities of daily living, but those with cognitively demanding jobs often find work increasingly difficult.

Over many years, cognitive impairment eventually progresses to frank dementia in most patients with HD. Unlike Alzheimer dementia, HD dementia is largely "subcortical," marked by slow thought processes, executive dysfunction, and problems with attention and sequencing [25, 26]. Episodic memory, though impaired, is relatively well preserved when compared to Alzheimer's disease (AD), as is language function. The MMSE is ineffective as a screening instrument in HD; the MoCA is considerably more sensitive in this population [27] as it contains more items evaluating executive function and attention. The Luria test (fist–edge–palm) requires good motor sequencing and executive function, so it is impaired particularly early in HD.

Individuals with HD often show striking lack of insight into their own cognitive and motor symptoms, even when these are obvious to others [28]. This might reflect dysfunction of striatal neurons receiving prominent frontal lobe inputs.

Psychiatric disorder

For many HD patients and their families, behavioral problems are the most vexing. These range from affective illness to anxiety disorders to delusional behavior and rarely hallucinations [29, 30]. Psychiatric features and their severity vary tremendously and do not correlate with chorea or dementia [29]. Psychiatric problems are especially problematic in juvenile-onset cases [31].

Most patients experience some behavioral symptoms prior to their diagnosis [32–34]; most common are depression, obsessive–compulsive behaviors, irritability, and outbursts [32, 33]. Personality changes may occur for years prior to the diagnosis, though this may be apparent to families only in retrospect.

Up to 50% of patients are depressed at some point in the disease [35]. Depression often responds very well to treatment, typically SSRI antidepressants. Apathy is also fairly common, though more difficult to treat. Compulsive behaviors in HD may resemble the cognitive rigidity and perseveration typical of frontal lobe disorders and probably reflect striatal dysfunction.

There is a high rate of suicide in gene-positive individuals, both after diagnosis and prediagnosis [36, 37]. Factors increasing suicide risk include being single, lacking children, living alone, being depressed, and showing manifest HD signs [36].

Clinical heterogeneity

There is a remarkable range of ages of onset and symptom features in HD. CAG repeat length is a major factor, correlating inversely with age of onset [38–41]. For the more common smaller repeat lengths (<45), however, there is a much larger variance in age of onset. Other genetic and environmental factors, yet unknown, must also contribute to age of onset.

Repeat length also influences motor phenotype, as early-onset disease is more likely to present with prominent dystonia and bradykinesia, though this may reflect the impact of the mutant allele on developing brains. It is unclear whether repeat length influences the rate of disease *progression*; whereas some studies have not [39], other studies have [42] found correlations. Age may have been a confounder; a more recent analysis showed a stronger correlation between longer repeats and faster decline after adjusting for age [43]. Familial aggregation of certain symptoms (e.g., psychosis) occurs in HD, and this likely reflects genetic modifiers.

Differential diagnosis

Mimics of HD are seen occasionally in clinical practice [44, 45]. The differential diagnosis for chorea alone is extensive and includes acquired entities such as hyperthyroidism, polycythemia vera, lupus, antiphospholipid antibody syndrome, HIV/AIDS, poststreptococcal chorea, anticholinergic and stimulant drug effects, and levodopa-induced dyskinesias in PD. Most such entities can be excluded by history, physical examination, or simple blood tests.

More difficult to distinguish are a few inherited neurodegenerative diseases that might resemble HD. These include dominant disorders such as the polyglutamine diseases, SCA17 and DRPLA; Huntington's disease-like 1 (HDL1), due to a mutation in the gene for the prion protein; HDL2, which is another expanded repeat disorder that closely resembles HD and is quite rare; and the neurodegeneration with brain iron accumulation (NBIA) disease spectrum. Recessive and X-linked disorders in the neuroacanthocytosis family might mimic HD. Molecular diagnoses are available for all these diseases. Because it is treatable, Wilson's disease must be considered in any nonelderly person (<50 years of age) presenting with a movement and cognitive disorder, though a chorea-dominant phenotype is uncommon.

Because HD is the most common progressive choreiform disorder, the simplest strategy is to first test for the HD mutation. This should be performed even if there is no apparent family history; there may be a new mutation, early death, or missing information on a parent, nonpaternity, or undisclosed adoption. If HD is excluded, more extensive testing would then be needed. Establishing an accurate diagnosis is crucial for both patient and family; the implications are vastly different for a dominant versus a recessive disorder, and an accurate diagnosis is required for presymptomatic testing of unaffected adult family members over the age of 18.

If there is a confirmed family history of HD (i.e., an affected parent or sibling with an established genetic diagnosis), mutation testing is generally not required in a patient presenting with motor abnormalities that are unequivocally characteristic of HD. A note of caution, however, is that mild motor anomalies, including subtle chorea, cannot be assumed to be diagnostic of HD simply on the basis of a known family history. Even mutation-negative relatives sometimes appear hyperkinetic, perhaps from behavioral imprinting.

Neuroimaging findings

Currently, neuroimaging is of limited value in the clinical diagnosis of HD. Individuals with many years of manifest HD typically demonstrate obvious caudate atrophy on CT or MRI, altering the contour of and enlarging the lateral ventricles.

Volumetric MRI analyses, performed in ongoing large prospective studies of at-risk subjects, reveal that the most clearly

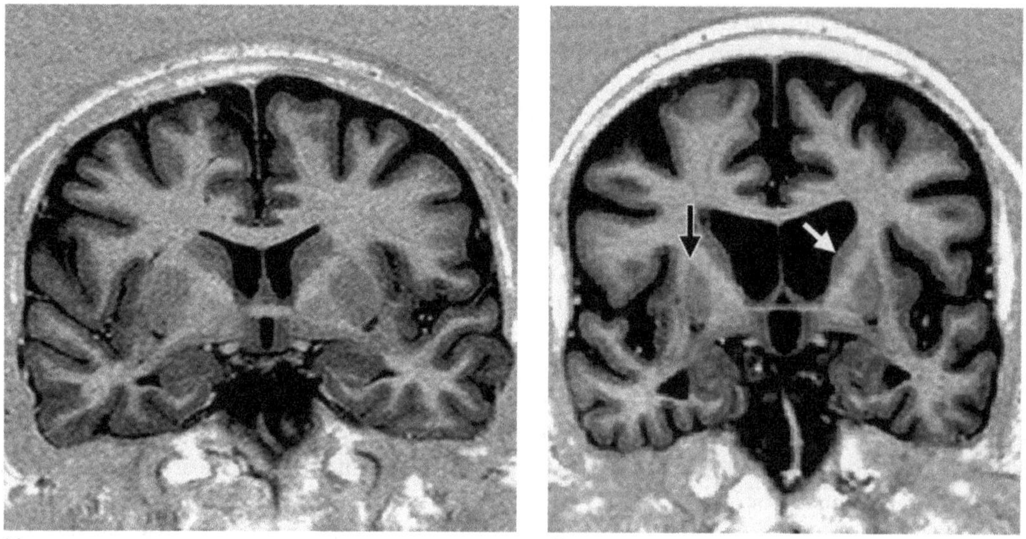
(a) (b)

Figure 8.1 Coronal T1-weighted brain MRI in Huntington's disease. (**a**) Healthy control. (**b**) HD carrier with early-stage (stage 2) disease. MRI shows caudate (white arrow) and putaminal (black arrow) atrophy showing that there is enlargement of the lateral ventricles due to partial degeneration of the caudate nucleus. Source: Mascalchi [48] (TBC). Reproduced with permission of Radiological Society of North America.

measurable and progressive atrophy affects the striatum and global cerebral white matter [46, 47] (see Figure 8.1). These changes occur well before the earliest typical motor features. Cortical atrophy also occurs in asymptomatic subjects [20, 49, 50], changing quantitatively over relatively short intervals (2–3 years), consistent with histopathologic findings of early neocortical degeneration [51]. There is tremendous interest in developing such MRI analyses as biomarkers for use in future clinical trials with premanifest subjects.

PET studies have demonstrated early declines in striatal neurotransmitter markers, particularly dopamine receptors, that occur even in preclinical HD [52–54].

Pathophysiology and pathology

The *HTT* gene

The *HTT* gene on chromosome 4 encodes the protein huntingtin [55], a very large protein that is expressed widely in the CNS and in other tissues. In neurons, it is found largely in somatodendritic and axonal cytoplasm and interacts with many other proteins. Huntingtin is essential for early neuronal development, but its precise functions in adults are unclear. It appears to be important in processes as diverse as protein and vesicular transport, signaling, transcriptional regulation, and apoptosis [56]. How mutant huntingtin initiates neurodegeneration is still unknown, though a toxic gain-of-function mechanism occurring primarily at the protein level is very likely.

Biomarkers

There is tremendous interest in identifying reliable biomarkers to pinpoint HD onset, track its progression, and determine response to treatment. Existing markers are useful but clearly not sufficient; the best known is the Unified Huntington's Disease Rating Scale (UHDRS) [57]. This standardized clinical instrument has four major components: motor, cognition, behavior, and functional ability; it has been widely used in HD clinical trials and observational studies. A subset of the full UHDRS, perhaps supplemented with specific cognitive assessments, might someday constitute a straightforward battery of tests that reliably measures disease onset and progression. Other candidate biomarkers might directly measure an aspect of HD pathophysiology; examples include changes in brain imaging (reviewed earlier), metabolic/proteomic profiles [58, 59], or gene expression changes [60].

Neuropathology

Gross CNS pathology

Huntingtin is expressed by neurons throughout the CNS without dramatic regional differences. Despite this, there is a definite regional pattern to HD pathology [51]. Classically, HD is described as a striatal degeneration. This is only partly true; in advanced cases in which HD pathology has been best studied, widespread degeneration is apparent. Gross striatal atrophy is prominent, but thinning of the cortical mantle and low brain weights and volumes are well documented. Careful studies reveal neuronal loss in many regions including the neocortex, cerebellum, hippocampus, substantia nigra, and brainstem nuclei. There is also diffuse loss of cerebral white matter. These findings are consistent with the many clinical deficits in advanced HD, including pyramidal signs, ataxia, dysarthria, dysphagia, incoordination, and dementia.

Early in the disease, however, striatal degeneration occurs nonuniformly and disproportionately to other brain regions [61]; there are even subregional differences in HD pathology in the striatal complex, with neurodegeneration progressing in caudal to rostral and dorsal to ventral gradients. There is also early degeneration in the neocortex [51].

Striatal pathology

Initial explorations of HD striatal pathology suggested loss of intrinsic GABAergic and cholinergic neurons with relative sparing of extrinsic dopaminergic terminals.

Intrinsic striatal neurons themselves are differentially affected. There are 2 major populations: (i) aspiny interneurons whose projection arbors are restricted to the striatum and (ii) GABAergic medium spiny projection neurons whose primary axons synapse in targets downstream of the striatum. The best studied aspiny neurons are cholinergic, which are virtually spared in HD [62]. Striatal choline acetyltransferase (ChAT) levels decline markedly, however, suggesting significant striatal cholinergic interneuron dysfunction, even in the absence of degeneration. At least one other population of striatal interneurons, those cocontaining somatostatin and neuropeptide Y and expressing high levels of nitric oxide synthase, are relatively spared in HD [63–65]. Recent work has identified progressive depletion of parvalbuminergic interneurons; this is a possible explanation for the emergence of dystonia as HD advances [66].

Subpopulations of medium spiny projection neurons are defined by their primary projection targets, coexpressed neuropeptides, and neurotransmitter receptors. Relatively segregated pools of these neurons project to the external segment of the globus pallidus (GPe), internal segment of the globus pallidus (GPi), substantia nigra dopaminergic pars compacta (SNc), and substantia nigra GABAergic pars reticulata (SNr). Striato-GPe neurons express enkephalins, dopamine D2 receptors, and adenosine A2a receptors, whereas the other striatal projection neuron pools tend to express tachykinins and dopamine D1 receptors. Examination of postmortem HD material suggests a sequential pattern in degeneration of striatal projection neuron subpopulations. The early changes appear to be loss of striato-GPe neurons and perhaps striato-SNr neurons, whereas striato-GPi neurons are relatively spared until late [67–69].

This temporal order of neuronal loss correlates broadly with features of the natural history of HD. As basal ganglia inputs to the superior colliculus come from SNr, the early loss of striato-SNr projection neurons correlates nicely with early saccadic abnormalities. The evolution of involuntary movements in HD also has neuropathologic correlates. Initial degeneration of striato-GPe neurons results in the inhibition of the subthalamic nucleus. Diminished subthalamic activity is associated with chorea. In many patients, disease progression is associated with gradual worsening of chorea, which then peaks in intensity and gradually declines, only to be accompanied by worsening dystonia and bradykinesia. In these later stages, there is generalized loss of striatal projection neurons and probably neurons within other nuclei of the basal ganglia [70]. The striatum is composed of two chemical compartments: the striosome and the matrix. One study looked specifically at a marker of striosomal striatal projection neurons in a broad spectrum of HD postmortem specimens; there appeared to be a correlation between disordered mood and striosomal pathology [71].

Management

HD has no cure. Furthermore, there is no known therapy that slows the degeneration or the rate of clinical decline. This unmet need is a major area of HD research.

Symptomatic pharmacotherapy

HD symptoms respond variably to medications. Psychiatric symptoms, in general, are perhaps the most amenable to pharmacotherapy. Of motor symptoms, chorea is the most readily responsive. Cognitive symptoms and dementia are the least responsive.

Many patients with chorea do not notice it or are not impaired by it. In these cases, reassurance and education (especially of family members) are important. When chorea requires treatment because it affects a patient's quality of life, function, or safety, it responds best to medications that reduce dopaminergic neurotransmission. In the United States, dopamine receptor blockers have been most commonly prescribed. Examples include haloperidol, risperidone, and olanzapine. These agents have the advantage of augmenting treatment for depression and helping with irritability, outbursts, and psychosis. A disadvantage is that typical and atypical antipsychotics increase the risk of sudden cardiac death [72]. The other major option for chorea is the dopamine-depleting agent tetrabenazine, which reduces chorea in a dose-dependent manner [73]. This medication, however, depletes other catecholamines, including serotonin and norepinephrine, so is best avoided in individuals with significant depression, and it sometimes worsens dysphagia. All of these therapies might worsen gait and bradykinesia or cause somnolence. Other medications, such as amantadine, have been reported as modestly beneficial for chorea [74, 75]. Bradykinesia and rigidity in younger-onset individuals can respond to dopaminergic agents used in parkinsonism [76]. Myoclonus, which is rare in HD and sometimes mistaken for chorea, can respond to valproic acid [77].

There is a lack of clinical trials for psychiatric treatments in HD specifically [78]. Most experts agree that depression in HD often responds well to antidepressants, most commonly SSRIs. Obsessive–compulsive behaviors, anxiety, and agitation often respond to SSRIs. Mood stabilizers such as valproate and carbamazepine sometimes help with emotional lability and impulsivity. Buspirone sometimes helps with anxiety. Antipsychotics, both typical and atypical, are used to treat psychosis, delusions, agitation, and outbursts, but doses should be maintained at a minimum to reduce the risk of extrapyramidal side effects. Apathy is currently the target of an ongoing clinical trial of bupropion [79].

Thus far, limited trials of cognitive-enhancing agents used primarily in AD, such as memantine [80], rivastigmine [81], and donepezil [82], have shown only questionable benefit. A trial with latrepirdine (also known as dimebon) in HD recently showed no benefit in cognition or other disease aspects [83].

Nonpharmacologic management

Comprehensive care in HD draws from a range of professionals: primary care physicians, neurologists, psychiatrists, geneticists, physical and occupational therapists, speech pathologists, nutritionists, social workers, and counselors. Nondrug interventions are a critical part of HD management [84].

Physical and occupational therapy are important in HD care. Gait assist devices (such as walkers) and home safety improvements (hazard removal, grab bars, shower chairs, etc.) are also valuable. Speech therapists can evaluate and palliate dysarthria and dysphagia; options include exercises and food consistency modifications. Distractions should be minimized during mealtime so that patients can concentrate on the mechanics of eating and swallowing. Dietary consultation can be a valuable adjunct in dealing with weight loss; high-calorie supplements are often used.

Behavioral symptoms such as apathy and cognitive problems such as executive dysfunction can be ameliorated via structured daily schedules and regular routines. Daytime respite care provides a social outlet for some patients and relieves caregiver burden. Severe dysarthria, rigidity, and bradykinesia can make patients with advanced HD appear more cognitively impaired than they really are. This only adds to frustrations and outbursts from the patient. One should assume that recognition and comprehension are preserved even in advanced HD; clinicians and family members must avoid "talking over" the patient.

The efficacy of nonpharmacologic interventions is often limited by the patient's cognitive and behavioral impairments. As with many aspects of HD, the burden of maximizing benefits from supportive interventions falls on caregivers.

Preventive and neuroprotective approaches

Currently, no therapy is known to delay or prevent the onset of HD or slow its progression. This is a major area of research. High-dose creatine was well tolerated and attenuated the rate of cortical thinning in premanifest HD subjects [85]. Large multicenter clinical trials in manifest HD, for high-dose creatine and coenzyme Q10, are currently in progress.

The ultimate preventive therapy, of course, would involve suppression of the pathologic gene expression within cells. RNA interference (RNAi) paradigms are currently being developed in animals. In one recent study in HD mice, jugular administration of an RNAi construct, using an adeno-associated viral vector, reduced mutant huntingtin expression, atrophy, and inclusion formation within the brain [86]. A major concern with RNAi is the off-target suppression of other normal mRNAs, and work is underway to reduce this risk [87]. Another promising technique uses antisense oligonucleotides (ASO). Infusion of ASO into the cerebrospinal fluid in HD mice reduced huntingtin synthesis and even reversed the disease phenotype [88].

Summary

HD is a relentlessly progressive inherited polyglutamine neurodegeneration causing severe cognitive, motor, and psychiatric disability in the prime of life. It is ultimately fatal in the vast majority of cases. Whereas many of its clinical characteristics can be explained by pathology of the striatum and its connections to the frontal lobes, HD is no longer simply considered a basal ganglia disorder. Current treatment is limited to symptomatic pharmacotherapy for behavioral disturbance and chorea and other supportive cares. A major goal of current research is to identify disease-modifying therapy.

SCA17

Many patients with SCA will admit to cognitive problems, most commonly a slowing of thought processes and difficulty with multitasking [89]. Few, however, develop progressive cognitive impairment culminating in dementia. Among the SCAs, SCA17 is an exception to this general rule [90]. Originally described in Japan, SCA17 was the last of the nine polyglutamine diseases to be discovered [91] and is the rarest among them.

More than any other SCA, SCA17 manifests with widespread cortical, subcortical, and cerebellar dysfunction. Affected persons typically present in young to midadulthood with progressive gait and limb ataxia usually accompanied by significant cognitive impairment, psychiatric symptoms, and various extrapyramidal features including parkinsonism, tremor, dystonia, and occasional chorea [90, 92]; in some cases, SCA17 can be mistaken for HD. More than 80% of SCA17 patients experience significant cognitive deficits, and ataxia is not always a predominant feature. Indeed, behavioral and cognitive symptoms are often the first signs of disease, with frontal lobe signs (executive dysfunction, apathy) being most typical. Thus, SCA17 should be considered in patients with atypical dementia, especially when there is any sign of ataxia or a family history consistent with dominantly inherited ataxia.

An individual evaluated by one of us recently illustrates the atypical dementia that can occur in SCA17. A man in his late 40s was referred for apathy and progressive difficulty with executive function. He was no longer able to hold down a job due to worsening cognitive difficulties and loss of interest in almost all of his normal activities. A workup had been initiated elsewhere, but no diagnosis had been established. There was a family history of unspecified dementia in his deceased father and paternal uncle, but there was no known disease gene in the family.

His mental status exam revealed inattentiveness, depressed affect, bradyphrenia, executive dysfunction, and mild memory impairment. The neurological exam showed hypophonic dysarthria, slowed saccadic initiation, slowed finger opposition, difficulty with tandem gait, and increased deep tendon reflexes. His affected father, by report, did not have ataxia, but the patient's MRI showed global brain atrophy with prominent atrophy of the cerebellum (MRI not available, but please see Figure 8.2 for representative findings). This radiological

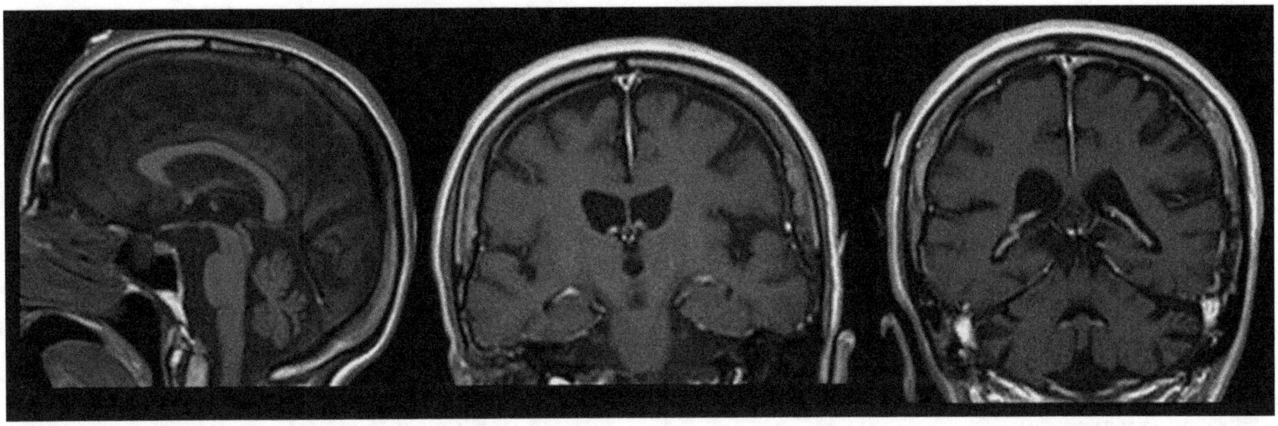

Figure 8.2 T1-weighted brain MRI images from SCA17 patients showing cerebellar atrophy of the vermis and cerebellar hemispheres. Source: Mariotti et al. [93] (TBC). Reproduced with permission of Springer.

finding, together with the slowly progressive limb and gait incoordination and the family history suggestive of a dominantly inherited disease, prompted us to perform gene testing for the SCA17 mutation. SCA17 gene analysis was the single gene test ordered in light of the patient's clinical presentation. The diagnosis of SCA17 was established by finding a CAG expansion of 46 repeats in the *TBP* gene (pathological repeats are greater than 42 CAGs in length). The patient and his mother were informed of this diagnosis and told that his affected father and uncle, in retrospect, must also have suffered from SCA17.

If the SCA17 gene test had instead been negative, we would have considered testing for another polyglutamine disease, DRPLA, because this disease rarely also can manifest in later adulthood with progressive cognitive impairment and cerebellar degeneration [94]. Other testable SCAs were not considered because they are unlikely to cause this patient's constellation of profound cognitive symptoms. The examination and MRI also did not strongly suggest HD as a potential cause. Thus, HD was not highest on the differential diagnosis, though it should be noted that rarely HD is associated with significant cerebellar atrophy.

As seen in many other repeat expansion diseases, SCA17 can show intrafamilial heterogeneity even between individuals with similar or identical repeat lengths. With few exceptions [95], the SCA17 expanded repeat is stably transmitted, thus most affected individuals within a family will share the same repeat length. We later evaluated the patient's affected cousin, who was similar in age and had an identical repeat number. He was also 6–7 years into the course of the disease with prominent limb dystonia but demonstrated far fewer cognitive difficulties.

The treatment of SCA17, a relentlessly progressive and fatal disease, is purely symptomatic at this point. Patients with depression or other psychiatric symptoms often respond to appropriate medications. In the case described previously, his depressive symptoms responded to an SSRI antidepressant, but he continued to display apathy and other frontal lobe features. Because dystonia and parkinsonism are frequent in SCA17, physicians should use caution in prescribing antipsychotics due to the increased potential for serious extrapyramidal side effects.

Fragile X-associated tremor/ataxia syndrome (FXTAS)

FXTAS can be considered the late-onset "cousin" to fragile X mental retardation syndrome, the most common heritable form of mental retardation. In fragile X syndrome, affected males have mental retardation because a fully expanded repeat (>200 repeats) mutation in a noncoding region of the *FMR1* gene silences expression (transcriptional inactivation) of a critical neurodevelopmental protein, FMRP. An intriguing observation made a decade ago is that the grandfathers of males with fragile X syndrome can develop a late-life neurodegenerative syndrome, FXTAS, characterized by progressive tremor, ataxia, and cognitive impairment [96–98]. Because of the particular genetics of fragile X, in which the disease-causing expansion enlarges over three generations, these affected males with FXTAS have a "premutation"-sized repeat (55–200 repeats) at the *FMR1* locus. Until FXTAS was described, premutations were thought not to cause disease.

For several reasons, FXTAS probably remains underrecognized: it was only recently discovered, is highly variable in presentation, and manifests late in life when other confounding neurological symptoms might obscure the recognition of FXTAS as a distinct syndrome. As its name suggests, most affected individuals develop a progressive ataxic gait disturbance with tremor and clumsiness accompanied by cognitive impairment. The cognitive deficits often, but not always, progress to subcortical dementia [99–101]. Because of its X-linked inheritance, FXTAS is more common in men than women. Because women carry two copies of the *FMR1* gene, female premutation carriers are less likely to develop the disease than are male carriers, who only have the premutation allele [102].

Approximately 45% of male carriers will develop FXTAS but only 10–15% of female carriers [103].

FXTAS should be considered as the cause of progressive cognitive impairment in elderly men who also have ataxia, with or without tremor, particularly if there is a family history of mental retardation. In a woman with these same symptoms, FXTAS should be considered if she has a history of a mentally retarded child and/or premature ovarian failure, which is also associated with the *FMR1* premutation. The most common features of disease are gait ataxia, action tremor, and executive dysfunction, with other frequent findings being parkinsonism, psychiatric symptoms (particularly mood and anxiety disorder), peripheral neuropathy, and autonomic dysfunction [96, 97]. The range of symptoms in FXTAS is quite wide, and more severe disease and more profound cognitive disturbance are associated with longer premutation repeats. There is a continuum from unaffected carriers to those with subtle subclinical involvement to those with full-blown dementia and movement disorder [104, 105].

A typical FXTAS case might be a man in his 60s who develops progressive unsteadiness accompanied by a shaking, clumsy hand when he attempts to write, hold a cup, or fasten buttons [106]. The kinetic tremor usually resembles benign essential tremor, but the accompanying ataxia is unusual for essential tremor. The ataxia and tremor are typically accompanied by cognitive disturbances and in some cases by parkinsonism or features reminiscent of the cerebellar form of multiple system atrophy (gait imbalance and mild autonomic dysfunction). The cognitive impairment in FXTAS is primarily frontal and subcortical, with prominent executive dysfunction being a hallmark [99, 100]. It has been described as similar to the frontal component of frontotemporal lobar degeneration, and indeed behavioral symptoms can occur in FXTAS. The brain MRI typically shows global brain atrophy, often with characteristic T2 hyperintensities in the middle cerebellar peduncles (the "MCP sign"; see Figure 8.3). Although the MCP sign suggests FXTAS, it is only seen in approximately 60% of cases and is more common in affected males [107]. Mood and anxiety disorders are higher in individuals with FXTAS than in "nonaffected" premutation carriers and higher in such carriers than in age-matched controls [108]. "Nonaffected" premutation carriers tend to show subtle, subclinical impairment in executive cognitive function, suggesting a forme fruste of the full-blown FXTAS disorder [99, 104].

The reader is reminded that the identification of a premutation in an elderly person has profound implications for his/her family. Because fragile X premutations in an affected male tend to expand into the full range upon transmission through his daughter to the next generation, the male grandsons of a premutation carrier are at high risk for having fragile X mental retardation syndrome.

The FMR1 premutation occurs at a relatively high frequency in the population. Thus, the discovery that the premutation leads to a neurodegenerative disease characterized by tremor and gait ataxia led to speculation that individuals with benign essential tremor, progressive supranuclear palsy, or MSA might prove to have the premutation as the cause of disease. Studies have shown, however, that the FXTAS premutation is not a common cause of essential tremor, PSP, or MSA [96, 97, 109]. In individuals with these disorders who do *not* have radiographic features suggestive of FXTAS or a family history of mental retardation, testing for the FXTAS mutation is of low yield and probably not warranted. The most common cause of slowly progressive ataxia in the absence of a family history of similar disease is the cerebellar subtype of multiple system atrophy (MSA-C). Unlike FXTAS, most individuals with MSA-C do not develop profound cognitive dysfunction

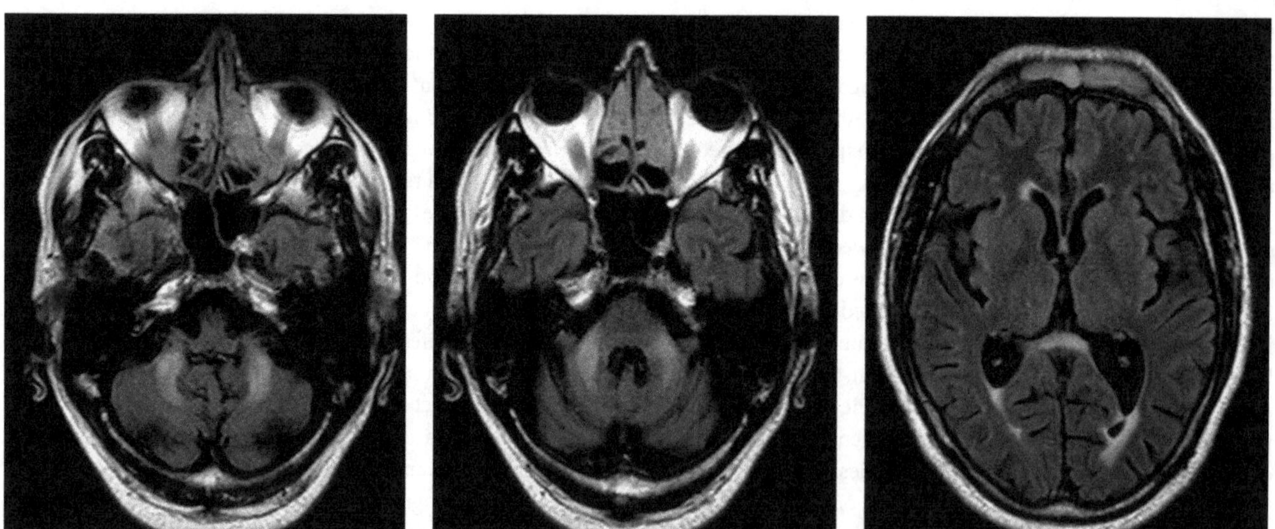

Figure 8.3 FLAIR MRI brain images of a 59-year-old asymptomatic male with the FXTAS premutation. Consecutive images of the posterior fossa highlight the characteristic bilateral signal abnormality of the middle cerebellar peduncles extending into cerebellar white matter. In addition, high FLAIR signal abnormalities are observed in the cerebri and in the splenium of the corpus callosum.

qualifying as dementia. In the elderly patient with clinical features consistent with MSA-C, no family history of mental retardation, and radiographic findings more suggestive of MSA than FXTAS (e.g., the presence of a pontine "hot cross bun" sign and absence of the MCP sign), we would not order genetic testing for the FXTAS premutation.

The pathophysiological mechanism by which the FMR1 premutation causes disease is still uncertain. Full expansion of the *FMR1* CGG repeat silences expression of the FMR1 protein. By contrast, the *FMR1* premutation actually leads to increased levels of the *FMR1* transcript and is thought to cause disease primarily at the RNA level [98]. FXTAS is one of several repeat expansion diseases in which the expanded repeat generates a toxic RNA species [110]. Nevertheless, FXTAS is distinct from other putative toxic RNA diseases in that brains examined at autopsy show prominent, widespread ubiquitin-positive inclusions, suggesting a superimposed proteinopathy as in polyglutamine diseases, PD, AD, and frontotemporal dementia (FTD) [111]. More research is needed to determine the precise pathophysiology in FXTAS and to determine the best approach toward preventive therapy.

Currently, treatment of FXTAS is purely symptomatic. Therapy for mood and anxiety with standard psychoactive medications can be effective, and the parkinsonism sometimes responds to dopaminergic therapy, though less robustly than in idiopathic PD. There is no effective therapy yet for the ataxia, and the action tremor often does not respond to standard treatment for essential tremor.

Summary

DNA repeat expansions cause a variety of neurologic disorders with motor problems, especially ataxia. Relatively few, however, result in cerebral degeneration that is widespread enough to cause progressive cognitive loss resulting in dementia. HD, SCA17, and FXTAS are the most notable exceptions. All three cause a movement disorder, a dementia with frontal/"subcortical" characteristics, and behavioral symptoms. HD and SCA17 present in the prime of life, devastating affected individuals and their families; HD, however, is much more common than SCA17. FXTAS is a disease of middle-aged to older men. Psychiatric symptoms due to these disorders often respond to pharmacotherapy, but the dementia lacks effective therapy. Ataxia is also difficult to treat, but chorea in HD does respond to medications. Genetic testing for each of these disorders is readily available and is highly sensitive and specific.

References

1 Burk K, Globas C, Bosch S, Graber S, Abele M, Brice A, et al. Cognitive deficits in spinocerebellar ataxia 2. *Brain* 1999 APR;**122**: 769–777.

2 Burk K, Globas C, Bosch S, Klockgether T, Zuhlke C, Daum I, et al. Cognitive deficits in spinocerebellar ataxia type 1, 2, and 3. *J Neurol* 2003 FEB;**250**(2):207–211.

3 Durr A, Smadja D, Cancel G, Lezin A, Stevanin G, Mikol J, et al. Autosomal dominant cerebellar ataxia type I in Martinique (French West Indies)—clinical and neuropathological analysis of 53 patients from three unrelated SCA2 families. *Brain* 1995 DEC;**118**:1573–1581.

4 Geschwind D, Perlman S, Figueroa C, Treiman L, Pulst S. The prevalence and wide clinical spectrum of the spinocerebellar ataxia type 2 trinucleotide repeat in patients with autosomal dominant cerebellar ataxia. *Am J Hum Genet* 1997 APR;**60**(4):842–850.

5 Huntington G. On chorea (Reprinted in the medical and surgical reporter: a weekly journal, vol 26, no. 15, April 13, 1872, pp. 317–321). *J Neuropsychiatry Clin Neurosci* 2003 WIN;**15**(1):109–112.

6 Evans SJW, Douglas I, Rawlins MD, Wexler NS, Tabrizi SJ, Smeeth L. Prevalence of adult Huntington's disease in the UK based on diagnoses recorded in general practice records. *J Neurol Neurosurg Psychiatry* 2013 OCT;**84**(10):1156–1160.

7 Fisher ER, Hayden MR. Multisource ascertainment of huntington disease in Canada: Prevalence and population at risk. *Mov Disord* 2014 JAN;**29**(1):105–114.

8 Bolt JMW. Huntington's Chorea in West of Scotland. *Br J Psychol* 1970;**116**(532):259–&.

9 Brothers CRD. Huntingtons Chorea in Victoria and Tasmania. *J Neurol Sci* 1964;**1**(5):405–420.

10 Young AB, Shoulson I, Penney JB, Starostarubinstein S, Gomez F, Travers H, et al. Huntingtons-disease in venezuela—neurologic features and functional decline. *Neurology* 1986 FEB;**36**(2):244–249.

11 Harper PS. The epidemiology of Huntingtons-disease. *Hum Genet* 1992 JUN;**89**(4):365–376.

12 Roos R, Hermans J, Vegtervandervlis M, Vanommen G, Bruyn G. Duration of Illness in Huntington's-disease is not related to age at onset. *J Neurol Neurosurg Psychiatry* 1993 JAN;**56**(1):98–100.

13 Kremer B, Goldberg P, Andrew SE, Theilmann J, Telenius H, Zeisler J, et al. A worldwide study of the Huntingtons-disease mutation—the sensitivity and specificity of measuring cag repeats. *N Engl J Med* 1994 MAY 19;**330**(20):1401–1406.

14 Ha AD, Jankovic J. Exploring the correlates of intermediate CAG repeats in Huntington Disease. *Postgrad Med* 2011 SEP;**123**(5): 116–121.

15 Almqvist EW, Elterman DS, MacLeod PM, Hayden MR. High incidence rate and absent family histories in one quarter of patients newly diagnosed with Huntington disease in British Columbia. *Clin Genet* 2001 SEP;**60**(3):198–205.

16 Falush D, Almqvist EW, Brinkmann RR, Iwasa Y, Hayden MR. Measurement of mutational flow implies both a high new-mutation rate for Huntington disease and substantial underascertainment of late-onset cases. *Am J Hum Genet* 2001 FEB;**68**(2):373–385.

17 Warby SC, Montpetit A, Hayden AR, Carroll JB, Butland SL, Visscher F, et al. CAG expansion in the Huntington disease gene is associated with a specific and targetable predisposing haplogroup. *Am J Hum Genet* 2009 MAR 13;**84**(3):351–366.

18 Obrien C, Miller C, Goldblatt D, Welle S, Forbes G, Lipinski B, et al. Extraneural metabolism in early Huntingtons-disease. *Ann Neurol* 1990 AUG;**28**(2):300–301.

19 Lasker AG, Zee DS, Hain TC, Folstein SE, Singer HS. Saccades in Huntingtons-disease—Initiation defects and distractibility. *Neurology* 1987 MAR;**37**(3):364–370.

20 Tabrizi SJ, Langbehn DR, Leavitt BR, Roos RAC, Durr A, Craufurd D, et al. Biological and clinical manifestations of Huntington's disease in the longitudinal TRACK-HD study: cross-sectional analysis of baseline data. *Lancet Neurol* 2009 SEP;**8**(9):791–801.

21 Landau ME, Cannard KR. EEG characteristics in juvenile Huntington's disease: a case report and review of the literature. *Epileptic Disord* 2003 SEP;**5**(3):145–148.

22 Feigin A, Kieburtz K, Bordwell K, Como P, Steinberg K, Sotack J, et al. Functional decline in Huntingtons-disease. *Mov Disord* 1995 MAR;**10**(2):211–214.

23 Djousse L, Knowlton B, Cupples LA, Marder K, Shoulson I, Myers RH, et al. Weight loss in early stage of Huntington's Disease. *Neurology* 2002 NOV 12;**59**(9):1325–1330.

24 Paulsen JS, Smith MM, Long JD, PREDICT HD Cognitive decline in prodromal Huntington Disease: implications for clinical trials. *J Neurol Neurosurg Psychiatry* 2013 NOV;**84**(11):1233–1239.

25 Paulsen JS, Butters N, Sadek JR, Johnson SA, Salmon DP, Swerdlow NR, et al. Distinct cognitive profiles of cortical and subcortical dementia in advanced illness. *Neurology* 1995 MAY; **45**(5):951–956.

26 Rohrer D, Salmon DP, Wixted JT, Paulsen JS. The disparate effects of Alzheimer's disease and Huntington's disease on semantic memory. *Neuropsychology* 1999 JUL;**13**(3):381–388.

27 Videnovic A, Bernard B, Fan W, Jaglin J, Leurgans S, Shannon KN. The montreal cognitive assessment as a screening tool for cognitive dysfunction in Huntington's disease. *Mov Disord* 2010 FEB 15;**25**(3): 402–404.

28 Hoth KF, Paulsen JS, Moser DJ, Tranel D, Clark LA, Bechara A. Patients with Huntington's disease have impaired awareness of cognitive, emotional, and functional abilities. *J Clin Exp Neuropsychol* 2007;**29**(4):365–376.

29 Paulsen JS, Ready RE, Hamilton JM, Mega MS, Cummings JL. Neuropsychiatric aspects of Huntington's disease. *J Neurol Neurosurg Psychiatry* 2001 SEP;**71**(3):310–314.

30 Caine ED, Shoulson I. Psychiatric syndromes in Huntingtons-disease. *Am J Psychiatry* 1983;**140**(6):728–733.

31 Ribai P, Nguyen K, Hahn-Barma V, Gourfinkel I, Vidailhet M, Legout A, et al. Psychiatric and cognitive difficulties as indicators of juvenile Huntington disease onset in 29 patients. *Arch Neurol* 2007 JUN;**64**(6):813–819.

32 Duff K, Paulsen JS, Beglinger LJ, Langbehn DR, Stout JC, Predict-HD investigators. psychiatric symptoms in Huntington's disease before diagnosis: the predict-HD study. *Biol Psychiatry* 2007 DEC 15;**62**(12):1341–1346.

33 Kirkwood SC, Siemers E, Viken R, Hodes ME, Conneally PM, Christian JC, et al. Longitudinal personality changes among presymptomatic Huntington disease gene carriers. *Neuropsychiatry Neuropsychol Behav Neurol* 2002 SEP;**15**(3):192–197.

34 Kirkwood SC, Siemers E, Viken RJ, Hodes ME, Conneally PM, Christian JC, et al. Evaluation of psychological symptoms among presymptomatic HD gene carriers as measured by selected MMPI scales. *J Psychiatr Res* 2002 NOV–DEC;**36**(6):377–382.

35 Paulsen JS, Nehl C, Hoth KF, Kanz JE, Benjamin M, Conybeare R, et al. Depression and stages of Huntington's disease. *J Neuropsychiatry Clin Neurosci* 2005 FAL;**17**(4):496–502.

36 Lipe H, Schultz A, Bird TD. Risk-Factors for suicide in Huntingtons-disease—a retrospective case-controlled study. *Am J Med Genet* 1993 DEC 15;**48**(4):231–233.

37 Almqvist EW, Bloch M, Brinkman R, Craufurd D, Hayden MR, A worldwide assessment of the frequency of suicide, suicide attempts, or psychiatric hospitalization after predictive testing for Huntington disease. *Am J Hum Genet* 1999 MAY;**64**(5):1293–1304.

38 Stine OC, Pleasant N, Franz ML, Abbott MH, Folstein SE, Ross CA. Correlation between the onset age of Huntingtons-disease and length of the trinucleotide repeat in It-15. *Hum Mol Genet* 1993 OCT;**2**(10):1547–1549.

39 Kieburtz K, Macdonald M, Shih C, Feigin A, Steinberg K, Bordwell K, et al. Trinucleotide repeat length and progression of illness in Huntingtons-disease. *J Med Genet* 1994 NOV;**31**(11):872–874.

40 Andrew SE, Goldberg YP, Kremer B, Telenius H, Theilmann J, Adam S, et al. The relationship between trinucleotide (cag) repeat length and clinical-features of Huntingtons-disease. *Nat Genet* 1993 AUG;**4**(4):398–403.

41 Ashizawa T, Wong LJC, Richards CS, Caskey CT, Jankovic J. Cag repeat size and clinical presentation in Huntingtons-disease. *Neurology* 1994 JUN;**44**(6):1137–1143.

42 Marder K, Sandler S, Lechich A, Klager J, Albert SM. Relationship between CAG repeat length and late-stage outcomes in Huntington's disease. *Neurology* 2002 NOV 26;**59**(10):1622–1624.

43 Rosenblatt A, Kumar BV, Mo A, Welsh CS, Margolis RL, Ross CA. Age, CAG repeat length, and clinical progression in Huntington's disease. *Mov Disord* 2012 FEB;**27**(2):272–276.

44 Rosenblatt A, Ranen NG, Rubinsztein DC, Stine OC, Margolis RL, Wagster MV, et al. Patients with features similar to Huntington's disease, without CAG expansion in huntingtin. *Neurology* 1998 JUL;**51**(1):215–220.

45 Schneider SA, Walker RH, Bhatia KP. The Huntington's disease-like syndromes: what to consider in patients with a negative Huntington's disease gene test. *Nat Clin Pract Neurol* 2007 SEP;**3**(9):517–525.

46 Aylward EH, Nopoulos PC, Ross CA, Langbehn DR, Pierson RK, Mills JA, et al. Longitudinal change in regional brain volumes in prodromal Huntington disease. *J Neurol Neurosurg Psychiatry* 2011 APR;**82**(4):405–410.

47 Tabrizi SJ, Scahill RI, Owen G, Durr A, Leavitt BR, Roos RA, et al. Predictors of phenotypic progression and disease onset in premanifest and early-stage Huntington's disease in the TRACK-HD study: analysis of 36-month observational data. *Lancet Neurol* 2013 JUL; **12**(7):637–649.

48 Mascalchi M. Huntington disease: volumetric, diffusion-weighted, and magnetization transfer MR imaging of brain. *Radiology* 2004; **232**:867–873.

49 Rosas HD, Liu AK, Hersch S, Glessner M, Ferrante RJ, Salat DH, et al. Regional and progressive thinning of the cortical ribbon in Huntington's disease. *Neurology* 2002 MAR 12;**58**(5):695–701.

50 Rosas HD, Hevelone ND, Zaleta AK, Greve DN, Salat DH, Fischl B. Regional cortical thinning in preclinical Huntington disease and its relationship to cognition. *Neurology* 2005 SEP 13;**65**(5):745–747.

51 Vonsattel JPG, DiFiglia M. Huntington disease. *J Neuropathol Exp Neurol* 1998 MAY;**57**(5):369–384.

52 van Oostrom JCH, Maguire RP, Verschuuren-Bemelmans CC, van der Duin LV, Pruim J, Roos RAC, et al. Striatal dopamine D2 receptors, metabolism, and volume in preclinical Huntington disease. *Neurology* 2005 SEP 27;**65**(6):941–943.

53 Weeks RA, Piccini P, Harding AE, Brooks DJ. Striatal D1 and D2 dopamine receptor loss in asymptomatic mutation carriers of Huntington's disease. *Ann Neurol* 1996 JUL;**40**(1):49–54.

54 Ginovart N, Lundin A, Farde L, Halldin C, Backman L, Swahn CG, et al. PET study of the pre- and post-synaptic dopaminergic markers for the neurodegenerative process in Huntington's disease. *Brain* 1997 MAR;**120**:503–514.

55 Macdonald ME, Ambrose CM, Duyao MP, Myers RH, Lin C, Srinidhi L, et al. A novel gene containing a trinucleotide repeat that is expanded and unstable on Huntingtons-disease chromosomes. *Cell* 1993 MAR 26;**72**(6):971–983.

56 Gil JM, Rego AC. Mechanisms of neurodegeneration in Huntington's disease. *Eur J Neurosci* 2008 JUN;**27**(11):2803–2820.

57 Kieburtz K, Penney JB, Como P, Ranen N, Shoulson I, Feigin A, et al. Unified Huntington's disease rating scale: reliability and consistency. *Mov Disord* 1996 MAR;**11**(2):136–142.

58 Dalrymple A, Wild EJ, Joubert R, Sathasivam K, Bjorkqvist M, Petersen A, et al. Proteomic profiling of plasma in Huntington's disease reveals neuroinflammatory activation and biomarker candidates. *J Proteome Res* 2007;**6**(7):2833–2840.

59 Gomez-Anson B, Alegret M, Munoz E, Sainz A, Monte GC, Tolosa E. Decreased frontal choline and neuropsychological performance in preclinical Huntington disease. *Neurology* 2007 MAR 20;**68**(12): 906–910.

60 Borovecki F, Lovrecic L, Zhou J, Jeong H, Then F, Rosas HD, et al. Genome-wide expression profiling of human blood reveals biomarkers for Huntington's disease. *Proc Natl Acad Sci U S A* 2005 AUG 2;**102**(31):11023–11028.

61 Vonsattel JP, Myers RH, Stevens TJ, Ferrante RJ, Bird ED, Richardson EP. Neuropathological classification of Huntingtons-disease. *J Neuropathol Exp Neurol* 1985;**44**(6):559–577.

62 Ferrante RJ, Beal MF, Kowall NW, Richardson EP, Martin JB. Sparing of acetylcholinesterase-containing striatal neurons in Huntingtons-disease. *Brain Res* 1987 MAY 12;**411**(1):162–166.

63 Graveland GA, Williams RS, Difiglia M. Evidence for degenerative and regenerative changes in neostriatal spiny neurons in Huntingtons-disease. *Science* 1985;**227**(4688):770–773.

64 Kowall NW, Ferrante RJ, Martin JB. Patterns of cell loss in Huntingtons-disease. *Trends Neurosci* 1987 JAN;**10**(1):24–29.

65 Shelbourne PF, Keller-McGandy C, Bi WL, Yoon S, Dubeau L, Veitch NJ, et al. Triplet repeat mutation length gains correlate with cell-type specific vulnerability in Huntington disease brain. *Hum Mol Genet* 2007 MAY 15;**16**(10):1133–1142.

66 Reiner A, Shelby E, Wang H, DeMarch Z, Deng Y, Guley NH, et al. Striatal parvalbuminergic neurons are lost in Huntington's disease: implications for dystonia. *Mov Disord* 2013 OCT;**28**(12):1691–1699.

67 Deng YP, Albin RL, Penney JB, Young AB, Anderson KD, Reiner A. Differential loss of striatal projection systems in Huntington's disease: a quantitative immunohistochemical study. *J Chem Neuroanat* 2004 JUN;**27**(3):143–164.

68 Albin RL, Reiner A, Anderson KD, Dure LS, Handelin B, Balfour R, et al. Preferential loss of striato-external pallidal projection neurons in presymptomatic Huntingtons-disease. *Ann Neurol* 1992 APR; **31**(4):425–430.

69 Reiner A, Albin RL, Anderson KD, Damato CJ, Penney JB, Young AB. Differential loss of striatal projection neurons in Huntington disease. *Proc Natl Acad Sci U S A* 1988 AUG;**85**(15):5733–5737.

70 Albin RL, Reiner A, Anderson KD, Penney JB, Young AB. Striatal and nigral neuron subpopulations in rigid Huntingtons-disease—implications for the functional-anatomy of chorea and rigidity-akinesia. *Ann Neurol* 1990 APR;**27**(4):357–365.

71 Tippett LJ, Waldvogel HJ, Thomas SJ, Hogg VM, van Roon-Mom W, Synek BJ, et al. Striosomes and mood dysfunction in Huntington's disease. *Brain* 2007 JAN;**130**:206–221.

72 Ray WA, Chung CP, Murray KT, Hall K, Stein CM. Atypical antipsychotic drugs and the risk of sudden cardiac death. *N Engl J Med* 2009 JAN 15;**360**(3):225–235.

73 Marshall FJ, Walker F, Frank S, Oakes D, Plumb S, Factor SA, et al. Tetrabenazine as antichorea therapy in Huntington disease—a randomized controlled trial. *Neurology* 2006 FEB 14;**66**(3):366–372.

74 Metman LV, Morris MJ, Farmer C, Gillespie M, Mosby K, Wuu J, et al. Huntington's disease—a randomized, controlled trial using the NMDA-antagonist amantadine. *Neurology* 2002 SEP 10;**59**(5): 694–699.

75 O'Suilleabhain P, Dewey RB. A randomized trial of amantadine in Huntington disease. *Arch Neurol* 2003 JUL;**60**(7):996–998.

76 Jongen PJH, Renier WO, Gabreels FJM. 7 cases of Huntingtons-disease in childhood and levodopa induced improvement in the hypokinetic—rigid form. *Clin Neurol Neurosurg* 1980;**82**(4): 251–261.

77 Saft C, Lauter T, Kraus PH, Przuntek H, Andrich JE. Dose-dependent improvement of myoclonic hyperkinesia due to valproic acid in eight Huntington's disease patients: a case series. *BMC Neurol* 2006 FEB 28;**6**:11.

78 Mestre TA, Ferreira JJ. An evidence-based approach in the treatment of Huntington's disease. *Parkinsonism Relat Disord* 2012 MAY;**18**(4):316–320.

79 Gelderblom H, Fischer W, McLean T, Saft C, Reilmann R, Suessmuth S, et al. ACTION-HD: A randomized, double-blind, placebo-controlled prospective crossover trial investigating the efficacy and safety of bupropion in Huntington's disease. *Neurotherapeutics* 2013 JAN;**10**(1):180–181.

80 Beister A, Kraus P, Kuhn W, Dose M, Weindl A, Gerlach M. The *N*-methyl-d-aspartate antagonist memantine retards progression of Huntington's disease. *J Neural Transm Suppl* 2004(**68**):117–122.

81 de Tommaso M, Difruscolo O, Sciruicchio V, Specchio N, Livrea P. Two years' follow-up of rivastigmine treatment in Huntington disease. *Clin Neuropharmacol* 2007 JAN–FEB;**30**(1):43–46.

82 Cubo E, Shannon KM, Tracy D, Jaglin JA, Bernard BA, Wuu J, et al. Effect of donepezil on motor and cognitive function in Huntington disease. *Neurology* 2006 OCT 10;**67**(7):1268–1271.

83 Kieburtz K, Landwehrmeyer GB, Cudkowicz M, Dorsey ER, Feigin A, Hunt V, et al. A randomized, double-blind, placebo-controlled study of latrepirdine in patients with mild to moderate Huntington disease. *JAMA Neurol* 2013 JAN;**70**(1):25–33.

84 Nance MA. Comprehensive care in Huntington's disease—A physician's perspective. *Brain Res Bull* 2007 APR 30;**72**(2–3):175–178.

85 Rosas HD, Doros G, Gevorkian S, Malarick K, Reuter M, Coutu J, et al. PRECREST: A phase II prevention and biomarker trial of creatine in at-risk Huntington disease. *Neurology* 2014 MAR 11; **82**(10):850–857.

86 Dufour BD, Smith CA, Clark RL, Walker TR, McBride JL. Intrajugular vein delivery of AAV9-RNAi prevents neuropathological changes and weight loss in Huntington's disease mice. *Mol Ther* 2014 APR;**22**(4):797–810.

87 Boudreau RL, Spengler RM, Davidson BL. Rational design of therapeutic siRNAs: minimizing off-targeting potential to improve the safety of RNAi therapy for Huntington's disease. *Mol Ther* 2011 DEC;**19**(12):2169–2177.

88 Kordasiewicz HB, Stanek LM, Wancewicz EV, Mazur C, McAlonis MM, Pytel KA, et al. Sustained therapeutic reversal of Huntington's disease by transient repression of huntingtin synthesis. *Neuron* 2012 JUN 21;**74**(6):1031–1044.

89 Kawai Y, Suenaga M, Watanabe H, Sobue G. Cognitive impairment in spinocerebellar degeneration. *Eur Neurol* 2009;**61**(5):257–268.

90 Toyoshima Y, Onodera O, Yamada M, Tsuji S, Takahashi H. Spinocerebellar ataxia type 17. 2005 Mar 29 [updated 2007 Aug 1]. In: Pagon RA, Bird TC, Dolan CR, Stephens K, editors. *GeneReviews* [Internet]. http://www.ncbi.nlm.nih.gov/bookshelf/br.fcgi?book=gene&part=sca17 (accessed August 10, 2015).

91 Nakamura K, Jeong SY, Uchihara T, Anno M, Nagashima K, Nagashima T, et al. SCA17, a novel autosomal dominant cerebellar ataxia caused by an expanded polyglutamine in TATA-binding protein. *Hum Mol Genet.* 2001 **10**(14):1441–8.

92 Bruni AC, Takahashi-Fujigasaki J, Maltecca F, Foncin JF, Servadio A, Casari G, et al. Behavioral disorder, dementia, ataxia, and rigidity in a large family with TATA box-binding protein mutation. *Arch Neurol.* 2004 **61**(8):1314–20.

93 Mariotti C, Alpini D, Fancellu R, Soliveri P, Grisoli M, Ravaglia S, et al. Spinocerebellar ataxia type 17 (SCA17): Oculomotor phenotype and clinical characterization of 15 Italian patients. *J Neurol* 2007 NOV;**254**(Issue 11):1538–1546.

94 Wardle M, Morris HR, Robertson NP. Clinical and genetic characteristics of non-Asian dentatorubral-pallidoluysian atrophy: a systematic review. *Mov Disord.* 2009 **24**(11):1636–40.

95 Rasmussen A, De Biase I, Fragoso-Benítez M, Macías-Flores MA, Yescas P, Ocho A, et al. Anticipation and intergenerational repeat instability in spinocerebellar ataxia type 17. *Ann Neurol.* 2007 **61**(6):607–10.

96 Leehey MA. Fragile X-associated tremor/ataxia syndrome: clinical phenotype, diagnosis, and treatment. *J Invest Med.* 2009 **57**(8):830–6.

97 Berry-Kravis E, Abrams L, Coffey SM, Hall DA, Greco C, Gane LW, et al. Fragile X-associated tremor/ataxia syndrome: clinical features, genetics, and testing guidelines. *Mov Disord.* 2007 **22**(14):2018–30.

98 Garcia-Arocena D, Hagerman PJ. Advances in understanding the molecular basis of FXTAS. *Hum Mol Genet.* 2010 **19**(R1):R83–9.

99 Brega AG, Goodrich G, Bennett RE, Hessl D, Engle K, Leehey MA, et al. The primary cognitive deficit among males with fragile X-associated tremor/ataxia syndrome (FXTAS) is a dysexecutive syndrome. *J Clin Exp Neuropsychol.* 2008 **30**(8):853–69.

100 Grigsby J, Brega AG, Leehey MA, Goodrich GK, Jacquemont S, Loesch DZ, et al. Impairment of executive cognitive functioning in males with fragile X-associated tremor/ataxia syndrome. *Mov Disord.* 2007 **22**(5):645–50.

101 Gonçalves MR, Capelli LP, Nitrini R, Barbosa ER, Porto CS, Lucato LT, et al. Atypical clinical course of FXTAS: rapidly progressive dementia as the major symptom. *Neurology.* 2007 **68**(21):1864–6.

102 Jacquemont S, Hagerman RJ, Leehey MA, Hall DA, Levine RA, Brunberg JA, et al. Penetrance of the fragile X-associated tremor/ataxia syndrome in a premutation carrier population. *JAMA.* 2004 **291**(4):460–9.

103 Rodriguez-Revenga L, Madrigal I, Pagonabarraga J, Xunclà M, Badenas C, Kulisevsky J, et al. Penetrance of FMR1 premutation associated pathologies in fragile X syndrome families. *Eur J Hum Genet* 2009 **17**:1359–62.

104 Grigsby J, Brega AG, Engle K, Leehey MA, Hagerman RJ, Tassone F, et al. Cognitive profile of fragile X premutation carriers with and without fragile X-associated tremor/ataxia syndrome. *Neuropsychology.* 2008 **22**(1):48–60.

105 Sévin M, Kutalik Z, Bergman S, Vercelletto M, Renou P, Lamy E, et al. Penetrance of marked cognitive impairment in older male carriers of the FMR1 gene premutation. *J Med Genet.* 2009 **46**(12):818–24.

106 Leehey MA, Berry-Kravis E, Min SJ, Hall DA, Rice CD, Zhang L, et al. Progression of tremor and ataxia in male carriers of the FMR1 premutation. *Mov Disord.* 2007 **22**(2):203–6.

107 Cohen S, Masyn K, Adams J, Hessl D, Rivera S, Tassone F, et al. Molecular and imaging correlates of the fragile X-associated tremor/ataxia syndrome. *Neurology.* 2006 **67**(8):1426–31.

108 Bourgeois JA, Seritan AL, Casillas EM, Hessl D, Schneider A, Yang Y, et al. Lifetime prevalence of mood and anxiety disorders in fragile X premutation carriers. *J Clin Psychiatry.* 2011 **72**(2):175–82

109 Kamm C, Healy DG, Quinn NP, Wüllner U, Moller JC, Schols L, et al. European multiple system atrophy study group. The fragile X tremor ataxia syndrome in the differential diagnosis of multiple system atrophy: data from the EMSA study group. *Brain.* 2005 **128**(Pt 8):1855–60.

110 Todd PK, Paulson HL. RNA-mediated neurodegeneration in repeat expansion disorders. *Ann Neurol.* 2010 Mar;**67**(3):291–300.

111 Greco CM, Berman RF, Martin RM, Tassone F, Schwartz PH, Chang A, et al. Neuropathology of fragile X-associated tremor/ataxia syndrome (FXTAS). *Brain* 2006 **129**(Pt 1):243–55

CHAPTER 9

Prion diseases and rapidly progressive dementias

Leonel T. Takada[1] **and Michael D. Geschwind**[2]
[1]University of Sao Paulo Medical School, Sao Paulo, Brazil
[2]University of California, San Francisco, San Francisco, CA, USA

Rapidly progressive dementias

Rapidly progressive dementias (RPDs) often are defined as disorders that cause progressive cognitive decline (usually with other signs and/or symptoms), in which the interval between the first symptom to the onset of dementia is typically over weeks to months, but almost always less than 2 years [1–6]. Some have defined rapidly progressive neurodegenerative diseases as those in which survival is less than 3 years [3, 4] as opposed to the 9–12 years typical for most neurodegenerative diseases, such as Alzheimer's disease (AD) and frontotemporal dementia (FTD) [7]. RPDs might also be thought of as conditions in which Jakob–Creutzfeldt disease (CJD), the prototypical RPD, is considered in the differential diagnosis.

CJD is the most frequent form of prion disease (PrD) and one of the most common etiologies of RPD [1, 3, 8, 9]. CJD and other PrDs therefore will be the primary focus of this chapter. RPDs can also be caused by a myriad of conditions, many of which are treatable, and thus the evaluation of RPDs is challenging not only for the variety of differential diagnoses but also for the sense of urgency to find a reversible or treatable cause. Potentially reversible conditions that cause RPDs are not infrequent, even at PrD centers [1, 8]. In our UCSF RPD program, whereas PrDs were diagnosed in 62% of the suspected CJD referrals, about 16% had potentially treatable causes (autoimmune, infectious, psychiatric, neoplastic/paraneoplastic, or toxic-metabolic) [1]. At the US National Prion Disease Pathology Surveillance Center (NPDPSC), although 68% of the 1106 autopsied cases were positive for PrDs, 6.1% had potentially treatable conditions (immune mediated, infectious, toxic-metabolic, or neoplastic) [8].

Many of the possible differential diagnoses for RPDs have been discussed in other chapters within this volume; thus, in this chapter, we will briefly discuss the diagnoses not previously covered and provide an algorithm for the clinical evaluation and diagnosis of RPDs.

Prion diseases

Introduction

PrDs are a group of neurodegenerative disorders caused by infectious proteins called prions. The term prion is derived from "proteinaceous infectious particle" and was coined by Stanley Prusiner [10], the 1997 Nobel Prize in Physiology or Medicine laureate for his work on identifying it as the causative agent of transmissible spongiform encephalopathies (TSE). PrD may occur in many species (viz., scrapie in sheep and goat, bovine spongiform encephalopathy [BSE] in cattle, chronic wasting disease in cervids, transmissible mink encephalopathy in minks, feline spongiform encephalopathy in cats, and exotic ungulate encephalopathy in greater kudu, nyala, and oryx) [11], but this chapter will focus on the human forms—for which we will use the single eponym, CJD, when referring to human prion diseases (hPrDs) in general.

CJD was first described in 1921 by the German neurologist and neuropathologist Alfons Jakob [12, 13], who felt his five cases resembled the one published by Hans Creutzfeldt 1 year prior. It is now known that Creutzfeldt's case was not PrD (only two of Jakob's cases are what we now consider CJD) [14]. For years, the disease was referred to as Jakob–Creutzfeldt or Jakob's disease. A prominent PrD researcher, C.J. Gibbs preferred to have the eponym match his own initials, so he began to call the disease Creutzfeldt–Jakob disease (CJD) [15], and the name has largely stuck, although it is historically inaccurate. In this chapter, we will use the eponym Jakob–Creutzfeldt disease but still keep the acronym CJD to avoid often and erroneous associations with the JC virus, causative agent of progressive multifocal leukoencephalopathy.

Currently, hPrDs are classified in three groups: sporadic (85–90% of cases), genetic (10–15%), and acquired (1–3%) [16, 17]. The sporadic forms are called sporadic CJD (sCJD). The genetic forms historically are subdivided into three categories—familial CJD (fCJD), Gerstmann–Sträussler–Scheinker (GSS) disease,

Non-Alzheimer's and Atypical Dementia, First Edition. Edited by Michael D. Geschwind and Caroline Racine Belkoura.
© 2016 John Wiley & Sons, Ltd. Published 2016 by John Wiley & Sons, Ltd.

and fatal familial insomnia (FFI)—and the acquired forms include kuru, iatrogenic CJD (iCJD), and variant CJD (vCJD).

The incidence (which in this case is comparable to mortality rate, because of the short disease duration in CJD) of sCJD is about 1–1.5 per million per year in most developed countries, with some variability from year to year and between countries [17, 18]. The mortality of genetic prion diseases (gPrDs) was calculated in a pooled data from the European countries, Canada, and Australia to be 0.17 per million per year, but with a wide range (0.01–1.07) [17]. The peak age of onset of sCJD occurs around a unimodal relatively narrow peak of about 68 years [19], with an age-of-onset range of 12–98 years [20, 21] (Geschwind, personal communication). CJD is rare in individuals younger than 30 years, and most of those cases are either acquired or genetic [18, 22]. There is no gender preference in sCJD, although there might be a female preponderance, possibly due to females living longer than men, creating a survival bias [18]. In the United States, an incidence 2.5 times higher in Caucasians compared to African Americans was found [18], but other interethnic comparison data is still lacking.

Pathophysiology

Prions

Gajdusek and colleagues were the first to demonstrate that human spongiform encephalopathies were transmissible [23] and, for a long time, slow viruses were thought to be the infective agents. Alper, Pattison, Griffith, and others postulated that the agent causing scrapie did not contain nucleic acid and actually might be a protein [24–27]. Prusiner and colleagues' groundbreaking work helped prove the concept that proteins could act as infections agents [10]. It is now generally accepted that PrDs are caused by the propagation of abnormally conformed infectious proteins called prions (also named PrP^{Sc}, for prion-related protein in which "Sc" comes from scrapie). The normal cellular prion-related protein (PrP^{C}, in which "C" stands for the normal cellular form) is a membrane-bound protein that is predominantly expressed in nervous tissue, but its physiologic function is not entirely known (although it probably plays a role in neuronal development and function) [28, 29]. Interestingly, recently, PrP^{C} has also been implicated in the metabolism of the amyloid-β peptide, one of the main proteins involved in AD pathogenesis [30]. Prion infectivity occurs through a mechanism in which the pathogenic PrP^{Sc} act as a template to convert PrP^{C} into PrP^{Sc} [11, 31], such that when PrP^{Sc}, which has mostly beta-pleated sheet structure, comes in contact with PrP^{C}, which has mostly alpha-helical structure, PrP^{C} is misfolded into the proteinase K-resistant PrP^{Sc}. This new PrP^{Sc} then becomes a template for the conversion of existing PrP^{C}, initiating an exponential, cascade reaction, which leads to neuronal injury and death.

PrDs are unique, as they can occur as sporadic, genetic, and infectious diseases [11]. Though the initial pathogenic step is not clear, sporadic PrD is thought to occur by spontaneous folding of PrP^{C} into PrP^{Sc} (or maybe through a somatic mutation in the PRNP gene) [10, 32]. In gPrD, it is believed that mutations in PRNP gene make PrP^{C} more susceptible to changing conformation into PrP^{Sc} [33]. In the orally acquired forms of PrD (such as kuru and vCJD), a currently accepted mechanism of neuroinvasion starts with the uptake of prions through the intestinal epithelium. Prions then accumulate in the lymphoid tissue before being transported via sympathetic and parasympathetic nerves to the central nervous system (CNS) [34].

Human PrP^{Sc} often is subclassified based on the fragment properties resulting from digestion by proteinase K and running on a Western blot into type 1 and type 2 [35]. Type 1 PrP^{Sc} fragments are approximately 21 kDa and type 2 are approximately 19 kDa in unglycosylated forms. Brains of patients with sCJD can have either or both types [36]. This has implications on clinical and pathological features, as will be briefly discussed below.

Genetics

In humans, the prion-related protein gene (*PRNP*) is located in chromosome 20p13 and is considerably conserved among mammals. Some interspecies sequence variation occurs, however, and might be responsible for the species barrier seen in some experiments on PrD transmissibility, as the differences between the infectious PrP^{Sc} and the host's PrP^{C} appear to influence infectivity and incubation period [32]. For example, the bank vole is very susceptible to prions from many species. Transgenic mice containing bank vole Prnp are much more susceptible than wild-type mice to prions from other species [37].

Only mutations in *PRNP* are known to cause gPrD [38, 39], and there are currently more than 40 known mutations in this gene [32, 40]. The majority of mutations are missense mutations, with the most common mutations being E200K (the most common worldwide), D178N, P102L, and V210I [41–43]. Stop codons, insertions (usually octapeptide repeat insertion (OPRI) mutations), and deletions of *PRNP* are less common causes of gPrD. The pattern of inheritance of gPrD is autosomal dominant and penetrance is usually 100%. Some mutations causing gPrD [44–46] do not have 100% penetrance, however [42]. Among E200K mutation carriers, for example, penetrance appears to be age dependent (i.e., 1% at age 40, close to 100% after the ninth decade of life); as such, it is not uncommon to find older asymptomatic mutation carriers [47, 48].

It is also known that variations (polymorphisms) in *PRNP* influence an individual's susceptibility to develop disease. The most acknowledged and important polymorphism is located in codon 129, which can have either valine (V) or methionine (M) as alleles (and so the three possible combinations are MM, MV, and VV). There is a clear overrepresentation of homozygotes (MM or VV) among PrD patients. Whereas in a normal Caucasian population about 50% are heterozygous (MV), 40% are MM, and <10% VV [49]; in every form of PrD, more than 65% of the patients are either MM or VV [17]. The particularities of codon 129 polymorphisms in each form of PrD will be discussed in the appropriate sections.

Sporadic Jakob–Creutzfeldt disease

Case 1

Mr. F was a 62-year-old right-handed man who started to complain of right foot numbness, and after about a month, he began having balance problems. Three months after onset, his family noticed he was more irritable, and he soon started to have memory problems. His gait continued to worsen and was accompanied by right hand cramps; his cognition also declined with time. During neurological examination (performed 6 months after onset), he was alert and cooperative, and his Mini-Mental State Examination score was 21/30. Neuropsychological testing revealed global cognitive impairment, with relative preservation of visuospatial functions. Neurological exam showed axial and appendicular ataxia, worse on the right. His gait was wide based, with mild postural instability. No involuntary movements were seen, and tone was increased in the upper limbs (right worse than left) only with activation. Motor and sensory examinations were otherwise unremarkable. Past medical history consisted of hypertension and hyperlipidemia. His family history was unremarkable and negative for dementia; his father died at the age of 58 from stroke and his mother had a sudden death at the age of 85. He had three siblings (one brother and two sisters) who were in good health. CSF analysis showed mildly increased protein levels (54 mg/dl; normal 14–45), 14-3-3 protein by Western blot was "ambiguous," and total tau protein level was normal. EEG showed diffuse slowing, but worse on left frontal region. MRI (Figure 9.1) showed restricted diffusion on the DWI and ADC map sequences in caudate nuclei and thalamus. No cortical ribboning was observed in repeated MRIs. Other ancillary testing was unremarkable. He died after 9 months after the onset of symptoms, and autopsy confirmed the diagnosis of probable CJD. It was presumed sporadic, although antemortem *PRNP* testing was done and the results were pending at the time of autopsy.

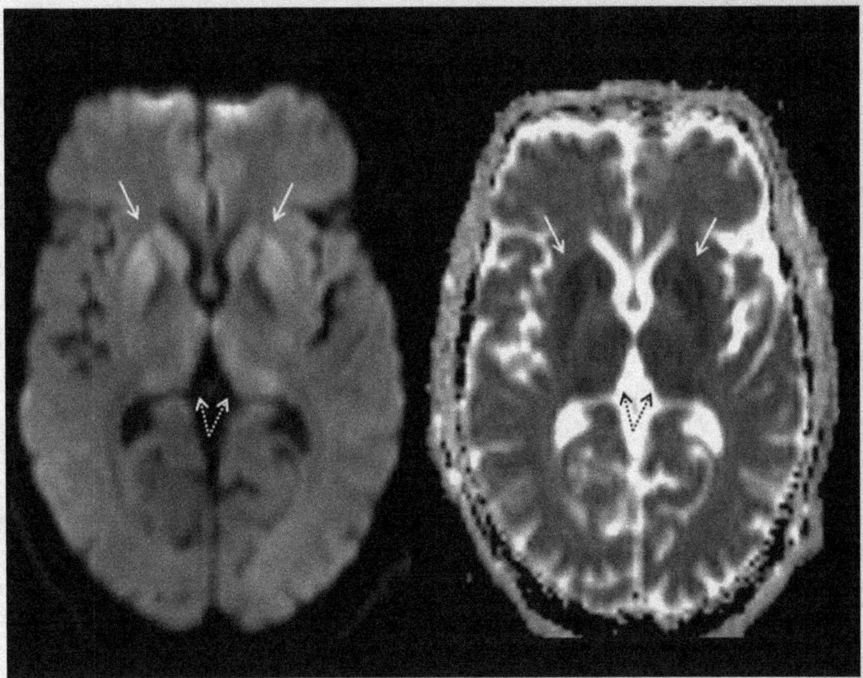

(a) (b)

Figure 9.1 Axial brain MRI of case 1. **(a)** DWI and **(b)** ADC MRI scans showing striatal (solid arrows) and medial-dorsal thalamic (dotted arrows) hyperintensities on DWI imaging, with corresponding ADC hypointensities (arrows) in a patient with probable sCJD.

Clinical features

The clinical presentation of sCJD is highly variable. In most cases, onset is subacute, although in a few cases onset may be acute or stroke-like [50]. In Mr. F's case, the first symptom was unspecific sensory changes, followed by cerebellar symptomatology. Cerebellar symptoms are the initial manifestation in about 20% of cases, as are constitutional symptoms (such as dizziness, headaches, sleep or eating changes, or fatigue) and behavioral symptoms (e.g., depression, irritability) [51]. In about 40% of patients, the initial symptom is cognitive (most commonly presenting as memory problems, executive dysfunction, and/or language impairment) [19, 51]. Visual changes (blurred vision, diplopia, oculomotor changes, visual hallucinations) occur as a first symptom in 10–15% of cases [19, 51, 52]. Extrapyramidal (i.e., parkinsonism, dystonia, myoclonus, chorea) and pyramidal motor symptoms are less frequently seen as the early or presenting manifestation but are more likely to be seen as the disease progresses. Parkinsonism in sCJD might manifest with supranuclear gaze palsy, early gait problems, and/or alien limb, sometimes resembling atypical parkinsonism [53]. Dystonia is rare in AD and dementia with Lewy bodies (DLB) but has been reported to be seen in as many as 20% of sCJD cases [54].

Myoclonus is rarely a presenting symptom but is seen during the clinical course in almost 90% of cases per one large retrospective study [19]. Myoclonus usually starts in a limb and eventually becomes generalized; sometimes, it is associated with periodic sharp wave complexes (PSWCs) on EEG [53]. Seizures (or even status epilepticus) are rarely described as an initial manifestation of sCJD but can occur, usually later, in the disease in a minority (~8–9%) of cases [19, 52, 55]. Clinically evident peripheral neuropathy (including cranial neuropathy) is uncommon in sCJD [56], even though PrP deposits may occasionally be found in the peripheral nerves [56, 57]; certain gPrDs, such as E200K among Libyan Jews, more commonly have neuropathy [58–60].

Symptoms usually follow a rapidly progressive course, and different manifestations are added to the symptomatology throughout the course of the disease. In Mr. F's case, cerebellar ataxia was soon followed by cognitive and behavioral changes, and the neurological examination revealed subtle extrapyramidal signs. The common final pathway of sCJD in most cases is the development of akinetic mutism, the terminal extrapyramidal manifestation [53]. Patients with sCJD and other PrDs usually die from aspiration pneumonia.

Median duration of disease is reported to be around 4–6 months (mean 7 months), and death occurs within 1 year in 90% of cases, with another 5% of patients dying in the second year of disease [19, 61]. Younger age of onset, female gender, and heterozygosity at *PRNP* codon 129 have been associated with longer survival in sCJD [61].

sCJD has been divided into six molecular subtypes based on the polymorphisms at codon 129 in the prion gene (MM, MV, or VV) and the type of protease-resistant prion (type 1 or 2) [35]. This classification, to some extent, separates sCJD cases based on their clinicopathological features. The MM1 and MV1 variants are the most frequent type (60–70% of cases) and are characterized by sCJD with a faster course, with a reported median survival of about 4 months. The VV2 type is characterized by ataxia with a later age of onset and short disease duration (about 6.5 months); the MV2 type is similar to the VV2 but has longer disease duration (17.1 vs. 6.5 months). The VV1 type is the less frequent variant and associated with the earliest age of onset. The MM2 type is further divided into cortical and thalamic type; the MM2 thalamic type is considered by some as the sporadic form of fatal insomnia. Since this classification scheme was established, it later was reported that type 1 and 2 prions often coexist in the same patient, so this classification scheme will need some revision. Preliminary analysis suggested that MM1/2 type phenotypically falls in between MM1 and MM2 subtypes [35, 36, 62, 63].

Amidst the great variability in clinical presentation, a few sCJD variants are recognized: the Heidenhain variant (less than 10% of sCJD cases; it is characterized by visual symptoms at presentation, such as visual hallucinations or distortions, cortical visual deficits, and/or oculomotor impairment; mostly MM1 [48, 64]), the Brownell–Oppenheimer variant (with ataxia as the presenting and dominant symptom, and lack of EEG PSWCs and deep nuclei hyperintensities [64]), a thalamic variant (sometimes referred to as sporadic fatal insomnia [sFI]; linked to MM2 [65, 66]), the panencephalopathic form (with significant or primary involvement of white matter; described primarily in Japan and only rarely seen in Caucasians [see following text, in neuroimaging] [67, 68]), and an amyotrophic form (with motor neuron disease findings) [69].

More recently, a new form of PrD was described, based on the finding that in a group of cases with similar clinical and neuropathological features, the PrP^{Sc} was more sensitive to proteinase K digestion. Those cases were termed as having variable proteinase-sensitive proteinopathy (VPSP) and are clinically characterized by having aphasia, ataxia, and parkinsonism as prominent manifestations and a longer disease course than sCJD [63, 70, 71].

Diagnostic criteria

The most commonly used diagnostic criteria are the ones proposed by the World Health Organization (WHO) in 1998 [72]. Those criteria do not take into consideration MRI findings (which are the most sensitive diagnostic test for PrD), and so, more recently, two other criteria have been published (see Table 9.1 for a review of all three).

Diagnostic criteria for sCJD are developed primarily for research purposes and aim to obtain the highest accuracy in predicting neuropathologically confirmed CJD. Because of that, the criteria are not particularly sensitive early in the disease course, and most cases will only fulfill diagnostic criteria later in the illness (e.g., akinetic mutism is one of the clinical criteria, despite being a late occurrence). The UCSF criteria for sCJD were first proposed in 2007, and they modified the WHO symptom criteria by substituting MRI for the CSF 14-3-3 protein [2, 73], separating visual and cerebellar symptoms from one another and adding the symptom of higher focal cortical signs. The UCSF CJD MRI criteria were updated in 2011 and are detailed in Table 9.2 [74].

Neuroimaging

Brain MRI is currently the most accurate method for the diagnosis of sCJD, with approximate sensitivity of 92–96% and specificity of 92–94% using diffusion-weighted imaging (DWI) [74, 75]. MRI changes can also be seen very early in the disease course (even though in some cases MRI abnormalities will only appear with repeated MRIs) [75], further enhancing its value for the diagnosis. MRI used for the diagnosis of CJD should always include DWI and apparent diffusion coefficient (ADC) sequences, as DWI findings are far more sensitive than FLAIR and/or T2 sequence abnormalities [74, 75].

There are three major patterns of DWI MRI hyperintensities in sCJD (Figure 9.2): cortical and deep nuclei (68% of cases), predominantly neocortical (24%), and predominantly deep nuclei (primarily the striatum; with or without thalamic changes—the pattern seen in Mr. F's case, Case 1) (5%) [74, 76]. The molecular classification of PrD seems to affect the pattern of MRI

Table 9.1 Diagnostic criteria for sporadic Jakob–Creutzfeldt disease.

WHO 1998 revised criteria [72]	UCSF 2007 criteria [73]	European criteria 2009* [188]
1. Progressive dementia 2. At least 2 of the following four features: a) Myoclonus b) Visual or cerebellar disturbance c) Pyramidal/ extrapyramidal signs d) Akinetic mutism 3. PSWCs on the EEG and/or a positive 14-3-3 CSF assay and a clinical duration to death<2 years 4. No alternative diagnosis on routine investigations	1. Rapidly progressive dementia with at least 2 of the following: a) Myoclonus b) Pyramidal/ extrapyramidal dysfunction c) Visual disturbance d) Cerebellar signs e) Akinetic mutism f) Other higher focal cortical sign† 2. Typical EEG or MRI 3. Routine investigations should not suggest an alternative diagnosis	1. Progressive dementia 2. At least 2 of the following four features: a) Myoclonus b) Visual or cerebellar disturbance c) Pyramidal or extrapyramidal signs d) Akinetic mutism 3. One of more of the following: a) Periodic discharges on the EEG b) A positive 14-3-3 CSF assay and a clinical duration to death<2 years c) High signal abnormalities in caudate nucleus and putamen or at least two cortical regions (temporal/ parietal/occipital, but not frontal, cingulate, insular, or hippocampal) either in DWI or FLAIR MRI d) No alternative diagnosis on routine investigations

* Clinical criteria as originally printed in [188] were erroneous, leaving out myoclonus and putting dementia as one of the four possible features.
† Higher focal cortical signs include such findings or symptoms as apraxia, neglect, acalculia, aphasia, etc.
CSF, cerebrospinal fluid; DWI, diffusion-weighted imaging; EEG, electroencephalogram; FLAIR, fluid-attenuated inversion recovery; MRI, magnetic resonance imaging; PSWCs, periodic sharp wave complexes.

Table 9.2 UCSF 2011 MRI criteria for sCJD.

MRI definitely CJD	DWI>FLAIR hyperintensities in: 1. Classic pathognomonic: cingulate, striatum, and >1 neocortical gyrus (often the precuneus, angular, superior, or middle frontal gyrus). Supportive for deep nuclei involvement: • Striatum with anterior-posterior gradient • Subcortical ADC hypointensity Supportive for cortical involvement: • Asymmetric involvement of midline neocortex or cingulate • Sparing of the precentral gyrus • ADC cortical ribboning hypointensity 2. Cortex only (>3 gyri); see supportive for cortex (above)
MRI probably CJD	1. Unilateral striatum or cortex≤3 gyri; see supportive for deep nuclei (above); see supportive for cortex (above) 2. Bilateral striatum or posteromesial thalamus; see supportive for deep nuclei (above)
MRI probably not CJD	1. Only FLAIR/DWI abnormalities in limbic areas, where hyperintensity can be normal (e.g., insula, anterior cingulate, hippocampi) and ADC map does not show restricted diffusion in these areas 2. DWI hyperintensities due to artifact (signal distortion); see other MRI issues (below) 3. FLAIR>DWI hyperintensities; see other MRI issues (below)
MRI definitely not CJD	1. Normal 2. Abnormalities not consistent with CJD
Other MRI Issues	1. In prolonged courses of sCJD (approximately >1 year), brain MRI might show significant atrophy with loss of DWI hyperintensity, particularly in areas previously with restricted diffusion 2. To help distinguish abnormality from artifact and obtain sequences in multiple directions (e.g., axial and coronal)

Source: Vitali et al. [74]. Reproduced with permission of Wolters Kluwer Health, Inc.
ADC, apparent diffusion coefficient; CJD, Creutzfeldt–Jakob disease; DWI, diffusion-weighted imaging; FLAIR, fluid-attenuated inversion recovery; sCJD, sporadic Creutzfeldt–Jakob disease

involvement [77]. Cortical hyperintensities (or cortical ribboning) can be seen in almost any neocortical region but with relative sparing of the precentral cortex [74]. Figure 9.2b shows an example of a predominantly cortical DWI in sCJD. Deep nuclei hyperintensities usually involve the striatum, often with an anterior-posterior gradient (i.e., the anterior caudate being more hyperintense than the posterior putamen) [74]. Involvement on MRI may be bilateral and symmetric, bilateral but asymmetric, and even completely unilateral. Limbic (i.e., insula, anterior cingulate, hippocampus) hyperintensities may be seen as an additional finding in up to 90% of sCJD cases (with the caveat that these regions are more frequently associated with artifacts and/or false-positive abnormalities), but predominant or isolated limbic abnormalities generally are not characteristic of sCJD and should make one consider a nonprion diagnosis (particularly infectious or autoimmune encephalitis and seizures) [74]. Whenever an area of hyperintensity is questioned to be false positive, adding coronal and sagittal acquisitioned images to the evaluation, as well as searching for correspondent ADC map hypointensities, may be helpful [74].

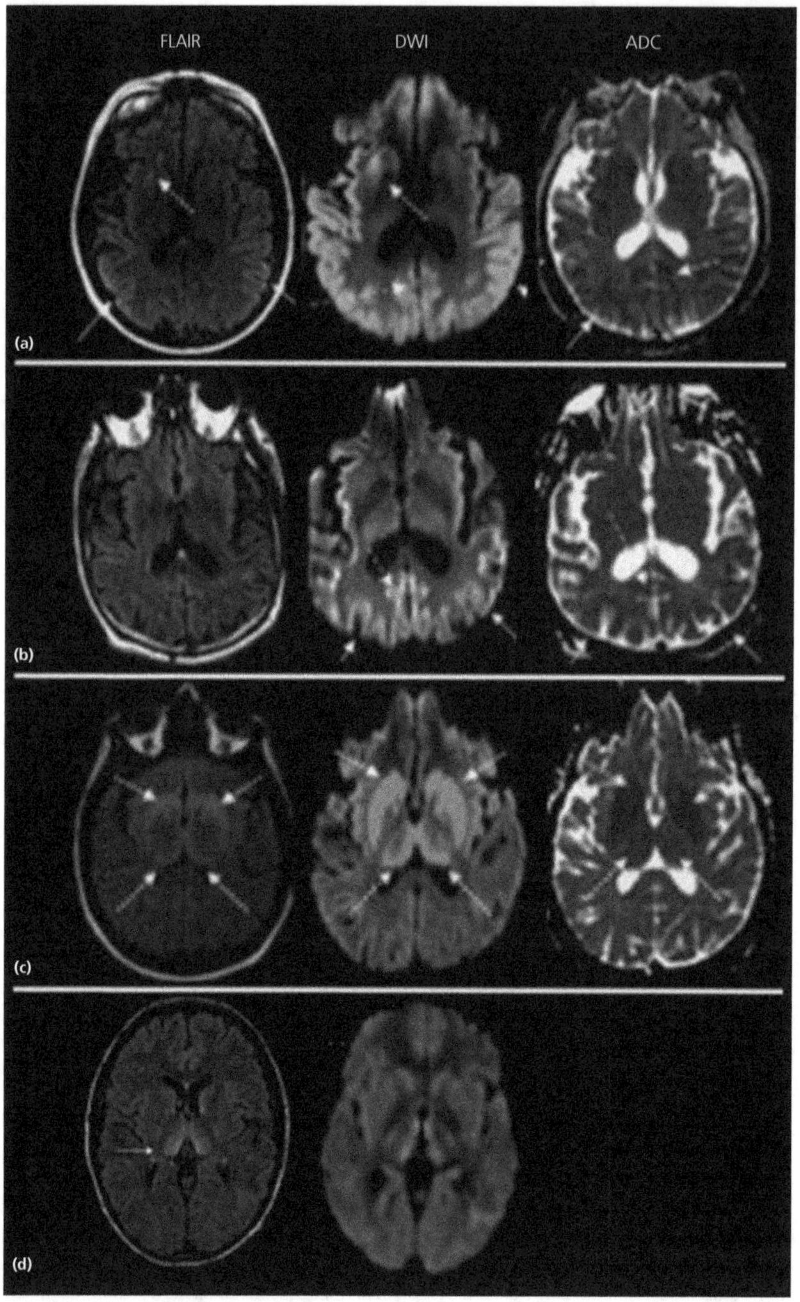

Figure 9.2 Axial brain MRI in sporadic CJD and variant CJD. (**a-c**) Each show a FLAIR, DWI and ADC sequences, whereas d shows only a FLAIR and DWI sequence. (**a**) Neocortical (solid arrow), limbic (dashed arrow) and subcortical (dotted arrow) DWI and FLAIR hyperintensities with corresponding ADC hypointensities in sporadic CJD. (**b**) Neocortical (solid arrow) and limbic (dashed arrow) DWI hyperintensities with corresponding ADC hypointensities in sporadic CJD. (**c**) Subcortical (dotted arrows) DWI and FLAIR hyperintensities, with corresponding ADC hypointensities in sporadic CJD. (**d**) Pulvinar sign (arrow) in variant CJD. ADC, apparent diffusion coefficient; CJD, Creutzfeldt–Jakob disease; DWI, diffusion-weighted imaging; FLAIR, fluid-attenuated inversion recovery; MRI, magnetic resonance imaging. Source: Adapted from Vitali et al. [74, 189]. Reproduced with permission of Wolters Kluwer Health, Inc.

The DWI hyperintensities have a pattern of water diffusion restriction (probably caused by vacuolation [78]), with corresponding hypointensities in the ADC maps. The ADC hypointensities are more easily identified in the deep nuclei but may also be found in cortical regions [74]. Cortical ribboning on DWI can also be seen in viral encephalitis, seizures, status epilepticus, hypo- and hyperglycemia (often with seizures), Wernicke's encephalopathy due to thiamine deficiency, and acute stroke (though usually associated with concomitant white matter abnormalities). Striatal or thalamic DWI hyperintensities with ADC hypointensities have also been described in extrapontine myelinolysis, Wilson's disease, Wernicke's encephalopathy, Bartonella infection, and hyperglycemia with seizures (as reviewed by Vitali et al. [74]) [79–81]. Mitochondrial disease, vasculitis, acute phase of hypoxic ischemic encephalopathy, posterior reversible leukoencephalopathy, and lymphoma may also be considered in the differential diagnosis of DWI hyperintensities [75, 82]. White matter abnormalities are typically absent in sCJD, except in the rare panencephalopathic form of CJD, which is associated with major white matter hyperintensities in T2-weighted MRI [83]. Many feel that the panencephalopathic form of sCJD merely occurs in patients with prolonged courses, often due to life-extending measures such as feeding tubes or intubation, and is due to Wallerian degeneration [67]. With the progression of disease, particularly in patients with disease duration of over 1 year, as atrophy progresses, DWI hyperintensities might fade away and be absent on later MRI scans [74].

Laboratory and EEG findings

Blood tests

There are no currently available clinical blood tests for the diagnosis of CJD. Blood tests, however, are always necessary to exclude other causes of RPD, as will be discussed in the following.

Cerebrospinal fluid

General cerebrospinal fluid (CSF) analysis is typically normal in sCJD, except mildly elevated protein (typically less than 75 mg/dl) is not uncommon. Although elevated protein (>75, <100 mg/dl), pleocytosis (>5 WBC cells), elevated IgG index, or the presence of oligoclonal bands rarely do occur in sCJD [84], their presence should lead to considering other conditions, particularly infectious or autoimmune disorders.

The most common CSF markers used in clinical practice are 14-3-3 protein, total tau (t-tau), and neuron-specific enolase (NSE) (S100β is used primarily in the United Kingdom [85]), but due to great variability in accuracy across studies, the clinical value of each marker is still not entirely clear. A large European study has found the sensitivity and specificity of the 14-3-3 to be 85 and 84%, t-tau (cutoff >1300 pg/ml) 86 and 88%, NSE 73 and 95%, and S100β 82 and 76%, respectively [86], and CSF markers collected later in the disease course seemed to be more sensitive than those collected earlier [87]. Among these three more common biomarkers, t-tau might be the best CSF diagnostic marker for sCJD, although there is still no complete agreement over its cutoff value, which tends to vary between 1150 and 1300 pg/ml. Combining markers also seem to increase their diagnostic value [85, 86].

The 14-3-3 protein is a nonspecific marker for neuronal injury and can be increased in non-PrD, such as cerebrovascular disease, metabolic and hypoxic encephalopathies, brain metastases and CNS infections, or even other neurodegenerative dementias [85, 88]. Overall, the 14-3-3 is not a very specific test; one large study found it to have about 40% specificity for CJD [63]. Among PrDs, 14-3-3 protein is not consistently elevated in genetic and iatrogenic forms [89]. A new assay for detecting prions, called real-time quaking-induced conversion (RT-QuIC), can detect very minute amounts of PrP^{Sc} by using in vitro conversion of PrP^{C} as a substrate [90]. The test is based on a combination of two methods for prion detection—a PCR-like method of amplifying prions called protein misfolding cyclic amplification (PMCA) [91] and an amyloid seeding assay [92]. The sensitivity and specificity of this assay in CSF for sCJD appear to be around 87 and 98%, respectively, based on preliminary studies [93, 94].

Electroencephalogram

A typical EEG in sCJD has sharp, or triphasic, waves (PSWCs) occurring about once every second. This EEG finding, however, is found in only about two-thirds of sCJD patients and usually only after serial EEGs and/or not until later stages of the illness [95]. Often, the only finding is focal or generalized slowing. PSWCs are relatively specific, but they can also be seen in other conditions, including toxic-metabolic and anoxic encephalopathies, progressive multifocal leukoencephalopathy, AD, Lewy body dementia, and Hashimoto's encephalopathy [96, 97].

Neuropathology

Mild atrophy usually is the only gross neuropathological finding in sCJD brains, and it is not always present. The typical neuropathological findings are neuronal loss, gliosis, and vacuolation (or spongiform changes), without inflammatory signs (Figure 9.3). Current diagnostic criteria for definite sCJD also require positive PrP^{Sc} tissue immunoreactivity [98, 99]. PrP amyloid plaques (or kuru plaques) are found in 5–10% of sCJD cases, particularly MV2 [65, 99]. These plaques are more characteristic of GSS, as will be discussed in the following section.

Genetic prion disease

> **Case 1 (continued)**
>
> Even though Mr. F's case was clinically and by brain pathology considered consistent with sporadic CJD, *PRNP* testing by blood test (and later from frozen brain tissue) later revealed an E200K–129M mutation. Upon receiving this information, his siblings requested to be tested for *PRNP* mutations. His older brother was found to carry the E200K mutation, but was asymptomatic at the age of 65, which is not that unexpected as the E200K mutation has approximately 60–96% penetrance, unlike most other *PRNP* mutations which have 100% penetrance [46, 47, 100].

Introduction to gPrD

gPrDs historically have been divided according to clinical and pathological characteristics into three forms: fCJD, GSS, and FFI. Identifying the prion gene, *PRNP*, has helped classify gPrDs more precisely by specific mutations, which include mostly point mutations, but also insertions (octapeptide repeats) and deletions [101]. A caveat to classifying patients by their *PRNP* mutation is that a single *PRNP* mutation can be associated with different phenotypes (and great variability even within a single family) [102]. Some of this variability depends on the codon 129 polymorphism but other unidentified factors as well.

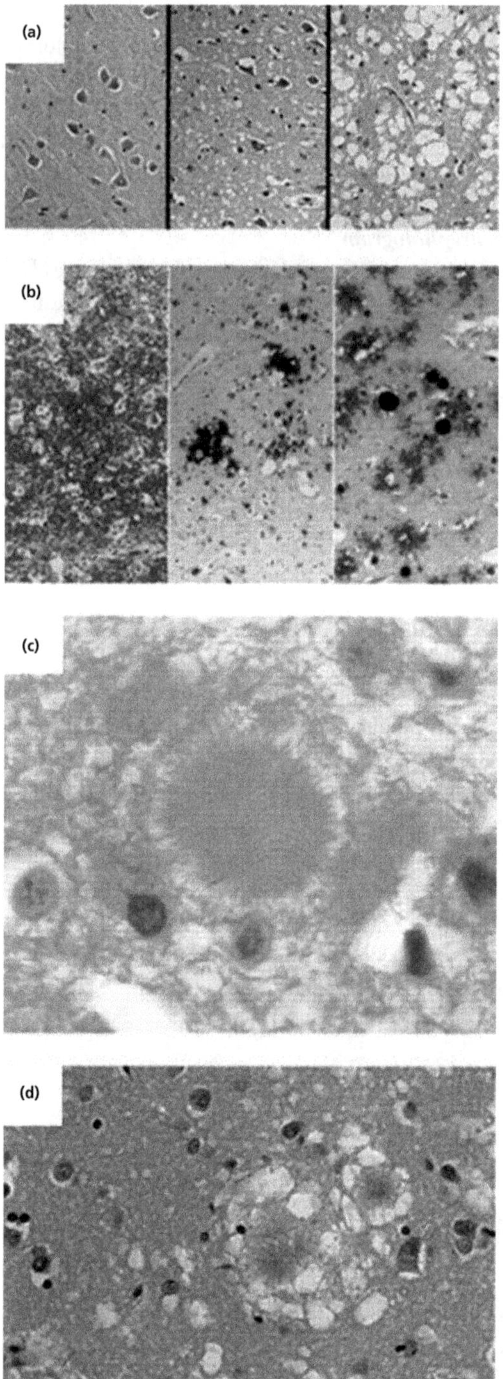

Figure 9.3 Neuropathological findings in prion diseases. **(a)** In sporadic CJD, some brain areas may have no (hippocampal end plate, left), mild (subiculum, middle), or severe (temporal cortex, right) spongiform change. Hematoxylin and eosin (H&E) stain. **(b)** Cortical sections immunostained for PrP^{Sc} in sporadic CJD: synaptic (left), patchy/perivacuolar (middle), or plaque type (right) patterns of PrP^{Sc} deposition. **(c)** Large kuru-type plaque, H&E stain. **(d)** Typical "florid" plaques in vCJD, H&E stain. Source: Adapted from Budka [98]. Reproduced with permission of Oxford University Press. (*See insert for color representation of the figure.*)

Another fundamental issue is that gPrDs are sometimes referred to as familial, but considering that up to 60% of the gPrD cases do not have a positive family history [42], the term "familial" can be misleading. We prefer not to use the term fCJD, as many patients with gCJD or gPrD, a family history of PrD is not known; this can be due to several reasons, including reduced penetrance or misdiagnosis [42, 46]. In those cases of negative family history, often there is a history of family members being (mis) diagnosed with more common neurodegenerative diseases such as AD or Parkinson's disease [42]. Other possibilities are incomplete or age-dependent penetrance [46, 103] (such as in case 1's, Mr. F's, brother and possibly his father, whose death from stroke may have occurred before he would develop CJD symptoms) or incomplete family history (the disease may even be kept secret from younger members of a family; M. Geschwind, personal experience).

Genetic Jakob–Creutzfeldt disease

The clinical features of gCJD are highly variable, and inter- and intrafamiliar variations may be seen (not only the mutation but also codon 129 polymorphism may affect presentation) [65]. As a group and in comparison to sCJD, gCJD is associated with a younger age of onset (typically <55 years; but onset may occur as late as the ninth decade) and longer clinical course [41, 48, 61]. Also, ancillary testing including CSF, EEG, and MRI may not be as sensitive or specific as in sCJD [41, 65, 104].

The E200K mutation is the most frequent *PRNP* mutation worldwide, and higher frequency of this mutation has been found among Libyan Jews and in Slovakia [105]. The clinical features (and neuropathological features) are highly variable, but in general comparable to sCJD, including age of onset and duration of disease [41]. Dementia and ataxia are the most frequently described symptoms, but vertical gaze palsy, polyneuropathy, and sleep changes have also been reported [60].

GSS

Mr. D (Case 2) had the prototypical GSS, which typically presents as a subacute progressive ataxic and/or parkinsonian disorder with later onset of cognitive impairment, and onset most commonly occurs in the fourth to sixth decades (but can occur as early as the twenties [41]). Because it is usually slower than sCJD or many other gPrDs, often with duration of about 5 years (range 3–8 or more years), the differential diagnoses of GSS are ataxic and/or parkinsonian conditions, such as multiple system atrophy, other atypical parkinsonian disorders, idiopathic Parkinson's disease, as well as ataxic disorders such as spinocerebellar ataxias or Huntington's disease. Pyramidal signs may also be found, and lower limb dysesthesia and areflexia may be other associated clinical features, especially in the P102L mutation [106, 107].

There is considerable phenotypic variability within and between mutations and families, and some cases may not even have ataxia as a main characteristic and rather present with early

Case 2

Mr. D. started complaining of balance problems at the age of 57. Symptom onset was gradual, and after a few months, his wife also started noticing an action tremor in his left hand. His gait problems progressed, and he also noticed a change in his voice (as if he had something in his mouth), as well as his handwriting. A neurological exam performed 2 years after symptom onset showed cerebellar ataxia (axial worse than appendicular) and preserved cognition. No pyramidal signs or other involuntary movements were appreciated at that time. An MRI done 2 years after onset was normal (Figure 9.4), and *PRNP* sequencing revealed a P102L mutation. Three years after symptom onset, he was wheelchair bound, and 4 years after onset, cognitive decline ensued. His father and paternal grandfather had progressive gait problems starting in their fifties. One of his four siblings was also affected by similar symptoms at the age of 48. Mr. D died after 5 years of disease, and his autopsy confirmed the diagnosis of GSS.

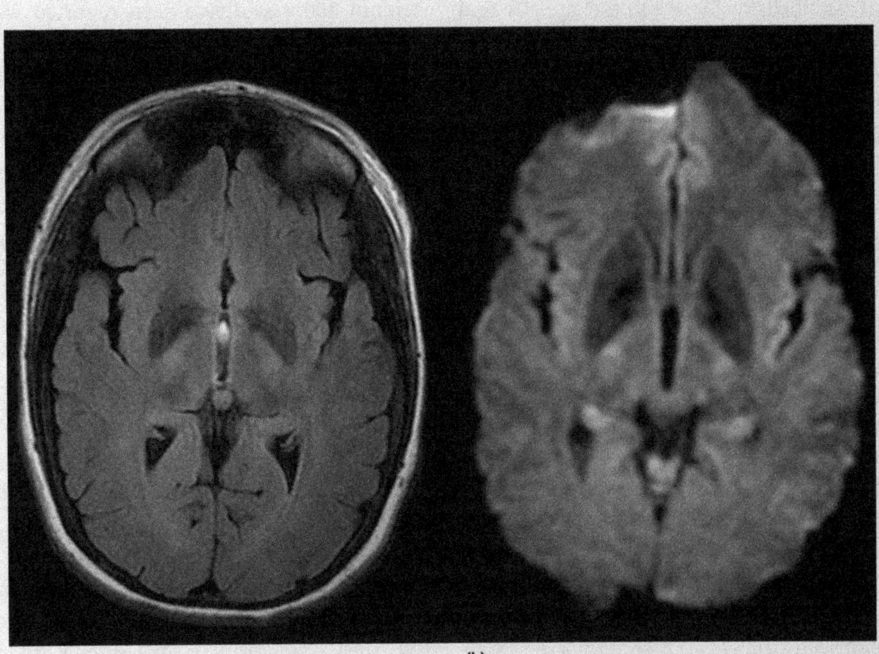

(a) (b)

Figure 9.4 Axial brain MRI of case 2 with GSS due to a P102L mutation in PRNP. (**a**) FLAIR and (**b**) DWI MRI scans show no clear abnormality. There is a suspicion of DWI hyperintensity in the bilateral posterior insula and posterior limb of bilateral hippocampi, which were not, however, hypointense on the ADC map (not shown). Cerebellum was also normal (not shown).

dementia and/or behavioral abnormalities [41, 48]. At least 15 *PRNP* mutations have been shown to cause GSS [102]. EEG in most cases does not show typical CJD findings, and CSF protein 14-3-3 is increased in about 50% of cases [42]. MRI scans are usually normal, and some degree of brain and cerebellar atrophy may be seen with the progression of disease [106]. Cortical ribboning or deep nuclei (striatal or thalamic) hyperintensities on T2/FLAIR or DWI are uncommon findings in GSS but have been reported [106, 108, 109]. Our own study found that limbic DWI or FLAIR hyperintensities can be found in some cases, but it was not clear that these were true diffusion restricted [74].

Classic neuropathological findings of GSS are its distinct large PrP^{Sc} amyloid plaques, called kuru plaques (Figure 9.3c), in association with pyramidal tract degeneration [48, 98, 99]. PrP^{Sc} amyloid plaques rarely are seen in other prion disorders, but their presence should make one consider *PRNP* testing. There is often gliosis but less vacuolation than classic sCJD [41]. GSS symptoms usually begin in the second to eighth decades (typically 20s–60s) with a mean duration of about 5 years [102], although a 15-year-old with a progressive motor and cognitive disorder beginning at age 10 was recently found by whole exome sequencing to have a de novo GSS mutation.

FFI

FFI is a rare disorder that usually begins with progressive, severe intractable insomnia that is present for several months before onset of other symptoms, such as dysautonomia, ataxia, or other motor symptoms, with cognitive problems appearing later in the course. Progressive insomnia is eventually associated with hallucinations. Onset usually occurs in the fifth and sixth decade with duration of around 12–18 months [48, 61]. Although brain MRI is usually normal, FDG-PET imaging reveals thalamic and cingulate hypometabolism, often even before disease onset. FFI is caused by a single *PRNP* point mutation, D178N, with codon 129 M on the same chromosome (cis) (patients with D178N-129V usually present with fCJD) [110]. The neuropathology of FFI is primarily characterized by thalamic gliosis and neuronal loss [48, 98].

Acquired prion disease

Kuru

Kuru ("to shake or tremble" in the Fore language) [111] was a form of PrD confined to the Fore ethnic group of Papua New Guinea and was transmitted through a practice in which deceased relatives were honored by ritualized cannibalism. The clinical presentation was of pure cerebellar ataxia (and relatively preserved cognition) and an illness duration of 6–36 months [112]. The practice of cannibalism stopped in the late 50s, and since then, the incidence of kuru decreased dramatically (from the more than 2700 cases identified between 1957 and 2004, only 11 occurred after 1996) [113]. The mean incubation period was estimated to be around 12 years, but with a wide range from 5 to 56 years (particularly longer in those heterozygous at codon 129) [113].

Iatrogenic Jakob–Creutzfeldt disease

More than 400 cases of iCJD have been reported, either from the use of cadaveric-derived human pituitary hormones, dura mater grafts, and corneal transplants, reuse of EEG implanted depth electrodes, and other neurosurgical equipments [114, 115]. The number of iCJD cases has been decreasing over the past years, probably due to increased surveillance and use of effective decontamination measures, but continuing surveillance is still necessary [114, 116].

The first recognized human-to-human transmission of CJD was reported in 1974, when a 55-year-old woman developed CJD 18 months after having inadvertently received a corneal transplant from a donor with CJD [117]. A second case associated with corneal transplant was reported years later, with an incubation period of 30 years [118]. In 1977, a report described two cases of iCJD caused by contaminated implanted stereotactic EEG electrodes that had been previously used in a CJD patient (incubation time of 16 and 18 months) [119]. Other neurosurgical instruments have also been implicated in iCJD cases [112], thus reinforcing the need of preventive measures when dealing with prions (see decontamination measures in the following).

Cadaveric human pituitary hormones (human growth hormones [hGH] and human pituitary gonadotropic [hPG] hormones) were used for medical treatment from the late 1950s until mid-1985, and more than 30 000 patients are thought to have received them. In 1985, a report first mentioned the association between CJD and hGH, leading to the suspension of human pituitary hormone. The cases of hGH iCJD (~200 worldwide) occurred mainly in France, the United Kingdom, and the United States, and the incubation period was calculated to be around 15 years (range 4–36 years) [114]. The clinical presentation usually was of pure cerebellar ataxia, with dementia occurring only late (if at all) in the disease progression [112]. As in other forms of iCJD, *PRNP* codon 129 homozygosity is a risk factor of hGH iCJD [120]. hGH iCJD risk varies from country to country; in the United States, no cases were reported from individuals that received hormones after 1977 (when purification methods were changed), whereas in France there was a strong clustering of cases that received hormone between 1982 and 1985 [121, 122]. In the early 1990s, four cases of iCJD associated with hPG were identified in Australia, in women who had received the hormone in the 1970s as an infertility treatment [114, 121, 123]. No cases of hPG iCJD have been reported in other countries.

The last major group of iCJD are those associated with cadaveric dura mater grafts, which was first recognized in 1987 [124]. Around 200 cases have been reported worldwide, and more than 60% occurred in Japan (but also in France, Spain, Germany, United Kingdom, and other countries) [114]. Lyodura© was the brand implicated in more than 90% of the cases, and no iCJD cases have been reported in patients who received the first dural graft in 1993 [112, 125]. The incubation period was calculated in the Japanese sample to range from 1.2 to 24.8 years, and the mean age of onset of symptoms was 55 years (range 15–80) [126]. Homozygosity at codon 129 (particularly M) is also a risk factor for this form of iCJD [114, 126].

Variant Jakob–Creutzfeldt disease

vCJD was first recognized in 1995 in the United Kingdom [127] and soon received worldwide attention for its association with BSE, or mad cow disease. As of June 2014, approximately 225 vCJD cases have been identified, most in the United Kingdom and France [128]. BSE is the only non-hPrD currently believed to be transmissible to humans, and it is thought that BSE occurred from the practice of feeding scrapie-infected sheep products to cattle. More than 180 000 cattle suffered from BSE, the vast majority in the United Kingdom [129]. Although the incidence of BSE has dramatically declined since 1992, a few isolated cases have still been reported over the past few years [129].

But how was BSE diseased cattle's meat consumption associated with vCJD? Since the first report of vCJD [127], a possible association between with BSE was raised due to the epidemiological temporal relationship between the two diseases. Compelling evidence soon came from experimental studies, in which similarities were found between BSE and vCJD PrP strains in mouse transmission studies, leading to the conclusion that they were caused by the same agent [130, 131].

It was later found out that vCJD could not only be acquired through contaminated beef consumption but also from blood product transfusion and there have been five cases reported so far with this association [132–136]. Four of those patients acquired vCJD from nonleukodepleted blood transfusions received before 1999, and one was a hemophiliac patient who received factor VIII in the 1990s from a contaminated batch. The incubation period ranged from 6 to 9 years in the three 129MM patients that died with definite vCJD. The other two patients (one acquired via blood transfusion, the other via factor VIII) were 129MV and died of nonneurological causes but had positive prion testing in their lymphoreticular system; it is not known whether they ever would have developed neurological PrD, although they were likely carriers. Because of this, additional measures were taken to prevent transmission of vCJD through blood products. Aside from donor selection and efforts toward developing methods to detect PrP in the blood, one of the main measures taken was universal leukoreduction of donated blood (which is being done since 1999 in the United Kingdom and later in the rest of Europe) [129]. In one study with hamsters, leukoreduction was shown to reduce TSE infectivity by 42% (comparing to whole blood) [137]. It is important to note that although transmission through blood products has been reported in vCJD, there are no known cases to date of transmission from sCJD patients through blood transfusion [138].

Codon 129 polymorphism is an important susceptibility factor for the development of vCJD, and almost every case reported so far has been 129MM (except for one symptomatic probable vCJD and the two presymptomatic blood product transfusion cases mentioned above) [139].

The clinical presentation of vCJD is different from sCJD in several ways. Patients with vCJD are usually younger, with a median age of onset around 27 (range 12–74) [140, 141]. The vast majority of cases occurred in persons younger than age 50; and among the patients in the United Kingdom, 12% died at age 20 or younger [142]. The mean disease duration is longer, about 14.5 months (vs. ~7 months for sCJD). Although psychiatric symptoms often occur early in sCJD [51], prominent psychiatric symptoms are often the initial symptoms in vCJD for several months (typically more than six) before obvious neurologic symptoms begin. The EEG only rarely shows the classic PSWCs and, if so, then only at the end stage of disease [143]. Brain MRI usually shows the "pulvinar sign," in which the pulvinar (posterior thalamus) is brighter than the anterior putamen on T2-weighted (and probably also on DWI) MRI (and was found in more than 85% of cases in the first exam) (Figure 9.2d) [144]; this finding is very rare in other hPrDs [145, 146]. Posterior thalamic hyperintensities have been reported in gCJD (in E200K mutations) and in sCJD, but in those cases, the basal ganglia are usually brighter than the posterior thalamus [147]. Diagnostic criteria for probable vCJD are shown in Table 9.3 and have reported sensitivity of 83% and specificity of 100% [140].

Definitive diagnosis of vCJD is based on neuropathologic evidence of the variant form of PrP^{Sc} in brain biopsy or autopsy. Because vCJD is acquired peripherally, PrP^{Sc} can be found in the lymphoreticular system, including tonsillar tissue [148]. Brain pathology of vCJD shows abundant PrP^{Sc} deposition, in particular multiple fibrillary PrP plaques surrounded by a halo of spongiform vacuoles ("florid" plaques) and other PrP plaques and deposits, especially prominent in the cerebellar molecular layer (Figure 9.3d) [98, 149].

From the blood product vCJD cases, it is now known that transmission from asymptomatic blood donors may occur years before the onset of symptoms, and so there is currently concern over the possibility of a second wave of vCJD in the future [150]. Exposed individuals with MV or VV genotype at codon 129 of the PRNP gene may also have longer incubation times, which could potentially increase the chance of a second wave. In an initial study in the United Kingdom, vCJD prions were found by immunostaining in 3 of 11 246 (~1 in 4000) appendix samples collected from 1995 to 2000 [151]. A more recent, larger study found that the rate of vCJD-affected appendices was 16 of 32 441 (~1 in 2000), about double the earlier study, suggesting an overall prevalence of 493 per million population [152]. Because the samples were anonymized, it is only possible to assume that there are asymptomatic persons in the UK population with vCJD prions in their lymphoreticular system (subclinically infected) who are at a minimum carriers of the disease. It is not clear what their risk is of developing symptomatic vCJD and/or transmitting it to others through medical/surgical procedures or blood products.

Table 9.3 Diagnostic criteria for vCJD.

Definite: IA and neuropathological confirmation of vCJD*
Probable: I and 4/5 of II and IIIA and IIIB or I and IVA.
Possible: I and 4/5 of II and IIIA

I
- A) Progressive neuropsychiatric disorder
- B) Duration of illness > 6 months
- C) Routine investigations do not suggest an alternative diagnosis
- D) No history of potential iatrogenic exposure
- E) No evidence of a familial form of TSE

II
- A) Early psychiatric features†
- B) Persistent painful sensory symptoms‡
- C) Ataxia
- D) Myoclonus or chorea or dystonia
- E) Dementia

III
- A) EEG does not show the typical appearance of sporadic CJD§ in the early stages of illness
- B) Bilateral pulvinar high signal on MRI scan

IV
- A) Positive tonsil biopsy¶

Source: Modified with permission from Heath et al. [140].
* Spongiform change and extensive prion protein deposition with florid plaques throughout the cerebrum and cerebellum.
† Depression, anxiety, apathy, withdrawal, and delusions.
‡ Includes frank pain and/or dysesthesias.
§ The typical appearance of the EEG in sporadic CJD consists of generalized triphasic periodic complexes at approximately 1 per second. These may occasionally be seen in the late stages of vCJD.
¶ Tonsil biopsy is not recommended routinely nor in cases with EEG appearances typical of sporadic CJD but may be useful in suspect cases in which the clinical features are compatible with vCJD and MRI that does not show bilateral pulvinar high signal.
EEG, electroencephalography; MRI, magnetic resonance imaging; TSE, transmissible spongiform encephalopathy; vCJD, variant Jakob–Creutzfeldt disease.

Treatment and management

In spite of all active efforts, there are no currently available drugs to change disease progression in hPrD, and so, symptomatic treatment is the only available option. Past efforts included quinacrine, an antimalarial drug, the antibiotic doxycycline, and the analgesic flupirtine, none of which recently have been shown to be effective in halting the progression of CJD [153–156]. Intraventricular pentosan polysulfate, an anticoagulant, was used in a few cases in the United Kingdom and in Japan, but its benefit is still uncertain. At best, it might prolong survival, but not affect disease progression and disability [157–160]. Symptomatic treatment may include the empirical use of SSRIs to treat depression and agitation, atypical antipsychotics (particularly quetiapine) to treat agitation and psychoses, and clonazepam to treat severe myoclonus or agitation.

Two other management points are fundamental. As mentioned before, a significant percentage of gPrD have no evident positive family history (and sporadic PrD and gPrD may be clinically indistinguishable), and so genetic testing should be considered for every PrD patient (genetic counseling is indispensable prior to testing for *PRNP* mutations). Also, family and caregiver education is paramount in the disease process. In some countries around the world, there are organizations (such as the CJD Foundation in the United States; www.cjdfoundation.org) specialized in providing the necessary information on the care of patients with PrD [161]. More on family and caregiver issues will be discussed in Chapter 15.

Prion decontamination and preventive measures

Decontamination of prions requires methods that will denature proteins, as prions resist normal inactivation methods used to kill viruses and bacteria. Typical methods for reducing the load of or inactivating prions include very high temperatures for prolonged periods, autoclaving at higher than normal temperatures, pressure, and time and with or without denaturing agents (many of which are caustic). Those measures often damage medical equipment and instrumentation [162]. WHO guidelines state that the preferred method is steam sterilization for at least 30 min at 132°C in a gravity displacement sterilizer. If a prevacuum sterilizer is used, they note 18 min at 134°C also is effective. Another option is 1M sodium hydroxide or 2% sodium hypochlorite for 1 h with 134°C autoclaving for at least 18 min. Nonfragile items may be immersed in 1N sodium hydroxide, a caustic solution, for 1 h at room temperature and then steam sterilized for 30 min at a temperature of 121°C [116, 163]. Due to the risk of transmission to subsequent patients, when feasible, many hospitals dispose of neurosurgical and other surgical equipment potentially exposed to prions by incineration. Our own medical center has developed its own policies and procedures for patients with suspected or confirmed hPrD, which are in some ways stricter than WHO guidelines, in part due to the large number of patients with PrD assessed at UCSF (http://infectioncontrol.ucsfmedicalcenter.org/sites/infectioncontrol.ucsfmedicalcenter.org/files/Sec%204.2%20Human%20Prion%20Policy.pdf).

Aside from prion decontamination, additional preventive measures have been taken (some of which have been commented above) to avoid further iCJD cases. Known pathogenic *PRNP* mutation carriers are asked not to donate blood, even though the actual risk of transmissibility in humans is unknown [164]. Patients who received potentially contaminated human pituitary hormones were likewise advised in some countries [123, 165]. Other issues involving those at-risk individuals are still unknown (such as the necessary precautions needed to avoid transmission after a general surgery), pointing out the need for further research.

Differential diagnosis of rapidly progressive dementias

Case 3

Mrs. W, a 59-year-old woman, with a past medical history of depression, began to have subacute onset of gait problems, followed after a month by apathy, myoclonic jerks in her upper limbs, and later dystonic posturing of her hands. Cognitive decline soon followed, and at the time of her evaluation (2 months after onset), she was wheelchair bound, would only speak a few words, and had a flexed posture of her trunk and dystonia in her hands, myoclonus in her face and upper limbs, as well as bilateral pyramidal signs. MRI showed gadolinium-enhancing bilateral basal ganglia hyperintensities (Figure 9.5), and biopsy of the lesions gave the diagnosis of large cell lymphoma. Her lymphoma was treated, and she had a slow but steady improvement; after a few weeks, she was able to walk again with assistance, and her cognition had improved markedly.

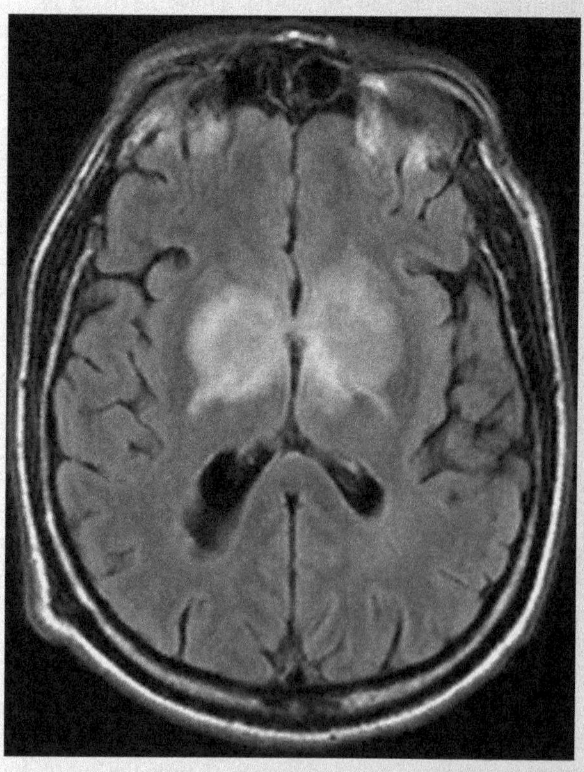

Figure 9.5 (Case 3)—Bilateral basal ganglia hyperintensities in axial FLAIR MRI scan with edema tracking along the limbs of the internal capsule. The lesions were gadolinium enhancing.

Table 9.4 Mnemonic acronym for RPD differential.

V	ascular
I	nfectious
T	oxic-metabolic
A	utoimmune
M	etastasis/neoplasm
I	atrogenic
N	eurodegenerative
S	ystemic/seizures/structural

Source: Adapted from Geschwind et al. [1]. Reproduced with permission of Wiley.

Differential diagnosis

The mnemonic acronym VITAMINS may be helpful in the clinical reasoning of RPD cases (Table 9.4), as it helps covering the most frequent causes of RPD [1, 2, 166]. The items vascular, infectious, toxic-metabolic, autoimmune (including paraneoplastic), neurodegenerative, and systemic causes are covered in other chapters of this book. Neoplasms will be briefly discussed here.

Neoplasms

CNS neoplasms—primary or secondary—usually present as mass lesions on brain MRI scans and so can be easily identified as the RPD etiology. There are a few rare conditions, however, in which MRI findings are not so obvious, such as primary CNS lymphoma (PCNSL), intravascular lymphomatosis (angiotropic large cell lymphoma), and gliomatosis cerebri [1].

PCNSLs represent 4% of the primary CNS tumors and were diagnosed in 0.7% of the cases referred with suspected CJD for autopsy at the NPDPSC (lymphomas represented more than 70% of their neoplastic cases) [8, 167]. They are predominantly diffuse large B-cell-type non-Hodgkin lymphomas, and the median age of onset is around 60 years [168, 169]. The CNS involvement may occur in the brain, leptomeninges, eyes, and spinal cord [170]. Immunodeficiency is the main risk factor, and focal neurological deficits are seen in 70% of cases (whereas neuropsychiatric symptoms in around 40%) [171]. When PCNSL manifests in the brain, it presents as a focal mass lesion (isohypointense or hyperintense on T2-weighted imaging, with homogeneous contrast enhancement [or with ring enhancement in immunocompromised patients] and little surrounding edema) in more than 50% of cases (and multifocal in other 25% of cases) [172, 173]. Most lesions are located in the cerebral hemispheres, thalamus, basal ganglia, and corpus callosum [174]. In case 3, the evolution of symptoms and basal ganglia hyperintensities were the reason why CJD was considered in the differential diagnosis. Contrast enhancement and edema, however, are not seen in CJD and led to further investigation with the ultimately diagnostic biopsy. DWI hyperintensities (sometimes with concomitant ADC hypointensities) may be seen due to ischemia and/or high cellularity [82]. In the context of RPD, those neuroradiological features must prompt the investigation of the nature of the lesion, usually through biopsy. There are, however, instances in which neuroradiological findings are far from straightforward, as in the case of lymphomatosis cerebri. It is a rare form of PCNSL that may present as a RPD [175, 176]. Brain MRI typically shows diffuse nonenhancing white matter hyperintensities, resembling leukoencephalopathy [173, 177]. Most of the PCNSL diagnosed at the NPDPSC were of this type [8].

Intravascular lymphomatosis (also called malignant angioendotheliomatosis or angiotropic large cell lymphoma) is a rare condition in which cutaneous and neurological symptoms (usually subacute dementia) are the most frequently reported (due to occlusion of small vessels). MRI findings include white matter hyperintensities, parenchymal masses, and stroke-like lesions, with variable contrast enhancement [178, 179]. Despite being rare, difficulty in diagnosis [180] probably led intravascular lymphomatosis to also be diagnosed in 0.7% of the cases autopsied at the NPDPSC [8].

Gliomatosis cerebri is a diffuse infiltrating glial tumor that can also manifest as a RPD [181]. Dementias, headaches, and seizures are the most commonly seen features, and brain MRI shows ill-defined white and gray matter hyperintensities in T2-weighted images. Contrast enhancement may be seen in around 50% of cases [182].

Psychiatric

Psychiatric disorders were diagnosed in 2% of nonprion RPD cases seen at the UCSF [1]. It is important, however, to highlight that many neurodegenerative disorders may be accompanied by neuropsychiatric symptoms, and so, even though conversion disorders, malingering, and psychosis may simulate RPD, a very low threshold to investigate the possibility of an underlying neurological cause must be kept. Psychiatric symptoms are often an early and prominent feature of many forms of PrD [51, 64, 183, 184] At the UCSF, psychiatric conditions causing RPD were more frequently seen in patients who self-diagnosed CJD [1].

Diagnostic algorithm

Obtaining a detailed history and physical examination is paramount in the evaluation of RPDs. From the history, important information, such as work-related exposure leading to lead intoxication, diarrhea narrowing the diagnosis to disorders such as Whipple's disease, or a prolonged ICU admission raising suspicion of extrapontine myelinolysis or Wernicke's encephalopathy, can be obtained. It is important to try to obtain the most accurate information on the specific timing of onset and initial symptoms. Not infrequently, symptoms (often noticed in retrospect) predate what was initially reported to be the first symptom in months (or even years), changing the list of possible differential diagnoses. From the physical examination, signs of hepatic failure can prompt a consideration of hepatic encephalopathy, Wilson's disease, or acquired hepatocerebral degeneration as possible etiologies; or a facial rash can suggest systemic lupus erythematosus.

Table 9.5 Clinical diagnosis algorithm.

Initial screening tests					
Blood	CBC, chemistry panel, liver function tests, RPR, rheumatological screen (ESR, ANA, CRP, ANCAs), thyroid function, vitamin B12, homocysteine, methylmalonic acid, HIV serology, Lyme disease serology, paraneoplastic/autoimmune antibodies panel				
Urine	Urine analysis				
CSF	Cell count and differential, protein, glucose, IgG index, oligoclonal bands, VDRL				
Brain MRI	With and without contrast. Include DWI and ADC sequences				
EEG	(Might be helpful)				
Review for potentially treatable causes					
Further testing based on initial screen					
Infectious	**Autoimmune**	**Neoplastic**	**Vascular**	**Toxic-metabolic or systemic**	**Degenerative**
Refer to Chapter 13	Refer to Chapter 10	Serum LDH and tumor markers, CSF cytology and flow cytometry, CT scan with and without contrast, whole-body PET scan, mammogram	Refer to Chapter 4	Refer to Chapters 11, 12 and 14 Low threshold to order serum ceruloplasmin/copper Screen for heavy metal intoxication (exposure?), other vitamin deficiency (B1, niacin), and porphyria Parathyroid or adrenal diseases	Refer to Chapters 3, 5–7 CSF Aβ, total and phospho-tau, 14-3-3, NSE
If negative, consider brain biopsy					

Source: Adapted from Geschwind et al. [1, 2]. Reproduced with permission of Elsevier.
ANA, antinuclear antibody; ANCA, antineutrophil cytoplasmic antibodies; anti-TG, antithyroglobulin antibody; anti-TPO, antithyroperoxidase antibody; CBC, complete blood count; CRP, C-reactive protein; CSF, cerebrospinal fluid; CT, computed tomography; EEG, electroencephalogram; ESR, erythrocyte sedimentation rate; NSE, neuron-specific enolase; PET, positron emission tomography; RPR, rapid plasma reagin; VDRL, Venereal Disease Research Laboratory test.

Following the history and exam, initial screening tests should be ordered (Table 9.5), including basic blood and urine tests, CSF analysis, and brain MRI, which help in narrowing possible diagnose (s). The initial screening and every step further in the investigation should focus primarily on finding potentially reversible causes of CJD. After the initial screen, some tests may be virtually diagnostic, such as a positive antibody in the setting of a case suggestive of one of the paraneoplastic or antibody-mediated limbic encephalopathy syndromes or typical MRI findings of sCJD in a patient whose other tests were negative for alternative causes. In some cases, however, the initial screen only helps to narrow the differential, and at this point, the VITAMINS mnemonic should be used again to direct further investigation.

If the secondary investigation suggests the possibility of inflammatory, infectious, or neoplastic causes and further investigation is still necessary to provide adequate treatment, a brain biopsy may be considered. Brain biopsies historically have been infrequently performed in the setting of dementia, and recently due to advances in the diagnosis of degenerative dementias (including CJD) and autoimmune disorders, biopsies perhaps are even less frequently required. Around 60–70% of brain biopsies were diagnostic in two dementia series [185–187] but changes in treatment due to the result occurred in only 11% of cases [186]. Biopsy-related complications (such as infection, seizures, and hemorrhage) were reported in 11–21% of procedures in one study [185], and so the risk–benefit ratio of a biopsy must be considered in each case. Due to concerns of prion infectivity of neurosurgical material and the greater ability to diagnose CJD with MRI, we feel that a brain biopsy should not be performed only to confirm a diagnosis of CJD, but rather to find another etiology for the dementia.

Summary

Assessing a case of RPD is usually a diagnostic challenge. The causes of RPD range from conditions in which the diagnosis is fairly straightforward (such as a neoplastic mass seen in an MRI scan) to fatal disorders such as CJD and also include potentially treatable causes (such as metabolic, infectious, or autoimmune) for which early diagnosis is invaluable. A detailed history and thorough physical exam are of utmost importance in the assessment of RPDs. Those evaluations, along with initial screening (including blood and urine tests, CSF analysis, and brain MRI) should either point to a diagnosis or narrow the differential. Further testing may be required to achieve a final diagnosis, but it is important to keep in consideration potentially reversible causes of RPD, which are found in about 10% of cases referred to PrD centers.

One of the most frequent causes of RPDs are PrDs. sCJD is the most frequent form of PrD and is characterized by RPD and pyramidal, extrapyramidal, cerebellar, and visual signs and symptoms. DWI Brain MRI is currently the most accurate test to diagnose CJD, but other tests are usually required in the clinical setting to rule out reversible causes. Other forms of PrDs include genetic (gCJD or fCJD, GSS, and FFI) and acquired/iatrogenic forms, which comprise 10–15% and 1–3% of PrD, respectively. There is no cure currently available for any PrDs, and sCJD is associated with a mortality rate of 90% within the first year.

Acronyms

AD	Alzheimer's disease
bvFTD	behavioral variant of frontotemporal dementia
CJD	Jakob–Creutzfeldt disease
CNS	central nervous system
CSF	cerebrospinal fluid
DWI	diffusion-weighted imaging
EEG	electroencephalogram
FFI	fatal familial insomnia
FLAIR	fluid-attenuated inversion recovery
gCJD	genetic CJD
gPrD	genetic prion disease
GSS	Gerstmann–Sträussler–Scheinker syndrome
iCJD	iatrogenic CJD
LBD	Lewy body dementia
MRI	magnetic resonance imaging
PCNSL	primary central nervous system lymphoma
PrD	prion disease
PrP	prion protein
PSWCs	periodic sharp wave complexes
RPD	rapidly progressive dementia
sFI	sporadic fatal insomnia
TSE	transmissible spongiform encephalopathies
vCJD	variant CJD
VD	vascular dementia

Acknowledgments

Dr. Geschwind's work regarding this chapter was supported by NIH R01 AG-AG031189, PO1-AG021601, and the Michael J. Homer Family Fund.

References

1 Geschwind MD, Shu H, Haman A, Sejvar JJ, Miller BL. (2008) Rapidly progressive dementia. *Ann Neurol* **64**:1, 97–108.

2 Geschwind MD, Haman A, Miller BL. (2007) Rapidly progressive dementia. *Neurol Clin* **25**:3, 783–807.

3 Josephs KA, Ahlskog JE, Parisi JE, Boeve BF, Crum BA, Giannini C, et al. (2009) Rapidly progressive neurodegenerative dementias. *Arch Neurol* **66**:2, 201–7.

4 Schmidt C, Wolff M, Weitz M, Bartlau T, Korth C, Zerr I. (2011) Rapidly progressive Alzheimer disease. *Arch Neurol* **68**:9, 1124–30.

5 Papageorgiou SG, Kontaxis T, Bonakis A, Karahalios G, Kalfakis N, Vassilopoulos D. (2009) Rapidly progressive dementia: causes found in a greek tertiary referral center in Athens. *Alzheimer Dis Assoc Disord* **23**:4, 337–46.

6 Sala I, Marquie M, Sanchez-Saudinos MB, Sanchez-Valle R, Alcolea D, Gomez-Anson B, et al. (2012) Rapidly progressive dementia: experience in a tertiary care medical center. *Alzheimer Dis Assoc Disord* **26**:3, 267–71.

7 Roberson ED, Hesse JH, Rose KD, Slama H, Johnson JK, Yaffe K, et al. (2005) Frontotemporal dementia progresses to death faster than Alzheimer disease. *Neurology* **65**:5, 719–25.

8 Chitravas N, Jung RS, Kofskey DM, Blevins JE, Gambetti P, Leigh RJ, et al. (2011) Treatable neurological disorders misdiagnosed as Creutzfeldt-Jakob disease. *Ann Neurol* **70**:3, 437–44.

9 Poser S, Mollenhauer B, Kraubeta A, Zerr I, Steinhoff B, Schroeter A, et al. (1999) How to improve the clinical diagnosis of Creutzfeldt-Jakob disease. *Brain* **122**:(Pt 12), 2345–51.

10 Prusiner SB. (1982) Novel proteinaceous infectious particles cause scrapie. *Science* **216**:4542, 136–44.

11 Prusiner SB. (1998) Prions. *Proc Natl Acad Sci U S A* **95**:23, 13363–83.

12 Jakob A. (1921) Concerning a disorder of the central nervous system clinically resembling multiple sclerosis with remarkable anatomic findings (spastic pseudosclerosis). Report of a fourth case. *Med Klin* **17**, 372–6.

13 Triarhou LC. (2009) Alfons Maria Jakob (1884–1931), neuropathologist par excellence. Scientific endeavors in Europe and the Americas. *Eur Neurol* **61**:1, 52–8.

14 Masters CL. (1989) Creutzfeldt-Jakob disease: its origins. *Alzheimer Dis Assoc Disord* **3**:1–2, 46–51.

15 Gibbs CJ, Jr. (1992) Spongiform encephalopathies—slow, latent, and temperate virus infections—in retrospect. In: Prusiner SB, Collinge J, Powell J, Anderton B, editors. *Prion Diseases of Humans and Animals.* Ellis Horwood, London, pp. 53–62.

16 Masters CL, Harris JO, Gajdusek DC, Gibbs CJ, Jr., Bernoulli C, Asher DM. (1979) Creutzfeldt-Jakob disease: patterns of worldwide occurrence and the significance of familial and sporadic clustering. *Ann Neurol* **5**:2, 177–88.

17 Ladogana A, Puopolo M, Croes EA, Budka H, Jarius C, Collins S, et al. (2005) Mortality from Creutzfeldt-Jakob disease and related disorders in Europe, Australia, and Canada. *Neurology* **64**:9, 1586–91.

18 Holman RC, Belay ED, Christensen KY, Maddox RA, Minino AM, Folkema AM, et al. (2010) Human prion diseases in the United States. *PLoS One* **5**:1, e8521.

19 Brown P, Cathala F, Castaigne P, Gajdusek DC. (1986) Creutzfeldt-Jakob disease: clinical analysis of a consecutive series of 230 neuropathologically verified cases. *Ann Neurol* **20**:5, 597–602.

20 Buganza M, Ferrari S, Cecchini ME, Orrico D, Monaco S, Zanusso G. (2009) The oldest old Creutzfeldt-Jakob disease case. *J Neurol Neurosurg Psychiatry* **80**:10, 1140–2.

21 Berman PH, Davidson GS, Becker LE. (1988) Progressive neurological deterioration in a 14-year-old girl. *Pediatr Neurosci* **14**:1, 42–9.

22 Corato M, Cereda C, Cova E, Ferrarese C, Ceroni M. (2006) Young-onset CJD: age and disease phenotype in variant and sporadic forms. *Funct Neurol* **21**:4, 211–5.

23 Gajdusek DC, Gibbs CJ, Alpers M. (1966) Experimental transmission of a Kuru-like syndrome to chimpanzees. *Nature* **209**:25, 794–6.

24 Pattison IH, Jones KM. (1967) The possible nature of the transmissible agent of scrapie. *Vet Rec* **80**:1, 2–9.

25 Alper T, Haig DA, Clarke MC. (1966) The exceptionally small size of the scrapie agent. *Biochem Biophys Res Commun* **22**:3, 278–84.

26 Alper T, Cramp WA, Haig DA, Clarke MC. (1967) Does the agent of scrapie replicate without nucleic acid? *Nature* **214**:5090, 764–6.

27 Griffith JS. (1967) Self-replication and scrapie. *Nature* **215**:5105, 1043–4.
28 Kanaani J, Prusiner SB, Diacovo J, Baekkeskov S, Legname G. (2005) Recombinant prion protein induces rapid polarization and development of synapses in embryonic rat hippocampal neurons in vitro. *J Neurochem* **95**:5, 1373–86.
29 Shmueli O, Horn-Saban S, Chalifa-Caspi V, Shmoish M, Ophir R, Benjamin-Rodrig H, et al. (2003) GeneNote: whole genome expression profiles in normal human tissues. *C R Biol* **326**:10–11, 1067–72.
30 Kellett KA, Hooper NM. (2009) Prion protein and Alzheimer disease. *Prion* **3**:4, 190–4.
31 Mallucci GR, White MD, Farmer M, Dickinson A, Khatun H, Powell AD, et al. (2007) Targeting cellular prion protein reverses early cognitive deficits and neurophysiological dysfunction in prion-infected mice. *Neuron* **53**:3, 325–35.
32 Colby DW, Prusiner SB. (2011) Prions. *Cold Spring Harb Perspect Biol* **3**:1, a006833.
33 van der Kamp MW, Daggett V. (2010) Pathogenic mutations in the hydrophobic core of the human prion protein can promote structural instability and misfolding. *J Mol Biol* **404**:4, 732–48.
34 Cobb NJ, Surewicz WK. (2009) Prion diseases and their biochemical mechanisms. *Biochemistry* **48**:12, 2574–85.
35 Parchi P, Castellani R, Capellari S, Ghetti B, Young K, Chen SG, et al. (1996) Molecular basis of phenotypic variability in sporadic Creutzfeldt-Jakob disease. *Ann Neurol* **39**:6, 767–78.
36 Cali I, Castellani R, Alshekhlee A, Cohen Y, Blevins J, Yuan J, et al. (2009) Co-existence of scrapie prion protein types 1 and 2 in sporadic Creutzfeldt-Jakob disease: its effect on the phenotype and prion-type characteristics. *Brain* **132**:Pt 10, 2643–58.
37 Watts JC, Giles K, Stohr J, Oehler A, Bhardwaj S, Grillo SK, et al. (2012) Spontaneous generation of rapidly transmissible prions in transgenic mice expressing wild-type bank vole prion protein. *Proc Natl Acad Sci U S A* **109**:9, 3498–503.
38 Hsiao K, Baker HF, Crow TJ, Poulter M, Owen F, Terwilliger JD, et al. (1989) Linkage of a prion protein missense variant to Gerstmann-Straussler syndrome. *Nature* **338**:6213, 342–5.
39 Goldgaber D, Goldfarb LG, Brown P, Asher DM, Brown WT, Lin S, et al. (1989) Mutations in familial Creutzfeldt-Jakob disease and Gerstmann-Straussler-Scheinker's syndrome. *Exp Neurol* **106**:2, 204–6.
40 Lloyd SE, Mead S, Collinge J. (2013) Genetics of prion diseases. *Curr Opin Genet Dev* **23**:3, 345–51.
41 Brown K, Mastrianni JA. (2010) The prion diseases. *J Geriatr Psychiatry Neurol* **23**:4, 277–98.
42 Kovacs GG, Puopolo M, Ladogana A, Pocchiari M, Budka H, van Duijn C, et al. (2005) Genetic prion disease: the EUROCJD experience. *Hum Genet* **118**:2, 166–74.
43 Lloyd S, Mead S, Collinge J. (2011) Genetics of prion disease. In: Tatzelt J, editor. *Prion Proteins*. Springer Berlin Heidelberg, pp. 1–22.
44 Rossi G, Giaccone G, Giampaolo L, Iussich S, Puoti G, Frigo M, et al. (2000) Creutzfeldt-Jakob disease with a novel four extra-repeat insertional mutation in the PrP gene. *Neurology* **55**:3, 405–10.
45 D'Alessandro M, Petraroli R, Ladogana A, Pocchiari M. (1998) High incidence of Creutzfeldt-Jakob disease in rural Calabria, Italy. *Lancet* **352**:9145, 1989–90.
46 Mitrova E, Belay G. (2002) Creutzfeldt-Jakob disease with E200K mutation in Slovakia: characterization and development. *Acta Virol* **46**:1, 31–9.
47 Spudich S, Mastrianni JA, Wrensch M, Gabizon R, Meiner Z, Kahana I, et al. (1995) Complete penetrance of Creutzfeldt-Jakob disease in Libyan Jews carrying the E200K mutation in the prion protein gene. *Mol Med* **1**:6, 607–13.
48 Mastrianni JA. (2010) The genetics of prion diseases. *Genet Med* **12**:4, 187–95.
49 Parchi P, Giese A, Capellari S, Brown P, Schulz-Schaeffer W, Windl O, et al. (1999) Classification of sporadic Creutzfeldt-Jakob disease based on molecular and phenotypic analysis of 300 subjects. *Ann Neurol* **46**:2, 224–33.
50 Hohler AD, Flynn FG. (2006) Onset of Creutzfeldt-Jakob disease mimicking an acute cerebrovascular event. *Neurology* **67**:3, 538–9.
51 Rabinovici GD, Wang PN, Levin J, Cook L, Pravdin M, Davis J, et al. (2006) First symptom in sporadic Creutzfeldt-Jakob disease. *Neurology* **66**:2, 286–7.
52 Will RG, Matthews WB. (1984) A retrospective study of Creutzfeldt-Jakob disease in England and Wales 1970–79. I: clinical features. *J Neurol Neurosurg Psychiatry* **47**:2, 134–40.
53 Maltete D, Guyant-Marechal L, Mihout B, Hannequin D. (2006) Movement disorders and Creutzfeldt-Jakob disease: a review. *Parkinsonism Relat Disord* **12**:2, 65–71.
54 Edler J, Mollenhauer B, Heinemann U, Varges D, Werner C, Zerr I, et al. (2009) Movement disturbances in the differential diagnosis of Creutzfeldt-Jakob disease. *Mov Disord* **24**:3, 350–6.
55 Espinosa PS, Bensalem-Owen MK, Fee DB. (2010) Sporadic Creutzfeldt-Jakob disease presenting as nonconvulsive status epilepticus case report and review of the literature. *Clin Neurol Neurosurg* **112**:6, 537–40.
56 Kovacs T, Aranyi Z, Szirmai I, Lantos PL. (2002) Creutzfeldt-Jakob disease with amyotrophy and demyelinating polyneuropathy. *Arch Neurol* **59**:11, 1811–4.
57 Ishida C, Okino S, Kitamoto T, Yamada M. (2005) Involvement of the peripheral nervous system in human prion diseases including dural graft associated Creutzfeldt-Jakob disease. *J Neurol Neurosurg Psychiatry* **76**:3, 325–9.
58 Neufeld MY, Josiphov J, Korczyn AD. (1992) Demyelinating peripheral neuropathy in Creutzfeldt-Jakob disease. *Muscle Nerve* **15**:11, 1234–9.
59 Antoine JC, Laplanche JL, Mosnier JF, Beaudry P, Chatelain J, Michel D. (1996) Demyelinating peripheral neuropathy with Creutzfeldt-Jakob disease and mutation at codon 200 of the prion protein gene. *Neurology* **46**:4, 1123–7.
60 Kovacs GG, Seguin J, Quadrio I, Hoftberger R, Kapas I, Streichenberger N, et al. (2011) Genetic Creutzfeldt-Jakob disease associated with the E200K mutation: characterization of a complex proteinopathy. *Acta Neuropathol* **121**:1, 39–57.
61 Pocchiari M, Puopolo M, Croes EA, Budka H, Gelpi E, Collins S, et al. (2004) Predictors of survival in sporadic Creutzfeldt-Jakob disease and other human transmissible spongiform encephalopathies. *Brain* **127**:10, 2348–59.
62 Polymenidou M, Stoeck K, Glatzel M, Vey M, Bellon A, Aguzzi A. (2005) Coexistence of multiple PrP^{Sc} types in individuals with Creutzfeldt-Jakob disease. *Lancet Neurol* **4**:12, 805–14.
63 Puoti G, Bizzi A, Forloni G, Safar JG, Tagliavini F, Gambetti P. (2012) Sporadic human prion diseases: molecular insights and diagnosis. *Lancet Neurol* **11**:7, 618–28.
64 Appleby BS, Appleby KK, Crain BJ, Onyike CU, Wallin MT, Rabins PV. (2009) Characteristics of established and proposed sporadic Creutzfeldt-Jakob disease variants. *Arch Neurol* **66**:2, 208–15.
65 Gambetti P, Kong Q, Zou W, Parchi P, Chen SG. (2003) Sporadic and familial CJD: classification and characterisation. *Br Med Bull* **66**:1, 213–39.

66 Mastrianni JA, Nixon R, Layzer R, Telling GC, Han D, DeArmond SJ, et al. (1999) Prion protein conformation in a patient with sporadic fatal insomnia. *N Engl J Med* **340**:21, 1630–8.
67 Jansen C, Head MW, Rozemuller AJ, Ironside JW. (2009) Panencephalopathic Creutzfeldt-Jakob disease in the Netherlands and the UK: clinical and pathological characteristics of nine patients. *Neuropathol Appl Neurobiol* **35**:3, 272–82.
68 Mizutani T, Okumura A, Oda M, Shiraki H. (1981) Panencephalopathic type of Creutzfeldt-Jakob disease: primary involvement of the cerebral white matter. *J Neurol Neurosurg Psychiatry* **44**:2, 103–15.
69 Worrall BB, Rowland LP, Chin SS, Mastrianni JA. (2000) Amyotrophy in prion diseases. *Arch Neurol* **57**:1, 33–8.
70 Zou WQ, Puoti G, Xiao X, Yuan J, Qing L, Cali I, et al. (2010) Variably protease-sensitive prionopathy: a new sporadic disease of the prion protein. *Ann Neurol* **68**:2, 162–72.
71 Head MW, Yull HM, Ritchie DL, Langeveld JP, Fletcher NA, Knight RS, et al. (2013) Variably protease-sensitive prionopathy in the UK: a retrospective review 1991–2008. *Brain* **136**:Pt 4, 1102–15.
72 WHO. Global surveillance, diagnosis and therapy of human transmissible spongiform encephalopathies: Report of a WHO consultation Geneva, Switzerland 9–11 February 1998. Geneva, Switzerland: World Health Organization, 1998 9–11 February. Report No. WHO/EMC/ZDI/98.9.
73 Geschwind MD, Josephs KA, Parisi JE, Keegan BM. (2007) A 54-year-old man with slowness of movement and confusion. *Neurology* **69**:19, 1881–7.
74 Vitali P, Maccagnano E, Caverzasi E, Henry RG, Haman A, Torres-Chae C, et al. (2011) Diffusion-weighted MRI hyperintensity patterns differentiate CJD from other rapid dementias. *Neurology* **76**:20, 1711–9.
75 Shiga Y, Miyazawa K, Sato S, Fukushima RS, Shibuya S, Sato Y, et al. (2004) Diffusion-weighted MRI abnormalities as an early diagnostic marker for Creutzfeldt-Jakob disease. *Neurology* **I63**, 443–9.
76 Young GS, Geschwind MD, Fischbein NJ, Martindale JL, Henry RG, Liu S, et al. (2005) Diffusion-weighted and fluid-attenuated inversion recovery imaging in Creutzfeldt-Jakob disease: high sensitivity and specificity for diagnosis. *AJNR Am J Neuroradiol* **26**:6, 1551–62.
77 Meissner B, Kallenberg K, Sanchez-Juan P, Collie D, Summers DM, Almonti S, et al. (2009) MRI lesion profiles in sporadic Creutzfeldt-Jakob disease. *Neurology* **72**:23, 1994–2001.
78 Geschwind MD, Potter CA, Sattavat M, Garcia PA, Rosen HJ, Miller BL, et al. (2009) Correlating DWI MRI with pathologic and other features of Jakob-Creutzfeldt disease. *Alzheimer Dis Assoc Disord* **23**:1, 82–7.
79 Halavaara J, Brander A, Lyytinen J, Setala K, Kallela M. (2003) Wernicke's encephalopathy: is diffusion-weighted MRI useful? *Neuroradiology* **45**:8, 519–23.
80 Niclot P, Guichard JP, Djomby R, Sellier P, Bousser MG, Chabriat H. (2002) Transient decrease of water diffusion in Wernicke's encephalopathy. *Neuroradiology* **44**:4, 305–7.
81 Schmidt C, Plickert S, Summers D, Zerr I. (2010) Pulvinar sign in Wernicke's encephalopathy. *CNS Spectr* **15**:4, 215–8.
82 Karaarslan E, Arslan A. (2008) Diffusion weighted MR imaging in non-infarct lesions of the brain. *Eur J Radiol* **65**:3, 402–16.
83 Matsusue E, Kinoshita T, Sugihara S, Fujii S, Ogawa T, Ohama E. (2004) White matter lesions in panencephalopathic type of Creutzfeldt-Jakob disease: MR imaging and pathologic correlations. *AJNR Am J Neuroradiol* **25**:6, 910–8.
84 Green A, Sanchez-Juan P, Ladogana A, Cuadrado-Corrales N, Sanchez-Valle R, Mitrova E, et al. (2007) CSF analysis in patients with sporadic CJD and other transmissible spongiform encephalopathies. *Eur J Neurol* **14**:2, 121–4.
85 Chohan G, Pennington C, Mackenzie JM, Andrews M, Everington D, Will RG, et al. (2010) The role of cerebrospinal fluid 14-3-3 and other proteins in the diagnosis of sporadic Creutzfeldt-Jakob disease in the UK: a 10-year review. *J Neurol Neurosurg Psychiatry* **81**:11, 1243–8.
86 Sanchez-Juan P, Green A, Ladogana A, Cuadrado-Corrales N, Sanchez-Valle R, Mitrovaa E, et al. (2006) CSF tests in the differential diagnosis of Creutzfeldt-Jakob disease. *Neurology* **67**:4, 637–43.
87 Sanchez-Juan P, Sanchez-Valle R, Green A, Ladogana A, Cuadrado-Corrales N, Mitrova E, et al. (2007) Influence of timing on CSF tests value for Creutzfeldt-Jakob disease diagnosis. *J Neurol* **254**:7, 901–6.
88 Deisenhammer F, Egg R, Giovannoni G, Hemmer B, Petzold A, Sellebjerg F, et al. (2009) EFNS guidelines on disease-specific CSF investigations. *Eur J Neurol* **16**:6, 760–70.
89 Pennington C, Chohan G, Mackenzie J, Andrews M, Will R, Knight R, et al. (2009) The role of cerebrospinal fluid proteins as early diagnostic markers for sporadic Creutzfeldt-Jakob disease. *Neurosci Lett* **455**:1, 56–9.
90 Atarashi R, Satoh K, Sano K, Fuse T, Yamaguchi N, Ishibashi D, et al. (2011) Ultrasensitive human prion detection in cerebrospinal fluid by real-time quaking-induced conversion. *Nat Med* **17**:2, 175–8.
91 Soto C, Saborio GP, Anderes L. (2002) Cyclic amplification of protein misfolding: application to prion-related disorders and beyond. *Trends Neurosci* **25**:8, 390–4.
92 Colby DW, Zhang Q, Wang S, Groth D, Legname G, Riesner D, et al. (2007) Prion detection by an amyloid seeding assay. *Proc Natl Acad Sci U S A* **104**:52, 20914–9.
93 McGuire LI, Peden AH, Orru CD, Wilham JM, Appleford NE, Mallinson G, et al. (2012) Real time quaking-induced conversion analysis of cerebrospinal fluid in sporadic Creutzfeldt-Jakob disease. *Ann Neurol* **72**:2, 278–85.
94 Peden AH, McGuire LI, Appleford NE, Mallinson G, Wilham JM, Orru CD, et al. (2012) Sensitive and specific detection of sporadic Creutzfeldt-Jakob disease brain prion protein using real-time quaking-induced conversion. *J Gen Virol* **93**:Pt 2, 438–49.
95 Steinhoff BJ, Zerr I, Glatting M, Schulz-Schaeffer W, Poser S, Kretzschmar HA. (2004) Diagnostic value of periodic complexes in Creutzfeldt-Jakob disease. *Ann Neurol* **56**:5, 702–8.
96 Seipelt M, Zerr I, Nau R, Mollenhauer B, Kropp S, Steinhoff BJ, et al. (1999) Hashimoto's encephalitis as a differential diagnosis of Creutzfeldt-Jakob disease. *J Neurol Neurosurg Psychiatry* **66**:2, 172–6.
97 Tschampa HJ, Neumann M, Zerr I, Henkel K, Schroter A, Schulz-Schaeffer WJ, et al. (2001) Patients with Alzheimer's disease and dementia with Lewy bodies mistaken for Creutzfeldt-Jakob disease. *J Neurol Neurosurg Psychiatry* **71**:1, 33–9.
98 Budka H. (2003) Neuropathology of prion diseases. *Br Med Bull* **66**, 121–30.
99 Venneti S. (2010) Prion diseases. *Clin Lab Med* **30**:1, 293–309.
100 Chapman J, Brown P, Goldfarb LG, Arlazoroff A, Gajdusek DC, Korczyn AD. (1993) Clinical heterogeneity and unusual presentations of Creutzfeldt-Jakob disease in Jewish patients with the PRNP codon 200 mutation. *J Neurol Neurosurg Psychiatry* **56**:10, 1109–12.

101 Mead S. (2006) Prion disease genetics. *Eur J Hum Genet* **14**:3, 273–81.
102 Kong Q, Surewicz WK, Petersen RB, Zou W, Chen SG, Gambetti P, et al. (2004) Inherited prion diseases. In: Prusiner SB, editor. *Prion Biology and Diseases*, 2nd edn. Cold Spring Harbor Laboratory Press, New York pp. 673–775.
103 Chapman J, Ben-Israel J, Goldhammer Y, Korczyn AD. (1994) The risk of developing Creutzfeldt-Jakob disease in subjects with the PRNP gene codon 200 point mutation. *Neurology* **44**:9, 1683–6.
104 Capellari S, Strammiello R, Saverioni D, Kretzschmar H, Parchi P. (2011) Genetic Creutzfeldt-Jakob disease and fatal familial insomnia: insights into phenotypic variability and disease pathogenesis. *Acta Neuropathol* **121**:1, 21–37.
105 Lee HS, Sambuughin N, Cervenakova L, Chapman J, Pocchiari M, Litvak S, et al. (1999) Ancestral origins and worldwide distribution of the PRNP 200K mutation causing familial Creutzfeldt-Jakob disease. *Am J Hum Genet* **64**:4, 1063–70.
106 Arata H, Takashima H, Hirano R, Tomimitsu H, Machigashira K, Izumi K, et al. (2006) Early clinical signs and imaging findings in Gerstmann-Straussler-Scheinker syndrome (Pro102Leu). *Neurology* **66**:11, 1672–8.
107 Webb TE, Poulter M, Beck J, Uphill J, Adamson G, Campbell T, et al. (2008) Phenotypic heterogeneity and genetic modification of P102L inherited prion disease in an international series. *Brain* **131**:Pt 10, 2632–46.
108 Park MJ, Jo HY, Cheon SM, Choi SS, Kim YS, Kim JW. (2010) A case of Gerstmann-Straussler-Scheinker disease. *J Clin Neurol* **6**:1, 46–50.
109 Irisawa M, Amanuma M, Kozawa E, Kimura F, Araki N. (2007) A case of Gerstmann-Straussler-Scheinker syndrome. *Magn Reson Med Sci* **6**:1, 53–7.
110 Goldfarb LG, Petersen RB, Tabaton M, Brown P, LeBlanc AC, Montagna P, et al. (1992) Fatal familial insomnia and familial Creutzfeldt-Jakob disease: disease phenotype determined by a DNA polymorphism. *Science* **258**:5083, 806–8.
111 Gajdusek DC, Zigas V. (1957) Degenerative disease of the central nervous system in New Guinea; the endemic occurrence of kuru in the native population. *N Engl J Med* **257**:20, 974–8.
112 Will RG. (2003) Acquired prion disease: iatrogenic CJD, variant CJD, kuru. *Br Med Bull* **66**, 255–65.
113 Collinge J, Whitfield J, McKintosh E, Beck J, Mead S, Thomas DJ, et al. (2006) Kuru in the 21st century—an acquired human prion disease with very long incubation periods. *Lancet* **367**:9528, 2068–74.
114 Brown P, Brandel JP, Preece M, Sato T. (2006) Iatrogenic Creutzfeldt-Jakob disease: the waning of an era. *Neurology* **67**:3, 389–93.
115 UK National CJD Surveillance Unit. *The National Creutzfeldt-Jakob Disease Surveillance Unit (NCJDSU)*. [electronic] Edinburgh: Western General Hospital; 2011 [updated August 2011; cited 2011 September 1, 2011]; Available from: http://www.cjd.ed.ac.uk/.
116 WHO. WHO guidelines on tissue infectivity distribution in transmissible spongiform encephalopathies; Report of the WHO consultation in Geneva 14–16 September 2005. Geneva, Switzerland: Quality and Safety of Plasma Derivatives and Related Substances Department of Medicines Policy and Standards Health Technology and Pharmaceuticals Cluster, World Health Organization, 2006 92-4-154701-4.
117 Duffy P, Wolf J, Collins G, DeVoe AG, Streeten B, Cowen D. (1974) Letter: Possible person-to-person transmission of Creutzfeldt-Jakob disease. *N Engl J Med* **290**:12, 692–3.
118 Heckmann JG, Lang CJ, Petruch F, Druschky A, Erb C, Brown P, et al. (1997) Transmission of Creutzfeldt-Jakob disease via a corneal transplant. *J Neurol Neurosurg Psychiatry* **63**:3, 388–90.
119 Bernoulli C, Siegfried J, Baumgartner G, Regli F, Rabinowicz T, Gajdusek DC, et al. (1977) Danger of accidental person-to-person transmission of Creutzfeldt-Jakob disease by surgery. *Lancet* **1**:8009, 478–9.
120 Brown P, Preece M, Brandel JP, Sato T, McShane L, Zerr I, et al. (2000) Iatrogenic Creutzfeldt-Jakob disease at the millennium. *Neurology* **55**:8, 1075–81.
121 Boyd A, Klug GM, Schonberger LB, McGlade A, Brandel JP, Masters CL, et al. (2010) Iatrogenic Creutzfeldt-Jakob disease in Australia: time to amend infection control measures for pituitary hormone recipients? *Med J Aust* **193**:6, 366–9.
122 Abrams JY, Schonberger LB, Belay ED, Maddox RA, Leschek EW, Mills JL, et al. (2011) Lower risk of Creutzfeldt-Jakob disease in pituitary growth hormone recipients initiating treatment after 1977. *J Clin Endocrinol Metab* **96**:10, E1666–9.
123 Healy DL, Evans J. (1993) Creutzfeldt-Jakob disease after pituitary gonadotrophins. *BMJ* **307**:6903, 517–8.
124 Centers Disease Control (CDC). (1987) Update: Creutzfeldt-Jakob disease in a patient receiving a cadaveric dura mater graft. *MMWR Morb Mortal Wkly Rep* **36**:21, 324–5.
125 Centers for Disease Control and Prevention (CDC). (2008) Update: Creutzfeldt-Jakob disease associated with cadaveric dura mater grafts—Japan, 1978–2008. *MMWR Morb Mortal Wkly Rep* **57**:42, 1152–4.
126 Yamada M, Noguchi-Shinohara M, Hamaguchi T, Nozaki I, Kitamoto T, Sato T, et al. (2009) Dura mater graft-associated Creutzfeldt-Jakob disease in Japan: clinicopathological and molecular characterization of the two distinct subtypes. *Neuropathology* **29**:5, 609–18.
127 Will RG, Ironside JW, Zeidler M, Cousens SN, Estibeiro K, Alperovitch A, et al. (1996) A new variant of Creutzfeldt-Jakob disease in the UK. *Lancet* **347**:9006, 921–5.
128 UK National CJD Surveillance Unit. Variant Creutzfeldt-Jakob disease Worldwide Current Data (June 2014). [electronic] Edinburgh: Western General Hospital; 2014 [updated June 2014; cited 2014 6/27/2014]; Available from: http://www.cjd.ed.ac.uk/documents/worldfigs.pdf.
129 Norrby E. (2011) Prions and protein-folding diseases. *J Intern Med* **270**: 1, 1–14.
130 Bruce ME, Will RG, Ironside JW, McConnell I, Drummond D, Suttie A, et al. (1997) Transmissions to mice indicate that "new variant" CJD is caused by the BSE agent. *Nature* **389**:6650, 498–501.
131 Scott MR, Will R, Ironside J, Nguyen HO, Tremblay P, DeArmond SJ, et al. (1999) Compelling transgenetic evidence for transmission of bovine spongiform encephalopathy prions to humans. *Proc Natl Acad Sci U S A* **96**:26, 15137–42.
132 Llewelyn CA, Hewitt PE, Knight RS, Amar K, Cousens S, Mackenzie J, et al. (2004) Possible transmission of variant Creutzfeldt-Jakob disease by blood transfusion. *Lancet* **363**:9407, 417–21.
133 Peden AH, Head MW, Ritchie DL, Bell JE, Ironside JW. (2004) Preclinical vCJD after blood transfusion in a PRNP codon 129 heterozygous patient. *Lancet* **364**:9433, 527–9.

134 Wroe SJ, Pal S, Siddique D, Hyare H, Macfarlane R, Joiner S, et al. (2006) Clinical presentation and pre-mortem diagnosis of variant Creutzfeldt-Jakob disease associated with blood transfusion: a case report. *Lancet* **368**:9552, 2061–7.

135 UK Health Protection Agency. *Variant CJD and blood products.* London: Health Protection Agency; 2007 [updated January 18, 2007; cited 2007 January 23]; Available from: http://www.hpa.org.uk/infections/topics_az/cjd/blood_products.htm.

136 Peden A, McCardle L, Head MW, Love S, Ward HJ, Cousens SN, et al. (2010) Variant CJD infection in the spleen of a neurologically asymptomatic UK adult patient with haemophilia. *Haemophilia* **16**:2, 296–304.

137 Gregori L, McCombie N, Palmer D, Birch P, Sowemimo-Coker SO, Giulivi A, et al. (2004) Effectiveness of leucoreduction for removal of infectivity of transmissible spongiform encephalopathies from blood. *Lancet* **364**:9433, 529–31.

138 Dorsey K, Zou S, Schonberger LB, Sullivan M, Kessler D, Notari Et, et al. (2009) Lack of evidence of transfusion transmission of Creutzfeldt-Jakob disease in a US surveillance study. *Transfusion* **49**:5, 977–84.

139 Kaski D, Mead S, Hyare H, Cooper S, Jampana R, Overell J, et al. (2009) Variant CJD in an individual heterozygous for PRNP codon 129. *Lancet* **374**:9707, 2128.

140 Heath CA, Cooper SA, Murray K, Lowman A, Henry C, MacLeod MA, et al. (2010) Validation of diagnostic criteria for variant Creutzfeldt-Jakob disease. *Ann Neurol* **67**:6, 761–70.

141 Heath CA, Cooper SA, Murray K, Lowman A, Henry C, Macleod MA, et al. (2011) Diagnosing variant Creutzfeldt-Jakob disease: a retrospective analysis of the first 150 cases in the UK. *J Neurol Neurosurg Psychiatry* **82**:6, 646–51.

142 Murray K, Ritchie DL, Bruce M, Young CA, Doran M, Ironside JW, et al. (2008) Sporadic Creutzfeldt-Jakob disease in two adolescents. *J Neurol Neurosurg Psychiatry* **79**:1, 14–8.

143 Binelli S, Agazzi P, Giaccone G, Will RG, Bugiani O, Franceschetti S, et al. (2006) Periodic electroencephalogram complexes in a patient with variant Creutzfeldt-Jakob disease. *Ann Neurol* **59**:2, 423–7.

144 Collie DA, Summers DM, Sellar RJ, Ironside JW, Cooper S, Zeidler M, et al. (2003) Diagnosing variant Creutzfeldt-Jakob disease with the pulvinar sign: MR imaging findings in 86 neuropathologically confirmed cases. *AJNR Am J Neuroradiol* **24**:8, 1560–9.

145 Petzold GC, Westner I, Bohner G, Einhaupl KM, Kretzschmar HA, Valdueza JM. (2004) False-positive pulvinar sign on MRI in sporadic Creutzfeldt-Jakob disease. *Neurology* **62**:7, 1235–6.

146 Haik S, Brandel JP, Oppenheim C, Sazdovitch V, Dormont D, Hauw JJ, et al. (2002) Sporadic CJD clinically mimicking variant CJD with bilateral increased signal in the pulvinar. *Neurology* **58**:1, 148–9.

147 Fulbright RK, Hoffmann C, Lee H, Pozamantir A, Chapman J, Prohovnik I. (2008) MR imaging of familial Creutzfeldt-Jakob disease: a blinded and controlled study. *AJNR Am J Neuroradiol* **29**:9, 1638–43.

148 Will R. (2004) Variant Creutzfeldt-Jakob disease. *Folia Neuropathol* **42** Suppl A, 77–83.

149 Ward HJ, Head MW, Will RG, Ironside JW. (2003) Variant Creutzfeldt-Jakob disease. *Clin Lab Med* **23**:1, 87–108.

150 Garske T, Ghani AC. (2010) Uncertainty in the tail of the variant Creutzfeldt-Jakob disease epidemic in the UK. *PLoS One* **5**:12, e15626.

151 Hilton DA, Ghani AC, Conyers L, Edwards P, McCardle L, Penney M, et al. (2002) Accumulation of prion protein in tonsil and appendix: review of tissue samples. *BMJ* **325**:7365, 633–4.

152 Gill ON, Spencer Y, Richard-Loendt A, Kelly C, Dabaghian R, Boyes L, et al. (2013) Prevalent abnormal prion protein in human appendixes after bovine spongiform encephalopathy epizootic: large scale survey. *BMJ* **347**, f5675.

153 Geschwind MD, Kuo AL, Wong KS, Haman A, Devereux G, Raudabaugh BJ, et al. (2013) Quinacrine treatment trial for sporadic Creutzfeldt-Jakob disease. *Neurology* **81**:23, 2015–23.

154 Haik S, Marcon G, Mallet A, Tettamanti M, Welaratne A, Giaccone G, et al. (2014) Doxycycline in Creutzfeldt-Jakob disease: a phase 2, randomised, double-blind, placebo-controlled trial. *Lancet Neurol* **13**:2, 150–8.

155 Geschwind MD. (2014) Doxycycline for Creutzfeldt-Jakob disease: a failure, but a step in the right direction. *Lancet Neurol* **13**:2, 130–2.

156 Otto M, Cepek L, Ratzka P, Doehlinger S, Boekhoff I, Wiltfang J, et al. (2004) Efficacy of flupirtine on cognitive function in patients with CJD: A double-blind study. *Neurology* **62**:5, 714–8.

157 Stewart LA, Rydzewska LH, Keogh GF, Knight RS. (2008) Systematic review of therapeutic interventions in human prion disease. *Neurology* **70**:15, 1272–81.

158 Whittle IR, Knight RS, Will RG. (2006) Unsuccessful intraventricular pentosan polysulphate treatment of variant Creutzfeldt-Jakob disease. *Acta Neurochir* **148**:6, 677–9.

159 Terada T, Tsuboi Y, Obi T, Doh-ura K, Murayama S, Kitamoto T, et al. (2010) Less protease-resistant PrP in a patient with sporadic CJD treated with intraventricular pentosan polysulphate. *Acta Neurol Scand* **121**:2, 127–30.

160 Tsuboi Y, Doh-Ura K, Yamada T. (2009) Continuous intraventricular infusion of pentosan polysulfate: clinical trial against prion diseases. *Neuropathology* **29**:5, 632–6.

161 Kranitz FJ, Simpson DM. (2009) Using non-pharmacological approaches for CJD patient and family support as provided by the CJD foundation and CJD insight. *CNS Neurol Disord Drug Targets* **8**:5, 372–9.

162 Brown SA, Merritt K, Woods TO, Busick DN. (2005) Effects on instruments of the World Health Organization—recommended protocols for decontamination after possible exposure to transmissible spongiform encephalopathy-contaminated tissue. *J Biomed Mater Res B Appl Biomater* **72**:1, 186–90.

163 Centers for Disease Control and Prevention. Guidelines for Environmental Infection Control in Health-Care Facilities: recommendations of CDC and the Healthcare Infection Control Practices. WHO, Geneva, Advisory Committee (HICPAC). MMWR 2003; 52 (No. RR-10): 1–48 2003 6 June.

164 Tateishi J, Kitamoto T. (1995) Inherited prion diseases and transmission to rodents. *Brain Pathol* **5**:1, 53–9.

165 Fradkin JE, Schonberger LB, Mills JL, Gunn WJ, Piper JM, Wysowski DK, et al. (1991) Creutzfeldt-Jakob disease in pituitary growth hormone recipients in the United States. *JAMA* **265**:7, 880–4.

166 Paterson RW, Takada LT, Geschwind MD. (2012) Diagnosis and treatment of rapidly progressive dementias. *Neurol Clin Pract* **2**:3, 187–200.

167 Hoffman S, Propp JM, McCarthy BJ. (2006) Temporal trends in incidence of primary brain tumors in the United States, 1985–1999. *Neuro Oncol* **8**:1, 27–37.

168 Abrey LE. (2009) Primary central nervous system lymphoma. *Curr Opin Neurol* **22**:6, 675–80.

169 Rubenstein J, Ferreri AJ, Pittaluga S. (2008) Primary lymphoma of the central nervous system: epidemiology, pathology and current approaches to diagnosis, prognosis and treatment. *Leuk Lymphoma* **49** Suppl 1, 43–51.

170 Bhagavathi S, Wilson JD. (2008) Primary central nervous system lymphoma. *Arch Pathol Lab Med* **132**:11, 1830–4.

171 Bataille B, Delwail V, Menet E, Vandermarcq P, Ingrand P, Wager M, et al. (2000) Primary intracerebral malignant lymphoma: report of 248 cases. *J Neurosurg* **92**:2, 261–6.

172 Gerstner ER, Batchelor TT. (2010) Primary central nervous system lymphoma. *Arch Neurol* **67**:3, 291–7.

173 Tang YZ, Booth TC, Bhogal P, Malhotra A, Wilhelm T. (2011) Imaging of primary central nervous system lymphoma. *Clin Radiol* **66**:8, 768–77.

174 Kuker W, Nagele T, Korfel A, Heckl S, Thiel E, Bamberg M, et al. (2005) Primary central nervous system lymphomas (PCNSL): MRI features at presentation in 100 patients. *J Neurooncol* **72**:2, 169–77.

175 Bakshi R, Mazziotta JC, Mischel PS, Jahan R, Seligson DB, Vinters HV. (1999) Lymphomatosis cerebri presenting as a rapidly progressive dementia: clinical, neuroimaging and pathologic findings. *Dement Geriatr Cogn Disord* **10**:2, 152–7.

176 Leschziner G, Rudge P, Lucas S, Andrews T. (2011) Lymphomatosis cerebri presenting as a rapidly progressive dementia with a high methylmalonic acid. *J Neurol* **258**:8, 1489–93.

177 Lewerenz J, Ding X, Matschke J, Schnabel C, Emami P, von Borczyskowski D, et al. (2007) Dementia and leukoencephalopathy due to lymphomatosis cerebri. *J Neurol Neurosurg Psychiatry* **78**:7, 777–8.

178 Martin-Duverneuil N, Mokhtari K, Behin A, Lafitte F, Hoang-Xuan K, Chiras J. (2002) Intravascular malignant lymphomatosis. *Neuroradiology* **44**:9, 749–54.

179 Heinrich A, Vogelgesang S, Kirsch M, Khaw AV. (2005) Intravascular lymphomatosis presenting as rapidly progressive dementia. *Eur Neurol* **54**:1, 55–8.

180 Vieren M, Sciot R, Robberecht W. (1999) Intravascular lymphomatosis of the brain: a diagnostic problem. *Clin Neurol Neurosurg* **101**:1, 33–6.

181 Slee M, Pretorius P, Ansorge O, Stacey R, Butterworth R. (2006) Parkinsonism and dementia due to gliomatosis cerebri mimicking sporadic Creutzfeldt-Jakob disease (CJD). *J Neurol Neurosurg Psychiatry* **77**:2, 283–4.

182 Vates GE, Chang S, Lamborn KR, Prados M, Berger MS. (2003) Gliomatosis cerebri: a review of 22 cases. *Neurosurgery* **53**:2, 261–71; discussion 71.

183 Wall CA, Rummans TA, Aksamit AJ, Krahn LE, Pankratz VS. (2005) Psychiatric manifestations of Creutzfeldt-Jakob disease: a 25-year analysis. *J Neuropsychiatry Clin Neurosci* **17**:4, 489–95.

184 Geschwind MD, Raudabaugh BJ, Haman A, Devereux G, Kramer JH, Miller BL. (2006) Neuropsychiatric features of Creutzfeldt-Jakob disease. *Neurology* **66**:5(Supplement 2), A56.

185 Schott JM, Reiniger L, Thom M, Holton JL, Grieve J, Brandner S, et al. (2010) Brain biopsy in dementia: clinical indications and diagnostic approach. *Acta Neuropathol* **120**:3, 327–41.

186 Warren JD, Schott JM, Fox NC, Thom M, Revesz T, Holton JL, et al. (2005) Brain biopsy in dementia. *Brain* **128**:Pt 9, 2016–25.

187 Josephson SA, Papanastassiou AM, Berger MS, Barbaro NM, McDermott MW, Hilton JF, et al. (2007) The diagnostic utility of brain biopsy procedures in patients with rapidly deteriorating neurological conditions or dementia. *J Neurosurg* **106**:1, 72–5.

188 Zerr I, Kallenberg K, Summers DM, Romero C, Taratuto A, Heinemann U, et al. (2009) Updated clinical diagnostic criteria for sporadic Creutzfeldt-Jakob disease. *Brain* **132**:Pt 10, 2659–68.

189 Vitali P, Migliaccio R, Agosta F, Rosen HJ, Geschwind MD. (2008) Neuroimaging in dementia. *Semin Neurol* **28**:4, 467–83.

CHAPTER 10
Autoimmune dementias

Andrew McKeon and Sean J. Pittock
Mayo Clinic, Rochester, MN, USA

Introduction

In the evaluation of a patient with cognitive decline, clinicians should consider the possibility of an autoimmune etiology on their list of differential diagnoses. The importance of not overlooking this possibility rests in the experience that these patients have a potentially immunotherapy-responsive, reversible disorder [1].

Traditionally, neurologists have usually considered autoimmune dementias within the framework of subacute-onset delirium and limbic encephalitis only. The development and widespread availability of neural antibody marker testing has changed this perspective so that other presenting symptoms such as personality change, executive dysfunction, and psychiatric symptoms are increasingly recognized in an autoimmune context. Clues that are helpful in identifying patients with an autoimmune dementia can be summarized within a triad of (i) suspicious clinical features (a subacute onset of symptoms, a rapidly progressive course, and fluctuating symptoms) and radiological findings, (ii) the detection of CSF or serological biomarkers of autoimmunity, and (iii) a response to immunotherapy (see Table 10.1 for Key Points). This rapidly evolving field is still in its infancy, and much of the clinical data, including that related to treatment and outcomes, is documented in single cases or small retrospective cases series only.

Nomenclature

Diagnostic terms often used to describe such patients include "autoimmune encephalopathy" (which implies delirium is present) and autoimmune dementias (where there is no delirium) and immunotherapy-responsive encephalopathy (as these patients typically have improvements after treatment with corticosteroids). For brevity's sake, we will refer to autoimmune cognitive impairment with or without encephalopathy as autoimmune dementia throughout this chapter. The nomenclature pertaining to autoimmune dementias can seem confusing. Disorders have been classified with respect to clinical phenotype (e.g., progressive encephalomyelitis with rigidity and myoclonus [aka PERM]) [2], eponym (Morvan's syndrome) [3], pathology (e.g., non-vasculitic autoimmune meningoencephalitis (NAIM)) [4], or associated antibody (e.g., the *N*-methyl-D-aspartate receptor (NMDAR) antibody-associated encephalitis) [5]. In some instances, there is more than one name in the literature for a particular disorder; both Hashimoto encephalopathy [6] and steroid-responsive encephalopathy associated with autoimmune thyroiditis (SREAT) [7] refer to the same entity: a triad of cognitive problems, thyroid antibodies detected serologically, and established clinical improvement with immunotherapy. While each description contributes something to our understanding of these disorders, from the standpoint of the practicing neurologist, immunotherapy responsiveness unites these and other autoimmune dementias.

Epidemiology

The incidence and prevalence of autoimmune dementias are unknown. They are thought to be rare but are likely under-recognized. An autoimmune or inflammatory cause of cognitive decline accounts for 20% of dementia in patients under 45 years of age [8].

Clinical features

Symptoms

Autoimmune dementias typically have a subacute onset with progression more rapid than would be expected for most neurodegenerative disorders, with the exception of Creutzfeldt–Jakob disease (CJD). While limbic encephalitis (a fluctuating confusional state accompanied by one or more of seizures, agitation, memory loss, and hallucinations) is the best recognized clinical presentation [9], other symptoms of dementia including apraxia, aphasia, behavioral change, and disturbances in orientation and

Non-Alzheimer's and Atypical Dementia, First Edition. Edited by Michael D. Geschwind and Caroline Racine Belkoura.
© 2016 John Wiley & Sons, Ltd. Published 2016 by John Wiley & Sons, Ltd.

Table 10.1 Key points for autoimmune dementias.

Key points
Clinical manifestations are diverse and often multifocal
Personal history or family history of autoimmunity or cancer might provide important diagnostic clues
Antibodies targeting nonneural antigens (e.g., thyroid, antinuclear) serve as clues for neurological autoimmunity, but do not provide a definitive diagnosis
Neural-specific autoantibodies serve as markers of neurologic autoimmunity and cancer
A trial of immunotherapy (steroids, IVIG, and/or plasma exchange) serves as a diagnostic test. Trials of multiple treatment types may be required
Autoimmune dementias are frequently relapsing and immunotherapy over years may be required

reasoning have been reported [10–12]. Delirium (impaired attention and consciousness) is a common, but not universal, presentation. Marked fluctuations in the clinical course and spontaneous remission suggest an autoimmune cause but can also be seen in patients with toxic and metabolic causes of dementia, in patients with psychogenic disorders, and in patients with depression.

A sleep history may also be informative. Patients with Ma2 antibody encephalitis might complain of hypersomnia [13]. Conversely, patients with voltage-gated potassium channel-complex autoimmunity often complain of insomnia [14]. Patients with sleep apnea syndrome (either central or obstructive) typically have fluctuating cognitive complaints related to a lack of restorative sleep rather than an autoimmune dementia [15].

Case 1

A 58-year-old man with a remote history of thyroid carcinoma, in remission, presented with acute onset of word-finding difficulty and memory problems when giving a presentation to colleagues at work. His evaluation included an MRI of head which demonstrated a left temporal T2 signal abnormality (Figure 10.1a) and an EEG which demonstrated left temporal epileptiform discharges. Neuropsychometric evaluation was remarkable for poor performance on mainly verbal memory scores. Serological evaluation revealed voltage-gated potassium channel (VGKC) complex antibodies, with value of 1.00 nmol/L (normal, ≤ 0.02 nmol/L). PET–CT imaging of body did not demonstrate any new carcinoma. He received intravenous methylprednisolone infusions (1000 mg) daily for 5 days, followed by weekly for 6 weeks. He improved considerably and was "90% better." At that stage, the methylprednisolone dosing interval was widened to one dose every other week. Within 2 weeks, he and his wife noted that he was regressing considerably with respect to memory. He also became emotionally labile and depressed. Repeat MRI imaging demonstrated atrophy of the left hippocampus and new T2 signal abnormality in the right hippocampus (Figure 10.1b). He was treated with seven exchanges of plasmapheresis over 14 days and noted marked improvements. These improvements continued over the next 3 months on prednisone 60 mg by mouth daily. In addition, azathioprine was initiated at 2.5 mg/kg/day as a remission-maintaining drug (mycophenolate mofetil, methotrexate, and hydroxychloroquine are alternatives in this situation; there is no evidence to support the use of one drug over the other). Surveillance neuropsychological evaluation revealed improvements in memory scores almost to within the normal range, although his MRI had not changed. He remained in remission as prednisone alone was tapered slowly over the following 6 months.

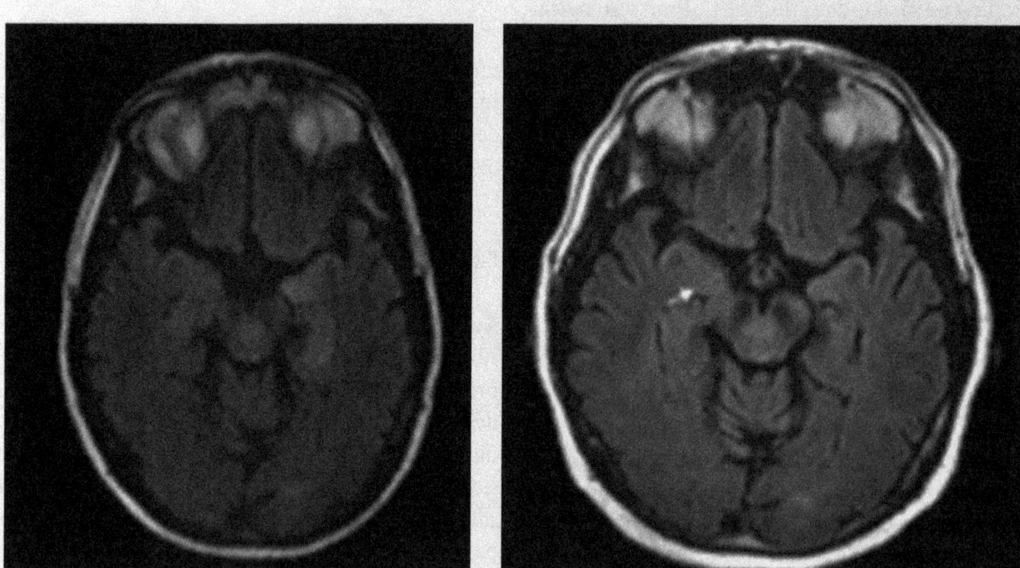

(a) (b)

Figure 10.1 Case 1: FLAIR axial MRIs (radiological orientation). **(a)** At initial symptom onset, T2 signal abnormality is seen in the left hippocampus. **(b)** After relapse, T2 signal is less prominent in the left hippocampus. New, subtle T2 signal abnormality is now seen in the right hippocampus (arrow). Bilateral temporal lobe atrophy is seen. See text.

Case 2

A 47-year-old woman presented with subacute onset of psychosis and severe headaches in 2001. Investigation revealed a lymphocytic pleocytosis on CSF (other CSF data was not available) and a normal MRI brain scan. After 3 months of persistent symptoms despite standard psychiatric treatments, she was treated with steroids empirically and improved significantly but had residual cognitive problems (impairments of verbal intellect, problem solving, visuospatial appreciation, memory and cognitive speed) preventing her return to work. She remained stable with moderate cognitive impairment from early 2002 until November 2009 when she had acute onset of confusion, worsening amnesia, agitation, crying, visual and auditory hallucinations, and behavioral disturbance. She also had one generalized seizure. Again, her CSF demonstrated a lymphocytic pleocytosis with 100 white cells, and oligoclonal bands were present. MRI imaging was unremarkable. CSF paraneoplastic evaluation sent to the Mayo Clinic Neuroimmunology Laboratory identified NMDAR antibodies (Figure 10.2). Evaluations for teratoma including clinical examination, pelvic ultrasound, PET imaging, and finally pathology (after bilateral salpingo-oophorectomy and hysterectomy) were all negative for cancer. She subsequently received intravenous methylprednisolone for 3 days and then five treatments of plasma exchange over 10 days and had marked improvements. The behavioral outbursts, crying, confusion, and agitation ceased. Her cognition improved back to her premorbid 2009 baseline of moderate generalized dysfunction. Maintenance therapy included a slow taper of oral prednisone over 9 months and ongoing maintenance of azathioprine (2.5 mg/kg/day).

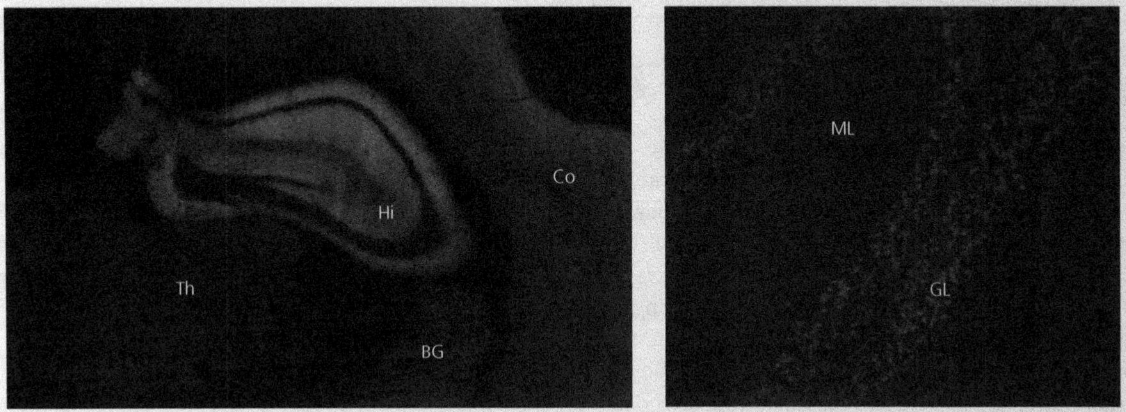

Figure 10.2 NMDAR antibody (relevant to Case 2). Indirect immunofluorescence staining pattern of patient's serum on a composite of mouse neural tissue, provided courtesy of Dr. Vanda A. Lennon, Neuroimmunology Laboratory, Mayo Clinic, Rochester, MN. Hippocampus (Hi) stains brighter than cerebral cortex (Co), basal ganglia (BG), and thalamus (Th). Granular layer (GL) of cerebellum also stains brightly, typical for NMDAR antibody; molecular layer (ML) is negative. (*See insert for color representation of the figure.*)

A fluctuating mental state accompanied by a sleep disorder and parkinsonism can be seen in diffuse Lewy body disease [16] (see Chapter 6).

In some disorders, characteristic noncognitive features are important also. For example, in a patient with a history of visual loss and hearing loss, in addition to cognitive symptoms, Susac's syndrome (an immunotherapy-responsive endotheliopathy) should be considered [17]. Other symptoms and signs common in Susac's syndrome include memory loss, psychiatric symptoms, and headache. Patients with mitochondrial disorders can also present with fluctuating encephalopathies and visual and hearing impairments.

Past and family history

This information is crucial. A history of cancer may be relevant, since an autoimmune, paraneoplastic dementia may be the herald of a recurrence of cancer. Patients with autoimmune dementia frequently have one or more coexisting autoimmune disorders, such as hypothyroidism, SLE, and rheumatoid arthritis. Likewise, a smoking history, review of systemic symptoms, and a family history of autoimmunity and cancer might be informative.

Examination findings

Impairments in one or more categories of attention, memory, reasoning, calculation, and praxis can be documented using brief bedside evaluations such as the MMSE [18], the Montreal Cognitive Assessment (MoCA; www.mocatest.org), or the Kokmen Short Test of Mental Status [19]. More extensive neuropsychological testing, however, is often required to fully characterize the degree of cognitive impairment. This serves both to document the abnormalities present and as a pretreatment baseline. Since autoimmune neurological disorders are often multifocal [20, 21], other neurologic symptoms and signs may accompany the cognitive impairment. These may include seizures, ataxia, brainstem signs, parkinsonism, myoclonus, tremor, myelopathy, or a peripheral nervous system disorder.

Differential diagnoses

Both potentially reversible etiologies (Table 10.2) and neurodegenerative causes for cognitive symptoms need to be considered. Unlike autoimmune dementias, neurodegenerative disorders, with the exception of prion diseases, are usually characterized by indolent onset and slow progression over years.

Table 10.2 Potentially reversible causes of cognitive impairment.

Potentially reversible causes of cognitive impairment	Examples
Cancer (neoplasia)	Primary CNS lymphoma (including intravascular and meningeal presentations)
Autoimmune encephalopathies and dementias	Immunotherapy-responsive disorders of presumed autoimmune etiology
Psychiatric illness	Anxiety, depression, psychosis
Toxic	Alcohol, opiates, cocaine, amphetamines, organic solvents
Inflammatory CNS disorders (other than autoimmune)	Multiple sclerosis, acute disseminated encephalomyelitis, neurosarcoidosis, neuro-Behçet's disease
Vasculopathies	CNS vasculitis, posterior reversible leukoencephalopathy (PRES), subdural hematoma, venous thrombosis
Endocrine	Disturbances in pituitary, thyroid, parathyroid, endocrine pancreatic, or adrenal function
Metabolic	Respiratory, renal or liver failure. Obstructive sleep apnea syndrome. Mitochondrial disorders* (e.g., MELAS)
Infection of the central nervous system	HSV, HHV-6, HIV, fungal (e.g., cryptococcus), mycobacterial, Whipple's disease, neurosyphilis
Nutritional deficiency	Vitamin B12, vitamin E, thiamine, folic acid,
Drugs	Benzodiazepines, antidepressants, antipsychotics, antiepileptics, analgesics
Seizure disorders	Nonconvulsive status epilepticus

The anagram CAPTIVE MINDS may aid memory.
* Mitochondrial diseases can remit, although they are not currently treatable or reversible.

Neurodegenerative disorders include Alzheimer disease, frontotemporal dementia, diffuse Lewy body disease, Parkinson's disease with dementia, progressive supranuclear palsy, and corticobasal degeneration (see Chapters 3, 5–7, and 9). Mitochondrial diseases can also lead to dementia but often have other distinguishing features, such as retinopathy, hearing loss, short stature, and/or neuropathy (www.genetest.org). Among the treatable causes to consider (Table 10.2) are some other idiopathic inflammatory disorders that are also immunotherapy responsive. Each has well-characterized clinical, radiologic, and pathologic diagnostic features and recommended treatments. Examples include multiple sclerosis, CNS vasculitis (also known as primary angiitis of the CNS), sarcoidosis, and neuro-Behçet's disease.

During an MS relapse, a patient may develop subacute cognitive symptoms with delirium and impaired attention, and subsequent improvements may occur during remission [22].

Headache and rapidly progressive dementia are two characteristic presentations of CNS vasculitis [23]. The diagnosis is aided by cerebral angiography and definitively proven by demonstrating multifocal inflammation and necrosis of small arteries, primarily in the leptomeninges; some have a coexisting amyloid angiopathy. This type of biopsy might be necessary to rule out intravascular lymphoma, which can have similar angiographic findings to CNS vasculitis [24].

Although noncognitive deficits (such as cranial neuropathies) are most common in CNS sarcoidosis, some patients may present with cognitive deficits [25]. The diagnosis often proves elusive in patients without systemic disease, and brain biopsy may be required to establish the pathological hallmark of an inflammatory infiltrate with noncaseating granulomas.

Behçet's disease is characterized by uveitis, oral aphthae, and genital ulcerations. Presentations of neuro-Behçet's disease may include a rapidly progressive subcortical dementia characterized by amnesia and a frontal dysexecutive syndrome [26]. In addition, patients can present with pyramidal tract, spinal cord, and sphincter dysfunction. Brain MRI often reveals focal or diffuse T2-weighted hyperintensities, particularly in the basal ganglia, thalamus, upper brainstem, and mesial temporal structures [26].

Rarer infiltrative, inflammatory disorders of the central nervous system, which may be steroid responsive, include Langerhans cell histiocytosis [27], crystal-storing histiocytosis [28], and lymphomatoid granulomatosis [29].

Neurological Testing

Defining abnormalities with objective tests: Neuropsychological testing, imaging, and EEG

There are several components to testing when evaluating a patient with autoimmune dementia. Some testing aids with documenting objective abnormalities, which serves as a baseline before a trial of treatment is undertaken. Resolution of neuropsychological, EEG, MRI (Figure 10.3), or functional imaging abnormalities after immunotherapy serves as an objective marker supporting patient-reported improvements.

Neuropsychological testing, in particular, provides a detailed assessment of deficits and can be very informative in mild cases where the abnormalities are subtle. In addition, other mitigating factors leading to cognitive complaints (such as depression) can be identified by a neuropsychologist. Unfortunately, there is a dearth of literature on the precise cognitive profile of patients with autoimmune dementia. Comprehensive cognitive testing, however, is probably best, including evaluation of memory, frontal-executive function, and processing speed [12].

MRI may reveal findings atypical for neurodegenerative disorders. Mesial temporal lobes are a common location for T2 signal abnormalities in autoimmune dementias. Large extratemporal abnormalities and subtle white matter or gyriform enhancement are sometimes observed [11, 30]. Gyriform T2 signal abnormalities are often seen in CJD but have also been observed in patients with autoimmune encephalopathies initially misdiagnosed with CJD [30]. Avid enhancement should raise concern for an alternative etiology such as a primary brain

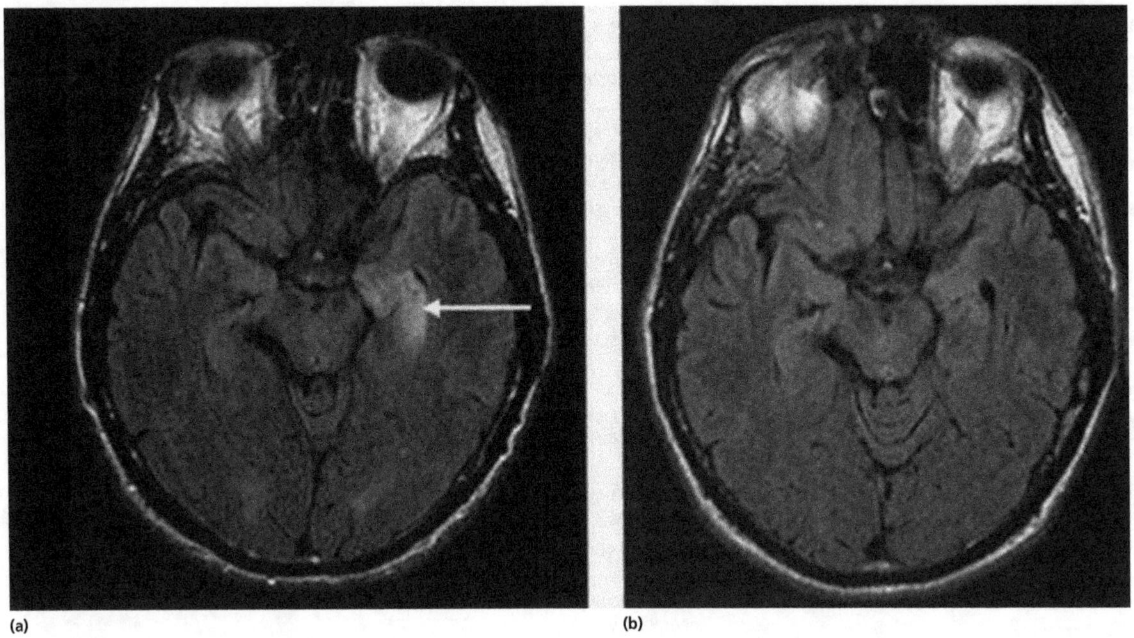

Figure 10.3 FLAIR axial MRIs in a patient with LGI1 ("VGKC") antibody and limbic encephalitis with left greater than right medial temporal lobe hyperintensities (a) that had radiologic and clinical improvements (b) after corticosteroid therapy. Source: McKeon et al. [1]. Reproduced with permission of Wolters Kluwer.

tumor or sarcoidosis. Other causes of large hemispheric T2 signal abnormalities include mitochondrial disorders and progressive multifocal leukoencephalopathy. Patients with Susac's syndrome typically have multifocal leptomeningeal enhancement and T2 signal abnormalities centered around the corpus callosum [17].

Functional imaging (PET or SPECT) may reveal areas of abnormal cerebral metabolism corresponding to clinical symptoms. These modalities are particularly useful in the absence of MRI or EEG abnormalities.

EEG may also help characterize the disorder and provide a pretreatment baseline. Common abnormalities include focal or bilateral mesial temporal abnormalities, but extratemporal abnormalities may also occur [11]. These can include generalized or focal (frontal, parietal, or occipital) slowing, or spike-and-slow-wave epileptiform discharges.

Routine CSF testing

CSF testing can be very informative for an autoimmune diagnosis. Findings supportive of an autoimmune etiology include an elevated CSF protein (>100 mg/dL), mild CSF pleocytosis, abnormal numbers of CSF-exclusive oligoclonal bands, and elevated IgG index and synthesis rate all support an autoimmune etiology. It should be emphasized that these findings are only supportive and not diagnostic of an autoimmune dementia, since any one of them can be detected in other disorders: elevated protein (any neurological disorder), pleocytosis (CNS infection), and elevated CSF oligoclonal bands (65% of multiple sclerosis patients [31], 7% of patients with neurodegenerative disorders [32], and 4% of CJD patients [33]).

Autoantibody testing

Nonneural autoantibodies

Seropositivity for nonneural antibodies may warrant further investigation for an autoimmune pathogenesis for dementia. Unfortunately, many of these commonly ordered tests including both organ (such as thyroid autoantibodies) and nonorgan-specific autoantibodies (such as antinuclear antibody or antibodies targeting the extractable nuclear antigen) lack specificity and are commonly encountered in the normal population. For example, the detection of thyroid autoantibodies in a patient with cognitive complaints should only raise suspicion of an autoimmune basis requiring further evaluation. The detection of antinuclear antibodies and double-stranded DNA antibodies in a patient with subacute-onset cognitive complaints will raise suspicion for lupus cerebritis (also known as CNS lupus; see Chapter 14). This poorly understood disorder is classified along with other manifestations including stroke and peripheral neuropathy under the umbrella of neuropsychiatric lupus. Common features include memory loss, headache, seizures, and movement disorders [34, 35]. There have been some reports of autoantibody markers of neuropsychiatric disease, but none have been confirmed to be of sufficient specificity to warrant clinical use [36, 37]. Similarly, no specific biomarker has been identified as a marker of autoimmune dementia occurring in patients with other nonorgan-specific autoimmune diseases, such as Sjögren's syndrome [38].

Neural autoantibodies

Detection of neural autoantibodies in serum or CSF serves two purposes: to inform the physician of a likely autoimmune etiology and to raise suspicion for a paraneoplastic cause (Table 10.3).

Table 10.3 Antibodies with specificity for neural antigens, accompanying cognitive and other neurological disorders, and oncological accompaniments.

Antibody specificity	Reported cognitive disorders	Other neurologic findings	Cancer association	References
VGKC complex	Limbic encephalitis, amnestic syndrome, executive dysfunction, personality change, disinhibition	Hypothalamic disorder, brainstem encephalitis, ataxia, extrapyramidal disorders, myoclonus, peripheral and autonomic neuropathy	Small cell lung carcinoma; thymoma; adenocarcinoma of breast, prostate	[39–43]
NMDA receptor	Amnestic syndrome	Anxiety, psychosis, seizures, extrapyramidal disorders	Teratoma, usually ovarian	[5]
GAD	Limbic encephalitis, other encephalitides	Stiff person syndrome, stiff person phenomena, ataxia, seizures, brainstem encephalitis, ophthalmoplegia, parkinsonism, myelopathy	Thymoma	[20]
AMPA receptor	Limbic encephalitis	Nystagmus, seizures	Thymic tumors, lung carcinomas, breast carcinoma	[44]
GABAB receptor	Encephalitis	Seizures	Small cell lung carcinoma	[45]
DPPX (subunit of Kv4.1 potassium channel)	Delirium, amnestic syndrome	Seizures, depression, cerebellar ataxia, myoclonus, stiffness, dysautonomia	B cell lymphoma, B-CLL	[46, 47]
mGluR5	Limbic encephalitis	—	Hodgkin lymphoma	[48]
ANNA-1 (anti-Hu)	Limbic encephalitis	Brainstem encephalitis, autonomic neuropathies, sensory neuronopathy	Small cell carcinoma	[49, 50]
ANNA-2 (anti-Ri)	Dementia, limbic encephalitis	Brainstem encephalitis, myelopathy, peripheral neuropathy	Small cell carcinoma or breast adenocarcinoma	[51]
ANNA-3	Limbic encephalitis	Brainstem encephalitis, myelopathy, peripheral neuropathy	Small cell carcinoma	[52]
AGNA (SOX1 antibodies)	Limbic encephalitis	Neuropathy, Lambert–Eaton syndrome	Small cell carcinoma	[53, 54]
PCA-2	Limbic encephalitis	Ataxia, brainstem encephalitis, Lambert–Eaton syndrome, peripheral and autonomic neuropathies	Small cell carcinoma	[55]
CRMP-5 IgG (anti-CV2)	Subacute-onset dementia, personality change, aphasia	Depression, chorea, ataxia, myelopathy, radiculopathy, neuropathy, Lambert–Eaton syndrome	Small cell carcinoma, thymoma	[56]
Amphiphysin	Limbic encephalitis, aphasia, other subacute-onset dementias	Stiff person phenomena, myelopathy, neuropathy	Breast adenocarcinoma, small cell carcinoma	[57]
Anti-Ma proteins (usually Ma2, sometimes Ma1)	Limbic encephalitis	Hypothalamic disorder, brainstem encephalitis	Testis, small cell carcinoma, other solid organ cancers	[58]
NMO-IgG	Reports of encephalopathies in children	Optic neuritis, transverse myelitis	Some reports of thymoma and other solid tumors	[59, 60]
Ganglionic AChR complex	Reports of reversible encephalopathies	Somatic and autonomic peripheral neuropathies	Adenocarcinomas, thymomas	[61]

Source: McKeon et al. [1]. Reproduced with permission of Wolters Kluwer.

The neurological associations of neural autoantibodies tend to be diverse and multifocal, although certain syndromic associations may apply. For example, limbic encephalitis is a classical neurological presentation accompanying ANNA-1 (anti-Hu) [49] and GABAB receptor antibody [45, 62]. Chorea and cognitive symptoms are well-recognized accompaniments of CRMP-5 IgG (anti-CV2 antibody) [56]. Dalmau et al. reported patients with NMDAR antibody [5] (Figure 10.2). These patients frequently reported to psychiatrists with psychosis and other psychiatric complaints early on (as in Case 2), only to develop florid encephalopathies and respiratory failure later on. The autoantibody nomenclature also evolves with increasing knowledge of antigen specificity. VGKC complex antibodies have been known as such because the radioligand used in the radioimmunoassay (^{125}I-α-dendrotoxin) binds to Kv1.1, Kv1.2, and Kv1.6 subunits of VGKCs [39, 40]. Recent data has identified leucine-rich glioma-inactivated 1 (LGI1, which might be coprecipitated with VGKCs) as the antigen targeted by antibodies from patients with limbic encephalitis seropositive by the ^{125}I-α-dendrotoxin immunoassay [41, 42]. There has been some controversy regarding the incidence of cancer among patients with VGKC antibodies. One small series of 10 patients reported no cancer among VGKC complex autoantibody seropositive patients [39]. Other authors have reported incidences ranging from 11 to 33% [41, 43, 63]. The identification of a marker of neural autoimmunity (regardless of target) should direct the physician toward a trial of immunotherapy.

The positive predictive values for cancer of individual antibodies vary from less than 30% for alpha 3 ganglionic AChR antibody [61] to over 80% for ANNA-1 (anti-Hu, pulmonary or extrapulmonary small cell in almost all cases) [49]. Since neurological presentations are often multifocal and diverse, comprehensive antibody testing is usually more informative than testing for one or two selected antibodies [21]. Also, a profile of seropositivity for multiple autoantibodies may be informative for cancer type. For example, in a patient presenting with a rapidly progressive dementia who has muscle acetylcholine receptor binding and modulating antibodies, striational antibody, alpha 3 ganglionic AChR, and CRMP-5 IgG (anti-CV2), those findings should raise a high suspicion for thymoma. Antibody testing on CSF is additionally helpful particularly when serum testing is negative. However, simultaneous testing on serum and CSF is recommended for some NMDAR antibody testing, since CSF is usually more informative.

Testing for cancer

When suspicious for a paraneoplastic cause because of risk factors from the history or because of specific serological or CSF finding, then a search for cancer is appropriate. A thorough physical examination and CT of chest, abdomen, and pelvis are commonly undertaken as primary screening tests in this setting. Other tests are appropriate also and may be required depending on the index of suspicion in an individual patient. Pelvic ultrasound (including transvaginal imaging) and gynecological examination are usually required to evaluate for ovarian carcinoma or teratoma. Mammography and breast examination are required to evaluate for breast carcinoma. Testicular ultrasound, prostate-specific antigen, and prostate examination by digital rectal examination are required to evaluate for testicular and prostate carcinomas, respectively. If neuroblastoma is suspected, and if CT imaging is negative, then imaging using radiolabeled metaiodobenzylguanidine (MIBG) should be considered. Endoscopic examination of the upper and lower gastrointestinal tracts and bronchial tree should also be considered where appropriate. PET–CT imaging increases the diagnostic yield for cancer by 20% in those patients who have had standard evaluations that have not revealed cancer [64].

Other tests aid the search for markers of autoimmunity and for cancer. Finally, it is important to exclude other causes of dementia, in particular other potentially reversible causes.

Treatment

There is no definitive evidence-based approach to treating autoimmune dementias. Much of the authors' practice emanates from small case series [12], individual case reports, and expert opinion [1, 65]. However, a rational approach can be applied to treatment. This can be done by using the acute trial of treatment to serve also as a "diagnostic test." If this is successful, then a maintenance phase of treatment can be embarked upon (Figure 10.4).

Acute therapy

A response to immunotherapy is both diagnostically and therapeutically important. The authors typically initiate a trial of high-dose IV corticosteroid therapy or high-dose intravenous immune globulin (IVIG). IVIG and plasma exchange are especially useful where corticosteroids are contraindicated, such as patients with type 1 diabetes mellitus or who are at risk for that disorder (Table 10.4). Plasma exchange may also be effective [66] where IVIG or corticosteroids have been poorly tolerated; only partial responsiveness to other immunotherapies has been

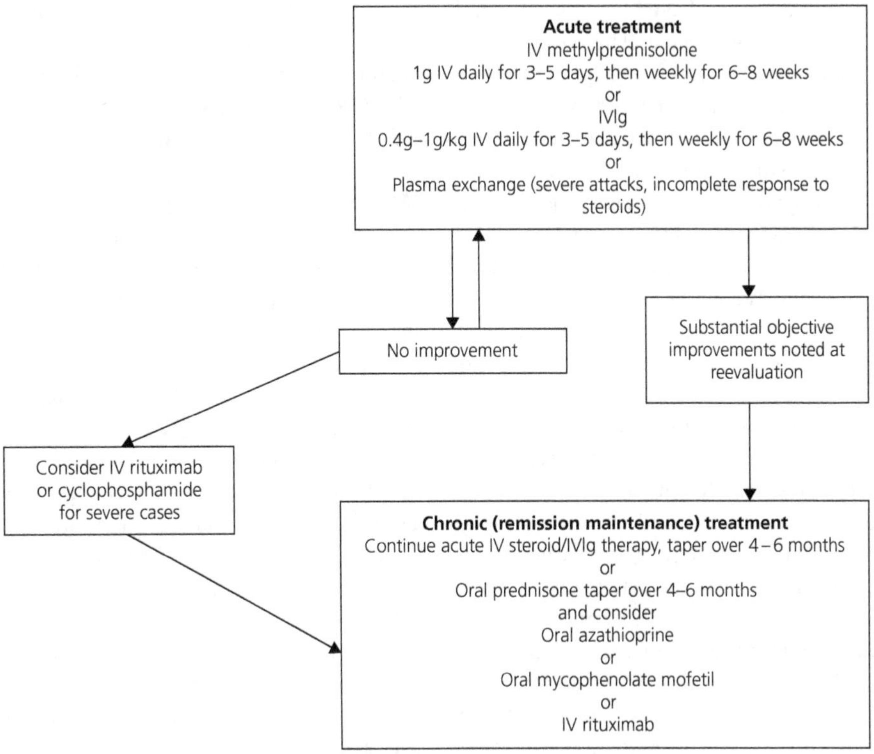

Figure 10.4 A nonevidence-based algorithm for the treatment of patients with suspected autoimmune dementias.

Table 10.4 Some commonly used therapies for autoimmune dementias.

Drug	Dose	Route	Frequency	Some common and severe side effects encountered	Therapeutic phase
Methylprednisolone	500–1000 mg or 15–30 mg/kg	IV	Daily for 3–5 days, followed by weekly for 4–8 weeks	Insomnia, increased appetite, psychiatric disturbance, Cushing's syndrome, skin thinning, diabetes, hypertension, cataracts, recurrent infections, osteoporosis, hip avascular necrosis. Addisonian crisis on rapid withdrawal of physiologic doses of corticosteroid	Acute and chronic
Prednisone	60 mg	PO	Daily for 3 months, then taper by 10 mg/d each month until at 10 mg, then taper by 1 mg/d each thereafter	Insomnia, increased appetite, psychiatric disturbance, Cushing's syndrome, skin thinning, diabetes, hypertension, cataracts, recurrent infections, osteoporosis, hip avascular necrosis. Addisonian crisis on rapid withdrawal of physiologic doses of corticosteroid	Acute and chronic
Immunoglobulin	0.4 g/kg	IV	Daily for 3 days, then alternate weeks for 6–8 weeks	Headache, aseptic meningitis, deep venous thrombosis, anaphylaxis, renal failure	Acute and chronic
Plasma exchange	1 exchange	IV (usually through a central line)	5–7 treatments, every other day over 10–14 days	Hypotension, electrolyte imbalance, infection, thrombosis, and pneumothorax related to central line	Acute
Azathioprine	1–2 mg/kg/d	PO	Two daily divided doses	Hypersensitivity reaction, rash, myelotoxicity	Chronic
Mycophenolate mofetil	500–2000 mg/d	PO	Two daily divided doses	Diarrhea, hypertension, myelotoxicity, CNS lymphoma, renal failure	Chronic
Cyclophosphamide	500–1000 mg/m²/mo (IV) 1–2 mg/kg/d (PO)	IV or PO	Monthly (IV) Daily (PO)	Alopecia, mucositis, infertility, myelotoxicity, hemorrhagic cystitis	Chronic

Source: McKeon et al. [1]. Reproduced with permission of Wolters Kluwer.

established, and further improvements can be expected; or where a rapid response is desired in critically ill patients.

After an initial trial of therapy (usually 6–12 weeks) has been completed, the patient should be reevaluated for subjective and objective evidence of clinical improvement. The reevaluations necessary (clinical, radiological, and electrophysiological) should ideally be completed at the same institution and by the same clinicians to try to avoid interrater variability and differences in testing techniques. This is of greatest importance for the neurological and neuropsychological evaluations. Having received corticosteroid therapy, patients frequently report increased energy and generally feel better, but without clear objective improvement. If one modality of treatment has been unsuccessful, then one or both of the other acute therapies can be tried sequentially to see if immunotherapy responsiveness is likely to occur.

In a Mayo Clinic study, predictors of immunotherapy responsiveness included a subacute onset, a fluctuating course, a short interval between symptom onset and treatment, the detection of a cation channel-specific autoantibody, and an inflammatory spinal fluid [12]. In the authors' experience, the earlier treatment with immunotherapy is initiated, the better the outcome. This is illustrated to some extent in the two described cases. In Case 1, the patient was promptly treated since the diagnosis of an autoimmune dementia was made within a week of symptom onset. Prompt resumption of treatment was also undertaken when he relapsed. The patient is now in remission with near normal cognition. The fortunes of Case 1 contrasts with Case 2 in which primary psychiatric diagnoses were considered for many months during the initial event in 2001 (several years before the NMDAR antibody was described by Dalmau and colleagues) [5]. Some improvements occurred with immunotherapy, but there were residual cognitive deficits. The second episode of neuropsychiatric symptoms in 2009 was recognized early as the NMDAR antibody-associated encephalopathy and was treated rapidly, with rapid return to her premorbid 2009 baseline.

Maintenance therapy

Objective improvements occurring during the acute phase of treatment include improved memory and thinking, a return to work, or resumption of living independently. The occurrence of any or all of these should prompt formulation of a long-term treatment strategy (Table 10.4), since approximately 80% of patients will have a relapse of cognitive symptoms once acute immunotherapy is discontinued [12]. The aims of maintenance therapy include maintaining remission and reducing dependence on corticosteroids, IVIG, and plasma exchange. These can be achieved by the addition of a steroid-sparing purine analog, usually administered orally on a daily basis (azathioprine, mycophenolate mofetil, methotrexate, hydroxychloroquine, or cyclophosphamide) or intravenously (cyclophosphamide). The authors use azathioprine or mycophenolate mofetil as first line treatments, since both have been used widely in myasthenia gravis and neuromyelitis optica. Careful monitoring of blood counts, liver, and renal function tests is necessary throughout treatment with these medications, particularly in the first 3 months.

Once one of these immunosuppressants has been established for 6–12 weeks, the interval between infusions of corticosteroids and IVIG can be gradually extended from weekly to every other week, to every 3 weeks, then monthly, and then discontinue. The overlap of maintenance immunosuppressant and corticosteroid (or IVIG) treatment required is usually 3 months for azathioprine and 6–8 weeks of mycophenolate mofetil. If at that stage the patient is still in remission, the maintenance immunosuppressive agent alone can be continued. In some patients, faster withdrawal of steroids or IVIG results in relapse, and in others, even slow tapering of these treatments is poorly tolerated. For this latter group, daily oral prednisone at a dose of 1 mg/kg/day, maintaining that dose for 3 months, with a slow taper over 6–9 months may be effective in maintaining remission. Withdrawal of chronic oral corticosteroids should be done cautiously (particularly for doses below 10 mg of prednisone/day) with guidance from an endocrinologist or internist, to avoid emergence of adrenocortical failure.

The optimum duration of maintenance immunosuppression for a patient with autoimmune dementia who has achieved remission is unknown. The authors generally recommend between 2 and 3 years of immunosuppression in those that have achieved remission before attempting to withdraw all immunotherapy.

Patients need to be thoroughly counseled regarding the side effects of therapies (Table 10.4). Patients commencing long-term corticosteroid therapy should have a bone density DXA scan at the baseline and take calcium 1500 mg/day and vitamin D 1000 IU/day [67]. These patients should also receive trimethoprim/sulfamethoxazole, one double-strength tablet three times per week as prophylaxis against *Pneumocystis carinii* pneumonia [68]. Prophylaxis against gastroduodenal ulceration and inflammation can also be considered in high-risk patients but is not mandatory.

Prognosis

Outcomes vary among patients with autoimmune dementias. Some patients achieve early (sometimes spontaneous) remissions, while others require lifelong immunosuppressant medication to maintain remission. In one study, 57% of patients who received chronic, maintenance immunosuppressive therapy experienced symptom relapse while reducing the dose of immunotherapy or increasing the interval between infusions of immune globulin and methylprednisolone [12]. Of those followed for 1 year or longer, 62% remained in remission long term.

Conclusion

The rapid identification of subacute cognitive decline as autoimmune dementia facilitates optimum treatment with immunotherapy and an expedited search for a limited stage of cancer in some patients. Clinical, neuropsychological, radiological, and electrophysiological evaluations, where appropriate, before and after a trial (or trials) of immunotherapy enable confirmation of the diagnosis in suspected cases. Chronicity of symptoms and relapsing courses are common. Long-term therapy with a combination of slowly tapered infusions of IVIG or corticosteroids and an oral immunosuppressant is done empirically but may permit long-term remission. Controlled studies are needed to determine the optimum treatments and duration of therapy.

References

1 McKeon A, Lennon, VA, Pittock, SJ. Immunotherapy responsive dementias and encephalopathies. *Continuum*. 2010;**16**(2):80–101.

2 Spitz M, Ferraz HB, Barsottini OG, Gabbai AA. Progressive encephalomyelitis with rigidity: a paraneoplastic presentation of oat cell carcinoma of the lung. Case report. *Arq Neuropsiquiatr*. 2004 Jun;**62**(2B):547–9.

3 Maselli RA, Agius M, Lee EK, Bakshi N, Mandler RN, Ellis W. Morvan's fibrillary chorea. Electrodiagnostic and in vitro microelectrode findings. *Ann N Y Acad Sci*. 1998 May 13;**841**:497–500.

4 Caselli RJ, Boeve BF, Scheithauer BW, O'Duffy JD, Hunder GG. Nonvasculitic autoimmune inflammatory meningoencephalitis (NAIM): a reversible form of encephalopathy. *Neurology*. 1999 Oct 22;**53**(7):1579–81.

5 Dalmau J, Gleichman AJ, Hughes EG, Rossi JE, Peng X, Lai M, et al. Anti-NMDA-receptor encephalitis: case series and analysis of the effects of antibodies. *Lancet Neurol*. 2008 Dec;**7**(12):1091–8.

6 Brain L, Jellinek EH, Ball K. Hashimoto's disease and encephalopathy. *Lancet*. 1966 Sep 3;**2**(7462):512–4.

7 Castillo P, Woodruff B, Caselli R, Vernino S, Lucchinetti C, Swanson J, et al. Steroid-responsive encephalopathy associated with autoimmune thyroiditis. *Arch Neurol*. 2006 Feb;**63**(2):197–202.

8 Kelley BJ, Boeve BF, Josephs KA. Young-onset dementia: demographic and etiologic characteristics of 235 patients. *Arch Neurol*. 2008 Nov;**65**(11):1502–8.

9 Graus F, Saiz A, Lai M, Bruna J, Lopez F, Sabater L, et al. Neuronal surface antigen antibodies in limbic encephalitis: clinical-immunologic associations. *Neurology*. 2008 Sep 16;**71**(12):930–6.

10 McKeon A, Marnane M, O'Connell M, Stack JP, Kelly PJ, Lynch T. Potassium channel antibody associated encephalopathy presenting with a frontotemporal dementia like syndrome. *Arch Neurol*. 2007 Oct;**64**(10):1528–30.

11 McKeon A, Ahlskog JE, Britton JA, Lennon VA, Pittock SJ. Reversible extralimbic paraneoplastic encephalopathies with large abnormalities on magnetic resonance images. *Arch Neurol*. 2009 Feb;**66**(2):268–71.

12 Flanagan EP, McKeon A, Lennon VA, Boeve BF, Trenerry MR, Tan KM, et al. Autoimmune dementia: clinical course and predictors of immunotherapy response. *Mayo Clin Proc*. 2010 Oct;**85**(10): 881–97.

13 Dalmau J, Graus F, Villarejo A, Posner JB, Blumenthal D, Thiessen B, et al. Clinical analysis of anti-Ma2-associated encephalitis. *Brain*. 2004 Aug;**127**(Pt 8):1831–44.

14 Cornelius JR, Lennon VA, Aston PA, McKeon A, Josephs KA, Silber MH. Sleep manifestation of Voltage-Gated Potassium Channel Autoimmunity. *Sleep* 2010;**33**:A283.

15 Engleman HM, Kingshott RN, Martin SE, Douglas NJ. Cognitive function in the sleep apnea/hypopnea syndrome (SAHS). *Sleep* 2000 Jun 15;**23** Suppl 4:S102–8.

16 McKeith IG, Dickson DW, Lowe J, Emre M, O'Brien JT, Feldman H, et al. Diagnosis and management of dementia with Lewy bodies: third report of the DLB Consortium. *Neurology*. 2005 Dec 27;**65**(12): 1863–72.

17 Susac JO, Egan RA, Rennebohm RM, Lubow M. Susac's syndrome: 1975–2005 microangiopathy/autoimmune endotheliopathy. *J Neurol Sci*. 2007 Jun 15;**257**(1–2):270–2.

18 Folstein MF, Folstein SE, McHugh PR. "Mini-mental state." A practical method for grading the cognitive state of patients for the clinician. *J Psychiatr Res*. 1975 Nov;**12**(3):189–98.

19 Kokmen E, Naessens JM, Offord KP. A short test of mental status: description and preliminary results. *Mayo Clin Proc*. 1987 Apr; **62**(4):281–8.

20 Pittock SJ, Yoshikawa H, Ahlskog JE, Tisch SH, Benarroch EE, Kryzer TJ, et al. Glutamic acid decarboxylase autoimmunity with brainstem, extrapyramidal, and spinal cord dysfunction. *Mayo Clin Proc*. 2006 Sep;**81**(9):1207–14.

21 Pittock SJ, Kryzer TJ, Lennon VA. Paraneoplastic antibodies coexist and predict cancer, not neurological syndrome. *Ann Neurol*. 2004 Nov;**56**(5):715–9.

22 Foong J, Rozewicz L, Quaghebeur G, Thompson AJ, Miller DH, Ron MA. Neuropsychological deficits in multiple sclerosis after acute relapse. *J Neurol Neurosurg Psychiatry*. 1998 Apr;**64**(4):529–32.

23 Scolding NJ, Joseph F, Kirby PA, Mazanti I, Gray F, Mikol J, et al. Abeta-related angiitis: primary angiitis of the central nervous system associated with cerebral amyloid angiopathy. *Brain*. 2005 Mar;**128**(Pt 3):500–15.

24 Calamia KT, Miller A, Shuster EA, Perniciaro C, Menke DM. Intravascular lymphomatosis. A report of ten patients with central nervous system involvement and a review of the disease process. *Adv Exp Med Biol*. 1999;**455**:249–65.

25 Hoitsma E, Faber CG, Drent M, Sharma OP. Neurosarcoidosis: a clinical dilemma. *Lancet Neurol*. 2004 Jul;**3**(7):397–407.

26 Al-Araji A, Kidd DP. Neuro-Behcet's disease: epidemiology, clinical characteristics, and management. *Lancet Neurol*. 2009 Feb;**8**(2): 192–204.

27 Grois N, Prayer D, Prosch H, Lassmann H. Neuropathology of CNS disease in Langerhans cell histiocytosis. *Brain*. 2005 Apr;**128** (Pt 4):829–38.

28 Kaminsky IA, Wang AM, Olsen J, Schechter S, Wilson J, Olson R. Central nervous system crystal-storing histiocytosis: neuroimaging, neuropathology, and literature review. *AJNR Am J Neuroradiol*. 2011 Feb;**32**(2):E26–8.

29 Rodriguez FJ, Gamez JD, Vrana JA, Theis JD, Giannini C, Scheithauer BW, et al. Immunoglobulin derived depositions in the nervous system: novel mass spectrometry application for protein characterization in formalin-fixed tissues. *Lab Invest*. 2008 Oct; **88**(10):1024–37.

30 Geschwind MD, Tan KM, Lennon VA, Barajas RF, Jr., Haman A, Klein CJ, et al. Voltage-gated potassium channel autoimmunity mimicking creutzfeldt-jakob disease. *Arch Neurol*. 2008 Oct;**65**(10):1341–6.

31 Zipoli V, Hakiki B, Portaccio E, Lolli F, Siracusa G, Giannini M, et al. The contribution of cerebrospinal fluid oligoclonal bands to the early diagnosis of multiple sclerosis. *Mult Scler*. 2009 Apr;**15**(4):472–8.

32 Janssen JC, Godbolt AK, Ioannidis P, Thompson EJ, Rossor MN. The prevalence of oligoclonal bands in the CSF of patients with primary neurodegenerative dementia. *J Neurol*. 2004 Feb;**251**(2): 184–8.

33 Green A, Sanchez-Juan P, Ladogana A, Cuadrado-Corrales N, Sanchez-Valle R, Mitrova E, et al. CSF analysis in patients with sporadic CJD and other transmissible spongiform encephalopathies. *Eur J Neurol*. 2007 Feb;**14**(2):121–4.

34 Borchers AT, Aoki CA, Naguwa SM, Keen CL, Shoenfeld Y, Gershwin ME. Neuropsychiatric features of systemic lupus erythematosus. *Autoimmun Rev*. 2005 Jul;**4**(6):329–44.

35 Joseph FG, Lammie GA, Scolding NJ. CNS lupus: a study of 41 patients. *Neurology*. 2007 Aug 14;**69**(7):644–54.

36 Weiner SM, Klein R, Berg PA. A longitudinal study of autoantibodies against central nervous system tissue and gangliosides in connective tissue diseases. *Rheumatol Int*. 2000;**19**(3):83–8.

37 Kimura A, Kanoh Y, Sakurai T, Koumura A, Yamada M, Hayashi Y, et al. Antibodies in patients with neuropsychiatric systemic lupus erythematosus. *Neurology*. 2010 Apr 27;**74**(17):1372–9.

38 Delalande S, de Seze J, Fauchais AL, Hachulla E, Stojkovic T, Ferriby D, et al. Neurologic manifestations in primary Sjogren syndrome: a study of 82 patients. *Medicine*. 2004 Sep;**83**(5):280–91.

39 Vincent A, Buckley C, Schott JM, Baker I, Dewar BK, Detert N, et al. Potassium channel antibody-associated encephalopathy: a potentially immunotherapy-responsive form of limbic encephalitis. *Brain*. 2004 Mar;**127**(Pt 3):701–12.

40 Thieben MJ, Lennon VA, Boeve BF, Aksamit AJ, Keegan M, Vernino S. Potentially reversible autoimmune limbic encephalitis with neuronal potassium channel antibody. *Neurology*. 2004 Apr 13;**62**(7):1177–82.

41 Lai M, Huijbers MG, Lancaster E, Graus F, Bataller L, Balice-Gordon R, et al. Investigation of LGI1 as the antigen in limbic encephalitis previously attributed to potassium channels: a case series. *Lancet Neurol*. 2010 Aug;**9**(8):776–85.

42 Irani SR, Alexander S, Waters P, Kleopa KA, Pettingill P, Zuliani L, et al. Antibodies to Kv1 potassium channel-complex proteins leucine-rich, glioma inactivated 1 protein and contactin-associated protein-2 in limbic encephalitis, Morvan's syndrome and acquired neuromyotonia. *Brain*. 2010 Sep;**133**(9):2734–48.

43 Tan KM, Lennon VA, Klein CJ, Boeve BF, Pittock SJ. Clinical spectrum of voltage-gated potassium channel autoimmunity. *Neurology*. 2008 May 13;**70**(20):1883–90.

44 Lai M, Hughes EG, Peng X, Zhou L, Gleichman AJ, Shu H, et al. AMPA receptor antibodies in limbic encephalitis alter synaptic receptor location. *Ann Neurol*. 2009 Apr;**65**(4):424–34.

45 Lancaster E, Lai M, Peng X, Hughes E, Constantinescu R, Raizer J, et al. Antibodies to the GABA(B) receptor in limbic encephalitis with seizures: case series and characterisation of the antigen. *Lancet Neurol* 2010 Jan;**9**(1):67–76.

46 Boronat A, Gelfand JM, Gresa-Arribas N, Jeong HY, Walsh M, Roberts K, et al. Encephalitis and antibodies to dipeptidyl-peptidase-like protein-6, a subunit of Kv4.2 potassium channels. *Ann Neurol*. 2013 Jan;**73**(1):120–8.

47 Tobin WO, Lennon VA, Komorowski L, Probst C, Clardy S, Aksamit A, Lucchinetti CF, Pittock SJ, Tippmann-Piekert M, Wirrell E, McKeon A. DPPX autoantibody: frequency, clinical accompaniments and outcomes. *Neurology* 2014;**82**:S40.001.

48 Lancaster E, Martinez-Hernandez E, Titulaer MJ, Boulos M, Weaver S, Antoine JC, et al. Antibodies to metabotropic glutamate receptor 5 in the Ophelia syndrome. *Neurology*. 2011 Nov 1;**77**(18):1698–701.

49 Lucchinetti CF, Kimmel DW, Lennon VA. Paraneoplastic and oncologic profiles of patients seropositive for type 1 antineuronal nuclear autoantibodies. *Neurology.* 1998 Mar;**50**(3):652–7.

50 Dalmau J, Furneaux HM, Gralla RJ, Kris MG, Posner JB. Detection of the anti-Hu antibody in the serum of patients with small cell lung cancer—a quantitative western blot analysis. *Ann Neurol.* 1990 May;**27**(5):544–52.

51 Pittock SJ, Lucchinetti CF, Lennon VA. Anti-neuronal nuclear autoantibody type 2: paraneoplastic accompaniments. *Ann Neurol.* 2003 May;**53**(5):580–7.

52 Chan KH, Vernino S, Lennon VA. ANNA-3 anti-neuronal nuclear antibody: marker of lung cancer-related autoimmunity. *Ann Neurol.* 2001 Sep;**50**(3):301–11.

53 Sabater L, Titulaer M, Saiz A, Verschuuren J, Gure AO, Graus F. SOX1 antibodies are markers of paraneoplastic Lambert-Eaton myasthenic syndrome. *Neurology.* 2008 Mar 18;**70**(12):924–8.

54 Graus F, Vincent A, Pozo-Rosich P, Sabater L, Saiz A, Lang B, et al. Anti-glial nuclear antibody: marker of lung cancer-related paraneoplastic neurological syndromes. *J Neuroimmunol.* 2005 Aug;**165**(1–2):166–71.

55 Vernino S, Lennon VA. New Purkinje cell antibody (PCA-2): marker of lung cancer-related neurological autoimmunity. *Ann Neurol.* 2000 Mar;**47**(3):297–305.

56 Yu Z, Kryzer TJ, Griesmann GE, Kim K, Benarroch EE, Lennon VA. CRMP-5 neuronal autoantibody: marker of lung cancer and thymoma-related autoimmunity. *Ann Neurol.* 2001 Feb;**49**(2):146–54.

57 Pittock SJ, Lucchinetti CF, Parisi JE, Benarroch EE, Mokri B, Stephan CL, et al. Amphiphysin autoimmunity: paraneoplastic accompaniments. *Ann Neurol.* 2005 Jul;**58**(1):96–107.

58 Dalmau J, Gultekin SH, Voltz R, Hoard R, DesChamps T, Balmaceda C, et al. Ma1, a novel neuron- and testis-specific protein, is recognized by the serum of patients with paraneoplastic neurological disorders. *Brain.* 1999 Jan;**122** (Pt 1):27–39.

59 McKeon A, Lennon VA, Lotze T, Tenenbaum S, Ness JM, Rensel M, et al. CNS aquaporin-4 autoimmunity in children. *Neurology.* 2008 Jul 8;**71**(2):93–100.

60 Pittock SJ, Lennon VA. Aquaporin-4 autoantibodies in a paraneoplastic context. *Arch Neurol.* 2008 May;**65**(5):629–32.

61 McKeon A, Lennon VA, Lachance DH, Fealey RD, Pittock SJ. Ganglionic acetylcholine receptor autoantibody: oncological, neurological, and serological accompaniments. *Arch Neurol.* 2009 Jun;**66**(6):735–41.

62 Jeffery OJ, Lennon VA, Pittock SJ, Gregory JK, Britton JW, McKeon A. GABAB receptor autoantibody frequency in service serologic evaluation. *Neurology.* 2013 Sep 3;**81**(10):882–7.

63 Klein CJ, Lennon VA, Aston PA, McKeon A, O'Toole O, Quek A, et al. Insights from LGI1 and CASPR2 potassium channel complex autoantibody subtyping. *JAMA Neurol.* 2013 Feb;**70**(2): 229–34.

64 McKeon A, Apiwattanakul M, Lachance DH, Lennon VA, Mandrekar JN, Boeve BF, et al. Positron emission tomography-computed tomography in paraneoplastic neurologic disorders: systematic analysis and review. *Arch Neurol.* 2010 Mar;**67**(3): 322–9.

65 Vernino S, Geschwind M, Boeve B. Autoimmune encephalopathies. *Neurologist.* 2007 May;**13**(3):140–7.

66 Hussain NS, Rumbaugh J, Kerr D, Nath A, Hillis AE. Effects of prednisone and plasma exchange on cognitive impairment in Hashimoto encephalopathy. *Neurology.* 2005 Jan 11;**64**(1):165–6.

67 Recommendations for the prevention and treatment of glucocorticoid-induced osteoporosis: 2001 update. American college of Rheumatology Ad Hoc Committee on Glucocorticoid-Induced Osteoporosis. *Arthritis Rheum.* 2001 Jul;**44**(7):1496–503.

68 Green H, Paul M, Vidal L, Leibovici L. Prophylaxis for Pneumocystis pneumonia (PCP) in non-HIV immunocompromised patients. *Cochrane database of Syst Rev.* 2007(3):CD005590.

CHAPTER 11

Toxic and metabolic dementias

Michelle Mattingly[1], Katie Osborn[2] and Leon Prockop[1]
[1] University of South Florida, Tampa, FL, USA
[2] Geisel School of Medicine at Dartmouth, Hanover, NH, USA

Introduction

Toxic and metabolic forms of dementia (TMD) are critical to identify as they are often treatable, if not curable, unlike most other dementias discussed in this book. Cognitive impairment might be a direct consequence of medical illness or metabolic perturbations. Although technically not dementia, delirium should always be considered as an etiology of cognitive impairment. First, we discuss toxic causes of dementia, followed by a review of major metabolic etiologies of cognitive impairment.

Toxic dementias

Exposure to toxic substances, either acutely or chronically, can lead to dementia. Table 11.1 includes a list of several toxic agents that might cause dementia [1]. This section of the chapter will focus on three agents that are among the most common causes of toxic cognitive dysfunction—carbon monoxide, ethanol, and lead.

Carbon monoxide

Carbon monoxide (CO) is a leading cause of death from poisoning in the United States and is responsible for 40 000 emergency department visits and 5000 to 6000 deaths per year [2]. CO is a tasteless, odorless, nonirritating but highly toxic gas, which makes it difficult to detect. Therefore, the true incidence of CO poisoning is unknown.

CO is a by-product of the incomplete combustion of hydrocarbons. Common sources of CO exposure include intentional suicides as well as unintentional exposures from home heating, automobile exhaust, and smoke inhalation [2]. CO poisoning may occur as a result of a building fire or from fuel-powered generators and heaters, particularly in poorly ventilated spaces. The latter commonly occurs during winter storms, earthquakes, and hurricanes following a power outage.

Case presentation (reprinted with permission from Prockop [3])

Chronic CO exposure

VB, a 39-year-old woman, and SB, her 8-year-old daughter, had lived in an apartment for several years without incident. In the fall of 1998, both suffered recurrent illnesses characterized by lethargy, headache, and occasional vomiting diagnosed as "flu" when medical assistance was sought. On several occasions, they stayed with friends while recuperating. Symptoms cleared quickly, only to recur on resuming residence in the apartment. VB, an educator, noted new learning dysfunction. SB's previously high grades declined. Suspecting an environmental toxin, VB summoned local health officials who found 106 ppm CO in a random apartment air sample. Although they vacated the apartment, headaches, malaise, and intellectual problems persisted such that VB discontinued efforts toward a PhD degree. SB experienced low school grades and had a B rather than a prior A average. On neurological examination, both were within normal limits except for cerebellar dysfunction characterized by loss of check with rebound in both with mild truncal ataxia in VB. Neuropsychological tests in VB demonstrated moderate to severe cognitive deficits, especially those involving executive functions. In SB, neuropsychological tests yielded scores from borderline to severe impairment in nonverbal sequences, complex copying, visuospatial judgment, and organization. Compared to premorbid estimated levels of functioning, both showed deficits involving higher-order cognitive functioning, reading comprehension, and qualitative conceptualization. MRI and MRS in both were normal.

Clinical symptoms/features

The brain and the heart are most susceptible to CO toxicity due to their high metabolic rates. Clinical symptoms of CO poisoning tend to be nonspecific and can mimic a variety of common disorders. Symptoms range in severity from mild, flu like (simulating a viral infection) to more severe leading to coma and

Non-Alzheimer's and Atypical Dementia, First Edition. Edited by Michael D. Geschwind and Caroline Racine Belkoura.
© 2016 John Wiley & Sons, Ltd. Published 2016 by John Wiley & Sons, Ltd.

Table 11.1 Toxic causes of dementia (differential diagnosis).

Agent	Occupational or Other exposure	Syndrome	
		Acute	*Chronic*
METALS			
Arsenic	Pesticides, pigments, paint, electroplating, seafood, smelter, semiconductors	Encephalopathy with dementia	Neuropathy
Bismuth	Over ingestion of bismuth salicylates (e.g., PeptoBismol®)	Encephalopathy, ataxia, myoclonus	Possible irreversibility, death
Lead	Solder, lead shot, illicit whiskey, insecticides, auto body shop, storage battery manufacture, smelter, paint, water pipes, gasoline sniffing	Encephalopathy with dementia	Encephalopathy, neuropathy, motor neuron disease- like syndrome
Manganese	Iron industry, welding, mining, smelter, fireworks, fertilizer, dry cell batteries	Encephalopathy	Parkinsonism
Mercury	Thermometers, other gauges, dental office (amalgams), felt hat manufacture, electroplating, photography	Headache, tremor with dementia	Neuropathy, encephalopathy with dementia, tremor
Tin	Canning industry, solder, electronics, plastics, fungicides	Delirium	Encephalomyelopathy with dementia
RECREATIONAL ABUSE			
Nitrous oxide	Dental offices	Encephalopathy with dementia	B_{12}-deficient myelopathy
ENVIRONMENTAL/FOOD			
Ciguatera (from fish)		Sensory neuropathy with temperature inversion	
Shellfish		Acute neuropathy	
Carbon monoxide	Accidental or deliberate exposure in motor vehicles, faulty gasoline-fueled heaters	Anoxic encephalopathy with dementia	Encephalopathy, delayed neuropsychiatric syndrome, dementia
Methyl alcohol	Contaminated illicit whiskey	Retinal blindness	
SOLVENTS			
Carbon disulfide	Rayon manufacture, preservatives, textiles, rubber cement, varnish, electroplating	Encephalopathy with dementia	Neuropathy, Parkinsonism
Trichlorethylene	Paints, degreasers, spot removers, decaffeination, dry cleaning, rubber solvents	Narcosis	Encephalopathy, trigeminal neuropathy, dementia
Hexacarbons	Paints, paint removers, varnish, degreasers, rapid-drying ink, glues, cleaning agents, glues for making shoes in poorly vented cottage industry, glue sniffing, MNBK in plastics	Narcosis	Neuropathy, encephalopathy, ataxia, dementia
INSECTICIDES			
Organophosphates, carbamates	Manufacture, application	Cholinergic syndrome	Ataxia, neuropathy, myelopathy

death. The general symptoms of CO poisoning include headache, malaise, difficulty concentrating, dizziness, nausea, fatigue, and weakness. When not fatal, a wide spectrum of CO-induced encephalopathy ranges from reversible dysfunction to severe irreversible dementia. Table 11.2 lists some of the clinical signs and symptoms associated with CO poisoning and correlated carboxyhemoglobin (COHb) levels [2, 4].

Neurologic symptoms include dementia, cerebellar dysfunction, and parkinsonism [5]. A delayed neuropsychiatric syndrome may follow acute exposure by 3–240 days, with cognitive

Table 11.2 Clinical signs and symptoms associated with CO poisoning and correlated COHb levels.

Severity	COHb level	Signs and symptoms
Mild	<15–20%	Headache, nausea, vomiting, dizziness, blurred vision
Moderate	21–40*	Confusion, syncope, chest pain, dyspnea, weakness, tachycardia, rhabdomyolysis
Severe	41–59*	Palpitations, dysrhythmias, hypotension, myocardial ischemia, cardiac arrest, respiratory arrest, pulmonary edema, seizures, coma
Fatal	60+%	Death

* At moderate to severe levels of COHb poisoning the correlation between blood levels and symptomatology is poor.

and personality changes and psychotic behavior [5, 6]. This syndrome is characterized by a relapse of symptoms associated with CO poisoning, occurring after a transient period of improvement. Whereas the physical and cognitive symptoms associated with severe acute exposure are obvious, the cognitive sequelae of low-level exposure are more easily misdiagnosed or overlooked [7].

Affective and personality changes following CO exposure are occasionally more prominent and/or life changing than cognitive impairment. Depression, anxiety, obsessive-compulsive behaviors, delusions and hallucinations, violent outbursts, fear, elated mood, apathy, lack of motivation, and irritability are commonly reported symptoms [8, 9]. Depression and anxiety likely result from a combination of factors that include neural injury and psychological reactions to the physical and cognitive sequelae that occur following CO poisoning.

Neurologic exam

Although not necessarily specific to CO intoxication, common neurological exam findings may include abnormalities on the Romberg test, impaired heel–toe gait, dysdiadochokinesis, and poor performance on finger nose testing and serial sevens. Impaired fine movements, nystagmus, ataxia, compromised mental status examination, impaired reflexes, and intention tremor may also present. In severe cases, a tonic disorder or decerebrate rigidity associated with increased deep tendon reflexes and extensor plantar responses may be observed. Cortical blindness may be transitory and characterized by visual loss but intact pupillary reactions to light. Visual field defects, paracentral scotomas, decreased light sensitivity, and decreased dark adaption have been reported [10]. Flame-shaped superficial retinal hemorrhages have been reported in long-term, subacute CO poisoning but are nonspecific [11]. Papilledema can be evident on funduscopic examination. The classic cherry-red discoloration of the skin and cyanosis are rare.

Neuropsychological findings

Cognitive impairment occurs in 15–49% of individuals exposed to CO [12]. No consistent pattern of cognitive deficits following CO poisoning has been observed, but impaired memory, attention, information processing speed, and executive function are common sequelae. Persistent cognitive dysfunction lasting more than one month appears to occur in 25–50% of individuals with associated loss of consciousness or COHb levels greater than 25% [13–16]. Even those individuals with less severe and lower level CO poisoning might develop cognitive impairments [17].

Neuroimaging

In general, neuroimaging demonstrates evidence of morphologic damage that correlates to that reported in postmortem pathological studies. A distinct constellation of brain and MRI abnormalities includes globus pallidus lesions, white matter changes, and diffuse low-density lesions throughout the brain. Abnormalities in the globus pallidus is common on both CT and MRI studies. Cerebral edema might occur early and sometimes predicts poor outcome (e.g., death or severe permanent damage). Globus pallidus changes do not always predict outcome. Diffuse deep white matter MRI abnormalities correlate better with clinical status and prognosis; these changes are probably related to hypoxia/ischemia associated with CO toxicity [18–20].

The brain MRI might appear normal in some cases of dementia caused by CO exposure; in such circumstances, brain MRS abnormalities are often present. As MRS examines brain metabolites, the abnormal MRS often reflects decreased *n*-acetylaspartase in the basal ganglia bilaterally [3].

Laboratory findings

Ambient air levels of CO should be obtained as soon as possible after CO exposure. The Centers for Disease Control and Prevention (CDC) [21] guidelines indicate the key to confirming the diagnosis in measuring the patient's COHb level, which can be tested either in whole blood or exhaled air. COHb level should be obtained immediately as the half-life of COHb is 4–5 h. Normal levels are <2% nonsmokers and 5–13% for smokers. An elevated COHb level of ≥2% for nonsmokers or >12% for smokers strongly supports a diagnosis of CO poisoning. Pulse oximetry is unreliable for the diagnosis of CO intoxication because it is unable to distinguish oxyhemoglobin from COHb. A thorough and accurate assessment of clinical symptoms and CO exposure history is critical to determine the type and intensity of treatment as COHb levels do not correlate well with severity of illness, outcomes, or response to treatment.

Pathophysiology and pathology

CO toxicity is caused by impaired oxygen delivery and use, leading to cellular hypoxia. Inhalation results in CO binding rapidly to Hb, leading to the formation of COHb. The oxygen-carrying capacity of the blood decreases, causing tissue hypoxia. The affinity of Hb for CO is 210 times its affinity for oxygen, and CO easily displaces oxygen from Hb. COHb also impairs the release of oxygen from Hb by increasing oxygen binding to Hb, resulting in decreased oxygen delivery to cells. CO also might directly cause mitochondrial damage [22].

The neuropathology of CO toxicity has been well described in postmortem studies [23] and in acute cases, includes petechial hemorrhages of the white matter, in particular involving the corpus callosum. In cases surviving more than 48 h, there is multifocal necrosis involving globus pallidus, hippocampus, pars reticularis of the substantia nigra, laminar necrosis of the cortex, and loss of Purkinje cells in the cerebellum, along with white matter lesions. The typical pallidum lesions are well defined—bilateral globus pallidus macroscopic infarctions, usually asymmetrical, extending anteriorly, superiorly, or into the internal capsule. Occasionally, only a small linear focus of necrosis is found at the junction of the internal capsule and the internal nucleus of the globus pallidus. Less commonly, hemorrhages in the hippocampus are seen. CO intoxication usually spares the hypothalamus, walls of the third ventricle, thalamus, striatum, and brainstem. Myelin damage is constant and ranges from discrete, perivascular foci in the corpus callosum, the internal–external capsule and the optic tracts usually seen in comatose patients who died within 1 week, to extensive periventricular demyelination and axonal destruction observed in comatose patients with longer survival, sometimes leading to formation of plaques of demyelination [5].

Treatment

Tissue hypoxia is the major outcome of CO intoxication; therefore, based on chemical and pathophysiological data, oxygen is the "natural antidote" [24].

The CDC [21] recommends the following guidelines for the management of CO poisoning:

- Administer 100% oxygen until the patient is symptom free, usually about 4–5 h. Serial neurologic exams should be performed to assess progress and to detect the signs of developing cerebral edema.
- Consider hyperbaric oxygen therapy (HBO) when the patient has a COHb level of more than 25–30%; there is evidence of cardiac involvement, severe acidosis, transient or prolonged unconsciousness, neurological impairment, abnormal neuropsychiatric testing; or the patient is ≥36 years in age. HBO is also administered at lower COHb (<25%) levels if suggested by clinical condition and history of exposure.

Although some nonrandomized studies indicate that HBO reverses both the acute and delayed effects of CO poisoning, other data are conflicting. Therefore, it is not clear whether HBO influences the rates of either late sequelae or morbidity. It is generally agreed that HBO hastens resolution of symptoms and is usually indicated [25–29].

Ethanol

Ethanol is a specific type of alcohol, and the only type that can be consumed. Within this section ethanol and alcohol will both be used to refer to the effects of Ethanol, given that alcohol is the more frequently used term. Ethanol intoxication is the consequence of an accumulation of it and its metabolites in the bloodstream that occurs faster than can be metabolized by the liver. In the United States, roughly 10% of adults meet diagnostic criteria for an alcohol abuse or dependence disorder. Of those, approximately 50% who become dependent exhibit neurocognitive impairments when assessed 3–4 weeks following abstinence [30]. A variety of dementia symptoms and neurological dysfunction can occur after ethanol ingestion [31] (Table 11.3).

Clinical and neurologic symptoms/features

Ethanol acts as a central nervous system depressant (Table 11.4). Acute overconsumption can lead to tremors, seizures, hallucinations, ataxia, neuropathy, stroke, stupor, respiratory depression, coma, and death. Visual findings may include suppression of

Table 11.3 Major dementia issues in alcoholics (sometimes nutritional).

Disorder	Clinical features	Probable deficiency
Wernicke syndrome	Dementia with lethargy, inattentiveness, apathy, and amnesia Ophthalmoparesis Gait ataxia	Thiamine
Korsakoff syndrome	Dementia, mainly amnesia, with or without confabulation	Thiamine
Cerebellar degeneration	Gait ataxia; limb coordination relatively preserved	Probably thiamine plus other vitamins plus ethanol neurotoxicity
Polyneuropathy	Distal limb sensory loss and weakness; less often autonomic dysfunction	Probably thiamine plus other vitamins plus ethanol neurotoxicity
Amblyopia	Optic atrophy, decreased visual acuity, central scotomas; total blindness rare.	Probably thiamine plus other vitamins plus ethanol neurotoxicity

Table 11.4 Metabolic causes of dementia (differential diagnosis).

Disorder	Clinical features
Endocrine	
1. Thyroid	
(a) Hypo	Encephalopathy, dementia
(b) Hyper	Dementia
2. Pituitary	
(a) Hypo	Encephalopathy, dementia
(b) Hyper	Visual disturbances/increased LCP
3. Adrenal	
(a) Hypo	Lethargy, fatigue, dementia
(b) Hyper	Seizures, dementia
Hepatic	Encephalopathy, dementia
Cardiac/pulmonary/hypoxia	Encephalopathy, dementia
Vitamin deficiency	Encephalopathy, dementia, peripheral neuropathy
Electrolyte disturbances	Encephalopathy, dementia
Glucose derangement	Encephalopathy, seizures, dementia, peripheral neuropathy

rapid eye movement during sleep, slow saccadic eye movements, and interrupted jerky pursuit movements. Gait and balance disturbances are also common and may persist after detoxification [32, 33]. Chronic overconsumption can cause liver damage, as well as severe withdrawal symptoms, including seizures, hallucinations, and autonomic dysfunction (i.e., delirium tremens) [34].

Ethanol affects cognition both directly and indirectly. Ethanol is a direct neurotoxin and when sufficiently abused may lead to dementia. Ethanol, or possibly the components of alcohol, such as certain compounds in red wine including resveratrol, however, appear to have neuroprotective properties and reduce the risk of dementia, including Alzheimer's type, when ingested in low-to-moderate amounts [35]. Further, both abstaining from and chronically abusing alcohol are associated with elevated risks of dementia. The relationship between drinking behavior and risk for dementia is described as a J-curve, meaning those who abstain from alcohol completely appear to develop dementia at higher rates than those who regularly drink moderate amounts of alcohol (e.g., up to three glasses of alcohol per day), whereas individuals who chronically abuse alcohol are also at high risk of developing dementia [36]. There is evidence of the beneficial effects of light-moderate, nonbinge consumption of alcohol, as well as experimental demonstration that moderate alcohol exposure can initiate cytoprotective mechanisms [37]. Intoxication, withdrawal, brain trauma, central nervous system infection, hypoglycemia, alterations in bodily systems (e.g., immune, hormonal), cerebellar degeneration, polyneuropathy, fetal alcohol syndrome, hepatic failure, and Marchiafava–Bignami disease are indirect effects of alcohol abuse, as are pellagra and Wernicke–Korsakoff disorder, resulting from nutritional deficiencies [31].

Neuropsychological findings

The precise etiology of neuropsychological impairment in alcohol abusers is controversial. Acute impairment tends to correlate reasonably well with BAC. Acute neuropsychological dysfunction is evident when BAC exceeds 50 mg/dL (see Table 11.5). The chronic effects of alcohol on the brain have been well studied. Alcohol dementia is characterized by gradually progressive, multidomain cognitive dysfunction with prominent neuropsychological deficits on tasks measuring visuospatial skills, abstraction, learning, and memory [30]. Language skills and global intellectual functioning remain relatively intact with chronic alcohol consumption. In contrast, Wernicke–Korsakoff syndrome, a brain disorder produced by thiamine deficiency, is characterized primarily by acute to subacute onset of severely impaired short-term recall, confabulation (fabrication), oculomotor abnormalities, and gait ataxia, with relatively preserved long-term memory and global intellectual functions. There can also be comorbidity of alcohol dementia and Wernicke–Korsakoff resulting in global cognitive impairment [30].

Table 11.5 Central nervous system (CNS) effects after ethanol ingestion as a function of blood-alcohol content (BAC).

mg/dL	Typical presentation
20–50	Tranquility, mild sedation, mild fine motor coordination deficits
50–100	Judgment impairment, further coordination deficits
100–150	Unsteady gait, nystagmus, slurring of speech, behavioral inhibition, impaired memory
150–300	Delirium and lethargy
300–400	Unconsciousness in the alcohol-naïve; chronic consumers may still appear unaffected in context of extreme tolerance
≥400	Potentially fatal

Cognitive impairment due to alcohol abuse likely reflects the combination of acute and chronic brain damage including alcohol intoxication, vitamin deficiency, metabolic disorders, and cerebrovascular diseases. The increased likelihood of psychopathology and head trauma/brain injury in individuals who abuse alcohol further complicate the diagnosis and prognosis. Ethanol-related dementia is believed to represent approximately 10% of all dementia cases [38].

Neuroimaging

Chronic alcohol consumption is associated with cerebral atrophy of both grey and white matter with preferential involvement of the frontal lobes [7]. Reports indicate that alcoholic patients with dementia have reduced numbers of neurons in the superior frontal cortex [39]. Cerebellar atrophy, particularly of the vermis, is also common. These pathological changes are confirmed by computed tomography (CT) or MRI brain imaging [40]. Research has indicated that drinking cessation might lead to a reduction in cerebral atrophy [41, 42], accompanied closely by improved cognition; amnesia associated with Wernicke–Korsakoff's is generally permanent, however [31].

Biomarkers/laboratory findings

Symptoms associated with acute ethanol or alcohol toxicity tend to progress proportionally to the amount ingested, which is measured directly via BAC level. Although there is some inter-individual variability, O'Connor [34] provides the guidelines for expected effects by BAC in Table 11.5.

Diagnosis is typically clinical, but in cases of acute intoxication, BAC should also be measured, and blood glucose level should be checked to rule out hypoglycemia. In chronic alcohol abuse, complete blood count (CBC), magnesium (Mg), liver function tests, and prothrombin time/partial prothrombin time (PT/PTT) should be ordered. In cases of alcohol withdrawal, the clinician should rule out of other central nervous system injuries or infections [34].

Several blood markers have been used to assess the effects of chronic alcoholism in clinical practice. These include elevated serum gamma-glutamyltransferase (GGT) and aminotransferase (ALT, AST) levels and mean corpuscular volume (MCV). These have poor specificity and limited sensitivity to determine postmortem evidence of chronic alcohol use, however [43]. New markers include carbohydrate-deficient transferrin (CDT), fatty acid ethyl esters (FAEES), fatty acid methyl esters (FAMEs), ethyl glucuronide (EtG), phosphatidylethanol (PEth), 5-hydroxytryptophol to 5-hydroxyindole-3-acetic acid (5-HTOL/5-HIAA) ratio, sialic acid, beta-hexosaminidase, blood acetate, acetaldehyde adducts, and dolichol [44].

Pathophysiology and pathology

Ethanol neurotoxicity likely has several mechanisms, including glutamate excitotoxicity and oxidative stress, which is sometimes exacerbated by thiamine deficiency [45–48]. The neuropathological correlates of alcoholism have been well documented via autopsy studies [45, 49–53]. In general, findings support the tendency for individuals with alcohol dependence to exhibit reductions in brain weights and increased pericerebral spaces consistent with hydrocephalus ex vacuo, as well as pronounced neuronal loss in the mammillary bodies, thalamus, basal forebrain, dorsal and medial raphe, and cerebellar vermis.

Treatment

Interested readers should refer to Table 11.6 for a brief overview of the medical management of ethanol intoxication and withdrawal [31].

There are a variety of inpatient and outpatient therapeutic alcohol treatment programs available in most countries, including the United States. Relapse rates are high, however, and psychotherapeutic treatment should follow medical detox.

Lead

Lead is a natural, abundantly occurring metal used frequently in manufacturing and industry, and it has been extensively researched as a neurotoxicant [54]. Lead neurotoxicity can be due to acute or chronic exposure. Acute lead encephalopathy in children, attributed to pica or ingestion of flaking lead-containing paint, was first reported in 1904 [1]. Lead poisoning, however, is among the oldest occupational illnesses and remains a common cause of metal poisoning today.

Clinical symptoms/features and neurologic exam findings

Acute lead exposure may involve the rapid onset of nausea, headaches, cognitive changes, and emotional dysregulation. Medical symptoms can include hypertension, abdominal pain, constipation, and joint/muscle pains. Chronic exposure, which is more typical of industrial workplace environments, reflects more prominent neurodegeneration and psychiatric manifestations.

Table 11.6 Medical management strategies for ethanol intoxication and withdrawal.

Medication	Mechanism of action	Effects	Side effects/risks
Disulfiram	Interferes with metabolism of acetaldehyde (intermediary product in the oxidation of alcohol)	Alcohol consumption within 12 h of taking disulfiram leads to facial flushing, suffusion of conjunctivae, throbbing headache, tachycardia, hyperpnea, sweating, vomiting, and potentially fainting and collapse, all of which typically lasts up to 3 h. These intense discomforts discourage alcohol consumption	Adherence rates are poor; contraindicated for patients who are pregnant
Naltrexone	Opioid antagonist	Decreases relapse rate and number of drinking days during relapse	Adherence rates are modest; contraindicated in patients with acute hepatitis or liver failure
Acamprosate	Synthetic analog of y-aminobutyric acid	May decrease relapse rate and number of drinking days during relapse	
Nalmefene	Opioid antagonist	May decrease relapse rate and number of drinking days during relapse	Still currently under study
Topiramate	Anticonvulsant/antiepileptic drug (AED)	May decrease relapse rate and number of drinking days during relapse	Still currently under study; some problems with memory and general neurocognitive functioning have been reported
Magnesium supplementation	Metal ion; necessary cofactor in thiamin-dependent metabolism	Correction of electrolyte abnormalities and thiamin deficiency	IV/IM administration should continue for at least 3–5 days; advanced disease necessitates hospitalization
Thiamine	Vitamin B1	Prevent Wernicke–Korsakoff syndrome and symptoms of severe withdrawals or delirium tremens	IV delivered; should remain in ICU over course of symptoms
Diazepam, lorazepam, chlordiazepoxide, carbamazepine oxazepam, etc.	Benzodiazepines	Counteracts and/or prevents withdrawal symptoms, especially delirium tremens and seizures with withdrawal from severe dependence	Can cause intoxication and dependence; for short-term management of withdrawal. For patients with significant liver problems, short acting benzodiazepines (e.g., lorazepam) or one metabolized by glucuronidation (e.g., oxazepam)
Phenobarbital	Barbiturate; sedative hypnotic	Acts as potential substitute when benzodiazepines are ineffective	Respiratory depression a risk with concomitant use

Lead-exposed workers frequently complain of fatigue, headaches, restlessness, irritability, and poor emotional control [55–57]. There is some evidence that chronic lead exposure may impair postural balance and speed of peripheral nerve function, as well as contributing to forearm extensor weakness. Psychosis with hallucinations, restlessness, and nightmares are typical psychological symptoms produced by organic lead exposure [55, 58]. Delirium, convulsion, and coma might even occur in high concentration exposure. In sum, the deleterious effects of lead on the brain range from mild cognitive decline to encephalopathy, parkinsonism, and dementia [59].

Although acute toxicity is rare, chronic toxicity causes both central and peripheral effects, the former more common in children and the latter in adults. Adults with chronic lead exposure and blood lead levels from 25 to 60 μg/dL often experience irritability, headache, and depressed mood, with signs of impaired visual–motor dexterity and reaction times. Even more overt effects, for example, weakness and atrophy of peripheral muscles with wrist drop, occur with long-term blood levels of 60 μg/dL or more. Peripheral neuropathy is usually accompanied by blood lead levels greater than 70 μg/dL. Chronic exposure over months or years adversely affects calcium-dependent enzyme systems, ATPases, and mitochondrial oxidative phosphorylation and cell growth; interferes with heme synthesis, membrane integrity, and steroid metabolism; and causes motor axon degeneration and demyelination [60]. Additional potential consequences include anemia, reduced sperm count, renal failure, chronic encephalopathy, delayed motor and sensory nerve conduction, hearing loss, and gout.

Neuropsychological findings

Lead exposure is considered a significant risk factor for accelerated cognitive decline [61, 62]. A consistent pattern of neurocognitive deficits associated with lead exposure has not been identified, although visuospatial and visual memory impairments are frequently reported as the most prominent declines [63, 64]. A cross-sectional study of workers in a leaded glass plant found deficits in psychomotor speed, motor strength, and verbal memory [56]. Other studies, however, have found no or few abnormal cognitive deficits in exposed persons, which may be due to moderately low exposure or current blood levels. Leaded fuels contain multiple neurotoxic substances; therefore, the neuropsychological deficits likely result from a combination of triethyl lead, solvents, and possible hypoxia [65]. Chronic exposure to lead tends to be more harmful to cognition than acute exposure as bone lead levels predicted poorer cognitive performance, whereas blood lead level did not [66]. Anxiety, depression, phobia, and antisocial behavior are linked to lead exposure [67].

Laboratory findings

Lead introduced into the bloodstream is excreted at a clearance rate of 1–3 mL/min in urine and bile with a half-life of approximately 30 days. The remaining lead binds to red blood cells, is distributed throughout soft tissues of the body, and accumulates in bone [68]. Lead's half-life in the bones ranges from 20 to 30 years. Blood lead levels are more reflective of acute exposure, whereas bone lead levels better reflect cumulative exposure over time [69].

Whole-blood lead concentration is the most reliable diagnostic test because urinary lead levels increase and decrease more rapidly than blood levels in response to changes in lead exposure. Mean whole-blood level in adults without known exposure to occupational hazard is less than 5 μg/dL. Standard recommendations now consider levels safe up to 30 μg/dL; some consider a higher limit of 50 μg/dL to be safe. Workers are monitored closely if levels exceed 40 μg/dL. The upper limit of normal measurement for lead in urine is 150 μg/dL creatinine [1].

Pathophysiology and pathology

Lead interferes with multiple enzyme systems in the body with primary targets to include the heme synthesis enzymes, thiol-containing antioxidants, and enzymes (superoxide dismutase, catalase, glutathione peroxidase, glucose 6-phosphate dehydrogenase, and antioxidant molecules like GSH). The induction of oxidative stress, intensification of apoptosis of neurocytes, and interference with Ca(2+)-dependent enzymes are all mechanisms of lead neurotoxicity [70]. Edema, capillary disruption, proliferation of glia, and diffuse anoxic injury are all postmortem pathological findings in lead toxicity [71].

Treatment

Treatment combines decontamination of the exposure source, supportive care, and the use of chelating agents; the primary focus of treatment for lead exposure, however, is to reduce the level of circulating lead in the bloodstream. In affected people, chelation therapy should commence at levels of ≥40 μg/dL. Supportive care might include treatment of increased ICP by standard use of IV mannitol and glucocorticoids, the latter because the pathophysiology of lead encephalopathy involves capillary leak. For chelation of patients with lead encephalopathy, calcium disodium edentate, or calcium ethylenediaminetetraacetic acid (EDTA), should be administered at 30 mg/kg every 24 h. Some advocate initiating chelation with a single dose of dimercaprol (British anti-Lewisite [BAL]), 4–5 mg/kg deep intramuscularly. Alternatively, meso-2,3-dimercaptosuccinic acid (DMSA or succimer) is advocated for treatment of moderately severe chronic lead intoxication [1]. Although cessation of lead exposure and chelation effectively lower blood lead levels, thereby reducing pharmacological effects of lead, they show no therapeutic benefit against potential morphological changes in brain during neurodevelopment [72].

Metabolic dementias

Cognitive impairment might be a direct consequence of medical illness or metabolic perturbations. For patients with potential endocrine disease, and liver or kidney failure, certain blood tests are essential to rule out metabolic causes for dementia. For example, it is important to obtain thyroid function studies because hypo- and hyperthyroidism are potentially reversible causes of cognitive impairment. Vitamin B_{12} deficiency is associated with hematologic, neurologic, and psychiatric manifestations. It is linked to memory decline, irritability, and dementia in some cases. Elevated levels of methylmalonic acid and/or homocysteine levels might indicate early vitamin B_{12} deficiency or suggest other metabolic pathway abnormalities [73–75]. Potential intoxication from illicit substance or other iatrogenic medications as a cause for cognitive dysfunction should be considered. Getting an accurate medication history and urine and/or blood tests might confirm such intoxication.

A variety of hormone abnormalities have been linked to cognitive impairment or dementia. Much attention has been focused on sex hormones, steroid hormones derived primarily from the gonads, including estrogens (e.g., 17β-estradiol and estrone), progestogens (e.g., progesterone), and androgens (e.g., testosterone and dihydrotestosterone). Thyroid hormone deficiency is a well-known cause of dementia. Psychological stress—linked to excess secretion of cortisol, a glucocorticoid produced within the adrenal cortex—has also been considered a theoretical contributor to dementia, but clinical implications are unclear. Sex hormones, glucocorticoids, and thyroid hormone are all members of a nuclear receptor superfamily. These hormones function primarily as intracellular ligand-activated transcription factors, which bind to hormone-responsive DNA elements to modulate expression of target genes. Receptors for estrogen, progesterone, androgen, cortisol, and thyroid hormone are found in human brain, expressed in subsets of neuronal or glial cells with unique topographically restricted distributions. A review of the full breadth of metabolic disorders with associated neurocognitive sequelae is beyond the scope of this chapter and has been reviewed elsewhere [76]. This section will focus on three common metabolic issues that have been shown to cause dementia: thyroid dysregulation, hepatic dysfunction, and disorders of glucose metabolism.

Thyroid

The thyroid, a small gland of approximately 2 in.^{2} lying just below the Adam's apple, is integral to proper metabolic functioning, as it stimulates bodily tissues to produce proteins and manages intracellular oxygen consumption. Accordingly, it is involved in maintenance of heart, respiratory, and metabolic rates, as well as influencing growth, heat production, and reproductive and digestive functions [77].

Clinical symptoms/features

Hypothyroidism and hyperthyroidism (i.e., thyrotoxicosis) are among the most commonly diagnosed endocrine disorders. Thyroid hormone is essential for fetal brain development and continues to impact brain health throughout adulthood. The most common cause of hypothyroidism in the United States is an autoimmune condition known as Hashimoto's disease, in which lymphocytes accumulate in the thyroid and lead to a reduction in thyroid function. Hashimoto's disease can cause a host of symptoms associated with inadequate thyroid hormone secretion: fatigue, weight gain, depression, memory deficits, cold intolerance, and joint/muscle pains among others. Rates are much higher among women than men, and onset is most common among individuals between 30 and 50 years of age [78]. Conversely, Graves' disease is a common autoimmune disorder leading to overactivity of the thyroid gland. Graves' disease typically leads to anxiety, concentration difficulties, diplopia, irritability, weight loss, and tremor. It is also most common among women over the age of 20 [79].

Neuropsychological findings

Individuals with both hyperthyroidism and hypothyroidism can exhibit neuropsychological impairment. Decreased concentration, slowed reaction time, decreased complex visual processing and spatial organizational abilities, and poor constructional skills are the most common neuropsychological deficits observed in patients with hyperthyroidism or Graves' disease [80]. A majority of individuals concurrently meet the criteria for major depressive disorder and generalized anxiety disorder relative to other hospitalized medical patients. Hyperthyroidism can also cause physiologic tremors similar in appearance to essential tremors or cause preexisting essential tremors to worsen in severity [81].

Neuropsychological deficits, however, have not been found in all studies. Vogel, Elberling, Hording, and colleagues [82] found higher ratings in psychiatric measures prior to treatment but no differences on neuropsychological test performance in patients with Graves' disease. The authors further reported that after reaching a euthyroid level, previously reported psychiatric and cognitive impairments decreased considerably.

Research on the neurocognitive functioning of individuals with primary hypothyroidism indicates multiple areas of potential deficits. The most common neuropsychological deficits observed in hypothyroidism include reduced processing speed, diminished attention and concentration, impairments in learning and memory, executive dysfunction, and global cognitive deficits or dementia [83]. Similar to hyperthyroidism, hypothyroidism is associated with frontal systems compromise and high potential for psychiatric comorbidities [83, 84].

Neuroimaging

Stern and colleagues proposed that the cognitive deficits present in hyperthyroidism reflect frontal systems dysfunction (i.e., frontal cortex and associated subcortical structures) [85–87]. Bhatara and colleagues found reduced cerebral metabolism in the right frontal lobes of Graves' patients compared to healthy controls using MR spectroscopy [88]. Preliminary data obtained by Stern and colleagues suggests that patients with Graves' disease who have abnormal single-photon emission computed tomography (SPECT) scans demonstrate impaired performance on tests of verbal list learning, planning and organization, visuospatial skills, perseveration, and mild to moderate depressive symptoms [89]. PET scanning has demonstrated generalized decrease in regional cerebral blood flow and in cerebral glucose, suggesting no specific localized deficits in overall reduction brain activity [90]. SPECT studies have also reflected diffuse cerebral hypoperfusion in hypothyroid individuals [91]. SPECT findings associated with hyperthyroidism tend to show bilateral temporoparietal defects similar to what is often observed with Alzheimer's disease. Accordingly, Graves' disease is an important treatable/reversible differential diagnostic consideration that can be easily overlooked for patients who present with clinical and radiological findings suggestive of "possible" Alzheimer's disease [92].

Treatment

Thyroid dysregulation represents a treatable yet sometimes overlooked cause for dementia in adults. Neurocognitive symptoms are improved by maintaining thyroid levels within the normal ranges; some research, however, suggests medical treatment of hypothyroidism is associated with partial and inconsistent patterns of neurocognitive recovery [93]. Thyroxine treatment does not appear to improve cognitive function in otherwise healthy patients with subclinical hypothyroidism [84].

Dementia associated with hyperthyroidism responds well to treatment with a beta-blocker, resulting in improved behavioral and attention-related cognitive functioning, along with enhanced tracer uptake in the frontal region of the brain. Subsequent methimazole intervention has been shown to further improve memory and visuoconstructional skills [92].

Hepatic disorders

Cirrhosis is not an isolated liver disorder but can have consequences for the whole body as well as on brain functioning. The impact of liver failure on the brain is evident in mental status and/or behavioral changes. These neurological and/or psychiatric consequences of liver failure are collectively termed hepatic encephalopathy (HE).

HE is a common neuropsychiatric complication in patients with hepatic insufficiency from acute liver failure or cirrhosis or from portosystemic shunting even in the absence of intrinsic liver disease. Symptom presentation is diverse and ranges in severity. HE results in a diminished quality of life, a poorer prognosis in patients with underlying liver cirrhosis [94], and is an independent predictor of mortality in patients with acute-on-chronic liver failure [95, 96]. In its most severe form, it can lead to coma or death. Mortality is extremely high in overt HE with cerebral edema, and temporizing measures are often found to be inadequate [97]. Mortality at 1 year for patients with severe HE in intensive care unit (ICU) is 54% [98].

Clinical symptoms/features

The onset of neurological symptoms in chronic HE is usually insidious. Patients with HE may present with subtle and mild alterations in intellectual abilities, cognitive functions, emotional and behavioral regulation, and psychomotor/fine motor skills, possible indications of emerging encephalopathy. Confusion, disorientation, and poor coordination are common [99]. Personality changes, decreased energy level, impaired sleep–wake cycle, impaired cognition, diminished consciousness, asterixis, hemiplegia, and loss of motor control may also be presenting symptoms.

Minimal hepatic encephalopathy (MHE) refers to the subclinical stage of HE, in which routine clinical neurological and mental status examinations are normal, but subtle deficits can be documented on comprehensive neuropsychological testing. Subclinical manifestations of HE can be found in upward of 50% of cirrhotic patients without overt encephalopathy [100]. The mildest form of HE, MHE, is associated with a significant compromise of quality of life, which is predictive of the onset of overt HE and is associated with a poorer prognosis for outcome [101].

Diagnostic criteria

There is no consensus on the diagnostic criteria for HE; a 1998 consensus group at the 11th World Congress of Gastroenterology in Vienna, however, proposed a standardized nomenclature for HE that characterizes both the type of hepatic abnormality and the duration/characteristics of neurological complications [102]. Diagnosis requires the exclusion of other causes of altered mental status. Overt HE consists of neurological and psychiatric abnormalities that can be detected by bedside clinical tests, whereas minimal HE can only be distinguished by specific psychometric tests due to lack of findings of clinical exam. Overt HE occurs in at least 30–45% of patients with cirrhosis and in 10–50% of patients with transjugular intrahepatic portosystemic shunts [103, 104].

Neurological exam

Clinical diagnosis of overt HE is based on the combination of impaired mental status and impaired neuromotor function, such as hyperreflexia, hypertonicity, and asterixis [105]. Parkinsonian-like symptoms, such as rigidity and tremors, as well as the aforementioned symptoms of confusion, disorientation, impaired sleep–wake cycle, impaired cognition, diminished consciousness, choreoathetoid movements, Babinski sign, transient focal symptoms, hemiplegia, and loss of motor control may also be evident on a neurologic examination. Exam may also show loss of facial expression, speech disturbances, and visual misperceptions (visual agnosia, macropsia, distortion and prolongation of the images, spatial disorientation, and a predominance of visual hallucinations). Rarely, auditory, tactile, olfactory, and gustatory hallucinations also have been reported [105].

Neuropsychological findings

Neuropsychological impairment has been well documented in patients with cirrhosis and end-stage liver disease [102, 106]. Neuropsychological testing in HE reflects deficits in attention, working memory, processing speed, visuomotor abilities, speeded fine motor movements, and executive function. In contrast, verbal abilities including verbal memory tend to be relatively preserved in HE and particularly in MHE. Several studies have demonstrated that many patients diagnosed with cirrhosis without clinical signs of encephalopathy perform poorer on neuropsychological tests when compared to healthy controls [107–113]. Schomerus [114] demonstrated that 60% of the cirrhotic patients with no clinical signs of HE were considered unable to drive, and driving capacity was questionable in 25%.

Cognitive impairment in persons with chronic liver disease was assumed to be a consequence of cirrhosis-associated HE until recently. Conditions such as portal-systemic shunting, however, also can result in cerebral dysfunction, thought to be an outcome of high ammonia concentration and astrocyte swelling, hallmarked by decreased recent memory, fluctuating consciousness, and disorientation [115, 116]. There is growing evidence of cognitive deficits in many patients with hepatitis C virus (HCV) infection prior to the development of cirrhosis that appear unrelated to markers of liver dysfunction, viral load, or genotype [117–123].

Hilsabeck and colleagues [120] found that a significant percentage of patients with chronic HCV experience cognitive deficits such as compromised attention, learning, psychomotor speed, and mental flexibility. Impaired cognitive test performance was also evident in up to 50% of individuals who have not yet developed cirrhosis, depending on the neuropsychological test administered. Testing revealed sustained attention and concentration; slowed processing speed were the most challenging tasks for these patients whereas visuoconstructional skills were within normal limits. Problems with learning, psychomotor speed, and mental flexibility are also present [120]. Greater neuropsychological impairment was present in those individuals with greater levels of fibrosis suggesting that the longer one experiences chronic hepatic injury, the more likely they are to develop neurocognitive impairment. In summary, HCV and other chronic liver diseases adversely affects cognition, particularly attention and concentration, even in the absence of cirrhosis early in the disease process. Depression is a common comorbidity with approximately 25% of HCV-infected patients meeting diagnostic criteria for concurrent depression [124, 125] and 50–60% reporting clinically significant depressive symptoms on self-report [126].

Neuroimaging

Classic MR imaging abnormalities in HE include bilateral and symmetric high signal intensity in the globus pallidus on T1-weighted images, which is likely a reflection of increased tissue concentrations of circulating manganese, and "an elevated glutamine/glutamate peak coupled with decreased myo-inositol and choline signals on proton MR spectroscopy, representing disturbances in cell volume homeostasis secondary to brain hyperammonemia" [127]. White matter abnormalities can be detected with MR imaging techniques such as magnetization transfer ratio measurements, fluid-attenuated inversion recovery sequences, and diffusion-weighted images [127]. These MR imaging abnormalities are believed to reflect mild diffuse brain edema, which seems to play an essential role in the pathogenesis of HE.

Laboratory findings

Diagnosis of HE requires exclusion of other causes of altered mental status. Laboratory abnormalities typically include evidence of electrolyte disturbances (such as hyponatremia and hypokalemia) and hepatic biochemical and synthetic dysfunction. Arterial and venous ammonia levels correlate with the severity of HE up to a certain point. Gastrointestinal bleeding, renal failure, hypovolemia, extensive muscle use, urea cycle disorder, parenteral nutrition, urosepsis, and the use of certain drugs (e.g., valproic acid) are additional nonhepatic causes of hyperammonemia that need to be excluded. Clinical presentation and clinical response to treatment are most important. Other laboratory tests of liver and renal function, electrolytes, glucose, cultures, and drug screening should be considered to assess for precipitating causes of HE.

Pathophysiology and pathology

The pathogenesis of HE is not well defined; it is believed, however, to involve alterations in various neurotransmitter systems within the brain. Involvement of the γ-aminobutyric acid (GABA) receptor complex in HE, in particular the benzodiazepine receptor site, as well as increased serotonin turnover has been postulated [128]. Patients with liver failure or portal-systemic shunt surgery have increased circulation of ammonia entering the brain through the blood–brain barrier. This leads to the accumulation of glutamine in brain astrocytes and brain swelling. Benzodiazepine-like agonists, inflammatory cytokines, manganese, and neurosteroids may play a role [129–132].

Treatment

Acute management of HE should focus on providing supportive care, identifying and treating any precipitating causes, reducing nitrogenous load in the gut, and assessing the need for long-term therapy and liver transplant evaluation. Pharmacological treatment of HE includes the use of nonabsorbable disaccharides such as lactulose and lactitol and antibiotics such as rifaximin [133].

Oral dose of lactulose for acute overt HE begins at 10–30 g (15–45 mL) every 1–2 h until a bowel movement occurs. Readjustment to 10–30 g (15–45 mL) two to four times daily is then recommended as the next step, titrated and continued indefinitely to induce two to three soft bowel movements daily. Nasogastric tube or rectal administration as an enema (300 mL in 1 L of water ever 6–8 h) can be used for comatose patients until the patient awakes and can start oral therapy. Rifaximin (550 mg twice daily) can be used to treat HE [134].

Correction of precipitating factors is critical. Increased nitrogen load (e.g., gastrointestinal bleed, infection, excess dietary protein), decreased toxin clearance (e.g., hypovolemia, renal failure, constipation, portosystemic shunt, medication noncompliance, acute-on-chronic liver failure), and altered neurotransmission (e.g., sedating medication, alcohol, hypoxia, hypoglycemia) are the most common precipitating factors for HE that need to be evaluated and treated if present.

Glucose

One of the most common metabolic diseases resulting in blood glucose imbalance is diabetes mellitus. The overwhelming majority of diabetes diagnoses fall into one of two broad etiopathogenetic categories: (i) Type 1 diabetes is characterized by a halting of insulin secretion secondary to an autoimmune pathogenic process in which pancreatic islet cells are destroyed. (ii) Type 2 diabetes is a much more prevalent condition in which a resistance develops to insulin, and pancreatic islet cells are unable to produce enough additional insulin to sufficiently compensate. Although both types of diabetes are present across the lifespan, Type 1 tends to be diagnosed during late adolescents or early adulthood, whereas Type 2 is more prevalent among older adults [135].

Clinical symptoms/features

The varied and complex complications associated with both Type 1 and Type 2 diabetes have been well documented [136]. This list ranges across a host of neurological and nonneurological problems, including but not limited to retinopathy with or without vision loss, nephropathy/renal failure, autonomic and peripheral neuropathy, cardiovascular complications, cerebrovascular disease, sexual dysfunction, affective disorders, and gastrointestinal issues.

The impact of hypoglycemia and hyperglycemia on the nervous system has been well studied [137]. Recent studies have focused on the effects of hypoglycemia and older individuals with Type 2 diabetes mellitus (DM2) [138]. The link between diabetes and cognitive decline is obscured by coexisting depression, hypertension, and cardio- and cerebrovascular diseases.

As the primary source of energy for neurons is glucose, brain hypoglycemia is very harmful to brain function and might cause permanent cognitive dysfunction leading to dementia, depending on the severity of hypoglycemia. Depending on the level of hypoglycemia, seizures also occur, which might be additionally detrimental to brain function [139]. Well-controlled studies, however, of the threshold for the development of seizures secondary to hypoglycemia are lacking.

Neuropathology

Impaired glucose tolerance might increase the occurrence of pathological changes associated with vascular dementia [140]. The pathological vascular damage changes may be the anatomical basis for the increased risk of cognitive impairment or dementia in DM2 [141]. Hyperglycemia is common among acute ischemic stroke patients [142]. It is also well known that hyperglycemia adversely affects the outcome of cerebral infarction [143, 144]; this association has been documented in recent stroke treatment trials [145].

The link between hyperglycemia in diabetes mellitus and dementia is obscured by other comorbidities associated with DM2, including depression, hypertension, and cardio- and cerebrovascular diseases. Impaired glucose tolerance appears to increase the occurrence of the pathological changes associated with vascular dementia and Alzheimer's Disease [140]. Pathological vascular damage changes, however, might be the anatomical basis for the increased risk of dementia in DM2 [141].

Recent studies have focused upon the effects of hypoglycemia on older people DM2 [146]. Infection-related hypoglycemia, especially in institutionalized demented patients, is a significant health-care problem that may aggravate dementia [147].

Neuropsychological findings

Diabetes-associated cognitive deficits have been observed by physicians and researchers since as early as the 1920s [148]. Diabetes is associated with accelerated cognitive decline and structural brain abnormalities, and deficits have been observed across a range of neuropsychological domains [149]. Cukierman et al. [150] reviewed prospective data relating to diabetes and cognitive function over time and found that people with diabetes have a greater rate of decline in cognitive function. Specifically, they found a 1.5-fold greater risk of cognitive decline and a 1.6-fold greater risk of future dementia when compared to individuals without diabetes. In the Framingham study [151], individuals with diabetes were more likely than were nondiabetics to obtain scores below the 25th percentile on more tests. Specific areas of decline have been observed in implicit memory, processing speed, psychomotor speed and efficiency, sustained attention, cognitive flexibility, and visual attention and perception [152]. The frequency of reported differences in neuropsychological performance among diabetic patients does not appear to account, however, for severe hypoglycemic episodes [153].

Neuroimaging

A burgeoning body of neuroimaging research is documenting the effects of glucose imbalance and diabetes on structural brain integrity [154–158]. Cortical and subcortical atrophy have been noted along with microvascular disease and other subcortical white matter abnormalities. In general, brain atrophy tends to be modest and other abnormalities usually subtle in nature, although earlier onset of DM has been shown to correlate with more severe findings on MRI.

Treatment

The benefits of maintaining normal blood glucose levels for minimizing neurocognitive and medical symptoms and lessening risks for complications among patients with diabetes have been well verified through randomized controlled trials and large-scale cohort studies [159–161]. Experimental animal studies also indicate THAT optimal glycemic control may lower risk for developing poststroke dementia [162]. Furthermore, decreased mortality is achieved by normalizing blood sugar after a stroke [163]. Therefore, normalization of blood glucose after a stroke is an appropriate clinical goal, and in general, current treatment for Type 1 and Type 2 diabetes emphasizes maintenance of normal blood glucose levels in order to achieve optimal neurological, medical, and neuropsychological functioning.

Summary

The role of toxic and metabolic disorders in dementia is quite complex. Because the effects of these conditions are so diverse and often little specific clinical evidence is available, animal models have helped provide additional evidence for the likely effects in humans. In this chapter, three specific toxic causes of dementia and three specific metabolic causes of cognitive impairment and dementia have been addressed in some detail. It is critical to consider toxic and metabolic causes in every patient with cognitive impairment, especially because early diagnosis and treatment might lead to improvement and perhaps even reversal of the dementia or cognitive decline.

References

1 Prockop LD, Rowland LP: Occupational and environmental neurotoxicology. In: *Merritt's Neurology*. 12 edn. Edited by Rowland LP, Pedley TA. Philadelphia: Lippincott Williams & Wilkins; 2010: 1174–1200.

2 Ernst A, Zibrak JD: Carbon monoxide poisoning. *New England Journal of Medicine* 1998, **339**(22):1603–1608.

3 Prockop LD: Carbon monoxide brain toxicity: Clinical, magnetic resonance imaging, magnetic resonance spectroscopy, and neuropsychological effects in 9 people. *Journal of Neuroimaging* 2005, **15**:144–149.

4 Tomaszewski C: Carbon monoxide. In: *Goldfrank's Toxicologic Emergencies*. 7 edn. Edited by Goldfrank LR, Flomenbaum NE, Lewis NA, Howland MA, Hoffman RS, Nelson LS. New York: McGraw-Hill; 2002: 1478–1497.

5 Prockop LD: Carbon monoxide. In: *Clinical Neurotoxicology*. Edited by Dobbs MR. Philadelphia: Saunders/Elsevier; 2009: 500–514.

6 Chang KH, Han MH, Kim HS, Wie BA, Han MC: Delayed encephalopathy after acute carbon monoxide intoxication: MR imaging features and distribution of cerebral white matter lesions. *Radiology* 1992, **184**(1):117–122.

7 Seger D, Welch L: Carbon monoxide controversies: Neuropsychological testing, mechanism of toxicity and hyperbaric oxygen. *Annals of Emergency Medicine* 1994, **24**:242–248.

8 Chang CC, Chang WN, Lui CC, Wang JJ, Chen CF, Lee YC, Chen SS, Lin YT, Huang CW, Chen C: Longitudinal study of carbon monoxide intoxication by diffusion tensor imaging with neuropsychiatric correlation. *Journal of Psychiatry & Neuroscience* 2010, **35**(2):115–125.

9 Hopkins RO, Weaver LK: Carbon monoxide controversies: Neuropsychologic testing, mechanisms of toxicity, and hyperbaric oxygen. *Annals of Emergency Medicine* 1995, **25**:272–273.

10 Crocker P: Carbon monoxide poisoning—The clinical entity an its treatment: A review. *Military Medicine* 1984, **149**:257–259.

11 Kelley JS, Sophocleus GJ: Retinal hemorrhages in subacute carbon monoxide poisoning. Exposures in homes with blocked furnace flues. *Journal of the American Medical Association* 1978, **239**(15): 1515–1517.

12 Myers RA, DeFazio A, Kelly MP: Chronic carbon monoxide exposure: A clinical syndrome detected by neuropsychological tests. *Journal of Clinical Psychology* 1998, **54**(5):555–567.

13 Min SK: A brain syndrome associated with delayed neuropsychiatric sequelae following acute carbon monoxide intoxication. *Acta Psychiatrica Scandinavica* 1986, **73**(1):80–86.

14 Raphael JC, Elkharrat D, Jars-Guincestre MC, Chastang C, Chasles V, Vercken JB, Gajdos P: Trial of normobaric and hyperbaric oxygen for acute carbon monoxide intoxication. *Lancet* 1989, **19**(2): 414–419.

15 Gorman DF, Clayton D, Gilligan JE, Webb RK: A longitudinal study of 100 consecutive admissions for carbon monoxide poisoning to the Royal Adelaide Hospital. *Anaesthesia & Intensive Care* 1992, **20**(3):311–316.

16 Weaver LK, Hopkins RO, Chan KJ, Churchill S, Elliott G, Clemmer TP, Orme JF, Thomas FO, Morris AH: Hyperbaric oxygen for acute carbon monoxide poisoning. *New England Journal of Medicine* 2002, **347**:1057–1067.

17 Amitai Y, Zlotogorski Z, Golan-Katzav V, Wexler A, Gross D: Neuropsychological impairment from acute low-level exposure to carbon monoxide. *Archives of Neurology* 1988, **55**(6):845–848.

18 Murata S, Asaba H, Naritomi H, Hiraishi K, Sakai T: Magnetic resonance imaging findings on carbon monoxide intoxication. *Journal of Neuroimaging* 1993, **3**(2):128–131.

19 Tom T, Abedon S, Clark RI, Wong W: Neuroimaging characteristics in carbon monoxide toxicity. *Journal of Neuroimaging* 1996, **6**:161–166.

20 Prockop LD, Nardu KA: Brain CT and MRI findings after carbon monoxide toxicity. *Journal of Neuroimaging* 1999, **9**:175–181.

21 Bronstein A, Clower JH, Iqbal S, Yip FY, Martin CA, Chang A, Wolkin AF, Bell J: Carbon monoxide exposures—United States, 2000–2009. *Center for Disease Control (CDC) Morbidity and Mortality Weekly Report (MMWR)* 2011, **60**(30):1014–1017.

22 Miro O, Casodemont J, Marrientos A, Urban-Marquez A, Candellach F: Mitochondrial cytochrome c oxide inhibition during acute carbon monoxide poisoning. *Pharmacology & Toxicology* 1998, **82**(4):199–202.

23 Lapresle J, Fardeau M: The central nervous system and carbon monoxide poisoning. II. Anatomical study of brain lesions following intoxication with carbon monoxide (22 cases). *Progress in Brain Research* 1967, **24**:31–74.

24 Elkharrat D: Indications of normobaric and hyperbaric oxygen therapy in acute CO intoxication. In: Proceedings satellite meeting IUTOX. Dijon, France: VIIIth International Congress of Toxicology; 1998.

25 Tibbles PM, Edelsberg JS: Hyperbaric-oxygen therapy. *New England Journal of Medicine* 1996, **334**:1642–1648.

26 Van Meter KW, Weiss L, Harch PG, Andrews LC, Simanonok JP, Staab PK, Gottlieb SF: Should the pressure be off or on with use of oxygen in the treatment of carbon monoxide poisoned patients? *Annals of Emergency Medicine* 1994, **24**(2):283–288.

27 Thom SR, Taber RI, Mediguren II, Clark JM, Hardy KR, Fisher AB: Delayed neuropsychological sequelae after carbon monoxide poisoning: prevention by treatment with hyperbaric oxygen. *Annals of Emergency Medicine* 1995, **25**:479–486.

28 Weaver LK, Hopkins RO, Larson-Lorh V, Howe S, Haberstock D: Double blind, controlled, prospective, randomized clinical trial (RCT) in patients with acute carbon monoxide (CO) poisoning: Outcome of patients tested with normobaric oxygen or hyperbaric oxygen (HBO2), an interim report. *Undersea & Hyperbaric Medicine* 1995, **22**:14.

29 Tibbles PM, Perotta PL: Treatment of carbon monoxide poisoning: A critical review of human outcome studies comparing normobaric oxygen with hyperbaric oxygen. *Annals of Emergency Medicine* 1994, **24**:269–276.

30 Rourke SB, Grant I: The neurobehavioral correlates of alcoholism. In: *Neuropsychological Assessment of Neuropsychiatric and Neuromedical Disorders.* 3 edn. Edited by Grant I, Adams KM. New York: Oxford University Press; 2009: 398–454.

31 Brust JCM: Alcoholism. In: *Merritt's Neurology.* 12 edn. Edited by Rowland LP, Pedley TA. Philadelphia: Lippincott Williams & Wilkins; 2010: 1076–1084.

32 Sullivan EV, Fama R, Rosenbloom MJ, Pfefferbaum A: A profile of neuropsychological deficits in alcoholic women. *Neuropsychology* 2002, **16**(1):74–83.

33 Sullivan EV, Rosenbloom MJ, Pfefferbaum A: Pattern of motor and cognitive deficits in detoxified alcoholic men. *Alcoholism, Clinical and Experimental Research* 2000, **24**(5):611–621.

34 O'Connor PG: Alcohol. In: *Merck Manual.* Whitehouse, Station: Merck Sharp & Dohme Corp.; 2015, http://www.merckmanuals.com/professional/special-subjects/drug-use-and-dependence/alcohol. Accessed September 10, 2015.

35 Brust JCM: Ethanol and cognition: Indirect effects, neurotoxicity and neuroprotection: A review. *International Journal of Environmental Research in Public Health* 2010, **7**(4):1540–1557.

36 Ruitenberg A, van Swieten JC, Witteman JCM, Mehta KM, van Duijn CM, Hofman A, Breteler MMB: Alcohol consumption and risk of dementia: The Rotterdam study. *The Lancet* 2002, **359**(9303): 281–286.

37 Collins MA, Neafsey EJ, Mukamal KJ, Gray MO, Parks DA, Das DK, Korthuis RJ: Alcohol in moderation, cardioprotection, and neuroprotection: Epidemiological considerations and mechanistic studies. *Alcoholism, Clinical and Experimental Research* 2009, **33**(2): 206–219.

38 Gupta A, Warner J: Alcohol-related dementia: A 21st-century silent epidemic? *The British Journal of Psychiatry* 2008, **193**(5):351–353.

39 Harper C, Kril J, Daly J: Are we drinking our neurones away? *British Medical Journal (Clinical Research Ed.)* 1987, **294**(6571):534–536.

40 Bergman H, Borg S, Hindmarsh T, Idestrom CM, Mutzell S: Computed tomography of the brain and neuropsychological assessment of male alcoholic patients and a random sample from the general male population. *Acta Psychiatrica Scandinavica Supplementum* 1980, **286**:77–88.

41 Carlen PL, Wilkinson DA, Wortzman G, Holgate R: Partially reversible cerebral atrophy and functional improvement in recently abstinent alcoholics. *Canadian Journal of Neurological Sciences* 1984, **11**(4):441–446.

42 Carlen PL, Wortzman G, Holgate R, Wilkinson DA, Rankin JC: Reversible cerebral atrophy in recently abstinent chronic alcoholics measured by computed tomography scans. *Science* 1978, **200**(4345):1076–1078.

43 Neumann T, Spies C: Use of biomarkers for alcohol use disorders in clinical practice. *Addiction* 2003, **98**(Suppl 2):81–91.

44 Rainio J, De Giorgio F, Bortolotti F, Tagliaro F: Objective postmortem diagnosis of chronic alcohol abuse: A review of studies on new markers. *Legal Medicine (Tokyo)* 2008, **10**(5):229–235.

45 Harper C, Matsumoto I: Ethanol and brain damage. *Current Opinion in Pharmacology* 2005, **5**(1):73–78.

46 Tsai G, Coyle JT: The role of glutamatergic neurotransmission in the pathophysiology of alcoholism. *Annual Review of Medicine* 1998, **49**:173–184.

47 Chandler LJ, Newsom H, Sumners C, Crews F: Chronic ethanol exposure potentiates NMDA excitotoxicity in cerebral cortical neurons. *Journal of Neurochemistry* 1993, **60**:1578–1581.

48 Gotz ME, Janetsky B, Pohli S, Gottschalk A, Gsell W, Tatschner T, Ransmayr G, Leblhuber F, Gerlach M, Reichmann H et al: Chronic alcohol consumption and cerebral indices of oxidative stress: Is there a link? *Alcoholism, Clinical and Experimental Research* 2001, **25**:717–725.

49 Harper C: The neuropathology of alcohol-specific brain damage, or does alcohol damage the brain? *Journal of Neuropathology and Experimental Neurology* 1998, **57**(2):101–110.

50 Harper C, Dixon G, Sheedy D, Garrick T: Neuropathological alterations in alcoholic brains. Studies arising from the New South Wales tissue resource centre. *Progress in Neuropsychopharmacology and Biological Psychiatry* 2003, **27**(6):951–961.

51 Harper C, Kril J: Corpus callosal thickness in alcoholics. *British Journal of Addiction* 1988, **83**:577–580.

52 Torvik A: Brain lesions in alcoholics: Neuropathological observations. *Acta Medica Scandinavica* 1987, **717**:47–54.

53 Torvik A, Lindboe CF, Rogde S: Brain lesions in alcoholics: A neuropathological study with clinical correlations. *Journal of the Neurological Sciences* 1982, **56**:233–248.

54 White RF, Janulewicz PA: Neuropsychological, neurological, and neuropsychiatric correlates of exposure to metals. In: *Neuropsychological Assessment of Neuropsychiatric and Neuromedical Disorders.* Edited by Grant I, Adams KM. New York: Oxford University Press; 2009: 350–365.

55 Hanninen H: Behavioral effects of occupational exposure to mercury and lead. *Acta Neurologica Scandinavica* 1982, **92**:167–175.

56 Pasternak G, Becker CE, Lash A, Bowler R, Estrin WJ, Law D: Cross-sectional neurotoxicology study of lead-exposed cohort. *Journal of Toxicology Clinical Toxicology* 1989, **27**(1–2):37–51.

57 Barth A, Schaffer AW, Osterode W, Winker R, Konnaris C, Valic E, Wolf C, Rudiger HW: Reduced cognitive abilities in lead-exposed men. *International Archives of Occupational and Environmental Health* 2002, **75**(6):394–398.

58 Jarup L: Hazards of heavy metal contamination. *British Medical Bulletin* 2003, **68**(1):167–182.

59 Feldman RG: *Occupational and Environmental Neurotoxicology.* Philadelphia: Lippincott-Raven Publishers; 1999.

60 Rosin A: The long-term consequences of exposure to lead. *The Israel Medical Association Journal* 2009, **11**(11):689–694.

61 Wright RO, Tsaih SW, Schwartz J, Spiro III A, McDonald K, Weiss ST, Hu H: Lead exposure biomarkers and mini-mental status exam scores in older men. *Epidemiology* 2003, **14**(6):713–718.

62 Weisskopf MG, Wright RO, Schwartz J, Spiro III A, Sparrow D, Aro A, Hu H: Cumulative lead exposure and prospective change in cognition among elderly men: The VA normative aging study. *American Journal of Epidemiology* 2004, **160**(12):1184–1193.

63 Khalil N, Morrow LA, Needleman H, Talbott EO, Wilson JW, Cauley JA: Association of cumulative lead and neurocognitive function in an occupational cohort. *Neuropsychology* 2009, **23**(1):10–19.

64 Schwartz BS, Stewart WF, Bolla KI, Simon PD, Bandeen-Roche K, Gordon PB, Links JM, Todd AC: Past adult lead exposure is associated with longitudinal decline in cognitive function. *Neurology* 2001, **56**(2):283.
65 Poklis A, Burkett CD: Gasoline sniffing: A review. *Clinical Toxicology* 1977, **11**(1):35–41.
66 Shih RA, Glass TA, Bandeen-Roche K, Carlson MC, Bolla KI, Todd AC, Schwartz BS: Environmental lead exposure and cognitive function in community-dwelling older adults. *Neurology* 2006, **67**(9):1556–1562.
67 Carpenter DO, Nevin R: Environmental causes of violence. *Physiology and Behavior* 2010, **99**(2):260–268.
68 Mason LH, Harp JP, Han DY: Pb neurotoxicity: Neuropsychological effects of lead toxicity. *BioMed Research International* 2014, **2014**:8 pages.
69 Rabinowitz MB: Toxicokinetics of bone lead. *Environmental Health Perspectives* 1991, **91**:33–37.
70 Nemsadze K, Sanikidze T, Ratiani L, Gabunia L, Sharashenidze T: Mechanics of lead-induced poisoning. *Georgian Medical News* 2009, **172–173**:92–96.
71 Environmental Protection Agency EPA: *Air Quality for Lead.* Washington, DC: Office of Research and Development, Office of Health and Environmental Assessment, Environmental Criteria and Assessment Office; 1986.
72 Gover RA: Results of lead research: Prenatal exposure and neurological consequences. *Environmental Health Perspectives* 1996, **104**(10):1050–1054.
73 Oh RC, Brown DL: Vitamin B12 Deficiency. *American Family Physician* 2003, **67**(5):979–986.
74 Sloan JL, Johnston JJ, Manoli I, Chandler RJ, Krause C, Carrillo-Carrasco N, . . . Venditti, CP: Exome sequencing identifies ACSF3 as a cause of combined malonic and methylmalonic aciduria. *Nature Genetics* 2011, **43**(9):883–886.
75 Boxer AL, Kramer JH, Johnston K, Goldman J, Finley R, Miller BL: Executive dysfunction in hyperhomocysteinemia responds to homocysteine-lowering treatment. *Neurology* 2005, **64**(8):1431–1434.
76 Lezak M: Metabolic and endocrine disorders. In: *Neuropsychological Assessment. Volume*, 3 edn. Edited by Lezak MD. New York: Oxford University Press; **1995**: 274–276.
77 Hershman JM: Overview of the thyroid gland. In: *Merck Manual.* Whitehouse Station: Merck Sharp & Dohme Corp.; 2015, http://www.merckmanuals.com/professional/endocrine-and-metabolic-disorders/thyroid-disorders/hyperthyroidism. Accessed September 10, 2015.
78 Pyzik A, Grywalska E, Matyjaszek-Matuszek B, Roliński J: Immune disorders in Hashimoto's thyroiditis: What do we know so far? *Journal of Immunology Research* 2015, **2015**:979167.
79 Bahn RS, Burch HB, Cooper DS, Garber JR, Greenlee MC, Klein I, Laurberg P, McDougall IR, Montori VM, Rivkees SA et al: Hyperthyroidism and other causes of thyrotoxicosis: Management guidelines of the American Thyroid Association and American Association of clinical endocrinologists. *Endocrinology Practice* 2011, **17**(3):456–520.
80 Trzepacz PT, McCue M, Klein I, Levey GS, Greenhouse J: A psychiatric and neuropsychological study of patients with untreated Graves' disease. *General Hospital Psychiatry* 1988, **10**(1):49–55.
81 Revuelta GJ, Weiner WJ, Factor SA: Hyperkinetic movement disorders. In: *Neurology for the Non-Neurologist.* 6 edn. Edited by Weiner WJ, Goetz CG, Shin RK, Lewis SL. Philadelphia: Lippincott Williams & Wilkins; 2010: 241–286.
82 Vogel A, Elberling TV, Hording M, Dock J, Rasmussen AK, Feldt-Rasmussen U, Perrild H, Waldermar G: Affective symptoms and cognitive functions in the acute phase of Graves' thyrotoxicosis. *Psychoneuroendocrinology* 2007, **32**(1):36–43.
83 Wekking EM, Appelhof BC, Fliers E, Schene AH, Huyser J, Tijssen JG, Wiersinga WM: Cognitive functioning and well-being in euthyroid patients on thyroxine replacement therapy for primary hypothyroidism. *European Journal of Endocrinology* 2005, **153**(6): 747–753.
84 Jorde R, Waterloo K, Storhaug H, Nyrnes A, Sundsfjord J, Jenssen TG: Neuropsychological function and symptoms in subjects with subclinical hypothyroidism and the effect of thyroxine treatment. *Journal of Clinical Endocrinology and Metabolism* 2006, **91**(1):145–153.
85 Stern RA, Robinson B, Thorner AR, Arruda JE, Prohaska ML, Prange Jr. AJ: A survey study of neuropsychiatric complaints in patients with Graves' disease. *Journal of Neuropsychiatry and Clinical Neuroscience* 1996, **8**(2):181–185.
86 Stern RA, Prange Jr. AJ: Neuropsychiatric aspects of endocrine disorders. In: *Comprehensive Textbook of Psychiatry.* Volume **1**, 6 edn. Edited by Kaplan HI, Saddock BJ. Baltimore: Williams & Wilkins; 1995: 241–251.
87 Somerville JG, Tremont G, Stern RA: The Boston qualitative scoring system as a measure of executive functioning in Rey-Osterrieth complex figure performance. *Journal of Clinical and Experimental Neuropsychology* 2000, **22**(5):613–621.
88 Bhatara VS, Tripathi RP, Sankar R, Gupta A, Khushu S: Frontal lobe proton magnetic-resonance spectroscopy in Graves' disease: A pilot study. *Psychoneuroendocrinology* 1998, **23**(6):605–612.
89 Tremont G, Stern RA, Westervelt HJ, Bishop CL, Davis JD: Neurobehavioral functioning in thyroid disorders. *Medicine and Health Rhode Island* 2003, **86**(10):318–322.
90 Constant EL, de Volder AG, Ivanoiu A, Boi A, Labar D, Seghers A, Cosnard G, Melin J, Daumerie C: Cerebral blood flow and glucose metabolism in hypothyroidism: A positron emission tomography study. *Journal of Clinical Endocrinology and Metabolism* 2001, **86**(8):3864–3870.
91 Kinuya S, Michigishi T, Tonami N, Aburano T, Tsuji S, Hashimoto T: Reversible cerebral hypoperfusion observed with Tc-99 m HMPAO SPECT in reversible dementia caused by hypothyroidism. *Clinical Nuclear Medicine* 1999, **24**(9):666–668.
92 Fukui T, Hasegawa Y, Takenaka H: Hyperthyroid dementia: Clinicoradiological findings and response to treatment. *Journal of Neurosurgical Sciences* 2001, **184**(1):81–88.
93 Dugbartey A: Neurocognitive aspects of hypothyroidism. *Journal of the American Medical Association* 1998, **158**(13):1413–1418.
94 Bustamante J, Rimola A, Ventura PJ, Navasa M, Cirera I, Reggiardo V, Rodes J: Prognostic significance of hepatic encephalopathy in patients with cirrhosis. *Journal of Hepatology* 1999, **30**(5):890–895.
95 Steward CA, Malinchoc M, Kim WR, Kamath PS: Hepatic encephalopathy as a predictor of survival in patients with end-state liver disease. *Liver Transplantation* 2007, **13**(10):1366–1371.
96 Garg H, Kumar A, Garg P, Sharma B, Sharma C, Sarin SK: Clinical profile and predictors of mortality in patients of acute-on-chronic liver failure. *Digestive and Liver Disease* 2012, **44**(2):166–171.
97 Detry O, DeRoover A, Honore P, Meurisse M: Brain edema and intracranial hypertension in fulminant hepatic failure: Pathophysiology and management. *World Journal of Gastroenterology* 2006, **12**(46): 7405–7412.

98 Fichet J, Mercier E, Genee O, Garot D, Legras A, Dequin PF: Prognosis and 1-year mortality of intensive care unit patients with severe hepatic encephalopathy. *Journal of Critical Care* 2009, **24**(3):364–370.

99 Prakash R, Muller KD: Mechanisms, diagnosis and management of hepatic encephalopathy. *National Review of Gastroenterology and Hepatology* 2010, **7**(9):515–525.

100 Li YY, Nie YQ, Sha WH, Zeng Z, Yang FY, Ping L, Jia L: Prevalence of subclinical hepatic encephalopathy in cirrhotic patients in China. *World Journal of Gastroenterology* 2004, **10**(16):2397–2401.

101 Randolph C, Hilsabeck R, Kato A, Kharbanda P, Li YY, Mapelli D, Ravdin LD, Romero-Gomez M, Stracciari A, Weissenborn K et al: Neuropsychological assessment of hepatic encephalopathy: ISHEN practice guidelines. *Liver International* 2009, **29**(5):629–635.

102 Ferenci P, Lockwood A, Mullen K, Tarter R, Weissenborn K, Blei AT: Hepatic encephalopathy—Definition, nomenclature, diagnosis, and quantification: Final report of the working party at the 11th World Congresses of Gastroenterology, Vienna, 1998. *Hepatology* 2002, **35**(3):716–721.

103 Poordad FF: The burden of hepatic encephalopathy. *Alimentary Pharmacology & Therapeutics* 2007, **25**(1):3–9.

104 Prasad S, Dhiman RK, Duseja A, Chawla YK, Sharma A, Agarwal R: Lactulose improves cognitive functions and health related quality of life in patients with cirrhosis who have minimal hepatic encephalopathy. *Hepatology* 2007, **45**:549–559.

105 Sherlock S, Summerskill WHJ, White RF, Phear EA: Portal-systemic encephalopathy: Neurological complications of liver disease. *Lancet* 1954, **2**:453–457.

106 Amodio P, Montagnese S, Gatta A, Morgan MY: Characteristics of minimal hepatic encephalopathy. *Metabolic brain disease* 2004, **19**(3–4):253–267.

107 Zeegen R, Drinkwater JE, Dawson AM: Method for measuring cerebral dysfunction in patients with liver disease. *British Medical Journal* 1970, **2**:633–636.

108 Elithorn A, Lunzer M, Weinman J: Cognitive deficits associated with chronic hepatic encephalopathy and their response to levodopa. *Journal of Neurology, Neurosurgery, and Psychiatry* 1975, **38**:794–798.

109 Gilberstadt SJ, Gilberstadt H, Zieve L, Buegel B, Collier RO, McClain CJ: Psychomotor performance defects in cirrhotic patients without overt encephalopathy. *Archives of Internal Medicine* 1980, **140**:519–521.

110 Hegedus A, Tarter RE, Van Thiel DH, Schade RR, Gavaler JS, Starzl TE: Neuropsychiatric characteristics associated with primary biliary cirrhosis. *International Journal of Psychiatry in Medicine* 1984, **14**(4):303–314.

111 Rikkers L, Jenko P, Rudman D, Friedes D: Subclinical hepatic encephalopathy: Detection, prevalence, and relationship to nitrogen metabolism. *Gastroenterology* 1978, **75**:462–469.

112 Tarter RE, Hegedus AM, Van Thiel DH, Schade RS, Gavaler JS, Starzl TE: Nonalcoholic cirrhosis associated with neuropsychological dysfunction in the absence of overt evidence of hepatic encephalopathy. *Gastroenterology* 1984, **86**:1421–1427.

113 McCrea M, Cordoba J, Vessey G, Blei AT, Randolph C: Neuropsychological characterization and detection of subclinical hepatic encephalopathy. *Archives of Neurology* 1996, **53**:758–763.

114 Schomerus H: Differential diagnosis of acute cerebral disorders in alcoholism and cirrhosis. *Internist (Berl)* 1981, **22**(9):555–561.

115 Cordoba J, Raguer N, Flavia M, Vargas V, Jacas C, Rovira AJ: T2 hyperintensity along the corticospinal tract in cirrhosis relates to functional abnormalities. *Hepatology* 2003, **38**:1026–1033.

116 Shawcross D, Jalan R: The pathophysiologic basis of hepatic encephalopathy: Central role for ammonia and inflammation. *Cellular and Molecular Life Sciences* 2005, **62**:2295–2304.

117 Forton DM, Allsop JM, Main J, Foster GR, Thomas HC, Taylor-Robinson SD: Evidence for a cerebral effect of the hepatitis C virus. *Lancet* 2001, **358**:38–39.

118 Forton DM, Thomas HC, Murphey CA, Allsop JM, Foster GR, Main J, Wesnes KA, Taylor-Robinson SD: Hepatitis C and cognitive impairment in a cohort of patients with mild liver disease. *Hepatology* 2002, **35**:433–439.

119 Kramer L, Bauer E, Funk G, Hofer H, Jessner W, Steindl-Munda P, Wrba F, Madl C, Gangl A, Ferenci P: Subclinical impairment of brain function in chronic hepatitis C infection. *Journal of Hepatology* 2002, **37**:349–354.

120 Hilsabeck R, Perry W, Hassanein TI: Neuropsychological impairment in patients with chronic hepatitis C. *Hepatology* 2002, **35**(2):440–446.

121 Hilsabeck R, Hassanein TI, Carlson MC, Ziegler EA, Perry W: Cognitive functioning and psychiatric symptomatology in patients with chronic hepatitis C. *Journal of the International Neuropsychological Society* 2003, **9**:847–854.

122 McAndrews MP, Farcnik K, Carlen PL, Damyanovich A, Mrkonjic M, Jones S, Heathcote EJ: Prevalence and significance of neurocognitive dysfunction in hepatitis C in the absence of correlated risk factors. *Hepatology* 2005, **41**:801–808.

123 Fontana RJ, Bieliauskas LA, Back-Madruga C, Lindsay KL, Kronfol Z, Lok ASF, Padmanabhan L, The HALT-C Trial Group A: Cognitive function in hepatitis C patients with advanced fibrosis enrolled in the HALT-C trial. *Journal of Hepatology* 2005, **43**:614–622.

124 Dwight MM, Kowdley KV, Russo JE, Ciechanowski PS, Larson AM, Katon WJ: Depression, fatigue, and functional disability in patients with chronic hepatitis C. *Journal of Psychosomatic Research* 2000, **49**(5):311–317.

125 Fontana RJ, Moyer CA, Sonnad S, Lok ASF, Sneed-Pee N, Walsh J, Klein S, Webster S: Comorbidities and quality of life in patients with interferon-refractory chronic hepatitis C. *American Journal of Gastroenterology* 2001, **96**(1):170–178.

126 Johnson ME, Fisher DG, Fenaughty A, Theno SA: Hepatitis C virus and depression in drug users. *American Journal of Gastroenterology* 1998, **93**(5):785–789.

127 Rovira AJ, Alonso J, Cordoba J: MR imaging findings in hepatic encephalopathy. *American Journal of Neuroradiology* 2008, **29**:1612–1621.

128 Fitz JG: Hepatic encephalopathy, hepatopulmonary syndromes, hepatorenal syndrome, coagulopathy, and endocrine complications of liver disease. In: *Sleisenger and Fordtran's Gastrointestinal and Liver Disease: Pathophysiology/Diagnosis/Management.* 7 edn. Edited by Feldman M, Friedman LS, Sleisenger MH. Philadelphia: Saunders; 2002: 1543–1565.

129 Butterworth RF: Pathogenesis of hepatic encephalopathy and brain edema in acute liver failure. *Journal of Clinical and Experimental Hepatology* 2015, **5**(Suppl 1):S96–S103.

130 Mladenović D, Hrnčić D, Petronijević N, Jevtić G, Radosavljević T, Rašić-Marković A, Puškaš N, Maksić N, Stanojlović O: Finasteride improves motor, EEG, and cellular changes in rat brain in

thioacetamide-induced hepatic encephalopathy. *American Journal of Physiology. Gastrointestinal and Liver Physiology* 2014, **307**(9): G931–940.

131 Kobtan AA, El-Kalla FS, Soliman HH, Zakaria SS, Goda MA: Higher grades and repeated recurrence of hepatic encephalopathy may be related to high serum manganese levels. *Biological Trace Element Research* 2015, DOI: 10.1007/s12011-015-0405-5, Online ISSN: 1559–0720.

132 Palomero-Gallagher N, Zilles K: Neurotransmitter receptor alterations in hepatic encephalopathy: A review. *Archives of Biochemistry and Biophysics* 2013, **536**(2):109–121.

133 Foster KJ, Lin S, Turck CJ: Current and emerging strategies for treating hepatic encephalopathy. *Critical Care Nursing Clinics of North America* 2010, **22**(3):341–350.

134 Liou IW: Diagnosis and management of hepatic encephalopathy. *Hepatitis C Online* 2013.

135 American Diabetes Association A: Diagnosis and classification of diabetes mellitus. *Diabetes Care* 2005, **28**:S37–S42.

136 American Diabetes Association A: Standards of medical care for patients with diabetes mellitus. *Diabetes Care* 2002, **25**:213–229.

137 Wilkinson DA, Prockop LD: Hypoglycemia: Effect on the nervous system. In: *Handbook of Clinical Neurology. Volume 27, Metabolic and Deficiency Diseases of the Nervous System*, Edited by Vinken PJ, Bruyn GW. Amsterdam: North Holland Publishing Co.; 1976: 53–78.

138 Whitmer RA, Kerter AJ, Yaffe K, Quesenberry Jr. CP, Selby JV: Hypoglycemic episodes and risk of dementia in older patients with type 2 diabetes mellitus. *Journal of the American Medical Association* 2009, **301**(15):1565–1572.

139 Buckingham B, Wilson DM, Lecher T, Hanas R, Kaiserman K, Cameron F: Duration of nocturnal hypoglycemia before seizures. *Diabetes Care* 2008, **31**(11):2110–2112.

140 Messier C: Impact of impaired glucose tolerance and type 2 diabetes on cognitive aging. *Neurobiology of Aging* 2005, **265**:S26–S30.

141 Korf ESC, White RF, Scheltens P, Launer LJ: Brain aging in very old men with type 2 diabetes. *Diabetes Care* 2006, **29**:2268–2271.

142 Decker DA, Royter V, Paletz L, Roberts P, Mirocha J, Waters M: Strict glycemic control improves functional outcomes in ischemic stroke. Unpublished data 2010.

143 Mazighi M, Amerenco P: Hyperglycemia: A predictor of poor prognosis in acute stroke. *Diabetes & Metabolism* 2001, **27**(6):718–720.

144 Parsons MW, Barber PA, Desmond PM, Baird TA, Darby DG, Byrnes G, Tress BM, Davis SM: Acute hyperglycemia adversely affects stroke outcome: A magnetic resonance imaging and spectroscopy study. *Annals of Neurology* 2002, **52**(1):20–28.

145 Ahmed N, Davalos A, Erikson N, Ford GA, Glahn J, Hennerici M, Mikulik R, Kaste M, Lees KR, Lindsberg PJ et al: Association of admission blood glucose and outcome in patients treated with intravenous thrombolysis. *Archives of Neurology* 2010, **67**(2):1123–1130.

146 Whitman RA, Kanter AJ, Yaffe K, Quesenberry Jr. CP, Selby JV: Hypoglycemic episodes and the risk of dementia in older people with type 2 diabetes mellitus. *Journal of the American Medical Association* 2009, **101**(15):1565–1572.

147 Aremza Z, Fidelman Z, Berner YN, Adunsky A: Infection related hypoglycemia in institutionalized demented patients. *Archives of Gerontology and Geriatrics* 2007, **45**:191–200.

148 Miles WR, Root HF: Psychological tests applied in diabetic patients. *Archives of Internal Medicine* 1922, **30**:767–777.

149 Dreary IJ, Crawford JR, Hepburn DA, Langan SJ, Blackmore LM, Frier BM: Severe hypoglycemia and intelligence in adult patients with insulin-treated diabetes. *Diabetes* 1993, **42**:341–344.

150 Cukierman T, Gerstein HC, Williamson JD: Cognitive decline and dementia in diabetes—Systematic overview of prospective observational studies. *Diabetologia* 2005, **48**(12):2460–2469.

151 Elias PK, Elias MF, D'Agostino RB, Cupples LA, Wilson PW, Silbershatz H, Wolf PA: NIDDM and blood pressure as risk factors for poor cognitive performance. *Francophone Studies Diabetes Care* 1997, **20**(9):1388–1395.

152 Cohen J: *Statistical Power Analysis for the Behavioral Sciences*, 2 edn. Hillsdale: Erlbaum; 1988.

153 Brands AMA, Kessels RPC: Diabetes and the brain: Cognitive performance in Type 1 and Type 2 diabetes. In: *Neuropsychological Assessment of Neuropsychiatric and Neuromedical Disorders.* 3 edn. Edited by Grant I, Adams KM. New York: Oxford University Press; 2009: 350–365.

154 Tiehuis AM, van der Graaf Y, Visseren FL, Vincken KL, Biessels GJ, Appelman APA, Kappelle J, Mali WPTM, SMART Study Group A: Diabetes increases atrophy and vascular lesions on brain MRI in patients with symptomatic arterial disease. *Stroke* 2008, **39**: 1600–1603.

155 Ferguson SC, Blane A, Wardlaw J, Frier BM, Perros P, McCrimmon RJ, Deary IJ: Influence of an early-onset age of type 1 diabetes on cerebral structure and cognitive function. *Diabetes Care* 2005, **28**(6):1431–1437.

156 Lobnig BM, Kromeke O, Optenhostert-Porst C, Wolf OT: Hippocampal volume and cognitive performance in longstanding Type 1 diabetic patients without macrovascular complications. *Diabetic Medicine* 2006, **23**:32–39.

157 Lunetta M, Damanti AR, Fabbri G, Lombardo M, Di Mauro M, Mughini L: Evidence by magnetic resonance imaging of cerebral alterations of atrophy type in young insulin-dependent diabetic patients. *Journal of Endocrinological Investigation* 1994, **17**:241–245.

158 Musen G, Lyoo IK, Sparks CR, Weinger K, Hwang J, Ryan CM, Jimerson DC, Hennen J, Renshaw PF, Jacobson AM: Effects of type 1 diabetes on gray matter density as measured by voxel-based morphometry. *Diabetes* 2006, **55**:326–333.

159 DCCT Research Group A: Effects of intensive diabetes therapy on neuropsychological function in adults in the diabetes control and complications trial. *Annals of Internal Medicine* 1996, **124**: 379–388.

160 Gaede P, Vedel P, Larsen N, Jensen GV, Parving HH, Pedersen O: Multifactorial intervention and cardiovascular disease in patients with type 2 diabetes. *New England Journal of Medicine* 2003, **348**:383–393.

161 Reichard P, Rosenqvist U: Nephropathy is delayed by intensified insulin treatment in patients with insulin-dependent diabetes mellitus and retinopathy. *Journal of Internal Medicine* 1989, **226**: 81–87.

162 Schurr A, Payne RS, Miller JJ, Tseng MT: Preischemic hyperglycemia-aggravated damage: Evidence that lactate utilization is beneficial and glucose-induced corticosterone release is detrimental. *Journal of Neuroscience Research* 2001, **1**(66):782–789.

163 Gentile NT, Seftchick MW, Huynh T, Kruus LK, Gaughan J: Decreased mortality by normalizing blood glucose after acute ischemic stroke. *Academic Emergency Medicine* 2006, **13**(2):174–180.

CHAPTER 12

Leukoencephalopathies/leukodystrophies

Gregory M. Pastores[1,2] and Swati A. Sathe[3]

[1] Mater Misericordiae University Hospital, Dublin, Ireland
[2] Yale University School of Medicine, New Haven, CT, USA
[3] Rutgers, The State University of New Jersey, New Jersey Medical School, Newark, NJ, USA

Introduction

The leukoencephalopathies encompass a group of heterogeneous disorders that can lead to cognitive problems as a consequence of brain white matter involvement. Many of the acquired leukoencephalopathies that cause cognitive decline such as inflammatory, vascular, infectious, neoplastic, and toxic diseases are covered elsewhere in the book. Our focus will be on the hereditary forms of white matter disorders, that is, leukodystrophies, in particular the adult-onset conditions leading to dementia as a predominant feature (Table 12.1). Strictly, the term leukodystrophy is applied to conditions which have a genetic basis, progressive course, and white matter involvement (Table 12.2) [1]. In several, the biochemical and/or molecular defect is known, enabling diagnostic confirmation, which then allows appropriate genetic counseling and prognostication.

The leukodystrophies are familiar to most in their so-called classic expression with onset usually in childhood. It must be recognized that there are late-onset presentations of almost every childhood leukodystrophy. In such cases, disease course is often insidious, and diagnosis can be significantly delayed. It is not uncommon for patients with late-onset leukodystrophy to be initially suspected and treated as primary or secondary progressive multiple sclerosis (MS) [2]. Given the complex clinical presentations and similarity with more common adult-onset white matter diseases, underdiagnosis of leukodystrophy is likely. A negative family history or low disease prevalence often complicates this issue.

Review of systems and laboratory assessments in patients with a leukodystrophy often show no indication of electrolyte imbalance, thyroid or liver disease, vitamin deficiency, brain mass, drug intoxication, or chronic infection. In most cases, cerebrospinal fluid (CSF) studies, including cell counts, glucose, and oligoclonal bands, also are normal. In metachromatic leukodystrophy (MLD) or globoid cell leukodystrophy (GLD), however, there is increased CSF protein levels; the diagnosis of these two lysosomal disorders can be confirmed by biochemical enzyme testing (*discussed in the following*) [3].

Although certain MRI features in leukodystrophy are quite characteristic, they might also suggest several alternate diagnoses. Those include white matter diseases such as MS, cerebrovascular diseases (e.g., Binswanger's disease), or chronic exposure to toxic substances (e.g., chemotherapy). The pattern and distribution of white matter changes on MRI in patients with a leukodystrophy might suggest a particular disorder or narrow the list of differential diagnoses [4]. Until proven otherwise, symmetrical changes consistent with white matter disease is indicative of a leukodystrophy. The differential diagnosis of a leukodystrophy can also be aided by incorporating the results of a neurological evaluation and genetic testing (see Table 12.3 for a review of clinical and MRI features associated with the disorders reviewed in this chapter). Figure 12.1 provides a framework for the clinical workup of a patient with suspected leukodystrophy or leukoencephalopathy.

The management of patients with most leukodystrophies currently unfortunately is primarily symptomatic. Hematopoietic stem cell transplantation and pharmacologic treatments are options in selected cases. For disorders that are potentially treatable, early diagnosis is critical for the best possible outcome.

Cerebral autosomal dominant arteriopathy with subcortical infarcts and leukoencephalopathy

Illustrative case history 1

A 41-year-old gentleman was seen because of migraine with aura since age 24 and multiple recurrent episodes of unilateral numbness and tingling, attributed to MS. Regarding the migraines, his visual auras were reported as bright spots and lines. Some episodes of headache were associated with confusion which typically occurred about half an hour after the onset of headache. During the headache, he is unable to recognize people he

Non-Alzheimer's and Atypical Dementia, First Edition. Edited by Michael D. Geschwind and Caroline Racine Belkoura.
© 2016 John Wiley & Sons, Ltd. Published 2016 by John Wiley & Sons, Ltd.

Table 12.1 Selected leukodystrophies.

Disorder	Cause
• Cerebral autosomal dominant arteriopathy with subcortical infarcts and leukoencephalopathy (CADASIL)	• Notch3 gene mutation (19q12)
• Adult-onset leukoencephalopathy with axonal spheroids and pigmented glia (ALSP): hereditary diffuse leukoencephalopathy with spheroids (HDLS) and pigmentary orthochromatic leukodystrophy (POLD)	• CSF1R gene mutation (5q32)
• Adult-onset autosomal dominant leukodystrophy (ADLD) with autonomic dysfunction	• *LMNB1* mutation (5q23)
• Adult polyglucosan body disease (APBD)	• Glycogen branching enzyme (*GBE1*) deficiency (3p16)
• Alexander disease	• Glial fibrillary acidic protein (*GFAP*) (17q21)
• Mitochondrial disorders, including mitochondrial encephalomyopathy, lactic acidosis, and stroke-like episodes (MELAS) and myoclonic epilepsy and ragged-red fibers (MERRF)	• MELAS (mtDNA A3243G); MERRRF (mtDNA A8344G)
• Lysosomal storage disorders, including metachromatic leukodystrophy (MLD), globoid cell leukodystrophy (GLD) and Fabry disease (FD)	• MLD (arylsulfatase A; 22q13), GLD (β-galactocerebrosidase; 14q21), FD (α-galactosidase A; Xq22)

Table 12.2 Clinical signs of a leukodystrophy.

- A period of normal development generally precedes the onset of neurological signs and symptoms
- Spasticity develops which is usually bilateral and symmetrical
- Other long-tract signs include motor weakness and ataxia
- Optic atrophy occurs late
- If peripheral myelin is affected, then neuropathy with loss of ankle reflexes is seen
- Seizures are uncommon but can be encountered
- Behavioral and cognitive changes can occur at any stage
- Environmental precipitants can quickly exacerbate an underlying metabolic disorder of myelin

knows and does not fully comprehend what is being said to him, his speech is affected, and he has word-finding difficulty. His problems usually resolve within hours, and he has partial memory for the episode.

At age 35, he suffered from an acute episode of numbness and clumsiness in the left face and arm with a field cut, with complete recovery. A brain MRI done at the time showed extensive white matter disease. He was diagnosed with MS after excluding HIV, Lyme disease, and lupus. He was treated with glatiramer acetate for 1 year without benefit, following which he was given interferon beta-1 for another year, again without clear benefit. Over the past 6 years since the first episode, he has had four additional episodes of left-sided numbness and clumsiness with left field cut.

Over the past 10–15 years, there has been a gradual decline in his memory and concentration. He keeps a diary to remember appointments and his schedule. Additionally, he has to pay close attention to his daily work routine as a machine operator to ensure that he correctly follows the sequence. There are also subtle changes in his personality such that he is more emotional and cries easily. His past medical history revealed major depression with suicidal ideation at age 24, elevated triglycerides (treated successfully with niacin), and no history of hypertension/diabetes/asthma or heart disease. His family history was remarkable for one older brother with migraine and episodes of arm and face numbness, attributed to MS. His father died at age 42 from bone cancer, and his mother, age 65, has hypertriglyceridemia, osteoarthritis, and cervical spondylosis. She has no history of migraine, stroke, or dementia.

On neurological examination, he was alert and oriented with fluent speech. Comprehension, repetition, and naming were intact. Three object recall was 2/3 (3/3 with cues). Neuropsychological testing showed impairment in attention, processing speed, and executive function, including deficits in timed measures and measures of error monitoring, but with spared memory. Cranial nerve, motor, and sensory examinations were normal. There was no pronator drift. Rapid alternating movements were accurate. There was no double simultaneous extinction. Deep tendon reflexes were bilaterally symmetric, 2+. Both plantars were flexor. Gait was normal and there were no cerebellar signs. His clinical course, brain MRI findings (Figure 12.2), and family history were deemed consistent with cerebral autosomal dominant arteriopathy with subcortical infarcts and leukoencephalopathy (CADASIL). The absence of optic nerve and spinal cord involvement on brain MRI, the absence of oligoclonal bands in the CSF, and the absence of hypertension are pertinent negative findings that help to distinguish cases of CADASIL from MS, small vessel disease, or primary angiitis of the nervous system. A significant proportion of patients with CADASIL often are initially diagnosed and treated for MS. Thus, evaluation of patients suspected to have MS should include careful consideration of red flags, which are features in the history, examination, or diagnostic tests that are not typical or suggestive of MS and may point toward the diagnosis of a leukodystrophy [5].

Background

CADASIL is included in this chapter although it is not a leukodystrophy in the conventional sense, but a vascular disease. Van Bogaert's description in 1955 of "Binswanger's disease with a rapid course in two sisters" probably depicts the first description of CADASIL. The acronym stands for cerebral autosomal dominant arteriopathy with subcortical infarcts and leukoencephalopathy, which essentially describes the key features of the disorder (i.e., hereditary small vessel disease leading to strokes

Table 12.3 Key features of leukodystrophies and leukoencephalopathies discussed in this chapter.

Disease	Age at (adult) onset	Key clinical features	Cognitive profile	Psychiatric findings	Distinguishing MRI features	Genetics	Diagnosis
CADASIL	30–50s; milder cases in 60s	Stroke/TIAs, migraines, confusional episodes, seizures	Slowed processing speed, frontal-executive deficits	Apathy, depression, lability	• Patchy, punctate WM lesions, approaching confluency. Anterior temporal lobe and external capsule often affected • Often mistaken for MS or ischemic vascular disease	AD	Notch3 gene mutation, GOM on skin biopsy with or without Notch3 immunostaining
HDLS (ALSP)	39 (±15 SD)	Dementia, stiffness, clumsiness, weakness, ataxia, extrapyramidal, and/or pyramidal dysfunction Rapid-onset cases reported Normal NCS, VEPs, SSEPs, and ERGs	Frontal syndrome with memory impairment, intellectual deterioration.	Often initial symptoms, depression, apathy, and blunting	• Moderate frontal-predominant atrophy, enlarged ventricles • Callosal and deep WM lesions (patchy, confluent, or diffuse depending on stage) • Might show punctate restricted diffusion in rapid-onset cases • Occipital involvement rare • Sparing of U-fibers and cerebellar WM • Cerebellar atrophy might occur	AD (reduced penetrance)	Clinical features, MRI/MRS, and brain pathology CSF1R gene mutation
POLD (ALSP)	43 (±13 SD)	Dementia, seizures, pyramidal (spastic paresis), ataxia, dysphagia, dysarthria. Normal NCS, VEPs, SSEPs, and ERGs	Frontal-executive	Mood disorder, apathy, disinhibition, aggressiveness, and euphoria; might present like Pick's. Psychosis less common	• Frontal-predominant atrophy and WM disease • PVWM disease • Pyramidal tract involvement	AD (reduced penetrance; possibly some sporadic cases)	Clinical features, MRI/MRS, and brain pathology
APBD	40s–60s	Tetrad: Urinary freq/urgency, gait disorder (spasticity), sensory > motor polyneuropathy, cognitive impairment. Less common EP, cerebellar ataxia, ALS, and cardiomyopathy. NCS – sensorimotor polyneuropathy	Dementia in approximately 60%; when present, involves memory loss	Not described. Possible depression	• Multiple, diffuse PVWM changes, including the mesencephalon and cerebellum, cavitations (not always present) • Spinal cord atrophy and cerebellar atrophy	AR, rare sporadic.	Sural n. biopsy PBs in myelinated axons, decreased GBE in WBCs and cultured fibroblasts, mutation(s) in GBE gene
ADLD	30s–40s	Early autonomic dysfunction, pyramidal (spasticity) and pseudobulbar signs, and cerebellar dysfunction such as action tremor NO peripheral neuropathy. Normal NCS, VEPs. SSEPs abnormal. Autonomic skin innervation	Absence of gross impairment	Absence of profound psychiatric features	• Early on: extensive, symmetrical, CSO WM involvement; sparing U-fibers and CC • Later: extensive symmetrical CSO, CR, CC, U-fibers, EC, IC, brainstem WM involvement • Sparing of optic radiations and cerebellar WM • Extensive cerebral atrophy with sparing pons and cerebellum • No cystic changes	AD (highly penetrant)	Duplication of *LMNB1* gene.

Adult-onset Alexander Disease	Teens to 60s	Common: pyramidal tract signs (spasticity and hyperreflexia), cerebellar signs (ataxia, nystagmus, dysmetria), urinary symptoms, bulbar/pseudobulbar signs (palatal myoclonus and dysphagia, dysphonia) Less common: dysautonomia, sleep apnea and RLS; poor fine motor skills. SEPs, VEPs, and BAERs often abnormal	Frontal-executive, memory	Not described	• Atrophy and T2 hyperintensity in the medulla and cervical cord • Mild–moderate, symmetric, cerebral WM hyperintensities • Abnormal contrast enhancement if onset age <40; absent if >40 onset • Supratentorial WM hyperintensities present if onset age <40, absent if onset > 40 onset	Usually sporadic; rare AD	GFAP gene mutation
MLD (adult onset)	(Adult form) Teens to 40s–50s.	Elevated CSF protein Peripheral neuropathy (might be subclinical in late-onset forms)	Progressive mental deterioration	Behavior/mood	Symmetric, confluent, T2 hyperintense WM, demyelinating appearance, often sparing of U-fibers	AR	Elevated urine sulfatide or ARSA gene mutation
GLD/ Krabbe (adult onset)	Variable; Includes those with subtly earlier symptoms, but diagnosed as adults versus adult onset after age 20, as late as 60s	Elevated CSF protein Peripheral neuropathy (might be subclinical in late-onset forms)	Progressive mental deterioration	Behavior/mood	Symmetric, confluent, T2 hyperintense WM, severe demyelination	AR	Very low GALC enzyme activity in leukocytes isolated from whole heparinized blood and cultured skin fibroblasts. In carriers, GALC assay often WNL; test for *GALC* gene mutation. Most common mutation in adult-onset Krabbe is c.857G>A mutation
Fabry	Teens to approximately 40s	Renal insufficiency, cardiomyopathy. Corneal and lenticular opacities Strokes, SIVD Acroparesthesias/pain might occur Female carriers often affected; variable presentation	Might occur poststroke	Depression	Consistent with ischemic vascular disease: PVWM disease, WM signal intensity abnormalities and single or multiple lacunar infarcts, large ischemic cerebral infarctions. Posterior thalamus involvement (pulvinar sign—T1 bright) might occur Tortuosity and dilatation of the larger vessels	X linked	Deficiency of the lysosomal hydrolases α-galactosidase A (AGAL); in females, AGAL might be normal, so need *GAL* gene mutation
X-ALD (adult onset)	Variable; AMN in 20s–middle age; female carriers might present >35 years old with mild disease	Spastic gait	Subacute decline. Cognitive deficits correlate with MRI findings. Might present as FTD	More common in childhood forms	Either caudorostral WM progression starting from initial parieto-occipital Involvement beginning in the splenium of CC (65% of cases) or a rostrocaudal progression starting frontally beginning in the genu of CC (35% of cases). Tract involvement in the corticospinal, spinothalamic, visual, and auditory pathways	X linked	Elevated VLCFAs (tissues, serum, and other fluids)—might be WNL in females, so check for ALDP gene mutation

AD, autosomal dominant; ALS, amyotrophic lateral sclerosis; ALSP, adult-onset leukoencephalopathy with axonal spheroids and pigmented glia; AMN, adrenomyeloneuropathy (form of X-ALD); AR, autosomal recessive; ARSA, arylsulfatase A; CC, corpus callosum; CSO, centrum semiovale; EC, external capsule; EP, extrapyramidal symptoms; ERG, electroretinogram; GALC, galactocerebrosidase; GBE, glycogen branching enzyme; GFAP, glial fibrillary acidic protein; IC, internal capsule; NCS, nerve conduction studies; PBs, polyglucosan bodies; PVWM, periventricular white matter; RLS, restless legs syndrome; SIVD, small vessel ischemic vascular disease; SSEPs, somatosensory evoked potentials; TIAs, transient ischemic attacks; VEPs, visual evoked potentials; VLCFAs, very-long-chain fatty acids; WM, white matter.

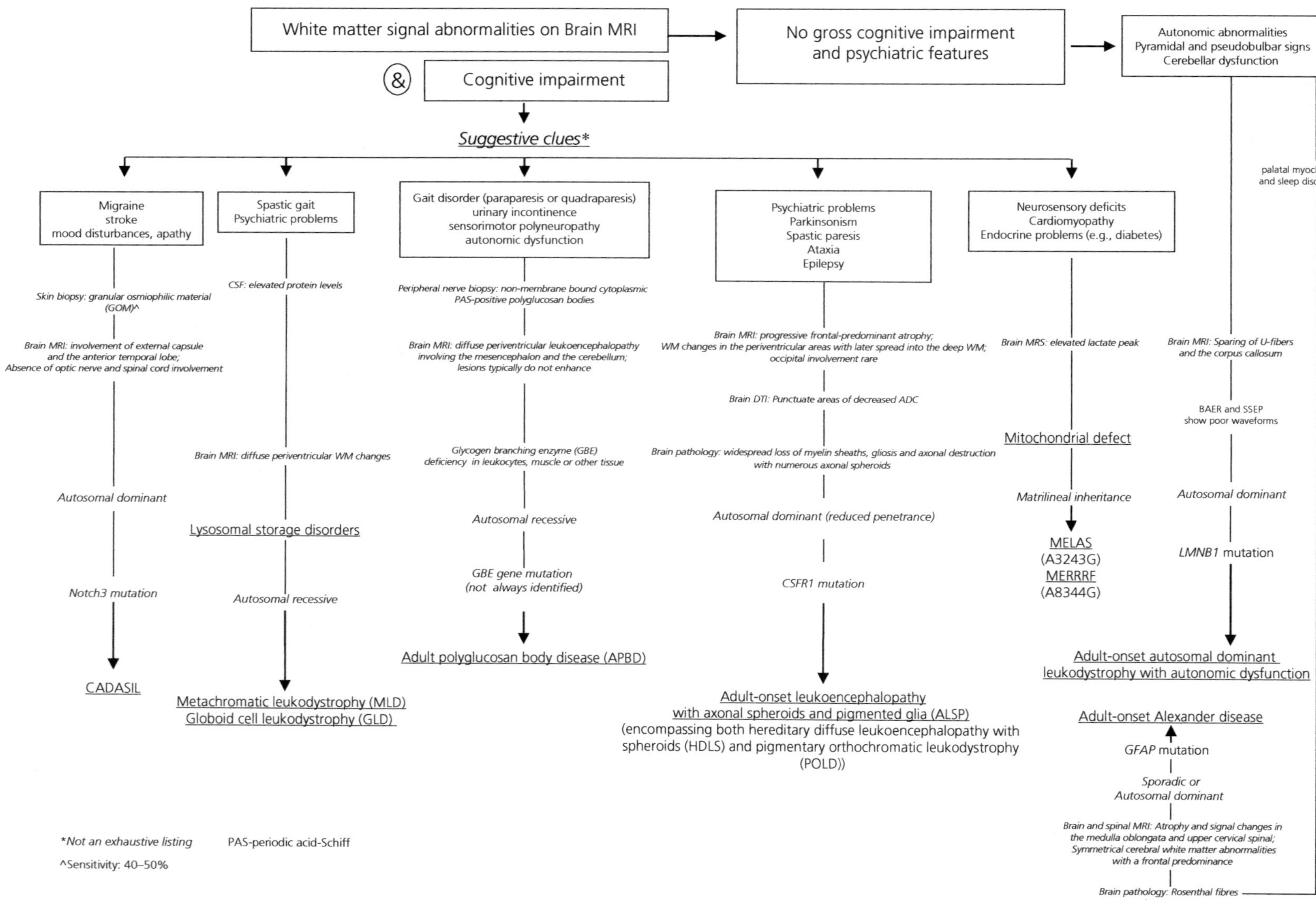

Figure 12.1 Flow chart listing selected leukodystrophies, their characteristic features, and mode of inheritance.

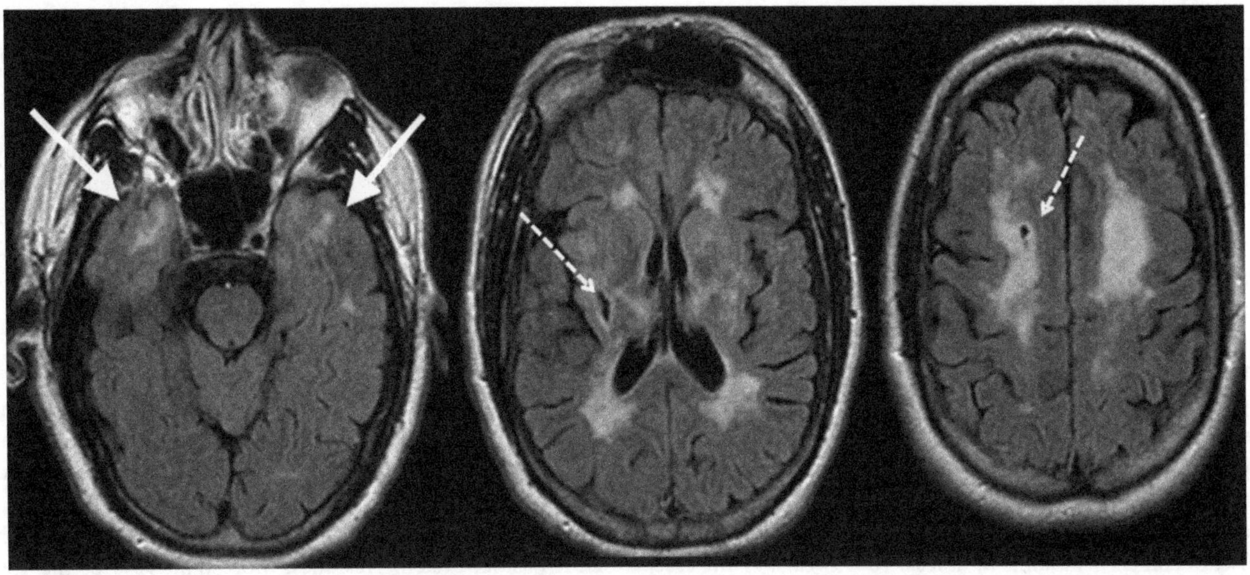

Figure 12.2 FLAIR brain MRI in a 50-year-old with CADASIL. Some classic MRI findings of CADASIL including T2-weighted medial temporal lobe hyperintensities (solid arrow), cavitations in the white matter (dashed arrows), and confluent white matter disease are shown.

and dementia). The overall prevalence of CADASIL is unknown, but one small study from Scotland provided an estimate of 4.14 cases per 100 000 [6].

Clinical presentation

Several main symptoms are described in CADASIL including migraine with aura, ischemic events (stroke), seizures, episodes of confusion (unexplained neurological episodes), mood disturbances, apathy, and cognitive impairment [7]. These symptoms occur in a successive manner over decades. Extraneurologic symptoms usually do not occur with CADASIL; this contrasts with Fabry disease (another entity associated with brain white matter changes, often erroneously attributed to MS). In Fabry disease, patients often develop renal insufficiency and cardiomyopathy prior to onset of the central nervous system (CNS) disease (*discussed in the following*).

Forty to 50% of patients with CADASIL have migraine with aura, which is usually the first symptom, with onset on average at age 30 years (range 6–48 years) [7]. The most common auras are visual and sensory; however, 50% of patients also have atypical attacks with basilar, hemiplegic, or prolonged aura, and some patients have very severe attacks with confusion, fever, meningitis, or coma.

Sixty to eighty five percent of patients with CADASIL suffer transient ischemic attacks (TIA) and ischemic strokes in the absence of other risk factors, at a mean age of 49 years (range 20–70 years) and at an estimated incidence of 10 episodes per 100 patient-years [7]. Ischemic events are almost invariably subcortical presenting as lacunar syndromes, for example, pure motor or sensory deficit, ataxic hemiparesis, and clumsy hand-dysarthria syndrome. Recurrent strokes over the years lead to significant morbidity with motor weakness, spasticity, gait difficulties, urinary urgency with or without incontinence, and pseudobulbar palsy.

Depressive episodes are described in 20% of cases, which may alternate with manic episodes [8]. Independent of depression, apathy is seen in about 40% of cases [9].

Cognitive impairment, the second most frequent clinical manifestation after migraine, follows a distinctive pattern of neuropsychological abnormalities similar to subcortical ischemic vascular dementia [10]. Executive dysfunction and attentional deficits are frequently impaired early in the course of the disease, often occurring as early as 35–50 years of age [11]. Cognitive dysfunction is accompanied by a narrowing range of interests. Patients with an overt stroke fare worse on tests of executive dysfunction [12].

Prominent areas of deficit are processing speed, for example, in timed measures of the Trail Making Test parts A and B (TMT-A and TMT-B) and a symbol digit test [10–12]. In patients with both early and advanced disease, TMT-B is abnormal, indicative of problems with processing speed and set shifting. Deficits are recorded frequently in verbal fluency, which has a strong executive component, especially in letter fluency more so than category or semantic fluency. Similarly, impairment in error monitoring on neuropsychological testing emphasizes the executive deficit [10–12].

On memory testing, there is often mild or worse impairment on both immediate and delayed free recall, but cued recall and recognition are often intact. This suggests that the encoding component of memory is relatively preserved. Memory problems are usually due to retrieval deficits, as is commonly found in small vessel disease-induced vascular cognitive impairment [12]. Visuospatial functions and abstract reasoning are largely preserved, particularly during early disease stages.

Lacunar infarcts, cerebral microbleeds, hippocampal volume, and brain atrophy are all shown to be independently associated with executive dysfunction when adjusted for age [13]. White matter hyperintensities appear to be less directly related to the cognitive decline. Cognitive decline progresses with age and at late stages involves verbal or visual memory, language, reasoning, and visuospatial abilities [10]. Severe aphasia, apraxia, or agnosia is rare.

Seizures, intracerebral hemorrhages, territorial infarcts (possibly coincidental), and extrapyramidal features are rarely reported [7].

Imaging

Typically, punctiform or nodular T2/FLAIR hyperintensities in periventricular areas and in the centrum semiovale are the first sign on MRI, which progress over decades to diffuse, extensive, and somewhat symmetrical hyperintensities, often with cavitations [7, 10]. White matter abnormalities probably precede the onset of clinical symptoms by at least 10–15 years; in any case, the brain MRI abnormalities are consistently seen by the age of 35. The frequency and severity of these T2 white matter abnormalities progress with age. MRI involvement of the external capsule and the anterior part of the temporal lobe is characteristic of CADASIL, helping to differentiate it from MS [7, 10].

Lacunar infarcts, which are often punctate or larger in size, appear later in life as T1 hypointense lesions in the same areas as the T2 signal changes [13]. Recent infarcts (within the past ~10 days) show hyperintensity (restricted diffusion) on diffusion-weighted MRI. With advancing age, microbleeds are commonly seen on gradient echo images. On diffusion tensor imaging (DTI), increased water diffusion is seen in the thalamus that may not be observed on standard T2/FLAIR neuroimaging. These DTI abnormalities are more strongly correlated with measures of executive dysfunction and clinical disability in comparison to T2 hyperintensities. Thus, diffusion histograms might be used as a marker of disease progression. In addition to white matter findings, global brain atrophy progresses three times more rapidly in patients with CADASIL compared to normal aging, and the extent of brain atrophy correlates with cognitive impairment and disability scales [14].

Pathology

Macroscopic neuropathological examination of the brain shows diffuse myelin pallor and rarefaction of white matter in periventricular areas and centrum semiovale, lacunar infarcts in white matter and basal ganglia, and dilated Virchow–Robin spaces [7, 10]. Neuronal apoptosis in the cortex correlates with the extent of subcortical ischemic lesion load.

Microscopically, the arteriopathy, characterized by thickening of the arterial wall causing luminal stenosis, deposition of nonamyloid granular osmiophilic material (GOM) in the media extending into the adventitia, and eventual disintegration of smooth muscle cells, is found in the small penetrating cerebral and leptomeningeal arteries. This in part explains the unusual pattern of white matter abnormalities seen in CADASIL. The endothelium is largely normal.

Extracellular GOM, located close to the cell surface of smooth muscle cells, is pathognomonic of CADASIL. Arteriopathy is found in other organs, such as the spleen, liver, kidneys, muscle, aorta, and skin, although clinical manifestations are restricted to the CNS. Therefore, a skin biopsy sample demonstrating this pathologic change is used for diagnosis; the sensitivity of this test is 40–50% [7, 10]. Immunostaining with NOTCH3 monoclonal antibody to detect the accumulation of NOTCH3 protein in the vessel wall is highly sensitive (85–95%) and specific (95–100%) [7, 10].

Molecular genetics

CADASIL, caused by mutations in the Notch3 gene encoded on chromosome 19q12, is inherited in an autosomal dominant manner. The Notch3 gene encodes a single-pass transmembrane receptor of 2321 amino acids with an extracellular domain containing 34 epidermal growth factor repeats (EGFR). Each EGFR has six cysteine residues. More than 95% of the 150 mutations described thus far are missense mutations found in exons 2–24, and that lead to addition or deletion of a cysteine residue in the EGFR [7, 10]. De novo mutations and homozygous mutations are rarely reported.

Molecular testing by screening exons 2–24 is the gold standard for the diagnosis of CADASIL; the test is 100% specific when a mutation involving cysteine residue is detected, and the sensitivity is close to 100%.

In asymptomatic adult first-degree family members of patients with CADASIL, genetic testing raises psychological and ethical concerns similar to other adult-onset autosomal dominant neurodegenerative disorders such as Huntington's disease. There is no recommendation to screen children, as currently there is no benefit in terms of treatment.

Mechanisms underlying symptoms

NOTCH3 is predominantly expressed in vascular smooth muscle cells of small arteries in particular. CADASIL mutations cause gradual accumulation of the extracellular domain of NOTCH3 protein in the form of microscopic aggregates around vascular smooth muscle cells and pericytes of brain arteries and capillaries, in close proximity to deposits of GOM [15]. Total loss of Notch3, however, does not cause CADASIL pathology. Evidence strongly suggests that CADASIL mutations act through gain of novel function mechanisms and that the change in the number of cysteine residues in NOTCH3 is the common denominator which affects the survival and function of vascular smooth muscle cells [15].

Chronic subcortical ischemia and compromised cerebral hemodynamics in addition to altered vasoreactivity resulting from structural and functional changes in brain arteries might lead to recurrent lacunar infarcts and microstructural alterations that ultimately cause cognitive decline, motor disability, cortical atrophy, and neuronal apoptosis [13]. The pathophysiology of mood disorders and migraine with aura is mostly unknown. Cortical morphology (i.e., depth and width of cortical sulci) in the mediofrontal and orbitofrontal areas, in contrast to cortical thickness, has been strongly and independently associated with apathy in CADASIL [16]. One recent study suggests that increased rapid-onset cortical plasticity may contribute to largely preserved cognitive and motor function in patients with CADASIL despite extensive ischemic small vessel disease [16].

Treatment

At present, there is no treatment for CADASIL. Migraine with aura is treated similarly to migraine in general population, with the exception that ergot derivatives and triptans are not considered safe in views of their vasoconstricting property [7, 10]. Usual prophylactic drugs such as antiepileptic drugs, tricyclic antidepressants, or antihypertensives can be used. Anecdotally, acetazolamide has been reported to be effective.

Secondary stroke prevention similar to noncardioembolic ischemic stroke is usually recommended: use of antiplatelet drugs and treatment of vascular risk factors. Use of anticoagulants is avoided because of the increased risk of intracerebral hemorrhage in the presence of cerebral microbleeds. Donepezil was tested in CADASIL patients with cognitive impairment. Inclusion criteria were a Mini-Mental State Examination score of 10–27 or a TMT-B time score that is at least 1.5 SD below the mean, after adjustment for age and education [17]. One hundred sixty-eight patients were followed for 18 weeks. No effect on the primary endpoint, using the cognitive subscale of the vascular Alzheimer's disease cognitive assessment scale (ADAS-Cog), was noted; improvements, however, were recorded on measures of executive functions [17]. Supportive measures such as physical therapy and rehabilitation, psychological support, and nursing care play an important role in the long-term management of elderly debilitated and demented individuals. Genetic counseling for asymptomatic members at risk of carrying the mutation is vital prior to testing.

Adult-onset leukoencephalopathy with axonal spheroids and pigmented glia: Hereditary diffuse leukoencephalopathy with spheroids and pigmentary orthochromatic leukodystrophy

Patients with hereditary diffuse leukoencephalopathy with spheroids (HDLS) and pigmentary orthochromatic leukodystrophy (POLD) manifest with behavioral changes, depression, dementia, epilepsy, and motor impairment including parkinsonism, spastic hemi-, para-, or tetraparesis, and/or ataxia [18, 19]. There has been compelling evidence from clinical presentation, imaging, and pathological studies that HDLS and familial POLD belong to the same disease spectrum. Comparative morphologic study of patients with HDLS and POLD shows no distinctive pathologic features [20]. This data and other literature suggest that HDLS and POLD should collectively be referred to as adult-onset leukoencephalopathy with axonal spheroids and pigmented glia (ALSP) [21]. Recent genetic analyses have confirmed that POLD and HDLS are due to mutations in the same gene, CSF1R, a tyrosine kinase receptor expressed on the surface of microglia, and to a lesser extent in neurons. Therefore, these two conditions likely are a single clinicopathologic entity [97, 98]. For historical reasons, we will discuss these two conditions separately but emphasizing their similarities.

POLD

Orthochromatic leukodystrophies (OLD) constitute a group of heterogeneous noninflammatory demyelinating disorders. The use of the term orthochromatic refers to characteristic birefringence, to distinguish the findings from metachromatic (leukodystrophy caused by arylsulfatase A deficiency, *discussed in the following*) in which granules take on a brown stain in the presence of acidic cresyl violet. Peiffer et al. divided OLD into four forms: (i) pure forms, (ii) special forms, (iii) OLD combined with phakomatoses and other disorders, and (iv) symptomatic forms [22]. The family described by Van Bogaert and Nyssen in 1936 with adult-onset OLD associated with pigmented macrophages and other glia (POLD) represents the pure forms of OLD [23]. To date, the majority of POLD cases are sporadic. Eight POLD families with recessive as well as, less commonly, dominant inheritance have been reported. The average age at onset (AAO) (±SD) was 43 ± 13 years with a life expectancy of 6 years from diagnosis [24]. Initial reported symptoms in POLD involve a frontotemporal phenotype with mood disorders; executive dysfunction; behavioral changes including disinhibition, aggressiveness, euphoria, and apathy; and variable memory impairment [24, 25]. Presentation consistent with a diagnosis of Pick's disease has been reported. Psychosis sometimes occurs. Cognitive decline, including memory impairment, but with frontal predominance occurs in most patients leading to end-stage dementia. Motor impairment follows and is commonly due to prominent pyramidal tract involvement producing spastic paraparesis, tetraparesis, or hemiparesis. Ataxia, dysphagia, and dysarthria have been reported [24, 25]. Seizures occur in most patients during the course of illness.

A few MRI studies show progressive frontal-predominant atrophy and white matter changes in the periventricular areas during the earlier periods which later spread into the deep white matter [24, 25] (Figure 12.3). SPECT (99mTc-ECD) showed frontoparietal hypoperfusion in one patient with POLD [26]. In one case, proton MRS enabled distinction of POLD from other disease processes such as ischemia, gliosis, or tumors, with metabolic derangements (e.g., decreased NAA/Cr ratio and increased Cho/Cr ratio that reflect demyelination accompanied with neuroaxonal loss) seen even in the normal-appearing white matter [26]. Brain pathology shows noninflammatory demyelination and axonal destruction with pigmented macrophages and other glia [24]. Ultrastructurally, the pigmented granules resemble lipopigment ceroid, with fingerprint, multilamellar, and granular morphology, not unlike that seen in ceroid lipofuscinosis; these findings suggest a disease process that might be

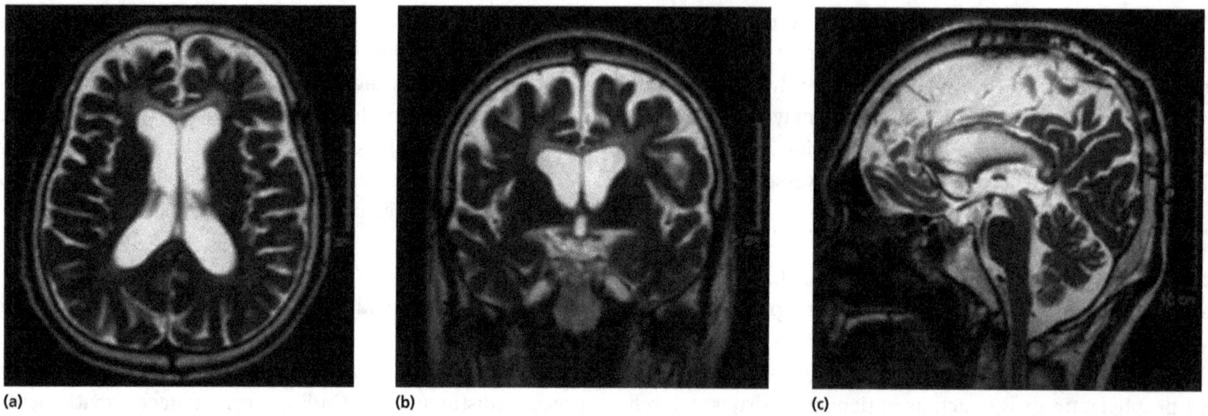

Figure 12.3 Brain MRI in ALSP/POLD. Axial (**a**), coronal (**b**), and sagittal (**c**) T2-weighted images of a case are presented. There is significant atrophy of the bilateral frontal lobes. There are areas of diffuse hyperintensity in the white matter of the bilateral frontal lobes and the corpus callosum. Note that there is substantial callosal atrophy, which is especially severe at the genu and body (**c**). A small focus of signal abnormality is identified within the splenium of the corpus callosum. Other parts of the brain appear to be relatively well preserved. Source: Itoh et al. [24]. Reproduced with permission of Springer.

due, in part, to oxidative damage [25]. The literature describes cases of POLD as sporadic (in the absence of a family history) or inherited in an autosomal recessive or dominant form.

The management of patients with POLD is largely symptomatic.

HDLS

Axelsson and colleagues, in 1984, described a large family with adult-onset autosomal dominant leukoencephalopathy characterized pathologically by the presence of numerous axonal dilations (spheroids) [27]. They coined the term hereditary diffuse leukoencephalopathy with axonal spheroids (HDLS). The average AAO in reported cases is 39 ± 15 years with the average life expectancy of 9 years from presentation [27, 28]. The initial symptoms are most commonly psychiatric, with depression presenting several years before other manifestations. Generalized convulsions, behavioral disturbances such as apathy and emotional blunting, mood disturbances, personality changes, and memory impairment, followed by emotional and intellectual deterioration occur. A frontal syndrome, mainly of the apathetic and emotionally blunted type, has been described in several patients [28]. Motor findings include stiffness, clumsiness, weakness, and gait difficulties due to parkinsonism, ataxia, pyramidal dysfunction, or a combination of these.

Brain imaging can help with the diagnosis of HDLS. Brain CT scans might be normal in the early stages but eventually shows moderate, frontal-predominant atrophy with enlarged lateral and third ventricles. MRI shows frontal-predominant atrophy with periventricular, callosal, and deep white matter lesions, which are patchy, confluent, or diffuse [29] (Figure 12.4). The variable imaging patterns described might reflect differences in disease stage among reported cases. Importantly, occipital involvement rarely occurs. Unlike most other leukodystrophies, diffusion imaging in at least two patients with a rapid form of HDLS showed multiple lesions with restricted diffusion (dark on ADC and bright on DWI/FLAIR) [30]. Fluorodeoxyglucose (FDG) PET in one patient with HDLS showed generalized hypometabolism, with asymmetric parietal predominance [31]. SPECT (99mTc-ECD) showed frontotemporal hypoperfusion in another patient with HDLS [32].

Electrophysiological studies have not been very helpful for diagnosis, as EEGs might be normal, but diffuse or paroxysmal slowing has been reported. No clear ictal or interictal epileptiform patterns were described despite epilepsy being a prominent symptom. Nerve conduction studies, visual evoked potentials (VEPs) and somatosensory evoked potentials (SEPs), and electroretinograms have been normal in HDLS and in POLD [33].

The pathologic hallmark of HDLS is widespread loss of myelin sheaths, gliosis, and axonal destruction [34]. Numerous axonal spheroids, containing phosphorylated neurofilaments, ubiquitin, amyloid precursor protein, and mitochondria, as well as autofluorescent sudanophilic lipid-laden macrophages are found predominantly in the frontal lobe, variably in the parietal or temporal lobes, and in the descending pyramidal tracts at the midbrain, brainstem, and spinal cord levels [35] (Figure 12.5). Neuronal loss and ballooned neurons are seen in the frontal cortex. U-fibers, cortical mantle, and the cerebellum are largely spared, but cerebellar atrophy sometimes occurs.

Several sporadic patients fulfill clinical and pathologic criteria for HDLS, except there is no family history [27, 28], although these cases were described prior to identifying the CSF1R gene as the cause of POLD and HDLS. It remains unknown whether these sporadic cases reflect reduced disease penetrance [98]. Among cases with a positive family history, the pattern of segregation has been consistent with autosomal dominant transmission.

Apart from symptomatic care, unfortunately, currently there is no treatment for either familial or sporadic HDLS.

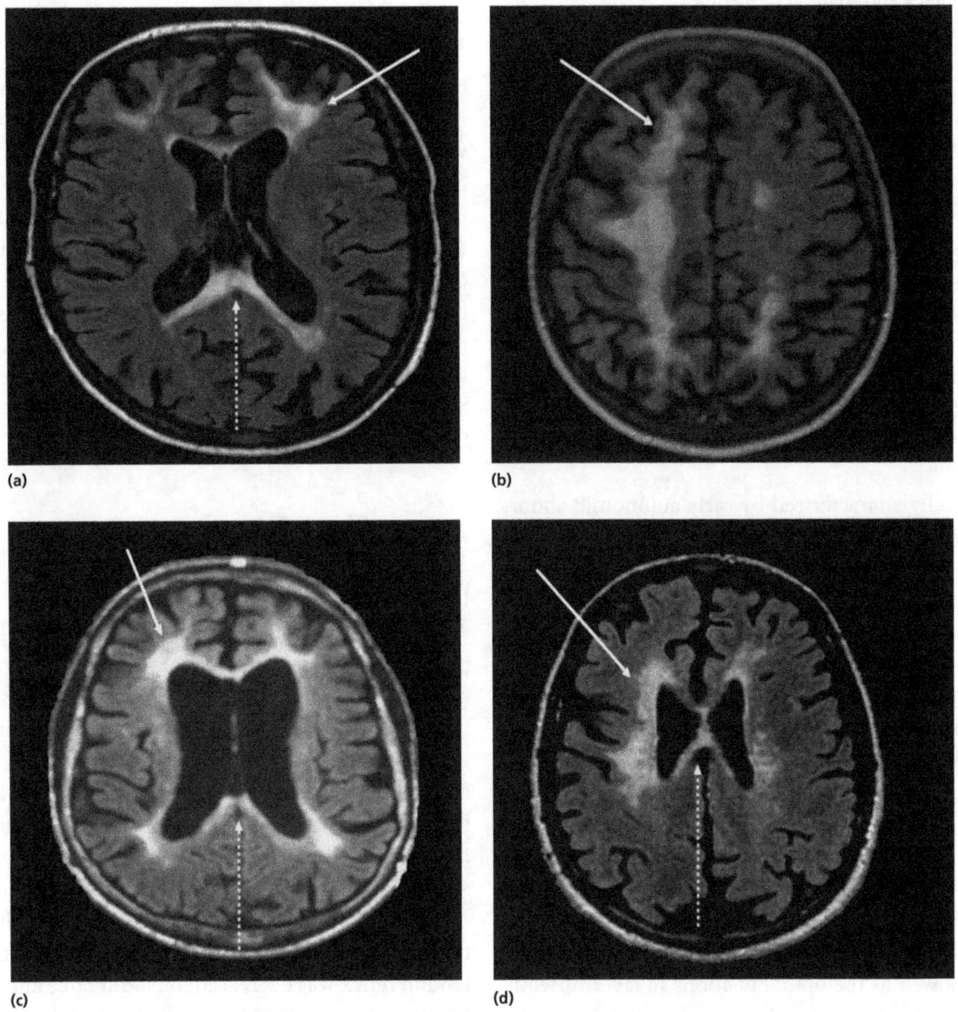

Figure 12.4 Magnetic resonance images (axial sections, T2-weighted) from four HDLS patients: **(a)** Patient 1 (MRI performed 1.2 years after start of symptoms); localized white matter lesions (arrow) in both frontal and parietal hemispheres involving the corpus callosum (arrow dashed). **(b)** Patient 2 (MRI performed 1.9 years after start of symptoms); confluent white matter lesions in both frontal and parietal hemispheres with cortical atrophy in the affected areas. **(c)** Patient 3 (MRI performed 3.5 years after start of symptoms); localized periventricular lesions (arrow) with corresponding frontoparietal atrophy and involvement of the corpus callosum (arrow dashed). **(d)** Patient 4 (MRI performed 2.5 years after start of symptoms); bilateral frontoparietal white matter changes (arrow) extending into the corpus callosum (arrow dashed). Source: Sundal et al. [99] (TBC). Reproduced with permission of Elsevier.

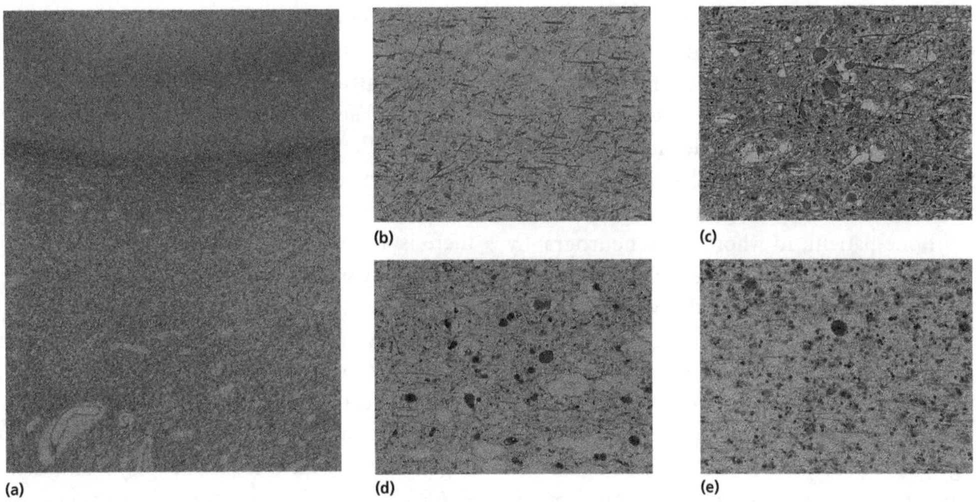

Figure 12.5 White matter lesions of the motor cortex from an ALSP/HDLS case. **(a)** Marked myelin loss of the subcortical white matter with spared U-fiber, KB staining. **(b–d)** Numerous axonal spheroids in the white matter lesion: **(b)** KB staining, **(c)** Bodian staining, and **(d)** immunohistochemistry for ubiquitin. **(e)** Abundant sudanophilic macrophages (*arrowhead*) in the white matter, Sudan III (*KB* Klüver–Barrera). *Bar* **(a)** 400 μm, **(b–e)** 90 μm. Source: Itoh et al. [24]. Reproduced with permission of Springer. (*See insert for color representation of the figure.*)

Adult-onset autosomal dominant leukodystrophy with autonomic dysfunction (*LMNB1* mutation)

Adult-onset autosomal dominant leukodystrophy (ADLD) was first described in an Irish-American family as a slowly progressive and fatal disorder simulating chronic progressive MS [36]. It is a highly penetrant, autosomal dominant, adult-onset disorder presenting in the fourth or fifth decade of life. The genetic basis of this disorder has been established as a tandem genomic duplication, which results in an extra copy of the gene encoding the nuclear lamina protein lamin B1 (*LMNB1*) on chromosome 5q23 [37].

ADLD is clinically characterized by early autonomic abnormalities, pyramidal and pseudobulbar signs, and cerebellar dysfunction such as action tremor, and symmetrical demyelination of the CNS [38]. In general, there is absence of gross cognitive impairment and psychiatric disorders; peripheral neuropathy is also not described [36–39].

In younger patients, brain MRI shows extensive involvement of the white matter of the centrum semiovale with mild enlargement of parietal sulci and lateral ventricles; U-fibers and the corpus callosum are spared. In the advanced stages of the disease, T2 hyperintense signal is symmetric involving the entire white matter of the centrum semiovale and corona radiata, corpus callosum, subcortical U-fibers, and the external and internal capsules [40]. The medulla oblongata, the pons, and the mesencephalon also show T2 hyperintense signal. The white matter of the cerebellum as well as the optic radiations (a layer of white matter immediately lateral to the trigone and occipital horns of lateral ventricles) is spared. Although there is marked cerebral atrophy, infratentorial structures, in particular the pons and cerebellum, are spared [40]. There is no evidence of necrosis or cystic changes on T1-weighted imaging and nor is there calcification on brain imaging, as seen in some other leukodystrophies. Brain MRI showing symmetrical demyelination serves to distinguish this entity from MS.

Nerve conduction studies and autonomic function studies are usually normal. In early stages of the disease, SEPs show poorly waveforms except wave and increased interpeak latencies [41]. In more advanced stages, there is loss of waveforms subsequent to wave I. VEPs show no significant abnormalities [41]. EEG shows mild nonspecific generalized slowing [42]. A selective sympathetic failure, sparing cardiovagal function has been shown in one patient, in whom microneurography revealed absent sympathetic activity [43]. The evaluation of autonomic innervation of skin annexes showed severely depleted and morphologically abnormal noradrenergic dopamine-β-hydroxylase (DβH) immunoreactive fibers with preserved cholinergic vasoactive intestinal polypeptide (VIP) immunoreactive fibers [43].

Neuropathology shows preservation of oligodendroglia with extensive demyelination and lack of astrogliosis and inflammation [39, 40]. As noted earlier, the molecular basis of ADLD has been shown to be duplication of *LMNB1*; this finding adds ADLD to the category of disease resulting from copy number variation, such as Charcot–Marie–Tooth disease type 1 (resulting from *PLP* duplication). An increase in cognate RNA and protein (lamin B1) levels has been found in the brain tissue of the affected patients bearing the duplication. Lamin B1 is a member of the intermediate filament family of proteins which serves a fundamental role within the nuclear envelope by anchoring the nucleus to the cytoskeleton [44].

There currently is no definitive treatment for ADLD. Symptomatic treatment of spasticity, urinary symptoms, and tremors is recommended.

Adult polyglucosan body disease

Illustrative case history 2

A 56-year-old gentleman sought neurological evaluation for progressive leg weakness. Review of systems revealed dizziness on sudden head movements for the past year, reduced concentration and recent memory problems, and urinary and bowel urgency and erectile dysfunction. On exam, he was noted to be alert, and mental function was preserved on orientation, attention, judgment, and immediate and recent memory, but was impaired on delayed recall memory and calculations (MMSE score: 22). Cranial nerve examination was normal. He had moderate motor weakness in the lower extremities, both proximally and distally. Sensation was intact in all modalities. Deep tendon reflex was decreased; bilateral knee and ankle jerk were nearly absent. Electrodiagnostic studies showed sensorimotor polyneuropathy. Autonomic testing revealed sweating abnormalities. A brain MRI showed diffuse white matter changes in bilateral deep parietal area (Figure 12.6). Family history revealed an older brother was wheelchair bound. Sural nerve biopsy revealed polyglucosan bodies in myelinated axons (Figure 12.7), enabling the diagnosis of adult polyglucosan body disease (APBD), which was confirmed following demonstration of decreased glycogen branching enzyme (GBE) activity in cultured fibroblasts.

Background

APBD is a late-onset autosomal recessive disorder caused by deficiency of the GBE and characterized by a gradual progressive involvement of both the CNS and peripheral nervous systems (PNS), with onset in the fifth to seventh decade [45, 46]. Although there is a great deal of heterogeneity, most patients develop a tetrad of symptoms including urinary incontinence (frequency and urgency), gait disorder (para- or quadriparesis), sensory greater than motor polyneuropathy, and cognitive impairment. Other symptoms also have been reported, though less commonly, including extrapyramidal symptoms, cerebellar ataxia, amyotrophic lateral sclerosis, and cardiomyopathy [45, 46]. When cognitive impairment exists, memory is almost always affected.

APBD should be suspected when patients present with late-onset progressive disease with PNS and CNS involvement, such

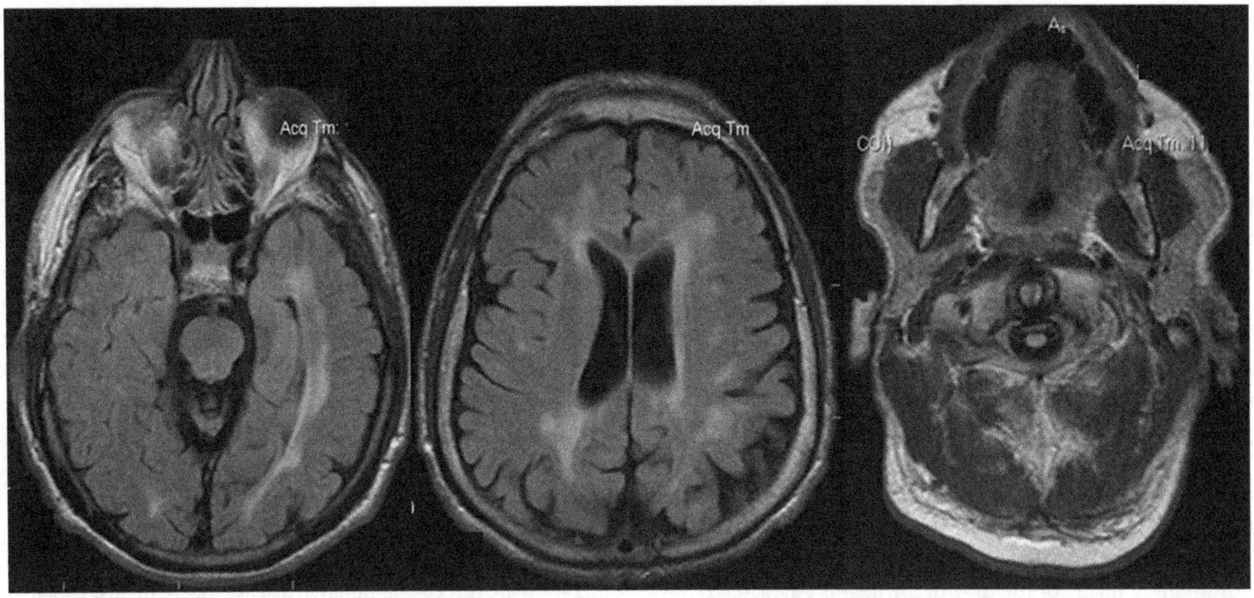

Figure 12.6 FLAIR Brain MRI of a 59-year-old man with APBD, showing periventricular, subcortical, and deep white matter signal abnormalities. Note the typical atrophic cervical spinal cord, typical of APBD.

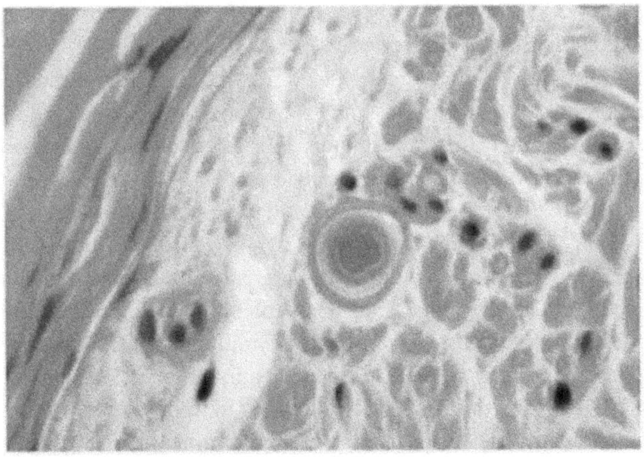

Figure 12.7 Sural nerve biopsy in APBD showing intra-axonal basophilic inclusions (polyglucosan bodies) in several nerve fascicles (light microscopy, H&E stain). Further investigations showed that the storage material is not membrane bound, is diastase resistant, and is PAS positive (not shown). (*See insert for color representation of the figure.*)

as progressive sensorimotor or pure motor peripheral neuropathy and spastic tetraparesis; neurogenic bladder is often a very early feature, followed several years later by the development of gait abnormalities and neuropathy. Dementia is seen rather late in the disease in about 60% of cases [47, 48]. Rarely, cognitive impairment precedes motor signs [49]. Brain MRI often shows diffuse periventricular leukoencephalopathy involving the mesencephalon and the cerebellum [50, 51]. Brain imaging in later stages also often reveal diffuse cerebral, cerebellar, and spinal cord atrophy. Cavitations in the white matter, as also seen in CADASIL, are often seen in APBD as well.

Recent studies suggest there is a secondary impairment of energy metabolism and disruption of methylation in these patients [52]. Pathologically, white matter degeneration in APBD might result from tissue damage involving axons and myelin [49]. Polyglucosan bodies (intracellular inclusions of amylopectin-like polysaccharide that has fewer branched points) are greatly increased in neurons and glia. It has been hypothesized that the accumulation of polyglucosan bodies, in addition to its deleterious effects on axonal integrity, may also induce direct or indirect myelin damage.

The diagnosis of APBD can be made in many cases by identification of a mutation in the glycogen branching enzyme (*GBE1*) gene, establishing decreased levels of GBE activity in blood leukocytes or cultured skin fibroblasts, and/or demonstration of nonmembrane-bound cytoplasmic periodic acid–Schiff-positive polyglucosan bodies in peripheral nerves, found most abundantly in myelinated nerve fibers [45]. Polyglucosan bodies are demonstrable in the sural nerve; however, some reports show that a skin biopsy also appears to be simple, reliable, and less invasive diagnostic tool [53]. Pathological findings are considered less diagnostic than identifying a mutation or by decreased GBE levels as polyglucosan bodies are also seen in other diseases such as progressive myoclonic epilepsy (Lafora bodies). At least eight different mutations found in *GBE* gene on 3p16 are associated with APBD. Most are homozygous, though compound heterozygotes have been identified. APBD has been shown to occur most frequently in patients of Ashkenazi Jewish origin, and in most such cases, a common missense (Tyr329Ser) mutation in the *GBE1* gene has been identified [54]. Curiously, there is overlap of mutations with glycogen storage disease type IV (GSD-IV), which presents as a fulminant fatal disease in infants and children [55]. It is not known why the same mutation can present so differently, but presumably due to the influence of epigenetic factors. In many patients, the disease is possibly sporadic, with no *GBE1* mutations identified.

Unfortunately, there is no effective therapy, except for symptomatic care. Clinical studies suggest that an anaplerotic diet therapy with the odd-carbon triglyceride (triheptanoin-C7TG) may interrupt the progression of symptoms and provide some functional recovery [52]. The discovery of a possible mouse model for APBD might hold promise for screening potential treatments [56].

Adult-onset Alexander disease

Alexander disease is a rare neurodegenerative disorder characterized by white matter degeneration and formation of cytoplasmic inclusions called Rosenthal fibers, which have been observed in astrocytes [57]. Adult-onset Alexander disease (AOAD) is associated with different clinical symptoms and brain MRI findings from infantile forms of the disorder, which is characterized by progressive psychomotor retardation with loss of developmental milestones, megalencephaly, and seizures [57]. Mutations in the gene encoding the glial fibrillary acidic protein (GFAP) have been found in patients with the infantile- and adult-onset variants [57, 58]. Age at onset and GFAP mutation site have been shown to be important clinical predictors [59].

Clinical features noted in adult patients found to have *GFAP* mutations include one or more of the following signs and symptoms: bulbar/pseudobulbar signs, including palatal myoclonus, dysphagia, and dysphonia; pyramidal tract signs, including spasticity and hyperreflexia; cerebellar signs, such as ataxia, nystagmus, and dysmetria; and dysautonomia [57–59]. Cognitive deficits in new learning and recent memory, executive functions, and fine motor dexterity and less apparent deficits in information processing and visual scanning speed were observed in a 21-year-old patient, followed from ages 15 to 21 [60]. A recent report on 12 Japanese patients showed behavioral problems and/or memory disturbance in three individuals, two of whom were said to have had parkinsonism and frontotemporal dementia or progressive supranuclear palsy until *GFAP* mutations were detected [61]. Interestingly, palatal myoclonus and sleep disorders (e.g., sleep apnea and restless legs syndrome), often observed in affected patients, were not observed in the Japanese cohort [61].

Atrophy and changes in signal intensity in the medulla oblongata and upper cervical spinal cord are considered diagnostic features of AOAD [62]. Symmetrical cerebral white matter abnormalities, of mild to moderate intensity and with a frontal predominance, can be found in the majority of cases. Supratentorial periventricular white matter abnormalities and abnormal contrast enhancement often are seen in adult-onset cases before age 40, but in cases with onset over 40 [58, 62], postcontrast enhancement is usually absent and mean diffusivity is not altered, except in areas showing abnormal white matter [62].

Prior to identification of *GFAP* mutations, the diagnosis of Alexander disease was based on the demonstration of Rosenthal fibers (intracellular inclusion bodies composed of aggregates of GFAP, vimentin, αβ-crystallin, and heat shock protein 27 found exclusively in astrocytes) on brain biopsy or at autopsy [57, 59]. Currently, the diagnosis is established when a *GFAP* sequence variant which has been previously reported as disease causing is found. In cases in which the identified sequence variant has not been previously described, the probability of causality is deemed high when there is involvement of a highly conserved site in the *GFAP* gene across species (orthologs) or in a similar domain motifs across other human intermediate filament proteins (paralogs) or studies in animals or cell culture systems have shown that the altered sequence leads to astrocyte dysfunction. The majority of cases occur sporadically; individuals with the slowly progressive adult form who have an affected parent have been described, indicative of autosomal dominant transmission [63].

Unfortunately, there is currently no specific treatment for any form of Alexander disease. Experimental approaches under consideration are directed at putative disease mechanisms, which are not fully elucidated; these include (i) reducing the initial insult arising from GFAP mutations (e.g., misfolded protein and the use of chaperones), (ii) enhancing protective stress responses, and (iii) minimizing detrimental downstream effects [64].

Mitochondrial disorders

Abnormalities on brain MRI, including white and/or gray matter involvement, and cognitive impairment often are encountered in adult patients with a mitochondrial disorder, although rarely as isolated features [65, 66]. Some commonly associated nervous system manifestations are migraine-like headache, sensorineural hearing loss, progressive external ophthalmoplegia, myopathy, and axonal neuropathy [65, 66]. Multisystem involvement might include hypothyroidism, diabetes mellitus, cardiomyopathy, cardiac conduction abnormalities, vomiting, gastrointestinal pseudo-obstruction, diarrhea, hepatopathy, anemia, leukopenia, thrombocytopenia, or renal insufficiency [65, 66].

Mitochondrial disorders are metabolic diseases, most frequently caused by a defect in the respiratory chain that leads to a decrease in the ability of the mitochondria to meet cellular energy demands. The mitochondria are involved in other cellular roles as well, including mitophagy and programmed cell death. Defects of mitochondrial function can arise as a result of mutations involving proteins encoded by mitochondrial or nuclear DNA (nDNA) [65, 66]. Mitochondrial dysfunction might also be implicated in the etiopathogenesis of Parkinson's disease, and mutations in several nuclear-encoded genes linked with inherited Parkinson's disease have been hypothesized to result in mitochondrial dysfunction [67].

A detailed discussion of mitochondrial disorders is beyond the scope of this review, which will focus on a selected subset of conditions associated with dementia to illustrate mode of disease presentation and its evolution.

Mitochondrial disorders present as either slowly or rapidly progressing single-organ or multisystem defects with onset at any time from birth to adulthood. The involvement of the CNS is estimated in 30–60% of patients [68, 69]. Most information about cognitive decline in mitochondrial diseases is derived from case reports or small case series. If systematically tested, however, cognitive impairment is frequent and more clearly evident on neuropsychological testing than might be anticipated from clinical examination alone [68, 69]. Cognitive impairment progresses with disease duration and occurs more frequently in patients with abnormal imaging.

Neuropsychiatric abnormalities are a frequent finding in mitochondrial disorders, although CNS problems are often found in the presence of other systemic features [68, 69]. Acute manifestations include impaired consciousness and alertness, acute or chronic confusional state, and hallucinations. Psychosis has been particularly described in patients with mitochondrial encephalomyopathy, lactic acidosis, and stroke-like episodes (MELAS) and rarely in Kearns–Sayre syndrome (KSS) [69, 70]. In a report on three adult patients exhibiting psychiatric symptoms as the core manifestations accompanied by various degrees of myopathic symptoms, skeletal muscle pathologic findings were compatible with mitochondrial myopathy in all cases [70]. In these cases, mutation analyses revealed mitochondrial DNA (mtDNA) deletion in skeletal muscles, but not in blood.

Cognitive dysfunction in the domains of abstract reasoning, verbal memory, visual memory, language, executive functions, calculation, attention, or visuospatial functions, with relative sparing of functional abilities, has been described and might be the initial manifestation of CNS involvement in patients with a mitochondrial disorder [63, 64]. Dementia may be a feature of MELAS; myoclonic epilepsy and ragged-red fibers (MERRF), Leigh syndrome; KSS; neuropathy, ataxia, and retinitis pigmentosa (NARP); Leber hereditary optic neuropathy (LHON); or Muir–Torre syndrome (MTS). Comorbidities associated with each of these individual mitochondrial disorders enable their differentiation.

In a small series of 36 patients with mitochondrial myopathies and encephalomyopathies, general cognitive dysfunction or focal deficits were detected in 61% of the patients, whereas moderate to severe deterioration was seen in 36% of the patients [70]. Seventy-eight percent of the patients with CNS involvement showed cognitive deficits of language, memory, or perception. These observations are consistent with the findings of a separate study involving 22 patients with chronic progressive external ophthalmoplegia (CPEO) or KSS [71]. In this, the latter patient cohort neuropsychological testing did not reveal signs that would suggest general intellectual decline or dementia, but provided evidence of specific focal neuropsychological deficits, suggesting particular impairment of visuospatial perception associated to parieto-occipital lobes and executive deficits associated to the prefrontal cortex [71]. It should be noted that secondary effects on cognition in patients with a mitochondrial disorder might also occur, due to the involvement of other organs (e.g., hyperglycemic encephalopathy due to uncontrolled diabetes or hypo- or hyperthyroid and hypoparathyroid encephalopathy) [65, 66].

Diagnosis of mitochondrial disorders

A patient already diagnosed with a mitochondrial disorder can develop cognitive dysfunction, in which case the etiology for dementia is evident. In cases wherein cognitive decline is the presenting feature, however, symptomatic involvement of two or more apparently unrelated organs (e.g., neurosensory and endocrine systems) raises the index of suspicion for a mitochondrial defect. Elevated blood and CSF lactate and pyruvate levels might provide a useful clue; attention must be paid, however, to the fact that uncontrolled seizures also cause elevated lactate levels and improper handling of the specimens (such as not keeping samples cold or analyzed expeditiously) artificially lowers lactate and pyruvate levels, possibly resulting in false-negative tests. Brain MR spectroscopy (MRS), especially of the stroke-like lesions in MELAS, often shows markedly reduced *N*-acetyl-aspartate, choline, creatine peaks, or an increased lactate peak [73]. SPECT studies may show hypoperfusion in temporal or occipital lobes [74].

Diagnostic confirmation may be obtained in patients with clinically defined syndromes by mutation analysis and demonstration of known mtDNA disease-causing defects [65, 66]. A muscle biopsy with estimation of enzymes involved in respiratory chain can sometimes detect mitochondrial dysfunction, but might not be abnormal in patients without significant muscle involvement. In contrast to point mutations in mtDNA, which can be often demonstrated in a peripheral blood sample, analysis for deletion-type mutation may require skeletal muscle biopsy [72].

Pathophysiology and molecular genetics of mitochondrial disorders

Mitochondria are intracellular organelles that change in number based on the substrate and oxygen requirements of the cell. Fundamental biological roles include provision of adenosine triphosphate (ATP), mediation of cell death by apoptosis, heat production by decoupling of the oxidative phosphorylation, and translation and transcription of mitochondrial genes [65, 66]. β-Oxidation, the citrate acid cycle, degradation of amino acids, parts of heme synthesis, steroid metabolism and uric acid cycle, mitochondrial protein synthesis, and reactions catalyzed by the pyruvate dehydrogenase complex (PDC) also occur in the mitochondria. The brain, skeletal muscles, and sensory organs that rely on mitochondrial aerobic metabolism are more frequently involved.

Human mtDNA is a 16.5-kb circular minichromosome encoding 37 genes, 13 of which code for subunits of the respiratory chain complexes I–V (excluding complex II), 22 encode tRNAs, and two encode rRNAs. A single mitochondrion contains 2–10 mtDNA copies [65, 66]. Thus, each cell houses up to several thousand mtDNA copies, as each cell contains hundreds of mitochondria. Fifty-four of the 67 respiratory chain proteins and 1000 other mitochondrial proteins are encoded by the nDNA.

mtDNA mutations such as large-scale rearrangements (partial deletions or duplications) can occur spontaneously, whereas point mutations are usually inherited from the mother (i.e., matrilineal inheritance as opposed to sex linked). Mitochondrial disorders caused by nDNA mutations follow a Mendelian pattern of inheritance. Random mutations in the mtDNA lead to coexistence of wild-type mtDNA and mutant mtDNA in a single cell or organ, a phenomenon known as heteroplasmy [65, 66]. A high proportion of the mutant mtDNA in an organ or a cell predicts a more severe phenotype. Phenotype in a mitochondrial disorder depends on the severity of the mutation, the affected gene, tissue distribution, cellular oxygen requirement, and threshold effect, which implies that if the load of mutant mtDNA copies exceeds a certain amount, the effect of a mutation can be no longer compensated for by wild-type mtDNA.

Recently, investigations undertaken in a 57-year-old woman with progressive neurodegeneration characterized by psychosis, dementia, and akinesia–rigidity revealed a novel mitochondrial transfer RNA (Phe) (MTTF) mutation [75]. Evaluations revealed neuropsychological features indicative of predominant frontal lobe dysfunction suggestive of progressive supranuclear palsy or Huntington's disease (subcortical dementia). Her brain MRI showed brainstem, cerebellar, and widespread cortical atrophy, but no evidence of white matter disease.

Therapy of mitochondrial disorders

Treatment of mitochondrial dementia includes general measures such as regular physiotherapy as tolerated by the individual, avoidance of stress, fasting, extreme temperature, or drugs known to induce secondary respiratory chain insufficiency [65, 66]. Use of ketogenic diet (65% fat) or substitution of fat by carbohydrates and supplementation of respiratory chain components such as coenzyme Q have also been recommended [65, 66]. Administration of metabolites or cofactors such as carnitine in order to restore secondarily lowered levels of free carnitine, creatine, thiamine, or riboflavin is recommended. Comorbid conditions such as seizures or endocrine abnormalities need appropriate control. The progressive course of cognitive involvement unfortunately is typically unaffected by these therapeutic approaches.

Lysosomal storage disorders

White matter signal abnormalities on brain MRI has been described in several lysosomal storage disorders (LSDs); although cognitive impairment can be a feature, it is often not the initial mode of presentation or the only clinical problem [3]. As with mitochondrial defects, LSDs are oligo- or multisystemic disorders; the pattern of organ involvement, however, is more a function of tissue substrate storage and not energy deficits, and symptoms bear no relationship to dietary intake or fasting [3]. Pertinent disorders include late-onset forms of MLD and GLD (Krabbe disease), Fabry disease, and other conditions.

Although not an LSD, X-linked adrenoleukodystrophy (ALD; a peroxisomal defect) is briefly described in this section.

MLD and GLD(Krabbe disease)

Behavioral abnormalities with modifications of mood, peculiar social reactions, and a progressive mental deterioration have been described in adult-onset MLD and Krabbe disease [79, 80], demyelinating leukodystrophies, caused by deficiency of the lysosomal enzymes hydrolase arylsulfatase A (ARSA) and β-galactocerebrosidase, respectively [81, 82]. Both disorders are inherited in an autosomal recessive manner. Peripheral neuropathy is common, due to peripheral myelin involvement; although in patients with late-onset forms of the disease, this finding may not be evident on presentation [83].

Brain MRI characteristics of MLD and GLD include prominent T2-weighted hyperintensity with T1-weighted hypointensity (relative to gray matter structures), consistent with demyelination [3]. The lesions found are frequently confluent, with a predominantly frontal and/or periventricular distribution (Figure 12.8).

Fabry disease

Fabry disease is an X-linked disorder caused by deficiency of the lysosomal hydrolases α-galactosidase A (AGAL). Although the classic features of disease occur in affected males, a significant proportion of carrier females (up to 70%) develop clinical problems; this likely due to X-inactivation of the normal chromosome and the fact that the signs and symptoms of disease among affected females, however, are highly variable and often milder and tend to occur at a later age [76]. In addition to problems related to cerebrovascular disease, patients usually suffer from progressive renal insufficiency and cardiomyopathy. Ophthalmic examination might show corneal and lenticular opacities in a verticillate (whorled) pattern [76]. An Italian study examining newborn blood spots found that adult-onset cases likely are highly underestimated and much more common than the classic younger-onset forms [90].

Although strictly not a leukodystrophy, brain MRI of adult patients with Fabry disease often show signal abnormalities, most of which are consistent with leukoaraiosis rather than demyelination [76, 77]. Patients with Fabry disease are estimated to have 20-fold higher risk of TIA or stroke compared to the general population. Signal abnormalities often are found in watershed regions, corresponding to brain vascular distribution, a finding that further suggests a role for ischemia in the disease process. White matter lesions on MRI, presumably ischemic, can be focal, multifocal, and confluent [76] (Figure 12.9). In spite of these findings, most affected individuals with Fabry disease reportedly do not have overt cognitive problems [76]. Dementia is rarely a presenting feature, although adult-onset cases presenting as vascular dementia cases have been reported [91, 92]. Patients with Fabry disease are at risk for cerebrovascular disease and might develop cognitive impairment following a stroke [78] or progressive small vessel ischemic vascular disease [91]. Cerebrovascular changes might be the only manifestation

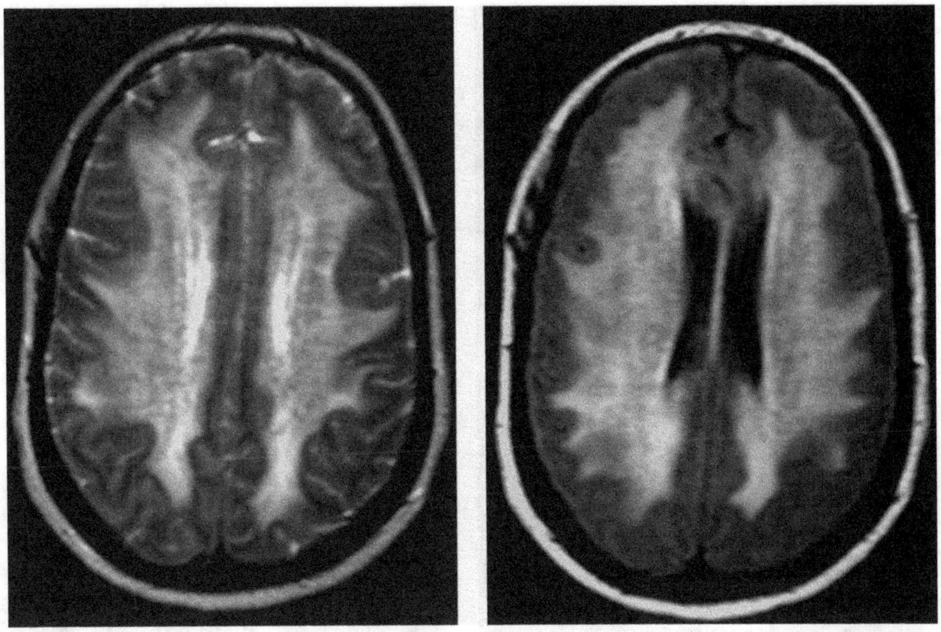

(a) (b)

Figure 12.8 Brain MRI in MLD. Axial T2 (**a**) and FLAIR (**b**) images show diffuse hyperintensity in the cerebral white matter with sparing of U-fibers. Source: Kanekar and Gustas [96]. Reproduced with permission of Elsevier.

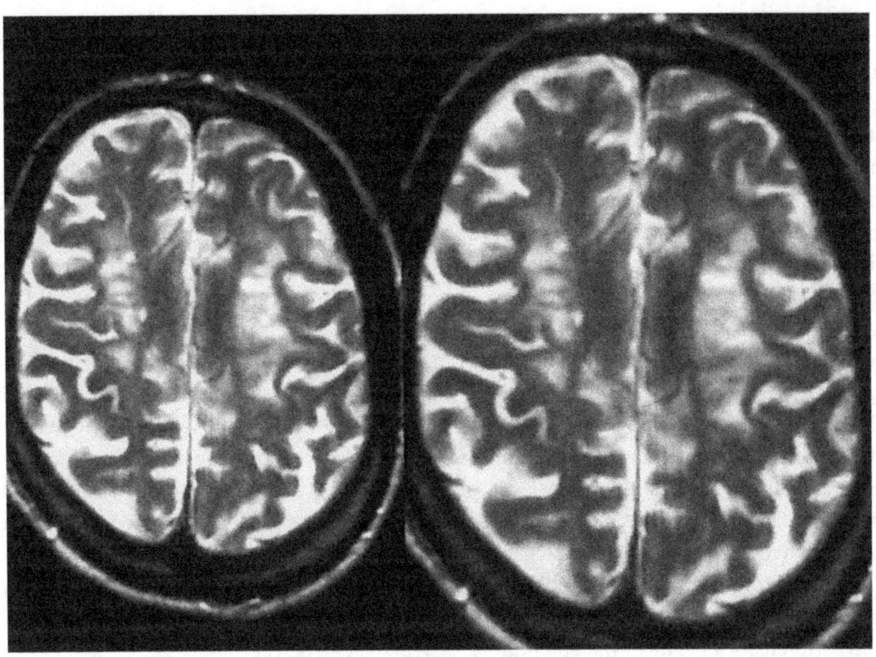

Figure 12.9 T2-weighted magnetic resonance images in a patient with Fabry disease, showing multifocal white matter hyperintensities approaching confluency. Source: Mohanraj et al. [92]. Reproduced with permission of BMJ Publishing Group.

of some patients in their 30s–40s, whereas others might be asymptomatic, but with cerebrovascular disease on MRI [91]. Fabry disease should be considered in patients with unexplained cerebrovascular disease [76, 91, 92]. A relatively specific MRI finding of Fabry disease appears to be T1 hyperintense lesions in the posterior thalamus and pulvinar, due to mineralization, occurring mostly in older (>30 years old) males with cardiomyopathy or renal disease (Figure 12.10) [76, 93–95].

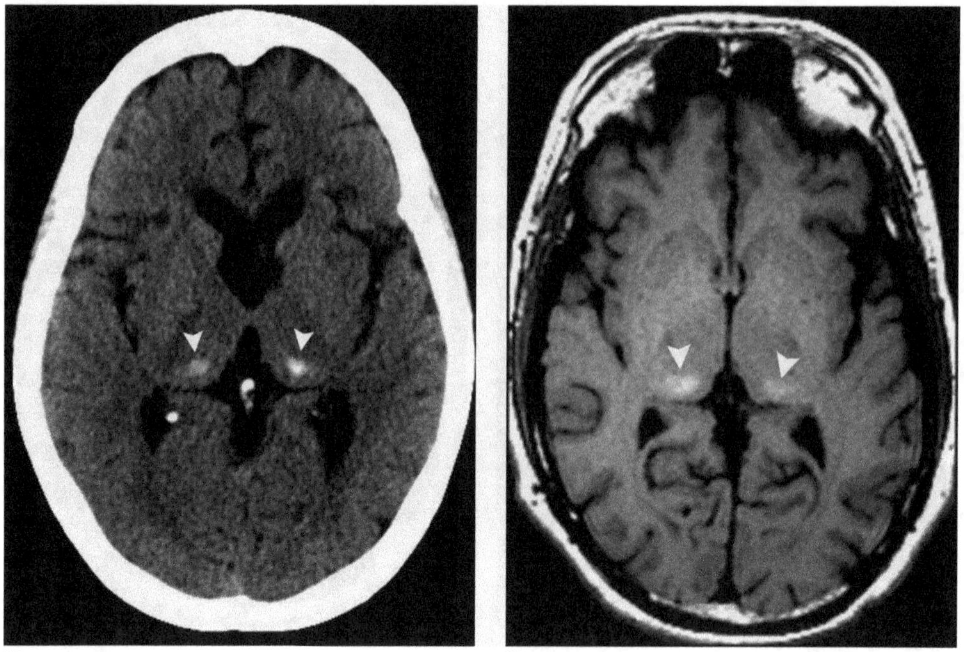

Figure 12.10 Fabry disease. Axial CT (**a**) scan at the level of deep gray matter nuclei shows calcification in the pulvinar nuclei of thalamus (arrowheads). Corresponding areas show hyperintensity on T1-weighted image (**b**). Source: Kanekar and Gustas [96]. Reproduced with permission of Elsevier.

ALD

X-linked ALD is caused by mutations in *ABCD1* gene, which encodes a peroxisomal membrane half-ATP-binding cassette transporter. A defect of ABCD1 (also known as ALDP, which stands for adrenoleukodystrophy protein) is associated with impaired peroxisomal beta-oxidation and accumulation of saturated very-long-chain fatty acids (VLCFA) in tissues and body fluids [84]. Affected individuals typically present with the childhood cerebral form (which manifests most commonly between ages 4 and 8 years), but onset in adulthood is well described [84]. The latter patients often have a spastic gait consistent from involvement of long tracts (adrenomyeloneuropathy), but do not always develop intellectual decline, but adult-onset forms might present as frontotemporal dementia [84]. Cognitive impairment or behavioral changes are more characteristic of the childhood cerebral form. Brain MRI in adult-onset cases of X-ALD have shown tract involvement in the corticospinal, spinothalamic, visual, and auditory pathways. Internal capsule and brainstem pyramidal involvement is common. More commonly, white matter hyperintensities begin in the splenium of the corpus callosum and move caudally–rostrally to the occipitoparietal cortex. T2 hyperintensities might also start in the genu of the corpus callosum and move frontally [84, 85].

Recently, Uchida and colleagues described a 46-year-old Japanese patient with adult-onset X-linked ALD who presented with topographic disorientation [86]. Intellectual function was relatively preserved and amnestic symptoms were absent. Brain MRI images revealed T2 signal hyperintensity along the occipitopontine tract and lateral lemnisci, but not in the corticospinal tract in the brainstem [86].

Diagnosis of LSDs

In the relevant clinical context, the diagnosis of MLD or Krabbe or Fabry disease might be established, based on the demonstration of deficient enzyme activity with several caveats. As 10–15% of the general population exhibit a pseudo-deficiency of ARSA activity, the enzymatic diagnosis of MLD requires demonstration of excess urine sulfatide excretion and/or presence of known defects in the cognate gene [81]. The diagnosis of Fabry disease in females with normal AGAL activity necessitates demonstration of a causal *AGAL* gene defect, as up to one-third of carrier females have residual enzyme activity which overlaps with that found in otherwise healthy individuals within the general population [76]. X-linked ALD is associated with elevated levels of VLCFA, although female carriers might have levels that overlap with values for the general population; thus, diagnosis of carrier females necessitates demonstration of an underlying *ALDP* gene defect [84].

Management

Hematopoietic stem cell transplantation for MLD, Krabbe disease, and X-linked ALD is available [87]. These therapeutic options might modify disease course, but often only when treatment is initiated in the early stages of the disease process. Dietary therapy with Lorenzo's oil (a 4:1 mixture of glyceryl trioleate and glyceryl trierucate) has been reported to slow progression in patients with X-linked ALD when initiated in the early stages of the disease process in children younger than 6 years of age and adrenomyeloneuropathy in patients without cerebral involvement [88]. Adrenal hormone replacement therapy is indicated in patients with X-linked ALD and adrenal insufficiency.

Enzyme replacement therapy is available for Fabry disease [89]. Adjunctive therapies for the primary and secondary prevention of stroke include antiplatelet agents and statins. Angiotensin-converting enzyme inhibitors or sartans are also prescribed in patients with proteinuria for its renoprotective properties.

Summary

Although infrequent to rare, the diagnosis of a leukodystrophy is important so as to avoid the often common situation wherein an affected individual is mistakenly considered to have and inappropriately treated as a case of primary or secondary chronic progressive MS or another disorder. Certain disorders in this class, whose incidence is likely significantly underestimated, include CADASIL, ALSP, and Fabry disease [90]. Table 12.3 presents a summary of key clinical, including MRI, differentiating features of several disorders discussed in this chapter. The diagnosis of a leukodystrophy, when confirmed by biochemical and/or molecular testing, enables appropriate genetic counseling, prognostication, and management.

References

1 Lyon G, Fattal-Valevski A, Kolodny EH. Leukodystrophies: clinical and genetic aspects. *Top Magn Reson Imaging.* 2006;**17**(4): 219–42.

2 Köhler W. Diagnostic algorithm for the differentiation of leukodystrophies in early MS. *J Neurol.* 2008;**255**(suppl 6):123–126.

3 Faust PL, Kaye EM, Powers JM. Myelin lesions associated with lysosomal and peroxisomal disorders. *Expert Rev Neurother.* 2010;**10**(9):1449–66.

4 Schiffmann R, van der Knaap MS. Invited article: an MRI-based approach to the diagnosis of white matter disorders. *Neurology.* 2009;**72**(8):750–9.

5 Brass SD, Smith EE, Arboleda-Velasquez JF, et al. Case records of the Massachusetts general hospital. case 12–2009. A 46-year-old man with migraine, aphasia, and hemiparesis and similarly affected family members. *N Engl J Med.* 2009;**360**(16):1656–65.

6 Razvi SS, Davidson R, Bone I, et al. The prevalence of cerebral autosomal dominant arteriopathy with subcortical infarcts and leucoencephalopathy (CADASIL) in the west of Scotland. *J Neurol Neurosurg Psychiatry.* 2005;**76**(5):739–41.

7 Chabriat H, Joutel A, Dichgans M, et al. CADASIL. *Lancet* 2009;**8**:643–53.

8 Valenti R, Pescini F, Antonini S, et al. Major depression and bipolar disorders in CADASIL: a study using the DSM-IV semi-structured interview. *Acta Neurol Scand* 2011 Mar; **124**:390–5.

9 Jouvent E, Reyes S, Mangin JF, et al. Apathy is related to cortex morphology in CADASIL. A sulcal-based morphometry study. *Neurology.* 2011;**76**(17):1472–7.

10 Dichgans M. Cognition in CADASIL. *Stroke* 2009; **40** (suppl 1): S45–S47.

11 Taillia H, Chabriat H, Kurtz A, et al. Cognitive alterations in non-demented CADASIL patients. *Cerebrovasc Dis* 1998;**8**: 97–101.

12 Peters N, Opherk C, Danek A, et al. The pattern of cognitive performance in CADASIL: A monogenic condition leading to subcortical ischemic vascular dementia. *Am J Psychiatry* 2005; **162**: 2078–2085.

13 Viswanathan A, Gschwendtner A, Guichard JP, et al. Lacunar lesions are independently associated with disability and cognitive impairment in CADASIL. *Neurology.* 2007;**69**(2):172–9.

14 O'Sullivan M, Jouvent E, Saemann PG, et al. Measurement of brain atrophy in subcortical vascular disease: a comparison of different approaches and the impact of ischaemic lesions. *Neuroimage.* 2008;**43**(2):312–20.

15 Joutel A. Pathogenesis of CADASIL: transgenic and knock-out mice to probe function and dysfunction of the mutated gene, Notch3, in the cerebrovasculature. *Bioessays.* 2011;**33**(1):73–80.

16 List J, Duning T, Meinzer M, et al. Enhanced rapid-onset cortical plasticity in CADASIL as a possible mechanism of preserved cognition. *Cereb Cortex.* 2011 Apr 29.

17 Dichgans M, Markus HS, Salloway S, et al. Donepezil in patients with subcortical vascular cognitive impairment: a randomised double-blind trial in CADASIL. *Lancet Neurol.* 2008;**7**(4):310–8.

18 Axelsson R, Röyttä M, Sourander P, et al. Hereditary diffuse leucoencephalopathy with spheroids. *Acta Psychiatr Scand Suppl* 1984;**314**:1–65.

19 Browne L, Sweeney BJ, Farrell MA. Late-onset neuroaxonal leucoencephalopathy with spheroids and vascular amyloid. *Eur Neurol.* 2003;**50**(2):85–90.

20 Ali ZS, Van Der Voorn JP, Powers JM. A comparative morphologic analysis of adult onset leukodystrophy with neuroaxonal spheroids and pigmented glia-a role for oxidative damage. *J Neuropathol Exp Neurol.* 2007;**66**(7):660–72.

21 Wider C, Van Gerpen JA, DeArmond S, et al. Leukoencephalopathy with spheroids (HDLS) and pigmentary leukodystrophy (POLD): a single entity? *Neurology.* 2009 Jun 2;**72**(22):1953–9.

22 Peiffer L. On non-metachromatic leukodystrophy. *Arch Psychiatr Nervenkr Z Gesamte Neurol Psychiatr* 1959;**199**:417–36.

23 Van Bogaert L, Nyssen R. Le type Tardif de la leucodystrophie progressive familiale. *Rev Neurol* 1936;**65**:21–45.

24 Itoh K, Shiga K, Shimizu K, et al. Autosomal dominant leukodystrophy with axonal spheroids and pigmented glia: clinical and neuropathological characteristics. *Acta Neuropathol.* 2006; **111**(1):39–45.

25 Constantinidis J, Wisniewski TM. The dominant form of the pigmentary orthochromatic leukodystrophy. *Acta Neuropathol.* 1991;**82**(6):483–7.

26 Sohn SY, Ko YJ, Hong JM, et al. A case of pigmentary orthochromatic leukodystrophy with findings of proton MR spectroscopy and serial brain MRIs. *J Neurol Sci.* 2010;**295**(1–2):23–6.

27 Axelsson R, Röyttä M, Sourander P, et al. Hereditary diffuse leucoencephalopathy with spheroids. *Acta Psychiatr Scand Suppl* 1984; **314**:1–65.

28 Mendes A, Pinto M, Vieira S, et al. Adult-onset leukodystrophy with axonal spheroids *J Neurol Sci* 2010;**297**(1–2):40–5.

29 Boissé L, Islam O, Woulfe J, et al. Neurological picture. Hereditary diffuse leukoencephalopathy with neuroaxonal spheroids: novel imaging findings. *J Neurol Neurosurg Psychiatry*. 2010;**81**(3): 313–4.

30 Maillart E, Rousseau A, Galanaud D, et al. Rapid onset frontal leukodystrophy with decreased diffusion coefficient and neuroaxonal spheroids. *J Neurol*. 2009;**256**(10):1649–54.

31 Kato K, Nishio A, Kato N, et al. Uptake of 18F-FDG in acute aortic dissection: a determinant of unfavorable outcome. *J Nucl Med*. 2010;**51**(5):674–81.

32 Freeman SH, Hyman BT, Sims KB, et al. Adult onset leukodystrophy with neuroaxonal spheroids: clinical, neuroimaging and neuropathologic observations *Brain Pathol*. 2009;**19**(1):39–47.

33 Van Gerpen JA, Wider C, Broderick DF, et al. Insights into the dynamics of hereditary diffuse leukoencephalopathy with axonal spheroids. *Neurology*. 2008;**71**(12):925–9.

34 Terada S, Ishizu H, Yokota O, et al. An autopsy case of hereditary diffuse leukoencephalopathy with spheroids, clinically suspected of Alzheimer's disease. *Acta Neuropathol*. 2004;**108**(6):538–45.

35 Lin WL, Wszolek ZK, Dickson DW. Hereditary diffuse leukoencephalopathy with spheroids: ultrastructural and immunoelectron microscopic studies. *Int J Clin Exp Pathol*. 2010;3(7):665–74.

36 Brussino A, Vaula G, Cagnoli C, et al. A family with autosomal dominant leukodystrophy linked to 5q23.2–q23.3 without lamin B1 mutations. *Eur J Neurol*. 2010;**17**(4):541–9.

37 Padiath QS, Saigoh K, Schiffmann R, et al. Lamin B1 duplications cause autosomal dominant leukodystrophy. *Nat Genet*. 2006;**38**(10):1114–23c.

38 Eldridge, R., Anayiotos CP, Schlesinger S, et al. Hereditary adult-onset leukodystrophy simulating chronic progressive multiple sclerosis. *N Engl J Med* 1984;**311**:948–953.

39 Schwankhaus JD, Katz DA, Eldridge R, et al. Clinical and pathological features of an autosomal dominant, adult-onset leukodystrophy simulating chronic progressive multiple sclerosis. *Arch Neurol* 1994 **51**:757–66.

40 Sundblom J, Melberg A, Kalimo H, et al. MR imaging characteristics and neuropathology of the spinal cord in adult-onset autosomal dominant leukodystrophy with autonomic symptoms. *AJNR Am J Neuroradiol*. 2009;**30**(2):328–35.

41 Schuster J, Sundblom J, Thuresson AC, et al. Genomic duplications mediate overexpression of lamin B1 in adult-onset autosomal dominant leukodystrophy (ADLD) with autonomic symptoms. *Neurogenetics*. 2011;**12**(1):65–72.

42 Quattrocolo G, Leombruni S, Vaula G, et al. Autosomal dominant late-onset leukoencephalopathy. Clinical report of a new Italian family. *Eur Neurol*. 1997;**37**(1):53–61.

43 Guaraldi P, Donadio V, Capellari S, et al. Isolated noradrenergic failure in adult-onset autosomal dominant leukodystrophy. *Auton Neurosci*. 2011;**159**(1–2):123–6.

44 Ji JY, Lee RT, Vergnes L, et al. Cell nuclei spin in the absence of lamin B1. *J Biol Chem*. 2007; **282**: 20015–26.

45 Gray F, Gherardi R, Marshall A, et al. Adult polyglucosan body disease (APBD). *J Neuropathol Exp Neurol*. 1988;**47**(4):459–74.

46 Klein CJ, Boes CJ, Chapin JE, et al. Adult polyglucosan body disease: case description of an expanding genetic and clinical syndrome. *Muscle Nerve*. 2004;**29**(2):323–8.

47 McDonald TD, Faust PL, Bruno C, et al. Polyglucosan body disease simulating amyotrophic lateral sclerosis. *Neurology*. 1993;**43**(4): 785–90.

48 Segers K, Kadhim H, Colson C, et al. Adult polyglucosan body disease masquerading as ALS with dementia of the Alzheimer type: an exceptional phenotype in a rare pathology. *Alzheimer Dis Assoc Disord*. 2012;**26**(1):96–9.

49 Rifai Z, Klitzke M, Tawil R, et al. Dementia of adult polyglucosan body disease. Evidence of cortical and subcortical dysfunction. *Arch Neurol*. 1994;**51**(1):90–4.

50 Bigio EH, Weiner MF, Bonte FJ, et al. Familial dementia due to adult polyglucosan body disease. *Clin Neuropathol*. 1997;**16**(4):227–34.

51 Berkhoff M, Weis J, Schroth G, et al. Extensive white-matter changes in case of adult polyglucosan body disease. *Neuroradiology*. 2001;**43**(3):234–6.

52 Roe CR, Bottiglieri T, Wallace M, et al. Adult polyglucosan body disease (APBD): Anaplerotic diet therapy (Triheptanoin) and demonstration of defective methylation pathways. *Mol Genet Metab*. 2010;**101**(2–3):246–52.

53 Vos AJ, Joosten EM, Gabreëls-Festen AA. Adult polyglucosan body disease: clinical and nerve biopsy findings in two cases. *Ann Neurol*. 1983;**13**(4):440–4.

54 Lossos A, Meiner Z, Barash V, et al. Adult polyglucosan body disease in Ashkenazi Jewish patients carrying the Tyr329Ser mutation in the glycogen-branching enzyme gene. *Ann Neurol*. 1998;**44**(6):867–72.

55 Tay SK, Akman HO, Chung WK, et al. Fatal infantile neuromuscular presentation of glycogen storage disease type IV. *Neuromuscul Disord*. 2004;**14**(4):253–60.

56 Raben N, Danon M, Lu N, et al. Surprises of genetic engineering: a possible model of polyglucosan body disease. *Neurology* 2001;**56**: 1739–45.

57 Johnson AB. Alexander disease: a review and the gene. *Int J Dev Neurosci*. 2002;**20**(3–5):391–4.

58 Pareyson D, Fancellu R, Mariotti C, et al. Adult-onset Alexander disease: a series of eleven unrelated cases with review of the literature. *Brain*. 2008;**131**(Pt 9):2321–31.

59 Prust M, Wang J, Morizono H, et al. GFAP mutations, age at onset, and clinical subtypes in Alexander disease. *Neurology*. 2011;**77**(13):1287–94.

60 Restrepo J, Bernardin L, Hammeke T. Neurocognitive decline in Alexander disease. *Clin Neuropsychol*. 2011 Oct **25**(7):1266–77.

61 Yoshida T, Sasayama H, Mizuta I, et al. Glial fibrillary acidic protein mutations in adult-onset Alexander disease: clinical features observed in 12 Japanese patients. *Acta Neurol Scand* 2011;**124**(2):104–8.

62 Farina L, Pareyson D, Minati L, et al. Can MR imaging diagnose adult-onset Alexander disease? *Am J Neuroradiol*. 2008;**29**(6): 1190–6.

63 Thyagarajan D, Chataway T, Li R, et al. Dominantly-inherited adult-onset leukodystrophy with palatal tremor caused by a mutation in the glial fibrillary acidic protein gene. *Mov Disord*. 2004;**19**(10):1244–8.

64 Messing A, Daniels CM, Hagemann TL. Strategies for treatment in Alexander disease. *Neurotherapeutics*. 2010;**7**(4):507–15.

65 Tuppen HA, Blakely EL, Turnbull DM, et al. Mitochondrial DNA mutations and human disease. *Biochim Biophys Acta*. 2010;**1797**(2): 113–28.

66 DiMauro S, Schon EA. Mitochondrial disorders in the nervous system. *Annu Rev Neurosci* 2008;**31**:91–123.

67 Jana S, Sinha M, Chanda D, et al. Mitochondrial dysfunction mediated by quinone oxidation products of dopamine: Implications in dopamine cytotoxicity and pathogenesis of Parkinson's disease. *Biochim Biophys Acta*. 2011;**1812**(6):663–73.

68 Finsterer J. Mitochondrial disorders, cognitive impairment and dementia. *J Neurol Sci.* 2009 Aug 15;**283**(1–2):143–8.

69 Finsterer J. Cognitive decline as a manifestation of mitochondrial disorders (mitochondrial dementia). *J Neurol Sci.* 2008 Sep 15; **272**(1–2):20–33.

70 Kartsounis LD, Troung DD, Morgan-Hughes JA, et al. The neuropsychological features of mitochondrial myopathies and encephalomyopathies. *Arch Neurol.* 1992;**49**(2):158–60.

71 Bosbach S, Kornblum C, Schröder R, et al. Executive and visuospatial deficits in patients with chronic progressive external ophthalmoplegia and Kearns-Sayre syndrome. *Brain.* 2003;**126**(Pt 5): 1231–40.

72 Kato M, Nakamura M, Ichiba M, et al. Mitochondrial DNA deletion mutations in patients with neuropsychiatric symptoms. *Neurosci Res.* 2011;**69**(4):331–6.

73 Tsujikawa T, Yoneda M, Shimizu Y, et al. Pathophysiologic evaluation of MELAS strokes by serially quantified MRS and CASL perfusion images. *Brain Dev.* 2010;**32**(2):143–9.

74 Gardner A, Salmaso D, Nardo D, et al. Mitochondrial function is related to alterations at brain SPECT in depressed patients. *CNS Spectr.* 2008;**13**(9):805–14.

75 Young TM, Blakely EL, Swalwell H, et al. Mitochondrial transfer RNA(Phe) mutation associated with a progressive neurodegenerative disorder characterized by psychiatric disturbance, dementia, and akinesia-rigidity. *Arch Neurol.* 2010;**67**(11):1399–402.

76 Schiffmann R. Fabry disease. *Pharmacol Ther.* 2009;**122**(1):65–77.

77 Buechner S, Moretti M, Burlina AP, et al. Central nervous system involvement in Anderson-Fabry disease: a clinical and MRI retrospective study. *J Neurol Neurosurg Psychiatry.* 2008;**79**(11): 1249–1254.

78 Fellgiebel A, Keller I, Marin D, et al. Diagnostic utility of different MRI and MR angiography measures in Fabry disease. *Neurology.* 2009;**72**(1):63–68.

79 Baumann N, Turpin JC, Lefevre M, et al. Motor and psycho-cognitive clinical types in adult metachromatic leukodystrophy: genotype/phenotype relationships? *J Physiol Paris.* 2002;**96**(3–4):301–6.

80 Sedel F, Baumann N, Turpin JC, et al. Psychiatric manifestations revealing inborn errors of metabolism in adolescents and adults. *J Inherit Metab Dis.* 2007;**30**(5):631–41.

81 Gieselmann V, Krägeloh-Mann I. Metachromatic leukodystrophy—an update. *Neuropediatrics.* 2010;**41**(1):1–6.

82 Pastores GM. Krabbe disease: an overview. *Int J Clin Pharmacol Ther* 2009;**47** Suppl 1:S75–81.

83 Franssen H. Electrophysiology in demyelinating polyneuropathies. *Expert Rev Neurother* 2008;**8**(3):417–431.

84 Ferrer I, Aubourg P, Pujol A. General aspects and neuropathology of X-linked adrenoleukodystrophy. *Brain Pathol.* 2010;**20**(4):817–30.

85 Smith SA, Golay X, Fatemi A, et al. Quantitative magnetization transfer characteristics of the human cervical spinal cord in vivo: application to adrenomyeloneuropathy. *Magn Reson Med.* 2009;**61** (1):22–7.

86 Uchida Y, Kimura E, Hirano T, et al. Identification of the occipitopontine tract using diffusion-tensor fiber tracking in adult-onset adrenoleukodystrophy with topographic disorientation. *Case Rep Neurol.* 2011;**3**(2):113–7.

87 Cartier N, Aubourg P. Hematopoietic stem cell gene therapy in Hurler syndrome, globoid cell leukodystrophy, metachromatic leukodystrophy and X-adrenoleukodystrophy. *Curr Opin Mol Ther* 2008;**10**(5):471–8.

88 Moser HW, Moser AB, Hollandsworth K, et al. "Lorenzo's oil" therapy for X-linked adrenoleukodystrophy: rationale and current assessment of efficacy. *J Mol Neurosci* 2007;**33**(1):105–13.

89 Lidove O, West ML, Pintos-Morell G, et al. Effects of enzyme replacement therapy in Fabry disease--a comprehensive review of the medical literature. *Genet Med.* 2010;**12**(11):668–79.

90 Spada M, Pagliardini S, Yasuda M, et al. High incidence of later-onset Fabry disease revealed by newborn screening. *Am J Hum Genet* 2006;**79**(1):31–40.

91 Mendez MF, Stanley TM, Medel NM, et al. The vascular dementia of Fabry's disease. *Dement Geriatr Cogn Disord* 1997;**8**(4):252–7.

92 Mohanraj R, Leach JP, Broome JC, et al. Neurological presentation of Fabry's disease in a 52 year old man. *J Neurol Neurosurg Psychiatry* 2002;**73**(3):340–2.

93 Burlina AP, Manara R, Caillaud C, et al. The pulvinar sign: frequency and clinical correlations in Fabry disease. *J Neurol* 2008;**255**(5):738–44.

94 Takanashi J, Barkovich AJ, Dillon WP, et al. T1 hyperintensity in the pulvinar: key imaging feature for diagnosis of Fabry disease. *AJNR Am J Neuroradiol* 2003;**24**(5):916–21.

95 Moore DF, Ye F, Schiffmann R, et al. Increased signal intensity in the pulvinar on T1-weighted images: a pathognomonic MR imaging sign of Fabry disease. *AJNR Am J Neuroradiol* 2003;**24**(6):1096–101.

96 Kanekar S, Gustas C. Metabolic disorders of the brain: part I. *Semin Ultrasound CT MR* 2011;**32**(6):590–614.

97 Rademakers R, Baker M, Nicholson AM, et al. Mutations in the colony stimulating factor 1 receptor (CSF1R) gene cause hereditary diffuse leukoencephalopathy with spheroids. *Nat Genet* 2012; **44**:200–205.

98 Nicholson AM, Baker MC, Finch NA, et al. CSF1R mutations link POLD and HDLS as a single disease entity. *Neurology* 2013;**80**: 1033–1040.

99 Sundal C, Lash J, Aasly J, et al. Hereditary diffuse leukoencephalopathy with axonal spheroids (HDLS): a misdiagnosed disease entity. *J Neurol Sci* 2012;**314**:130–137.

CHAPTER 13

Infectious causes of dementia

Cheryl A. Jay[1,2], Emily L. Ho[3,4] and John Halperin[5,6,7]
[1] University of California, San Francisco, San Francisco, CA, USA
[2] San Francisco General Hospital (SFGH), San Francisco, CA, USA
[3] University of Washington, Seattle, WA, USA
[4] Swedish Neuroscience Institute, Seattle, WA, USA
[5] Atlantic Neuroscience Institute, Summit, NJ, USA
[6] Sidney Kimmel Medical College of Thomas Jefferson University, Philadelphia, PA, USA
[7] Overlook Medical Center, Summit, NJ, USA

Introduction

Viruses, bacteria, fungi, and parasites most commonly reach the brain hematogenously during disseminated infection, although a few pathogens target specific neuronal or glial cells. Acute cerebral infections, such as community-acquired bacterial meningitis and most viral encephalitides, might begin with cognitive and personality dysfunction, but the rapid deterioration of alertness over subsequent hours to days causes little diagnostic confusion with most neurodegenerative disorders. Neuropsychological dysfunction is often a long-term, disabling complication of many acute brain infections.

Patients with subacute or chronic infections develop cognitive and behavioral disturbances in several settings. A few nonprion chronic cerebral infections, such as HIV-associated dementia (HAD) and general paresis, manifest primarily as either a rapidly progressive or a more indolent dementia. Memory and behavioral complaints, with or without abnormalities by neuropsychological testing, are common among patients with some chronic cerebral or systemic infections in which other clinical features predominate. Neuropsychological dysfunction often is the predominant feature in the early weeks and months of other nonacute brain infections, including the long list of pathogens that cause chronic meningitis. The general approach to such patients is beyond the scope of this chapter and has been the subject of reviews [1, 2]. The focus here will be infections whose manifestations overlap with neurodegenerative disorders, along with briefer discussions of the neuropsychological sequelae of acute cerebral infections.

Viruses

Human immunodeficiency virus (HIV)-associated dementia

Case: A young man with AIDS for 8 years and previously treated neurosyphilis presented to a clinic for evaluation of memory and gait difficulties for several weeks, on a background of a decreasing CD4+ T-cell count in the past year. He was not on antiretroviral therapy because of poor adherence related to active methamphetamine use. His physician noted him to be less jovial and talkative than usual. On examination, he had impaired reverse digit span and short-term memory. Reflexes were symmetrically diminished in the legs, with flexor plantar responses bilaterally. There was length-dependent sensory loss to the knees and wrists. Although Romberg's test was negative, he walked on a slightly broad base with impaired tandem gait.

Laboratory studies revealed a low CD4+ T-cell count at 98 cells/mm^3 (normal = 500–1500 cells/mm^3) with HIV viral load of greater than 200 000 copies/mL. Serum rapid plasma reagin (RPR) serology was 1:2 (1:1024 2 years previously prior to the treatment for neurosyphilis). CT was normal. MRI showed symmetric periventricular white matter abnormalities, compatible with HIV infection (Figure 13.1). CSF showed mildly elevated protein of 77 mg/dL (normal 15–45 mg/dl), glucose of 56 mg/dL, 7 RBC/mm^3, and a slight pleocytosis of 12 WBC/mm^3 (91% lymphocytes), with negative cryptococcal antigen and Venereal Disease Research Laboratory (VDRL) test. He was presumptively diagnosed with HAD, began combination antiretroviral therapy (cART), and was referred to drug rehabilitation (follow-up continued below).

Non-Alzheimer's and Atypical Dementia, First Edition. Edited by Michael D. Geschwind and Caroline Racine Belkoura.
© 2016 John Wiley & Sons, Ltd. Published 2016 by John Wiley & Sons, Ltd.

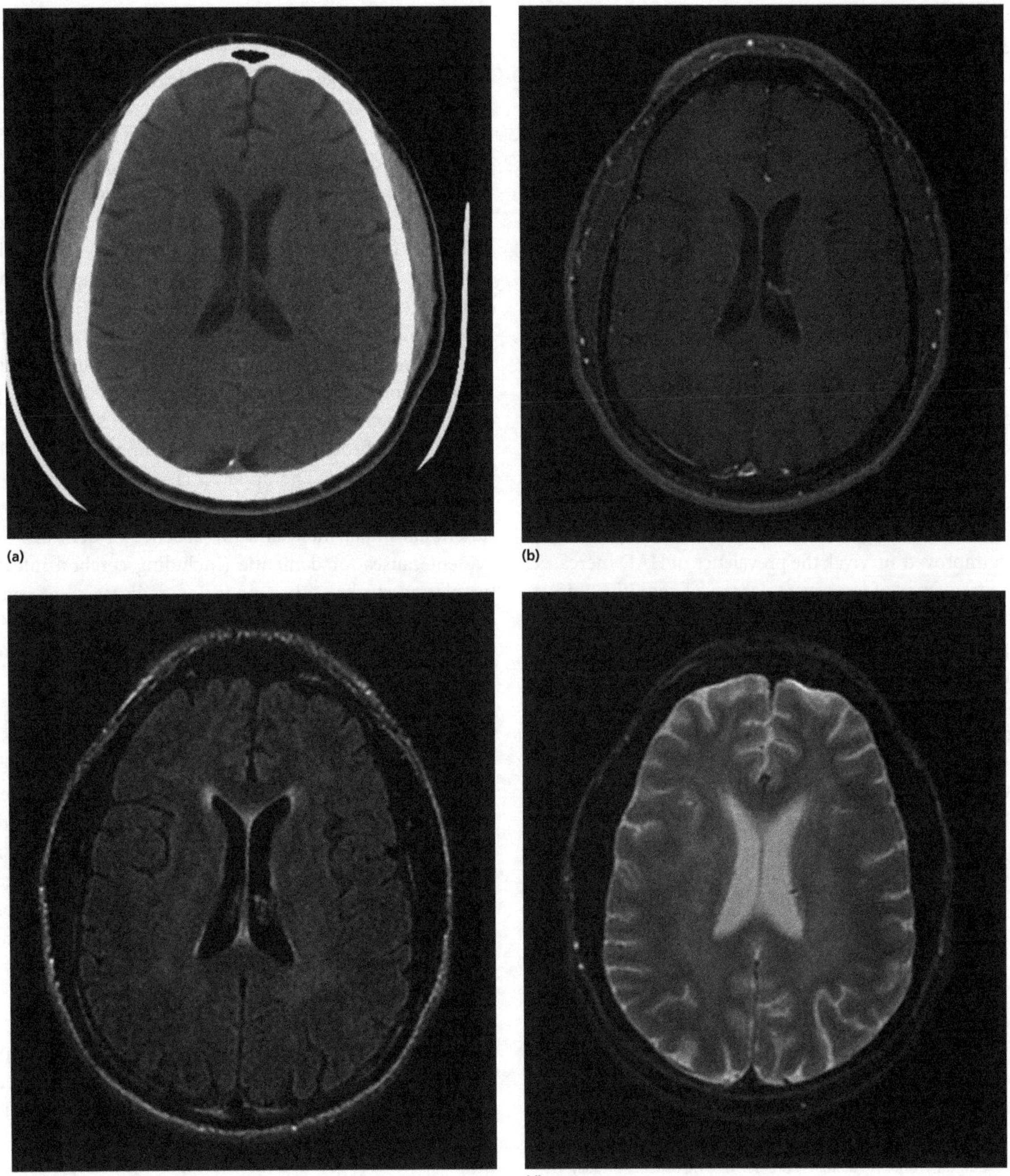

Figure 13.1 Neuroimaging in HIV-associated dementia studies obtained from a patient with untreated HIV infection, cognitive impairment, and gait disorder (see text). Noncontrast head CT (**a**) and T1-weighted brain MRI after gadolinium administration (**b**) are normal. FLAIR (**c**) and T2-weighted (**d**) images demonstrate ill-defined, symmetric white matter abnormalities, consistent with HIV-associated dementia.

Soon after outbreaks of opportunistic infections (OIs) in Los Angeles among men who have sex with men heralded the HIV/AIDS pandemic in 1981, the nervous system emerged as a major site of clinical involvement [3]. Manifestations included cerebral OIs and neoplasms from severe immunocompromise, peripheral neuropathy, and a dementing illness initially referred to as *subacute encephalitis* [3–5]. The clinical syndrome, termed *AIDS dementia complex* (ADC) [4], and its neuropathologic substrate [5] were defined further in 1986. *HIV encephalopathy* [6] and *AIDS-related dementia* [7] were other terms for the occasionally static but more characteristically progressive cognitive, motor, and behavioral impairments that characterized the syndrome before cART [4, 6, 7]. Typical early symptoms include apathy, slowed thinking, impaired memory, and gait difficulty; neurological examination might be normal or reveal psychomotor slowing, hyperreflexia (sometimes masked by concomitant distal symmetric polyneuropathy), and pathological reflexes [4, 7]. In untreated patients, these early features often progress over months to mutism, quadriparesis, and incontinence [4]. Occasional patients may present with psychosis or mania [4, 7]. The Memorial Sloan Kettering (MSK) scale for ADC (Table 13.1), a staging system devised for patient care and clinical research in the late 1980s [8], remains in use. Host risk factors for dementia in the pre-cART era included low CD4 count, hemoglobin, or body mass, as well as constitutional symptoms, advancing age, and elevated cerebrospinal fluid (CSF) HIV viral load [9, 10]. Before cART, dementia was common, affecting approximately half of the HIV-infected patients [11].

In 1991, the AIDS Task Force of the American Academy of Neurology (AAN) defined the criteria for HAD and a milder condition, *minor cognitive motor disorder (MCMD)* [12]. The advent of cART with at least three antiretroviral drugs, in the mid-1990s, dramatically improved the outlook for HIV+ patients with access to treatment. Death rates fell, as did the incidence of HAD along with neurologic and systemic OIs [13, 14]. With improved survival, the prevalence of HAD increased, as did the frequency of less severe degrees of cognitive impairment [9–11, 13]. Progression over months was less common in treated patients, suggesting that cART had beneficial effects on the natural history of HAD, including slowing down the course. Dementia is now seen at higher CD4 counts than in the pre-cART era [13]. Risk factors for cognitive impairment in patients on cART include advancing age, particularly older than 50 years of age, and possibly hepatitis C coinfection [10]. With

Table 13.1 Memorial Sloan Kettering scale for AIDS Dementia Complex (ADC).

Stage 0	Normal
Stage 0.5	Absent, minimal, or equivocal symptoms of cognitive or motor dysfunction characteristic of ADC Mild signs (snout reflex, slowed ocular or limb movements) without impairment of work or capacity to perform activities of daily living (ADL) Normal gait and strength
Stage 1	Able to perform all but the more demanding aspects of work or ADL Unequivocal evidence (symptoms, signs, neuropsychological testing) of functional intellectual or motor impairment Can walk without assistance
Stage 2	Cannot work or maintain more demanding aspects of daily life but able to perform basic self-care activities Ambulatory but may require single prop
Stage 3	Major intellectual incapacity (unable to follow news or personal events, sustain complex conversation; considerable slowing of all output) or motor disability (unable to walk unassisted, requiring walker or personal support, usually with slowing and clumsiness in arms)
Stage 4	Nearly vegetative, with rudimentary intellectual and social comprehension and responses; nearly or absolutely mute Paraparetic or paraplegic with double incontinence

Source: Price and Brew [8]. Reproduced with permission of Oxford University Press and Richard W. Price.

Requires documented HIV-1 infection and exclusion of other causes of acquired cerebral dysfunction, such as opportunistic infections and metabolic encephalopathies.

increasing numbers of older HIV+ patients, due in part to long-term survival on cART, distinguishing HAD and related conditions from age-related neurodegenerative disorders could become a more common clinical problem [15].

In 2007, a working group of the National Institute of Mental Health and the National Institute of Neurological Disorders and Stroke revised the AAN research nosology and associated diagnostic criteria, in part reflecting changes in clinical features and epidemiology in the era of cART [16]. This most recent update defined three conditions as comprising the *HIV-associated neurocognitive disorders* (HANDs): *asymptomatic neurocognitive impairment, mild neurocognitive disorder*, and *HIV-1-associated dementia*. The revised criteria emphasize acquired cognitive impairment, assessed by neuropsychological testing when possible, in at least two cognitive domains, typically impaired attention and learning with slowed information processing. The updated HAD criteria usually correspond to MSK stage score of two or greater. Significant functional impairment and the absence of delirium or other evident causes for dementia (including cerebral infection or neoplasm, stroke, other neurologic diseases, or substance abuse) are other key elements. The prevalence of HAND is approximately 50%, with a shift from HAD to milder forms in the era of cART [10, 16].

The differential diagnosis of cognitive impairment in patients with known HIV infection is broad. Substance abuse, psychiatric disorders, toxic-metabolic encephalopathies, neurosyphilis (discussed later in this chapter), and neurodegenerative disorders are considerations throughout the course of HIV disease. At CD4 counts below 200 cells/mm^3, cerebral malignancies and OIs are important and life-threatening diagnostic concerns [8–10]. Depression is common in HIV+ patients and can be difficult to distinguish from early HAD. Primary central nervous system (CNS) lymphoma in the setting of HIV classically causes altered mental status with focal cerebral dysfunction or headache, typically evolving over months. The predilection of this B-cell lymphoma for periventricular regions and the corpus callosum [9] means that patients with bifrontal involvement may present primarily with personality change and cognitive impairment with minimal visual or motor dysfunction, at least in the early stages. Progressive multifocal leukoencephalopathy, an infection of oligodendrocytes by JC virus, typically manifests as worsening lateralized visual or motor impairment, evolving over months, consistent with asymmetric hemispheric white matter involvement, or occasionally as progressive brainstem dysfunction, but presentation with dementia has been reported [17]. Cerebral toxoplasmosis is a common cerebral OI in the setting of HIV/AIDS. Most commonly, this protozoal infection presents with headache, fever, focal cerebral dysfunction, impaired alertness, and other features of expanding cerebral mass lesions, although rarer meningoencephalitic forms with unusually bland neuroimaging have resembled HAD [18]. Cryptococcal meningitis, another common cerebral OI in HIV+ patients, is discussed later in this chapter.

Cytomegalovirus (CMV) encephalitis sometimes presents as a rapidly progressive dementia, usually in very advanced AIDS, when CD4 count falls below 50 cells/mm^3 [9, 19, 20]. Nearly one-third of the patients with CMV encephalitis and concurrent HIV infection have evidence of brainstem or cerebellar dysfunction [20]. Concomitant myelitis, radiculitis, retinitis, esophagitis, hepatitis, or colitis can also be useful diagnostic clues, since these are other common sites of CMV infection [9, 20]. CSF findings of polymorphonuclear pleocytosis with hypoglycorrhachia, resembling bacterial meningitis, and neuroimaging revealing ventriculitis are also suggestive, although the absence of either or both does not exclude CMV encephalitis. CSF CMV polymerase chain reaction (PCR) is more specific than sensitive for the diagnosis. CMV encephalitis is fatal without treatment but, if caught early, might respond to ganciclovir or foscarnet [9, 20].

It should be emphasized that throughout the HIV/AIDS epidemic, dementia has been reported as the presenting manifestation of previously undiagnosed HIV infection [21, 22]. HIV testing is thus an appropriate part of the evaluation for patients with unexplained cognitive impairment.

HIV entry into the CNS has been demonstrated early in the course of infection, via infected monocytes [9–11, 23]. Occasionally, this is associated with typical aseptic meningitis but more commonly with asymptomatic mild lymphocytic CSF pleocytosis and elevated protein [9–11, 23–25]. Productive infection of neurons has not been demonstrated, suggesting that indirect mechanisms of brain injury, such as chronic inflammation or viral protein neurotoxicity, may underlie the myelin pallor and multinucleated giant cells seen in patients dying with HAD in the pre-cART era [5, 10, 23]. As the epidemiology and natural history of HANDs in the cART era have evolved, so also has the neuropathology, with more prominent inflammation in the brains of treated patients [10].

The diagnostic evaluation for HIV+ patients with cognitive dysfunction should include review of medications and screening for depression and substance use disorders, along with appropriate blood tests for thyroid disease, vitamin B_{12} deficiency, and neurosyphilis. Neuroimaging, with and without contrast when safe and feasible, to exclude multifocal OIs and malignancies typically reveals cerebral atrophy [9, 10]. MRI is superior to CT (Figure 13.1) in demonstrating symmetric, ill-defined, nonenhancing white matter hyperintensities on T2-weighted images [10], but these are neither necessary nor sufficient for a diagnosis of HAD. CSF protein often is mildly elevated; white cell count depends in part on CD4+ count [24, 25]. Pleocytosis is unusual among patients with CD4 counts below 50 cells/mm^3, regardless of treatment status [24]. At higher CD4+ counts, patients not on cART, with or without neurologic symptoms, may demonstrate mildly elevated CSF white count (<30 cells/mm^3). Pleocytosis normalizes within months of virologic control of HIV on cART, in concert with CSF HIV viral load falling near or below the limit of detection [11, 24, 25].

Small clinical studies in the pre-cART era demonstrated that zidovudine monotherapy, albeit at doses higher than typically used currently, slowed the progression of dementia [9, 23]. Zidovudine, unlike most other antiretrovirals in use at the time, achieved good CSF levels, generating debate about the degree to which CSF (and, it is assumed, cerebral) penetration is important in treating HAD [9, 10, 23, 26]. In addition to zidovudine, nevirapine and ritonavir-boosted indinavir penetrate well into the CNS, followed by abacavir, emtricitabine, delavirdine, efavirenz, and indinavir; boosted darunavir, fosamprenavir, or lopinavir; and maraviroc and raltegravir [10, 26]. Other antiretroviral drugs do not penetrate the CNS as well [9–11]. Patients who develop HANDs while not on cART should be started on therapy [9–11, 23]; whether patients who develop HANDs while on cART benefit from modifying the regimen toward drugs with good CNS penetration remains uncertain. Controlled trials of adjunctive antioxidant and neuroprotective agents have been disappointing [9, 10].

Case follow-up

The patient was begun on abacavir, lamivudine, zidovudine, and nevirapine, which led to an increased CD4+ T-cell count and a decrease in viral load to undetectable levels. Over the next year, his attention, memory, and gait improved. Subsequently, he suffered a relapse of his methamphetamine use, nonadherence with his antiretroviral regimen, and was lost to follow-up.

Subacute sclerosing panencephalitis

Subacute sclerosing panencephalitis (SSPE) is caused by cerebral infection with defective measles virus occurring long after acute measles infection [27–32]. Incidence estimates range from four to nearly 30 SSPE cases per 100 000 measles cases [27]. As a consequence of a preventable childhood infection, SSPE has become quite rare in countries with effective measles vaccination programs, and the diagnosis is easily missed [27, 28]. SSPE is typically a disease of childhood and adolescence, although adult-onset cases have been reported, with symptoms beginning as late as 49 years of age [28, 29].

Acute measles acquired very early in life increases the risk for SSPE, and pregnancy may also be a risk factor [27–29]. Symptoms begin months to decades after acute measles, which might not have been diagnosed, and include cognitive impairment, behavioral and personality changes, visual dysfunction, myoclonus, and seizures, usually developing over months [27, 28]. The myoclonus is typically generalized, without associated loss of consciousness and is common, but not always present [27, 28]. When myoclonus is present, the differential diagnosis includes prion disorders, corticobasal syndrome, dementia with Lewy bodies, hypoxia, thyrotoxic encephalopathy, and progressive myoclonic epilepsies such as mitochondrial cytopathies, Lafora's disease, neuronal ceroid lipofuscinoses, Unverricht–Lundborg syndrome, and the sialidoses [27]. In the absence of myoclonus, the clinical syndrome suggests a neurodegenerative disorder, making the recognition of SSPE especially challenging [30].

The diagnosis should be considered through middle age in patients with cognitive or behavioral decline, particularly associated with myoclonus. Neuroimaging may be normal in early SSPE. As the disease advances, subcortical and periventricular white matter and basal ganglia abnormalities may be seen, progressing to hemispheric, brainstem, and cerebellar atrophy [27]. EEG may be normal or nonspecifically slow in early disease but typically demonstrates synchronous, stereotyped high-voltage periodic complexes usually associated with myoclonic jerks in midstage SSPE [27]. Routine CSF studies may be entirely normal or show mild lymphocytic pleocytosis and protein elevation, with elevated CSF gamma globulin concentration [27, 28, 30]. Antimeasles antibodies are elevated in CSF and establish the diagnosis, in the appropriate clinical setting and with characteristic EEG abnormalities [27–31]. Brain biopsy might be necessary in rare cases, such as in very early or advanced disease, when EEG may not show periodic complexes [27].

Neuropathologic findings include parenchymal inflammation in hemispheres spreading to brainstem and spinal cord, with demyelination and neuronal and glial viral inclusions [27, 32]. The occipital lobes are often involved in early disease, perhaps accounting for visual symptoms, although retinitis or optic nerve involvement also occurs [27, 32].

Fulminant cases resembling acute viral encephalitis have been reported [29], but the typical course is progression to death over several years [27, 28]. Oral isoprinosine alone or in combination with alpha interferon (intramuscular, intravenous, or intrathecal) or ribavirin (intraventricular or intravenous) might prolong survival, with varying degrees of symptomatic improvement [27]. Myoclonus is managed with benzodiazepines and antiepileptic agents but can be refractory to treatment [27]. Previous concerns that the measles vaccine might cause SSPE have not been realized. Prevention with vaccination remains the best intervention for this devastating infection [27].

Hepatitis C

Seroprevalence rates for antibodies to hepatitis C virus (HCV), indicating exposure to the hepatotropic single-stranded RNA virus, are below 2% in most industrialized nations and higher in Africa (0.8% in Ethiopia to more than 15% in Rwanda and Egypt), Latin America (0.7% in Mexico to 11.2% in Bolivia), and parts of Asia (5.6% in Thailand, 6.2% in Vietnam, 10.7% in Mongolia) [33]. Most infected individuals develop chronic liver disease, which can progress to cirrhosis and hepatocellular carcinoma [33–35]. Extrahepatic disease is common, and neurologic complications include peripheral neuropathy and stroke, in addition to hepatic encephalopathy from portal hypertension [35]. Coinfection with HIV and HCV is common, as both viruses are transmissible by exposure to blood, including injection drug use [33].

Even in the absence of cirrhosis, fatigue and functionally limiting memory impairment are common complaints in early HCV disease [35–37]. Abnormal neuropsychological testing, particularly in attention and executive function, compared to controls has been reported in patients with HCV without cirrhosis in many, but not all, studies [36]. Proton magnetic resonance spectroscopy demonstrated elevated choline to creatine ratio in the basal ganglia of patients with HCV and histologically mild liver disease [37]. Selection of proper testing batteries, control for psychiatric comorbidities, and relevance of abnormal functional imaging are among many methodologic concerns in these studies [35, 36]. In the setting of HIV coinfection, HCV infection was associated with adverse effects on cognitive function in patients with advanced HIV disease [38], but not in the setting of well-controlled HIV infection [39] or hemophilia [40]. Interestingly, HCV is not strictly hepatotropic and can replicate in peripheral blood mononuclear cells [33, 41]. The identification in the brain of macrophages and microglia harboring HCV is reminiscent of the pathogenesis of HAD and related disorders [10, 41]. Treatment for HCV consists of ribavirin with alpha interferon, the latter of which can cause depression or cognitive impairment [36].

Cognitive sequelae of viral encephalitis

Viruses are common causes of acute infectious encephalitis, although extensive diagnostic evaluation often does not reveal the specific pathogen [42]. Herpesviruses, neurotropic double-stranded DNA viruses, are important diagnostic considerations year-round. Herpes simplex virus 1 (HSV-1) accounts for 5–10% of encephalitis cases in the United States [42–44]. Reactivation of latent HSV-1 in trigeminal ganglia most commonly causes labial vesicular lesions known as cold sores and, rarely, spreads proximally to the brain, resulting in HSV-1 encephalitis [44, 45]. In addition to fever, headache, and seizures, common presenting symptoms include behavioral and personality change and aphasia, consistent with involvement of one or both medial temporal lobes or orbitofrontal cortices [44, 45]. High-dose intravenous acyclovir lowered mortality to 28%, compared to 70% in historical controls [46]. Even with treatment, many survivors have persistent neuropsychological impairment including anterograde and retrograde amnesia, anomia, semantic memory deficit, executive dysfunction, mood disorders, and dementia [43–46].

Arbovirus (*ar*thropod-*bo*rne virus) infections occur classically as summer outbreaks and are important causes of encephalitis globally. West Nile virus, first isolated from an African patient in 1937, rapidly became endemic in North America after a 1999 outbreak in New York City [47]. The mosquito-borne virus most frequently causes the acute febrile illness known as West Nile fever and, occasionally, West Nile neuroinvasive disease involving the meninges, brain, or anterior horn cells [47, 48]. Impaired function or quality of life was noted 18 months after the acute illness in half or more patients after West Nile infection, even those without neuroinvasive disease [48]. Neuropsychological testing revealed psychomotor slowing [47]. Acute mortality for tick-borne encephalitis, the predominant European arbovirus, is low, but persistently impaired memory is a common long-term complication, with normal cognitive testing in only 10% of survivors and dementia evident in one-third [49].

Data are even more scant for neuropsychological outcomes from other forms of viral encephalitis [45]. Cognitive dysfunction tends to remain stable or improve slowly over time [50].

Bacteria

Neurosyphilis: General paresis

Case

A middle-aged man was brought to the emergency department for cognitive decline and personality change. His family described him as progressively disoriented, hostile, and moody for over several months. Earlier that week, he had struck his wife. The patient did not have any pain, incontinence, or a gait disorder. He took atenolol for hypertension and had no other medical problems and no previous psychiatric history. The patient worked as a kitchen assistant; did not use tobacco, alcohol, or illicit drugs; and had no family history of dementia. On examination, he was disheveled, mildly agitated, and afebrile, with normal vital signs and no meningismus. The neurologic exam was limited by the rare dialect that he spoke—he was oriented only to name, with normal speech and language, and impaired registration. Other exam findings included normal pupils, slightly brisk right patellar and bilateral ankle reflexes, flexor plantar responses, and normal proprioception and gait.

Electrolytes and liver and renal function tests were normal. Head CT showed marked generalized atrophy for his age, without hydrocephalus or mass lesion, with no additional abnormalities on MRI (Figure 13.2). Lumbar puncture showed normal opening pressure of 80 mm H_2O. CSF protein was elevated at 110 mg/dL and glucose was slightly low at 42 mg/dL (serum 82 mg/dL). Tube #1 of CSF showed 2500 RBC/mm^3 and 19 WBC/mm^3 (84% lymphocytes). Tube #4 showed 695 RBC/mm^3 and 12 WBC/mm^3 (84% lymphocytes). VDRL was 1:128 in serum and VDRL was 1:16 in CSF, confirming a diagnosis of neurosyphilis. Thyroid-stimulating hormone and vitamin B_{12} were normal, and HIV serology was negative. An EEG showed diffuse slowing. The patient underwent treatment for neurosyphilis with penicillin four million units intravenously every 4 h for 2 weeks. Behavioral symptoms were managed with risperidone, haloperidol, and lorazepam (case continued below).

The incidence of primary syphilis in the United States has risen in recent years, especially among men who have sex with men [51–54]. Caused by infection with the bacterium *Treponema pallidum* spp. *pallidum* (hereafter referred to as *T. pallidum*), the CNS may be involved at any stage of disease, from primary to tertiary syphilis [55]. Although manifestations of late symptomatic neurosyphilis include tabes dorsalis, meningovascular syphilis, and optic atrophy, it is general paresis of the insane, also known as dementia paralytica, a condition involving treponemal infection of the brain parenchyma, which is most likely to present with cognitive decline and neuropsychiatric symptoms [56].

First described by Antoine Laurent Jessé Bayle in 1822 as a syndrome consisting of severe mental dysfunction accompanied by other neurologic symptoms [57], general paresis occurs years after initial infection (ranging from 3 to 30 years, peak at 10–20 years). Previously, neurosyphilis accounted for large proportions of patients admitted to mental asylums (in the 1920s, more than 20% of such patients in the United States [58]). The search for treatment for this debilitating disease led to Julius Wagner-Jauregg being awarded the Nobel Prize in Medicine in 1927 for demonstrating that general paresis patients benefited from malaria therapy [59]. Although the prevalence of general paresis was reported to be approximately 5% of all cases of syphilis, since the advent of penicillin, general paresis has become very rare in developed countries [60].

Symptoms of general paresis include subacute, chronic, relapsing-remitting changes in personality, affect, and cognition. By history and on examination, patients have depression, mania, emotional lability, irritability, apathy, and/or, rarely, hallucinations [60]. Patients might also have delusions, disorientation, impaired memory (especially short term), impaired ability to calculate, poor judgment, lack of insight, and poor personal hygiene and grooming [56, 60–63, 63a]. In addition, there may be impaired speech (including aphasia and anomia), pupillary abnormalities (including the Argyll Robertson pupil), apraxia, ataxia, tremors, and abnormal reflexes (usually hyperreflexia) [56, 60–63, 63a]. Accompanying symptoms may include headaches, incontinence, and seizures [56, 61, 62]. Without treatment, patients progress invariably to vegetative degeneration and then death [56].

Given its myriad symptoms, general paresis is difficult to distinguish from many other psychiatric and dementing illnesses. In a case series from 1969 of 91 patients with neurosyphilis admitted to a psychiatric hospital, 28 patients (30.8%) had an initial diagnosis of depression, and 13 patients (14.3%) were initially diagnosed with "dementia" [63a]. Besides reactive treponemal serologic tests, features that help to differentiate general paresis from other causes of progressive dementia are the relatively early age of onset (most commonly between 30 and 50 years) and the fact that general paresis is fatal within months to a few years without treatment [56].

Diagnosing general paresis can be difficult given that there are no gold standard tests to diagnose CNS infection by *T. pallidum*. It is diagnosed by first making a diagnosis of syphilis and then a lumbar puncture from which diagnostic tests indicate neurosyphilis. The diagnosis of syphilis is made through the measurement of antibodies, termed "nontreponemal" and "treponemal." The "nontreponemal" antibodies, currently detected by the RPR and VDRL tests, react to phospholipids, such as cardiolipin. "Treponemal" antibodies are directed against *T. pallidum* polypeptides and are detected by the fluorescent treponemal antibody absorption (FTA-ABS) test or by agglutination in the *T. pallidum* hemagglutination (TPHA) or *T. pallidum* particle agglutination (TP-PA) tests. The development of enzyme immunoassays (EIA), chemiluminescence immunoassays (CIA), and rapid point-of-care tests [63b, 64a] which detect antitreponemal IgM and IgG antibodies, usually to

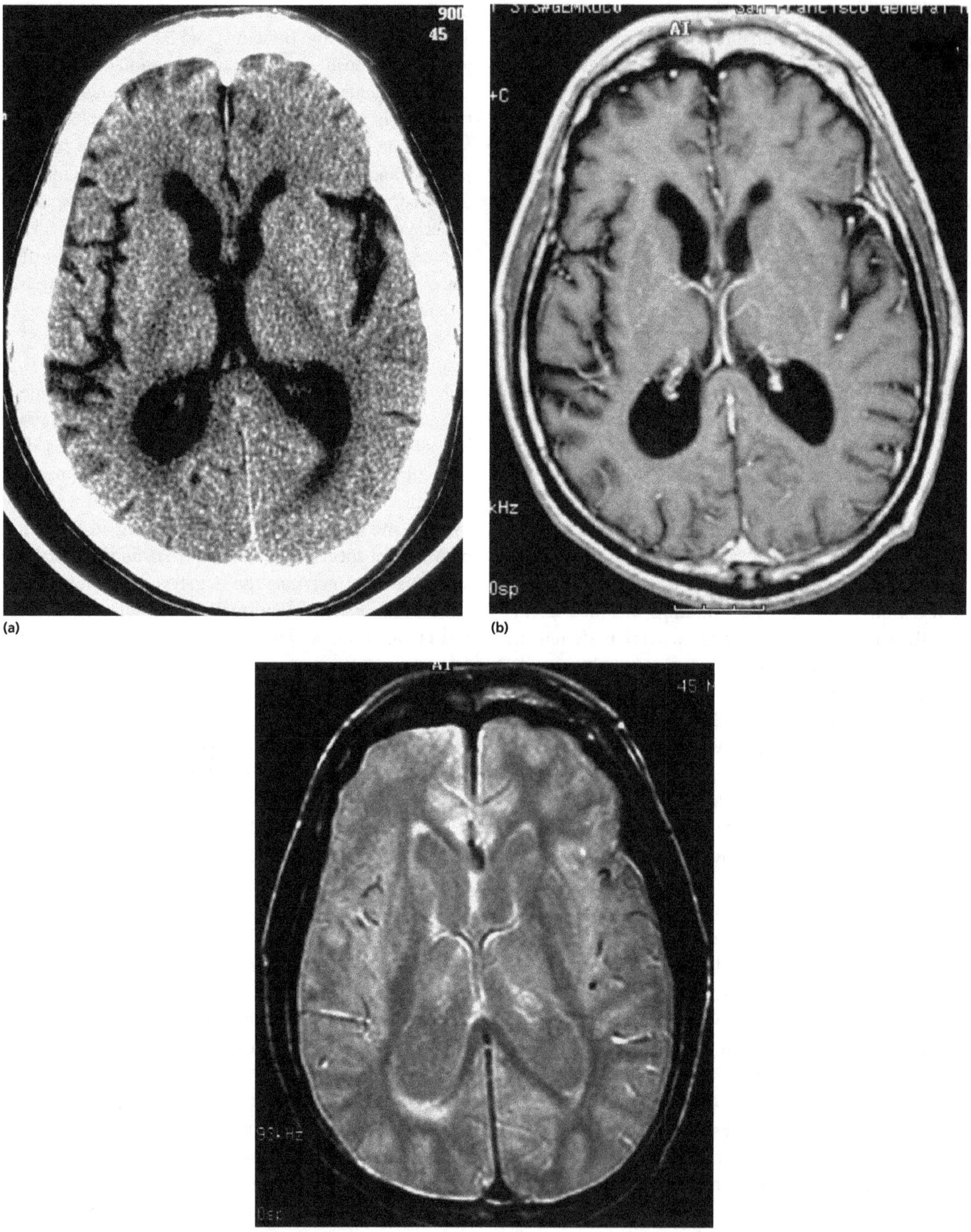

(a) (b) (c)

Figure 13.2 Neuroimaging in general paresis noncontrast head CT (**a**), postgadolinium T1-weighted (**b**), and proton density (**c**) MRI images obtained from a middle-aged patient with general paresis (see text) show severe cerebral atrophy for age.

recombinant *T. pallidum* proteins, has allowed some large laboratories in the United States to test for treponemal antibodies in an automated fashion. Importantly, measurements of treponemal antibodies may be falsely reactive due to antibodies induced by cross-reactive antigens in commensal treponemes or treponemes associated with periodontal disease or autoantibodies.

Traditionally in the United States, *T. pallidum* infection has been diagnosed serologically using a nontreponemal screening test, with reactive results confirmed using treponemal tests (FTA-ABS, TPHA, or TP-PA). RPR and VDRL, which are very sensitive for early syphilis, decrease after treatment, and a response to therapy is defined as a fourfold decrease in titers. Unfortunately, the nontreponemal tests are nonreactive in up to 30% of infected individuals with late syphilis even without treatment, complicating the ability to diagnose general paresis. In contrast, the treponemal tests are positive in all but the earliest cases of syphilis. These antibodies commonly remain positive permanently, even after treatment, however. With the availability of automated treponemal testing, new syphilis screening algorithms that begin with a treponemal test have become more common in the United States. This shift has caused significant confusion among clinicians, as the appropriate interpretation of reactive tests is unclear. The EIA and CIA tests are more sensitive than FTA-ABS or agglutination tests but have less specificity. Thus, reactive EIA/CIA results may be obtained in patients who are highly unlikely to have syphilis. In a patient with reactive EIA/CIA testing with no history of syphilis, nontreponemal testing should be performed. In patients with discordant test results (e.g., EIA+ and nonreactive RPR), a second treponemal test that has higher specificity (e.g., TP-PA) should be performed. Given that the treponemal antibodies are highly sensitive, there is no need for a lumbar puncture if a patient has a negative treponemal testing. If, however, clinical suspicion is high for late syphilis, a treponemal test should be obtained because in late syphilis, the nontreponemal tests, such as serum RPR, may be negative.

Once a diagnosis of syphilis is made and there is suspicion for neurosyphilis, based on clinical findings, a lumbar puncture should be performed to send CSF for diagnostic confirmatory tests. CSF laboratory abnormalities consistent with neurosyphilis include a lymphocytic pleocytosis, elevated protein, and/or positive CSF-VDRL. Laboratory tests for other conditions that may resemble general paresis, including thyroid function tests, should be unremarkable. HIV testing should also be conducted as there may be concurrent HIV infection. Neuroimaging often reveals no structural abnormalities other than atrophy of the frontal, temporal, and parietal lobes. There have been case reports, however, describing unilateral or bilateral medial temporal lobe T2 hyperintensity on MRI imaging, which were mistaken for HSV-1 encephalitis [64b, 65, 66]. These hyperintense regions resolve with treatment, but the atrophy is often irreversible [67].

According to the Centers for Disease Control, treatment with penicillin consists of intravenous penicillin G, 12–24 million units daily for 10 to 14 days, followed by penicillin G benzathine, 2.4 million units weekly for 1–3 weeks [68]. An alternative regimen is intramuscular procaine penicillin G, 2.4 million units once daily with oral probenecid, 500 mg four times daily, both for 10–14 days, followed by penicillin G benzathine, 2.4 million units weekly for 1–3 weeks [68]. Follow-up CSF evaluations should be conducted to confirm a decrease in CSF titers as well as normalization of pleocytosis and protein. CSF cell counts will normalize over weeks, while protein and CSF-VDRL may take months to normalize.

On neuropathology, a diffuse inflammatory process is seen in the cerebrum, meninges, and intraparenchymal blood vessels. There is a "coat-sleeve" lymphocytic and plasma cell infiltration of the capillaries, with thickening of the walls of small vessels, and degeneration of parenchymal cells with reactive gliosis [60]. This process eventually leads to gross parenchymal atrophy.

Case follow-up

Before his discharge to a skilled nursing facility, the patient's follow-up CSF showed glucose of 54 mg/dL, protein of 99 mg/dL, and 4 WBC/mm^3. CSF VDRL was still reactive, but reduced, at 1 : 8. On exam, the patient was oriented to name, place, and year, demonstrating clinical improvement after treatment.

Lyme disease

Case: An elderly, still practicing attorney from a Lyme-endemic area presented with 7 weeks of severe, intractable right upper quadrant pain. Extensive imaging and endoscopic evaluation were unrevealing. History revealed the pain to be dysesthetic and dermatomal. Mild memory and cognitive difficulty were attributed to high doses of narcotics and sleep deprivation. Lyme serology was seven times the negative cutoff; IgG Western blot was positive. CSF contained 49 WBC/mm^3, protein of 86 mg/dL, elevated IgG index, and strongly positive CSF Lyme serology, with the value equal to that in serum. Within a week of starting a 2 week course of ceftriaxone, the pain eased. One month after treatment, he was pain-free, off narcotics, but still fatigued and mildly forgetful. He then returned to his normal baseline but presented 3 years later with typical early Alzheimer's. Lyme ELISA was still positive but lower; Western blot had the same bands as previously. CSF was normal. He was diagnosed with Alzheimer's disease and not Lyme disease.

The neurologic manifestations of the disorder now known as Lyme disease were initially described in France in 1922 [69]. Following an unusual tick bite-associated rash, known as erythema migrans (EM), a patient developed the first 2 elements of the now classic triad of lymphocytic meningitis, painful radiculoneuritis, and cranial nerve palsy. In the 1950s [70], this syndrome was shown to be penicillin-responsive. In the 1970s, a cluster of cases of a juvenile rheumatoid arthritis-like disorder in Lyme CT, also associated with EM, was found to be caused by a novel tick-borne spirochete [71–73] named *Borrelia burgdorferi.* Shortly thereafter, this infection was also linked to the same neurologic triad [74]; *B. burgdorferi* was subsequently identified as the cause of the European syndrome as well [75]. The disorder is now known to be caused by a group of closely related spirochetes, known as *B. burgdorferi sensu stricto* (the only strain in the United States, also present in Europe), *B. garinii*, *B. afzelii*, and *B. spielmanii.*

The infection is a zoonosis, requiring the colocalization of a reservoir host (most commonly field mice), hard-shelled *Ixodes* ticks, large mammal hosts for the adult ticks (deer and bears in the United States, sheep in much of the rest of the world) and humans. This occurs only in areas with a moist temperate climate and significant vegetation. In the United States, approximately 95% of the cases occur along the eastern seaboard from Maine to Maryland and in the upper Midwest (Wisconsin, Minnesota) [76]; smaller clusters of cases occur elsewhere in the United States, including parts of California. The infection is transmitted to humans solely by bites of infected *Ixodes* ticks. These ticks only feed when the temperature is above about 50°F and must be attached for at least 24–48 h before there is a significant risk of infection.

Diagnosis generally requires three elements—likely exposure to infected ticks, serologic confirmation or EM, and a clinical disorder reasonably likely to be caused by the infection. Serologic testing, particularly with the recommended two-tier approach using Western blots in individuals found to have positive or borderline ELISA, is both sensitive and specific [77]. Because any antibody response takes time to reach measurable concentrations—typically 3 to 6 weeks—more than 50% of the patients with EM (which usually occurs within the first 30 days of infection) and even occasional patients with Lyme-associated meningitis or cranial neuritis will be seronegative. Also as with any serology, antibodies remain detectable long after the infection has resolved, so a positive serology can only be interpreted as evidence of past or present exposure, not active infection. Unfortunately, direct methods for spirochete detection (culture, PCR) have very low sensitivity. In patients with CNS infection (Lyme neuroborreliosis), nonspecific CSF markers of inflammation (leukocytes, protein) are almost always elevated. In many instances, there is local production of anti-*B. burgdorferi* antibody within the CNS, resulting in proportionately higher ELISA values in CSF than serum.

Over the years, anecdotal reports have raised the possibility of associations with many different neurologic disorders, including multiple sclerosis, motor neuron disease, Alzheimer's disease [78], and Parkinson's disease. All seem highly unlikely, but the fact that patients with Lyme disease often describe memory and cognitive difficulty has led to questions about a possible association with dementia. On very rare occasions, Lyme disease is associated with parenchymal inflammation in the brain or spinal cord. As in any encephalomyelitis, this is usually evident both on MRI scans and CSF examination. As in the patient described here, though, in virtually all patients, the cognitive symptoms are probably an epiphenomenon, identical to the toxic-metabolic encephalopathy [79] seen in many other inflammatory states. Just as in other instances, this may be more pronounced in individuals in the very early, even preclinical, throes of Alzheimer's. There is no evidence, however, to suggest that Lyme disease plays a causal role in this or any other neurodegenerative disease.

Whipple's disease

First described in 1907, Whipple's disease is a rare multisystem disorder in which weight loss and gastrointestinal and joint symptoms are common systemic manifestations [80, 81]. The identification of the Whipple's bacillus in pathologic specimens and antibiotic responsiveness of the condition supported an infectious etiology [80, 81]. The agent now known as *Tropheryma whipplei* was identified by molecular genetic techniques in 1992 [82] and cultivated in 2000 [83]. Incidence, prevalence, and risk factors are not known, although the typical affected patient is a middle-aged white male [80, 83]. Neurologic disease, predominantly cerebral, with occasional myelopathy or neuropathy, develops in approximately one-third of the cases and portends a poor outcome [80–84]. Whipple's disease is difficult to diagnose even with classic concomitant gastrointestinal and joint involvement. When confined to the CNS, it poses even greater diagnostic challenges [80, 81, 84].

In addition to weight loss, diarrhea, and arthralgia, common systemic features include anemia, lymphadenopathy, abdominal pain, skin darkening, and fever [80, 81, 84]. Cognitive and behavioral abnormalities are prominent cerebral features, commonly associated with supranuclear ophthalmoplegia [80, 81, 84, 85]. Other neurologic manifestations include depressed level of consciousness, ataxia, corticospinal tract signs, hypothalamic dysfunction, cranial neuropathies, myoclonus, seizures, cerebellar disorder, headache, and peripheral neuropathy [80, 81, 84, 85]. Oculomasticatory or oculofacial-skeletal myorhythmia (OMM, OFSM) is virtually pathognomonic but observed in only a minority of patients with neurologic involvement [80, 81, 84, 85].

Upper gastrointestinal endoscopy might reveal pale yellow duodenal or jejunal mucosa with dilated villi and ectatic lymphatics in advanced disease [80, 81]. In early disease, small intestinal biopsy reveals periodic acid–Schiff (PAS)-positive macrophages in lamina propria and is the preferred initial diagnostic test [81]. As noted earlier, OMM or OFSM is virtually pathognomonic for cerebral Whipple's disease; PAS-positive cells in CSF or brain biopsy or PCR for *T. whipplei* in CSF also establish the diagnosis (Table 13.2) [80, 81, 84, 85]. CSF glucose is usually normal; protein and cell count may be normal or mild to moderately elevated [84, 85].

If the characteristic movement disorder is absent, the differential diagnosis depends on the predominant systemic and neurologic features. When classic systemic manifestations are present, the differential diagnosis of neurologic Whipple's disease includes chronic inflammatory conditions such as connective tissue and collagen vascular disorders and neurosarcoidosis [81]. When systemic disease is absent or minimal, the diagnostic possibilities are broader still [84]. Patients with reversible dementia, rapidly progressive or chronic, and, in one instance, meeting consensus criteria for frontotemporal dementia (FTD) have been reported [86, 87].

Whipple's disease typically is fatal without treatment. The prognosis for CNS disease is poor, as is the response to retreatment. Regimens for systemic and neurologic disease typically involve an induction course with intravenous penicillin or ceftriaxone for 2 weeks followed by maintenance therapy for at least a year with trimethoprim/sulfamethoxazole or

Table 13.2 Diagnostic guidelines for CNS Whipple's disease.

Definite CNS Whipple's disease (one of the following)
1. Oculomasticatory or oculofacial-skeletal myorhythmia
2. Positive tissue biopsy
If histological or PCR analysis was not performed on CNS tissue, then the patient must also demonstrate neurological signs. If histological or PCR analysis was performed on CNS tissue, then the patient need not demonstrate neurological signs (i.e., asymptomatic CNS infection)
Positive polymerase chain reaction
Possible CNS Whipple's disease
Must have any one of four systemic symptoms, not due to another known etiology:
1. Fever of unknown origin
2. Gastrointestinal symptoms (steatorrhea, chronic diarrhea, abdominal distension, pain)
3. Chronic migratory arthralgias or polyarthralgias
4. Lymphadenopathy, night sweats, or malaise
Also must have any one of four neurological signs, not due to another known etiology:
1. Supranuclear vertical gaze palsy
2. Rhythmic myoclonus
3. Dementia with psychiatric symptoms
4. Hypothalamic manifestations

Source: Louis et al. [85]. Reproduced with permission of John Wiley & Sons Ltd. Small bowel biopsy with periodic acid–Schiff staining and electron microscopy is recommended for all patients with possible CNS Whipple's disease.

doxycycline with hydroxychloroquine, which cross the blood–brain barrier. Relapses can occur, however [80, 81]. Tetracycline, the initial drug of choice, was associated with relapse rates of approximately one-third, frequently in the nervous system, presumably due to the drug's poor CNS penetration [80, 81]. Given the rarity of Whipple's disease, the lack of high-quality randomized clinical trial data is not surprising. For CNS disease, there is class B-III evidence for ceftriaxone induction followed by maintenance with trimethoprim/sulfamethoxazole or cefixime [42].

Cognitive sequelae of acute bacterial meningitis

Neisseria meningitidis and *Streptococcus pneumoniae* cause most community-acquired acute bacterial meningitis in adults, with case fatality rates of 7–10% and 15–33%, respectively [88–90]. Neuropsychological assessment 6 months or more after the acute illness identified abnormalities, in particular cognitive slowing, in up to one-third of survivors [88–90]. Concentration, visuoconstructive, and memory abnormalities were observed in studies utilizing more detailed testing batteries, with sparing of language and praxis [91]. Abnormalities were more severe among survivors of pneumococcal than meningococcal meningitis [89, 90, 92, 93]. Despite animal studies suggesting adverse effects of adjunctive steroids on hippocampal neurons, dexamethasone, which reduces acute mortality in community-acquired bacterial meningitis, does not increase the risk for cognitive impairment among long-term survivors [90, 92]. Cognitive function was stable to gradually improving when tested as long as 8–10 years after the acute illness [90, 93].

Fungi

Cryptococcus neoformans is an encapsulated fungus that causes chronic meningoencephalitis, pneumonia, and occasionally symptomatic disease in the skin, eye, bones, or joints [94]. At-risk patients for *C. neoformans* infection include those with AIDS, especially when CD4 count falls below 100 cells/μL, or therapeutic immunosuppression. Much of the modern evidence base derives from these settings, especially HIV infection [95]. Presenting clinical syndromes vary and include rapidly progressive dementia, particularly when headache, photophobia, and neck stiffness are minimal or absent [94]. In HIV-associated cryptococcal meningitis, neuroimaging may demonstrate atrophy related to HIV disease or complications of advanced cryptococcal infection such as cerebral edema, hydrocephalus, or both. Routine CSF studies may be normal or reveal the expected chronic meningitis profile of high pressure, elevated protein, low glucose, and lymphocytic pleocytosis; measuring opening pressure is critical since intracranial hypertension portends poor outcome and may require management beyond antifungal therapy [95, 96].

Fungal CSF culture is the diagnostic gold standard. The high fungal load in HIV-positive patients makes CSF India ink stains sensitive in that setting [96]. CSF cryptococcal antigen testing is even more sensitive and highly specific. Serum cryptococcal antigen is usually positive and can be helpful when CSF cannot be obtained [9, 94, 96].

Rarely, *C. neoformans* meningitis occurs in apparently immunocompetent individuals, including several case reports of patients in their sixth decade of life or older with cognitive impairment over months to years [97–100]. In one of these reported cases, myoclonus and dementia, progressive over 2 months, prompted consideration of Creutzfeldt–Jakob disease [97]. Vascular dementia [98] and Alzheimer's disease [99, 100] were the initial diagnoses in patients with more protracted courses. CSF examination was critical to establishing the diagnosis.

First-line therapy for cryptococcal meningitis consists of an induction course of at least two weeks of amphotericin B with flucytosine, followed by 8 weeks of high-dose fluconazole, and 6–12 months of fluconazole maintenance [95]. Relapse is a major concern, and HIV-infected patients with persistently low CD4 count typically require long-term maintenance therapy. Additionally, patients with untreated HIV infection with cryptococcal meningitis are at risk to develop immune reconstitution inflammatory syndrome, which can resemble failure of antifungal therapy, in the days to months after beginning cART [94, 95]. Steroids might be helpful; the optimal timing of cART remains uncertain.

Parasites

Humans and pigs are hosts for the pork tapeworm *Taenia solium*, which is endemic in Central and South America and parts of Africa and Asia [101]. Ingestion of larvae causes the intestinal infection taeniasis, and ingestion of eggs causes cysticercosis, in which larval cysts disseminate, in particular to muscle and immunologic sanctuaries such as the eye and CNS [102]. Neurocysticercosis (NCC) is the most common parasitic CNS infection in the world and an important cause of epilepsy in developing countries [101, 103]. With increased travel to low-income countries and immigration, NCC occurs even in industrialized nations in which *T. solium* has been eliminated [101, 102]. Extraparenchymal forms of cerebral NCC are less common and include meningeal, intraventricular, and subarachnoid diseases, which typically present with signs and symptoms of intracranial hypertension from obstructive or communicating hydrocephalus or meningeal inflammation with arachnoiditis [102]. Parenchymal disease is the predominant form of NCC and may be asymptomatic. Seizures and epilepsy are the most common clinical manifestation, occurring in over half of the symptomatic patients [102, 104].

Cognitive impairment, with or without psychosis, has occasionally been reported as the presenting syndrome of NCC, typically in association with a high cyst burden on neuroimaging; cysticidal therapy was associated with significant, but incomplete, clinical improvement [105, 106]. Additionally, neuropsychiatric dysfunction is common in patients with NCC [104, 107, 108], diagnosed during evaluation for other cerebral disorders, most commonly epilepsy. In a recent study from Brazil, patients with NCC demonstrated impaired executive function, verbal and nonverbal memory, constructive praxis, and verbal fluency compared to controls (normal and with cryptogenic epilepsy); 12.5% met DSM-IV criteria for dementia [108].

Cerebral cysts initially evoke little host immune response and remain viable for months to years [101]. As cysts degenerate, the resulting inflammatory response can cause headache with focal or diffuse cerebral dysfunction. Neuroimaging captures this natural history and is the cornerstone of diagnosis (Figure 13.3) [101–103]. CT and MRI are both sensitive and specific in parenchymal disease. In the early vesicular phase, the scolex appears as a nodule surrounded by CSF density fluid without surrounding edema and with minimal or no enhancement, reflecting the lack of local immunity [102, 103]. Cyst degeneration and death, either naturally or with cysticidal therapy, evoke an inflammatory response evident on CT or MRI as surrounding edema, more viscous cyst fluid, and degeneration of the scolex with thin ring enhancement in the colloidal stage progressing to thicker enhancement in the nodular stage [101–103]. In the final calcified stage, dead cysts appear as nonenhancing calcified lesions without mass effect [101–103]. Parenchymal lesions may be seen in varying stages in an individual patient, occasionally with concomitant extraparenchymal disease, which is better demonstrated by MRI [104, 105]. The differential diagnosis includes other cerebral infections, particularly tuberculoma, and cerebral metastases [102, 103]. Serum and CSF antibody testing is available but often of limited clinical utility.

The use of cysticidal drugs such as albendazole or praziquantel in patients with parenchymal NCC remains controversial [101–103, 109, 110]. Cyst death may trigger intense inflammation and symptomatic increased intracranial pressure, requiring steroid therapy. This is of particular concern in patients with high lesion burden, as may occur in NCC patients presenting with dementia. In uncontrolled studies of such patients, cognitive function improved with albendazole and steroids [105, 106, 111]. Extraparenchymal disease often requires neurosurgical intervention, and epilepsy usually responds to appropriate medications. *T. solium* infection, in particular NCC, is a global health problem. Improvements in sanitation and public health infrastructure in endemic countries will be necessary to control this potentially eradicable infection [101, 102].

Summary

Table 13.3 presents a brief summary of the infections discussed in this chapter, including clinical presentation, diagnostic tests, and treatments. Dementia complicates HIV infection, especially advanced, untreated disease; milder, less progressive cognitive impairment is the more common syndrome in patients on cART. Neuropsychological dysfunction with myoclonus is the classic manifestation of SSPE, an infection with defective measles virus that occurs months to years after measles. Cognitive and mood disorders are reported by individuals with HCV, often accompanied by abnormalities in neuropsychological testing. Neuropsychological impairment is common after HSV encephalitis and tick-borne encephalitis, reported after West Nile infection, even in the absence of neuroinvasive disease, and poorly understood after other acute viral encephalitides. General paresis, the cerebral form of tertiary syphilis, was a common reason for admission to mental asylums a century ago but has become rare since the advent of penicillin. Another spirochete, *B. burgdorferi*, causes Lyme disease, which is not associated with neurodegenerative disorders and very rarely with encephalomyelitis. The bacillus *T. whipplei* causes Whipple's disease, whose protean manifestations include neuropsychological decline, variably associated with movement disorders, weight loss, abdominal symptoms, and joint pain. Acute bacterial meningitis leaves many survivors with permanent cognitive impairment. The fungus *C. neoformans* causes chronic meningitis predominantly in immunocompromised patients, including HIV/AIDS, but has been reported to cause dementia resembling neurodegenerative disorders in apparently immunocompetent elderly individuals. NCC, resulting from infection with *T. solium*, occasionally presents with dementia, which is sometimes also evident in patients with epilepsy, the most common neurologic manifestation of this parasitic infection. Many of these infections are fatal without treatment; appropriate antimicrobial therapy can arrest or reverse cerebral manifestations to varying degrees. A few infectious causes of dementia, such as SSPE and some forms of bacterial meningitis, are preventable by vaccines. Transmission of some other pathogens causing neuropsychological impairment can be attenuated by public health interventions including screening of blood products, mosquito control, insect repellants, and proper sanitation.

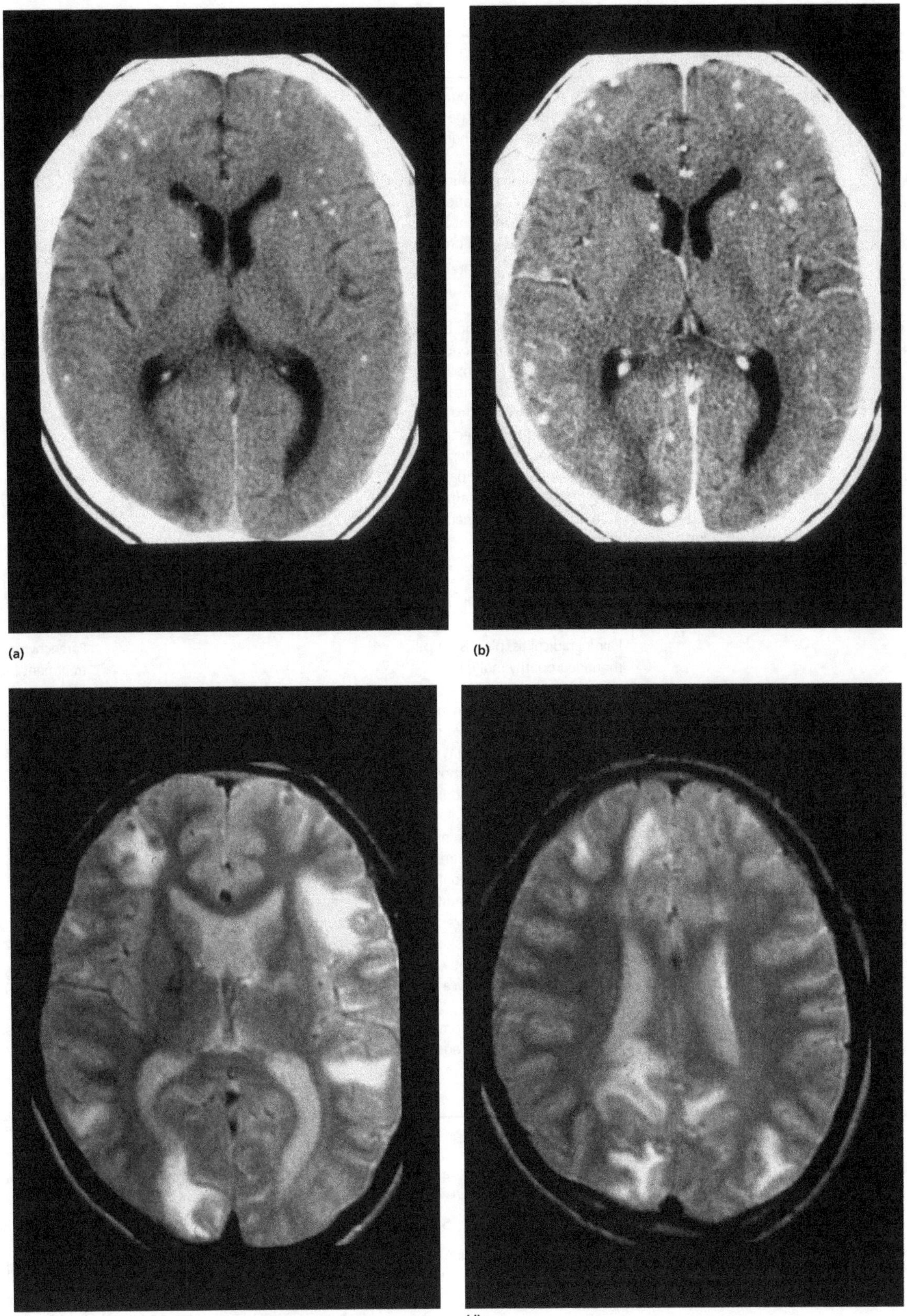

(a) (b) (c) (d)

Figure 13.3 Neuroimaging in neurocysticercosis noncontrast head CT (**a**) demonstrates numerous, punctate calcified lesions consistent with nonviable cysts and a small focus of low attenuation in the right occipital lobe, consistent with edema. Associated enhancement in these and other areas on the postcontrast study (**b**) is compatible with degenerating cysts. T2-weighted MRI studies (**c** and **d**) from the same patient more clearly demonstrate the extent of edema surrounding degenerating cysts. Reproduced with permission of Alisa D. Gean, MD.

Table 13.3 Neuropsychological impairment in cerebral infections.

	Pathogen	Clinical syndrome	Diagnosis	Treatment
Human immunodeficiency virus (HIV)-associated dementia	HIV (retrovirus)	Apathy, cognitive slowing, memory loss, gait disorder; may be presenting feature of undiagnosed HIV infection Progressive over months in up to half of the untreated patients; milder and more indolent in patients well controlled on antiretrovirals	Consider substance abuse, opportunistic infection, including CMV CD4 often < 200 cells/mm^3 in untreated patients MRI: symmetric, frontal predominant nonenhancing white matter disease CSF: normal or mildly elevated protein, lymphocytic pleocytosis	Combination antiretroviral therapy
Subacute sclerosing panencephalitis (SSPE)	Defective measles virus	Progressive cognitive and behavioral impairment with myoclonus and visual symptoms, developing months or years after measles	EEG: periodic complexes CSF: antimeasles antibodies, elevated gamma globulin levels	Oral isoprinosine, with or without parenteral or intrathecal alpha interferon or ribavirin
Hepatitis C virus (HCV)	HCV	Cognitive impairment accompanying HCV infection without associated cirrhosis	Consider substance abuse, HIV coinfection, liver disease	None
General paresis (of the insane)	*Treponema pallidum* (spirochete)	Progressive cognitive impairment, altered personality and affect accompanied by other neurologic deficits	CSF: lymphocytic pleocytosis, elevated protein, and/or positive CSF-VDRL	High-dose intravenous penicillin
Lyme meningoencephalomyelitis	*Borrelia burgdorferi* (spirochete)	Lymphocytic meningitis Single or multiple cranial neuropathies, particularly facial nerve Painful radiculitis, plexitis, or other mononeuropathy multiplex Rarely encephalomyelitis	Likely exposure + positive 2 tier serology (ELISA + Western blot) + abnormal CSF if CNS involved	Meningitis, cranial neuritis and PNS syndromes: oral doxycycline Parenchymal CNS or treatment failure IV ceftriaxone
Whipple's disease	*Tropheryma whipplei* (Whipple's bacillus)	Neuropsychologic impairment, supranuclear gaze palsy, or facial myorhythmias, with weight loss, GI, and joint symptoms; most frequently reported in middle-aged white men	Oculomasticatory or oculofacial-skeletal myorhythmia CSF: *T. whipplei* polymerase chain reaction Biopsy	Antibiotics, including long-term maintenance therapy (see text)
Cryptococcal meningitis	*Cryptococcus neoformans* (fungus)	Rare cause of dementia in elderly patients without obvious immune dysfunction (more commonly presents as chronic meningitis in HIV/AIDS or other immunosuppressed states)	CT or MRI: atrophy or may demonstrate hydrocephalus CSF: elevated protein, low glucose, lymphocytic pleocytosis, positive cryptococcal antigen or culture	Amphotericin B induction, followed by fluconazole maintenance
Neurocysticercosis	*Taenia solium* (parasite)	Rarely presents as dementia in patients from Latin America, Asia, or Africa Common cause of symptomatic epilepsy in patients from endemic areas; cognitive impairment may coexist	CT or MRI: multiple parenchymal lesions with varying combinations of enhancement, edema or calcification	Albendazole (or praziquantel), steroids

References

1 Ginsberg L, Kidd D. Chronic and recurrent meningitis. *Pract Neurol* 2008; **8**: 348–361.

2 Helbok R, Broessner G, Pfausler B, Schmutzhard E. Chronic meningitis. *J Neurol* 2009; **256**: 168–175.

3 Snider WD, Simpson DM, Nielsen S et al. Neurological complications of acquired immune deficiency syndrome: analysis of 50 patients. *Ann Neurol* 1983; **14**: 403–418.

4 Navia BA, Jordan BD, Price RW. The AIDS dementia complex: I. clinical features. *Ann Neurol* 1986; **19**: 517–24.

5 Navia BA, Cho ES, Petito CK, Price RW. The AIDS dementia complex: II. *Ann Neurol* 1986; **19**: 525–535.

6 Centers for Disease Control and Prevention. Revision of the CDC surveillance case definition for acquired immunodeficiency syndrome. *Morb Mortal Wkly Rep* 1987; **36** (suppl 1S): 3S–15S.

7 McArthur JC. Neurologic manifestations of AIDS. *Medicine* 1987; **66**: 407–437.

8 Price RW, Brew BJ. The AIDS dementia complex. *J Infect Dis* 1988; **158**: 1079–1083.

9 Singer EJ, Valdes-Sueiras M, Commins D, Levine A. Neurologic presentations of AIDS. *Neurol Clin* 2010; **28**: 253–275.

10 McArthur JC, Steiner J, Sacktor N, Nath A. Human immunodeficiency virus-associated neurocognitive disorders: mind the gap. *Ann Neurol* 2010; **67**: 699–714.

11 Ances BM, Ellis RJ. Dementia and neurocognitive disorders due to HIV-1 infection. *Semin Neurol* 2007; **27**: 86–92.

12 Janssen RS, Cornblath DR, Epstein LG et al. Nomenclature and research case definitions for neurological manifestations of human immunodeficiency virus type-1 (HIV-1) infection: report of a working group of the American Academy of Neurology AIDS task force. *Neurology* 1991; **41**: 778–785.

13 Sacktor N. The epidemiology of human immunodeficiency virus-associated neurological disease in the era of highly active antiretroviral therapy. *J Neurovirol* 2002; **8** (suppl 2): 115–121.

14 Monforte AD, Cinque P, Mocroft A et al. Changing incidence of central nervous system diseases in the EuroSIDA cohort. *Ann Neurol* 2004; **55**: 320–328.

15 Valcour V, Paul R. HIV infection and dementia in older adults. *Clin Infect Dis* 2006; **42**: 1449–1454.

16 Antinori A, Arendt G, Becker JT et al. Updated research nosology for HIV-associated neurocognitive disorders. *Neurology* 2007; **69**: 1789–1799.

17 Zunt JR, Tu RK, Anderson DM et al. Progressive multifocal leukoencephalopathy presenting as human immunodeficiency virus type 1 (HIV)-associated dementia. *Neurology* 1997; **49**: 263–265.

18 Arendt G, Hefter H, Figge C et al. Two cases of cerebral toxoplasmosis in AIDS patients mimicking HIV-related dementia. *J Neurol* 1991; **238**: 439–442.

19 Fiala M, Singer EJ, Graves MC et al. AIDS dementia complex complicated by cytomegalovirus encephalopathy. *J Neurol* 1993; **240**: 223–231.

20 Griffiths P. Cytomegalovirus infection of the central nervous system. *Herpes* 2004; **11** Suppl 2: 95A–104A.

21 Navia BA, Price RW. The acquired immunodeficiency syndrome dementia complex as the presenting or sole manifestation of human immunodeficiency virus infection. *Arch Neurol* 1987; **44**: 65–69.

22 Costello D, Davis J, Venna N. HIV infection with immunodeficiency presenting with subacute cognitive decline: recent illustrative cases. *CNS Spectr* 2007; **12**: 842–850.

23 Price RW, Spudich S. Antiretroviral therapy and central nervous system HIV-1 infection. *J Infect Dis* 2008; **197** Suppl 3: S294–S306.

24 Spudich SS, Nilsson AC, Lollo ND et al. Cerebrospinal fluid HIV infection and pleocytosis: relation to systemic infection and antiretroviral treatment. *BMC Infect Dis* 2005; **5**: 98.

25 Marra CM, Maxwell CL, Collier AC et al. Interpreting cerebrospinal fluid pleocytosis in HIV in the era of potent antiretroviral therapy. *BMC Infect Dis* 2007; **7**: 37.

26 Letendre S, Marquie-Beck J, Capparelli E et al. Validation of the CNS penetration-effectiveness rank for quantifying antiretroviral penetration into the central nervous system. *Arch Neurol* 2008; **65**: 65–70.

27 Garg RK. Subacute sclerosing panencephalitis. *J Neurol* 2008; **255**: 1861–1871.

28 Prashanth LK, Taly AB, Ravi V et al. Adult onset subacute sclerosing panencephalitis: clinical profile of 39 patients from a tertiary care centre. *J Neurol Neurosurg Psychiatry* 2006; **77**: 630–633.

29 Gagnon A, Bouchard RW. Fulminating adult-onset subacute sclerosing panencephalitis in a 49-year-old man. *Arch Neurol* 2003; **60**: 1160–1161.

30 Tan E, Namer IJ, Ciger A et al. The prognosis of subacute sclerosing panencephalitis in adults: report of 8 cases and review of the literature. *Clin Neurol Neurosurg* 1991; **93**: 205–209.

31 Frings M, Blaeser I, Kastrup O. Adult-onset subacute sclerosing panencephalitis presenting as a degenerative dementia syndrome. *J Neurol* 2002; **249**: 942–943

32 Mawrin C, Lins H, Koenig B et al. Spatial and temporal disease progression of adult-onset subacute sclerosing panencephalitis. *Neurology* 2002; **58**: 1568–1571.

33 Bostan N, Mahmood T. An overview about hepatitis C: a devastating virus. *Crit Rev Microbiol* 2010; **36**: 91–133.

34 Sene D, Limal N, Cacoub P. Hepatitis C virus-associated extrahepatic manifestations: a review. *Metab Brain Dis* 2004; **19**: 357–381.

35 Acharya JN, Pacheco VH. Neurologic complications of hepatitis C. *Neurologist* 2008; **14**: 151–156.

36 Forton DM, Taylor-Robinson SD, Thomas HC. Central nervous system changes in hepatitis C virus infection. *Eur J Gastroenterol Hepatol* 2006; **18**: 333–338.

37 Forton DM, Allsop JM, Main J et al. Evidence for a cerebral effect of the hepatitis C virus. *Lancet* 2001; **358**: 38–39.

38 Ryan EL, Morgello S, Isaacs K et al. Neuropsychiatric impact of hepatitis C on advanced HIV. *Neurology* 2004; **62**: 957–962.

39 Clifford DB, Smurzynski M, Park LS et al. Effects of active HCV replication on neurologic status in HIV RNA virally suppressed patients. *Neurology* 2009; **73**: 309–314.

40 Soogoor M, Lynn HS, Donfield SM et al. Hepatitis C virus infection and neurocognitive function. *Neurology* 2006; **67**: 1482–1485.

41 Laskus T, Radkowski M, Adair DM et al. Emerging evidence of hepatitis C virus neuroinvasion. *AIDS* 2005; **19** (suppl 3): S140–144.

42 Tunkel AR, Glaser CA, Bloch KC et al. The management of encephalitis: clinical practice guidelines by the Infectious Diseases Society of America. *Clin Infect Dis* 2008; **47**: 303–327.

43 Hokkanen L, Poutiainen E, Valanne L et al. Cognitive impairment after acute encephalitis: comparison of herpes simplex and other aetiologies. *J Neurol Neurosurg Psychiatry* 1996; **6**: 478–484.

44 Kaplan CP, Bain KP. Cognitive outcome after emergent treatment of herpes simplex encephalitis with acyclovir. *Brain Inj* 1999; **13**: 935–941.

45 Hokkanen L, Launes J. Cognitive outcome in acute sporadic encephalitis. *Neuropsychol Rev* 2000; **10**: 151–167.

46 Utley TFM, Ogden JA, Gibb A et al. The long-term neuropsychological outcome of herpes simplex encephalitis in a series of unselected survivors. *Neuropsychiatry Neuropsychol Behav Neurol* 1997; **10**: 180–189.

47 Gyure KA. West Nile virus infections. *J Neuropathol Exp Neurol* 2009; **68**: 1053–1060.

48 Sejvar JJ, Curns AT, Welburg L et al. Neurocognitive and functional outcomes in persons recovering from West Nile virus illness. *J Neuropsychol* 2008; **2**: 477–499.

49 Gustaw-Rothenberg K. Cognitive impairment after tick-borne encephalitis. *Dement Geriatr Cogn Disord* 2008; **26**: 165–168.

50 Hokkanen L, Launes J. Cognitive recovery instead of decline after acute encephalitis; a prospective follow up study. *J Neurol Neurosurg Psychiatry* 1997; **63**: 222–227.

51 Centers for Disease Control and Prevention. Outbreak of syphilis among men who have sex with men–Southern California, 2000. *MMWR Morb Mortal Wkly Rep* 2001; **50**: 117–120.

52 Centers for Disease Control and Prevention. Primary and secondary syphilis among men who have sex with men–New York City, 2001. *MMWR Morb Mortal Wkly Rep* 2002. **51**: 853–856.

53 Centers for Disease Control and Prevention. Internet use and early syphilis infection among men who have sex with men–San Francisco, California, 1999–2003. *MMWR Morb Mortal Wkly Rep* 2003. **52**: 1229–1232.

54 Centers for Disease Control and Prevention. Trends in primary and secondary syphilis and HIV infections in men who have sex with men–San Francisco and Los Angeles, California, 1998–2002. *MMWR Morb Mortal Wkly Rep* 2004. **53**: 575–578.

55 Klausner JD and Hook EW III eds. *Current diagnosis and treatment of sexually transmitted diseases*,1st ed. New York: McGraw-Hill, 2007.

56 Merritt HH, Adams RD, Solomon HC. *Neurosyphilis*, Oxford University Press: New York, 1946.

57 Brown EM. French psychiatry's initial reception of Bayle's discovery of general paresis of the insane. *Bull Hist Med* 1994; **68**: 235–53.

58 Brandst AM. *No magic bullet: a social history of venereal disease in the United States since 1880.* Oxford University Press: New York, 1987.

59 Brown, EM. Why Wagner-Jauregg won the Nobel Prize for discovering malaria therapy for general paresis of the insane. *Hist Psychiatry* 2000; **11**: 371–382.

60 Stokes JH, Beerman H, Ingraham HR. *Modern clinical syphilology*, 3rd ed. WB Saunders: Philadelphia, 1944

61 Hahn RD, Webster B, Weickhard G et al. Penicillin treatment of general paresis (dementia paralytica). *Arch Neurol Psychiatry* 1959; **81**: 557–90.

62 Storm-Mathisen A. General paresis; a follow-up study of 203 patients. *Acta Psychiatr Scand* 1969; **45**(2): 118–32.

63 (a) Dewhurst K. The neurosyphilitic psychoses today. A survey of 91 cases. *Br J Psychiatry* 1969; **115**: 31–8; (b) Herring AJ, Ballard RC, Pope V, et al. A multi-centre evaluation of nine rapid, point-of-care syphilis tests using archived sera. *Sex Transm Infect* 2006; **82** Suppl 5:v7–12.

64 (a) Mabey D, Peeling RW, Ballard R, et al. Prospective, multi-centre clinic-based evaluation of four rapid diagnostic tests for syphilis. *Sex Transm Infect* 2006; **82** Suppl 5:v13–6; (b) Gurses C, Bilgic B, Topcular B et al. Clinical and magnetic resonance imaging findings of HIV-negative patients with neurosyphilis. *J Neurol* 2007; **254**: 368–74.

65 Zhang SQ, Wan B, Ma XL, Zheng HM. Worsened MRI findings during the early period of treatment with penicillin in a patient with general paresis. *J Neuroimaging* 2008. **18**: 360–3.

66 Fadil H, Gonzalez-Toledo E, Kelley BJ, Kelley RE. Neuroimaging findings in neurosyphilis. *J Neuroimaging* 2006; **16**: 286–9.

67 Peng F, Hu X, Zhong X et al. CT and MR findings in HIV-negative neurosyphilis. *Eur J Radiol* 2008. **66**: 1–6.

68 Centers for Disease Control and Prevention. Sexually transmitted diseases treatment guidelines 2006. *MMWR Morb Mortal Wkly Rep* 2005; **55** (RR11): 22–35.

69 Garin C, Bujadoux A. Paralysie par les tiques. *J Med Lyon* 1922; **71**: 765–767.

70 Hellerstrom S. Erythema migrans Afzelius with meningitis. *Acta Derm Venereol* 1951; **31**: 227–234.

71 Steere AC, Malawista SE, Hardin JA et al. Erythema chronicum migrans and Lyme arthritis. The enlarging clinical spectrum. *Ann Intern Med* 1977; **86**: 685–698.

72 Benach JL, Bosler EM, Hanrahan JP et al. Spirochetes isolated from the blood of two patients with Lyme Disease. *N Engl J Med* 1983; **308**: 740–742.

73 Steere AC, Grodzicki RL, Kornblatt AN et al. The spirochetal etiology of Lyme Disease. *N Engl J Med* 1983; **308**: 733–740.

74 Reik L, Steere AC, Bartenhagen NH et al. Neurologic abnormalities of Lyme disease. *Medicine* 1979; **58**: 281–294.

75 Asbrink E, Hederstedt B, Hovmark A. The spirochetal etiology of acrodermatitis chronica atrophicans Herxheimer. *Acta Derm Venereol* 1984; **64**: 506–512.

76 Bacon RM, Kugeler KJ, Mead PS. Surveillance for Lyme Disease—United States, 1992–2006. *Morb Mortal Wkly Rep* 2008; **57**: 1–9.

77 Anonymous. Recommendations for test performance and interpretation from the second national conference on serologic diagnosis of Lyme Disease. *Morb Mortal Wkly Rep* 1995; **44**: 590–591.

78 Meer-Scherrer L, Chang Loa C, Adelson ME et al. Lyme disease associated with Alzheimer's disease. *Curr Microbiol* 2006; **52**: 330–332.

79 Halperin JJ, Krupp LB, Golightly MG, Volkman DJ. Lyme borreliosis-associated encephalopathy. *Neurology* 1990; **40**: 1340–1343.

80 Fenollar F, Puechal X, Raoult D. Whipple's disease. *N Engl J Med* 2007; **356**: 55–66.

81 Schneider T, Moos V, Loddenkemper C et al. Whipple's disease: new aspects of pathogenesis and treatment. *Lancet Infect Dis* 2008; **8**: 179–190.

82 Relman DA, Schmidt TM, MacDermott RP, Falkow S. Identification of the uncultured bacillus of Whipple's disease. *N Engl J Med* 1992; **327**: 293–301.

83 Raoult D, Birg ML, La Scola B et al. Cultivation of the bacillus of Whipple's disease. *N Engl J Med* 2000; **342**: 620–625.

84 Gerard A, Sabrot-Reynauld F, Liozon E et al. Neurologic presentation of Whipple disease. *Medicine* 2002; **81**:443–457.

85 Louis ED, Lynch T, Kaufmann P et al. Diagnostic guidelines in central nervous system Whipple's disease. *Ann Neurol* 1996; **40**: 561–568.

86 Rossi T, Haghighipour R, Haghighi M et al. Cerebral Whipple's disease as a cause of reversible dementia. *Clin Neurol Neurosurg* 2005; **107**: 258–261.

87 Benito-Leon J, Sedano LF, Louis ED. Isolated central nervous system Whipple's disease causing reversible frontotemporal-like dementia. *Clin Neurol Neurosurg* 2008; **110**: 747–749.

88 van de Beek D, Schmand B, de Gans J et al. Cognitive impairment in adults with good recovery after bacterial meningitis. *J Infect Dis* 2002; **186**: 1047–1052.

89 Weisfelt M, van de Beek D, Hoogman M et al. Cognitive outcome in adults with moderate disability after pneumococcal meningitis. *J Infect* 2006; **52**: 433–439.

90 Hoogman M, van de Beek D, Weisfelt M et al. Cognitive outcome in adults after bacterial meningitis. *J Neurol Neurosurg Psychiatry* 2007; **78**: 1092–1096.

91 Merkelbach S, Sittinger H, Schweizer I, Muller M. Cognitive outcome after bacterial meningitis. *Acta Neurol Scand* 2000; **102**: 118–123.

92 Weisfelt M, Hoogman M, van de Beek D et al. Dexamethasone and long-term outcome in adults with bacterial meningitis. *Ann Neurol* 2006; **60**: 456–468.

93 Schmand B, de Bruin E, de Gans J, van de Beek D. Cognitive functioning and quality of life nine years after bacterial meningitis. *J Infect* 2010; **61**: 330–334.
94 Chaykulkeeree M, Perfect JR. Cryptococcosis. *Infect Dis Clin North Am* 2006; **20**: 507–544.
95 Perfect JR, Dismukes WE, Dromer F et al. Clinical practice guidelines for the management of cryptococcal disease: 2010 update by the Infectious Diseases Society of America. *Clin Infect Dis* 2010; **50**: 291–322.
96 Jarvis JN, Harrison TS. HIV-associated cryptococcal meningitis. *AIDS* 2007; **21**: 2119–2129.
97 Steiner I, Polacheck I, Melamed E. Dementia and myoclonus in a case of cryptococcal encephalitis. *Arch Neurol* 1984; **41**: 216–217.
98 Aharon-Peretz J, Kliot D, Finkelstein R et al. Cryptococcal meningitis mimicking vascular dementia. *Neurology* 2004; **62**: 2135.
99 Ala TA, Doss RC, Sullivan CJ. Reversible dementia: a case of cryptococcal meningitis masquerading as Alzheimer's disease. *J Alzheimers Dis* 2004; **6**: 503–508.
100 Hoffmann M, Muniz J, Carroll E, De Villasante J. Cryptococcal meningitis misdiagnosed as Alzheimer's disease: complete neurological and cognitive recovery with treatment. *J Alzheimers Dis* 2009; **16**: 517–520.
101 Carpio A. Neurocysticercosis: an update. *Lancet Infect Dis* 2002; **2**: 751–762.
102 Garcia HH, Del Brutto OH. Neurocysticercosis: updated concepts about an old disease. *Lancet Neurol* 2005; **4**: 653–651.
103 Sinha S, Sharma BS. Neurocysticercosis: a review of current status and management. *J Clin Neurosci* 2009; **16**: 867–876.
104 Sotelo J, Guerrero V, Rubio F. Neurocysticercosis: a new classification based on active and inactive forms. *Arch Int Med* 1985; **145**: 442–445.
105 Singh S, Dhikav V, Agarwal N, Anand KS. An unusual cause of psychosis. *Lancet* 2004; **363**:1522.
106 Patel R, Jha S, Yadav RK. Pleomorphism of the clinical manifestations of neurocysticercosis. *Trans R Soc Trop Med Hyg* 2006; **100**: 134–141.
107 Forlenza OV, Filho AHGV, Nobrega JPS et al. Psychiatric manifestations of neurocysticercosis: a study of 38 patients from a neurology clinic in Brazil. *J Neurol Neurosurg Psychiatry* 1997; **62**: 612–612.
108 Ciampi de Andrade D, Rodrigues CL, Abraham R et al. Cognitive impairment and dementia in neurocysticercosis: a cross-sectional controlled study. *Neurology* 2010; **74**: 1288–1295.
109 Abba K, Ramaratnam S, Ranganathan LN. Antihelminthics for people with neurocysticercosis. *Cochrane Database Syst Rev* 2010; **3**: CD000215.
110 Baird RA, Wiebe S, Zunt JR et al. Evidence-based guideline: treatment of parenchymal neurocysticercosis. *Neurology* 2013; **80**: 1424–1429.
111 Ramirez-Bermudez J, Higuera J, Sosa AL et al. Is dementia reversible in patients with neurocysticercosis? *J Neurol Neurosurg Psychiatry* 2005; **76**: 1164–1166.

CHAPTER 14

Rheumatologic and other autoimmune dementias

Laura J. Julian[1] **and Christopher M. Filley**[2,3]

[1] University of California, San Francisco, San Francisco, CA, USA
[2] University of Colorado School of Medicine, Denver, CO, USA
[3] Denver VA Medical Center, Denver, CO, USA

Introduction

The intersection of rheumatology and neurology, particularly with respect to central nervous system (CNS) and cognitive manifestations, is undoubtedly complex and presents unique challenges for each specialty. For neurologists who most often see these patients in consultation, neurologic complications of rheumatic disease present the challenge of understanding and managing the complex interactions of the immune system with the nervous system. For rheumatologists, CNS complications of rheumatic diseases present some of the most difficult clinical problems as well as the most potentially disabling complications for their patients. The scope of this chapter will be limited to conditions that fall within the discipline of rheumatology and that can cause dementia or significant cognitive impairment. Systemic lupus erythematosus (SLE) is the rheumatologic disease whose neuropsychiatric manifestations have received the most attention from both clinicians and researchers, and a sizeable proportion of our discussion will be focused on this disorder. In addition, we will also discuss other rheumatic disorders with the propensity for producing neuropsychiatric sequelae, including the antiphospholipid antibody syndrome (APS), Sjögren's syndrome, the vasculitides, systemic sclerosis (scleroderma), sarcoidosis, and celiac disease.

The clinical information about CNS manifestations of rheumatologic disease is variable and in many cases sparse, reliant solely on case reports and case series. The CNS complications of these conditions can result in a range of cognitive effects, from relatively mild cognitive impairment to severe dementia. In the majority of these conditions, the cognitive loss is characterized by a loss in function compared to a previous level and has the potential to impair functioning in social, occupational, and educational domains while not meeting the severity level of dementia. For the purposes of this chapter, we define cognitive dysfunction conventionally as the presence of significant deficits in any cognitive domain, which can include learning and memory, executive function, language, visuospatial function, information processing speed, and simple and complex attention.

In the practice of rheumatology as well as neurology, there is a high likelihood of encountering patients with milder degrees of cognitive dysfunction that are disconcerting to the patient and disruptive to daily functioning, yet not always detectable in the general clinical encounter, particularly when other neurologic functions (e.g., motor, sensory) appear to be unaffected. Therefore, we emphasize in this chapter the benefit of employing a multidisciplinary approach to patient evaluation and treatment, specifically through the use of neuropsychological assessment. Neuropsychological testing can facilitate quantification of cognitive deficits that cannot be as thoroughly assessed in the clinical encounter, serve to track the course of cognitive functioning, and help determine the efficacy or toxicity of specific treatments on cognition. We recommend the use of neuropsychology as an integrated component of the clinical evaluation not only because subtle deficits may escape recognition in the clinical encounter but also because subjective complaints of cognitive decline by patients are not always objectively confirmed. This discordance among patient reports of cognitive dysfunction and performance on neuropsychological testing may stem from several sources, including the influence of psychological distress (e.g., depression) [1], the impact of fatigue, and the insensitivity of cognitive screening measures to more subtle alterations in cognition [2].

The diagnostic conundrum of rheumatologic disease in the neurologic setting

The neurologist typically becomes involved in the care of a rheumatologic patient under two primary circumstances. The first is in the context of a known and previously diagnosed rheumatologic condition after the onset and/or progression of

Non-Alzheimer's and Atypical Dementia, First Edition. Edited by Michael D. Geschwind and Caroline Racine Belkoura.
© 2016 John Wiley & Sons, Ltd. Published 2016 by John Wiley & Sons, Ltd.

CNS or peripheral nervous system involvement. The second, and more challenging scenario, is when the initial presentation of the patient to the neurologist occurs before the underlying rheumatologic condition is diagnosed. In this latter situation, there is no typical presentation, and the spectrum of potential neurologic presenting complaints is broad, ranging from headaches and malaise to stroke, transverse myelitis, peripheral neuropathy, and cognitive impairment. The majority of rheumatologic diagnoses are reached through a careful characterization of the patient's clinical syndrome using the history, physical examination, and laboratory testing and with the exclusion of nonrheumatologic conditions.

The use of laboratory studies for the diagnosis of rheumatologic conditions has become increasingly refined and remains a key feature of the diagnostic process. There are few if any rheumatologic conditions that can be definitively diagnosed through laboratory testing, however, and it remains important to understand the limitations of diagnostic tests and the potential problems with interpreting specific laboratory measures. For example, an essential feature of any rheumatologic panel is testing for antinuclear antibodies (ANA). Whereas this is a reasonable approach, as these autoantibodies are considered a hallmark of systemic autoimmune disease, it is important to consider that the sensitivity of a positive ANA for a specific autoimmune disease varies widely, from 48% in Sjögren's syndrome to 93% in SLE, and that many people in the general population with a positive ANA do not have an identifiable systemic disease [3]. Another example is the testing of antiphospholipid antibodies, which should be considered for the assessment of neurologic complications of SLE, primary APS, and Sneddon's syndrome. Whereas testing for such antibodies as anticardiolipin antibodies (AcL), beta-2-glycoprotein 1 antibodies, and the lupus anticoagulant (LAC) can provide clues to the pathogenesis of clotting disorders and cerebrovascular (CV) disease, only repeat testing at least 12 weeks after the initial testing can be used to make a definitive diagnosis of APS [4].

Consideration of a rheumatic condition in a patient presenting with a neurologic complaint requires a thorough evaluation of extraneurologic symptoms and manifestations as well as those involving the nervous system. For example, evaluation of constitutional symptoms, organ involvement, joint manifestations, skin rashes, and hematologic abnormalities can all be helpful. Table 14.1 lists the conditions reviewed in this chapter along with the range of neurologic features, primary nonneurologic features, and potential neurobehavioral sequelae. We will briefly describe each condition, discuss the major cognitive and/ or neurological manifestations, highlight specific diagnostic approaches and findings (including neuroimaging), and briefly discuss aspects of prognosis as well as interventions in clinical practice. To illustrate the complexity of diagnosis and treatment that may characterize rheumatologic patients with neurologic manifestations, the following case is presented.

Case report

A 75-year-old right-handed man was referred for 1 year of progressive cognitive decline. He had been noted to develop apathy, inattention, and poor memory, followed by gait disorder and incontinence of bladder and bowel. Brain magnetic resonance imaging (MRI) showed scattered ischemic white matter (WM) changes, and electroencephalography (EEG) showed frontal intermittent rhythmic delta activity. Three months after onset, cerebrospinal fluid (CSF) examination showed clear fluid with glucose 41 mg/dL, protein 117 mg/dL, 33 white blood cells (WBCs) per μL with lymphocytic predominance, and 14 red blood cells (RBCs) per μL. In addition, the CSF had evidence of low amyloid β42 (509 pg/mL) and high tau (709 pg/mL), resulting in an amyloid β42/tau ratio interpreted as consistent with Alzheimer's disease (AD). EEG at that time showed bilateral periodic lateralized epileptiform discharges. Other laboratory tests for reversible causes of dementia were unremarkable. Despite the inflammatory CSF, a diagnosis of probable AD was made. Cognition and neurologic status continued to worsen, and 5 months after disease onset, the score on the Mini-Mental State Examination (MMSE) [5] was 14, with poor orientation and attention and 1/3 word recall. At 8 months, the MMSE score was 9, with marked apathy and 0/3 word recall. At 10 months, he was nearly mute, had muscle rigidity, and could neither stand nor walk. The patient was then referred for a second opinion.

When examined at the University of Colorado Hospital Neurobehavior Clinic 1 year after disease onset, the patient was profoundly apathetic and the MMSE could not be administered. He had diffuse rigidity, the inability to stand or walk, and bilateral grasp reflexes. The CSF pleocytosis documented months before was recognized, and he was emergently admitted to the hospital for thorough evaluation. MRI scan showed ventricular enlargement and meningeal inflammation (Figure 14.1). CSF examination again showed lymphocytic pleocytosis, this time with 10 WBCs/μL, and elevated protein of 108 mg/dL; glucose was 45 mg/dL. An extensive workup for infectious disease and neoplasia was unrevealing, and the ANA was negative, but the perinuclear antineutrophil cytoplasmic antibody (P-ANCA) titer was positive at 1:320 with negative cytoplasmic ANCA (C-ANCA). Chest roentgenogram and pulmonary computed tomography (CT) showed mediastinal adenopathy and right lower lobe consolidation, and diagnostic possibilities including Wegener's granulomatosis and sarcoidosis were considered. Bronchoscopy was felt to be of low yield, however, and was not performed. The decision was then made to obtain brain biopsy, and tissue taken from the right frontal lobe and adjacent meninges showed meningeal inflammation with necrosis, histiocytes, and abundant plasma cells without vasculitis; there was no evidence of neuritic plaques, neurofibrillary tangles, or amyloid angiopathy. Treatment was initiated with insertion of a ventriculoperitoneal shunt and methylprednisolone for 5 days followed by prednisone. Rapid improvement occurred, and 6 weeks later, the patient was alert, fully oriented, and talkative; the MMSE score was 29, with only sentence writing impaired. Rigidity and

Table 14.1 Rheumatologic and related dementias and neurological characteristics.

Condition	Potential neurological manifestations	Primary extraneurological manifestations	Potential behavioral characteristics
Systemic lupus erythematosus	See Table 14.2; 19 identified peripheral and central nervous system manifestations (e.g., seizure, stroke, headache)	Any organ system (commonly dermatologic, renal, and musculoskeletal involvement)	Cognitive impairment Confusion/disorientation Depression and/or anxiety Psychosis
Antiphospholipid syndrome	Stroke Transient ischemic attack Migraine Seizures Chorea Transverse myelitis Guillain–Barré syndrome	Pregnancy morbidity Evidence of vascular thrombosis in any tissue or organ	Cognitive impairment Psychosis Depression
Sneddon's syndrome	Stroke Transient ischemic attack	Livedo reticularis	Cognitive impairment
Sjögren's syndrome	Transverse myelitis Meningoencephalitis Subarachnoid hemorrhage Migraines	Dryness of the eyes, mouth, and other mucous membranes	Cognitive impairment
Antineutrophil cytoplasmic antibody-associated vasculitides (e.g., Wegner's granulomatosis, Churg–Strauss syndrome)	Hemorrhagic stroke (especially in the context of uncontrolled hypertension) Peripheral nerve involvement	Wegner's granulomatosis Upper respiratory involvement (including inflammatory lesions in sinus regions) Other pulmonary involvement Renal involvement Churg–Strauss Syndrome Upper and lower respiratory Cardiac complications	Cognitive impairment Disorientation
Behcet's disease	Headache Dysarthria Cranial nerve findings Ataxia		Psychosis Confusion Cognitive impairment
Giant cell arteritis	Headache (especially in temporal regions) Cranial nerve involvement Neuro-ophthalmologic signs Neuropathy Stroke Transient ischemic attack	Ophthalmologic signs Polymyalgia Systemic symptoms (weight loss, fatigue, etc.) Medium vessel Scalp tenderness Temporal artery tenderness Jaw claudication Large vessel Claudication of arms, asymmetrical pulses	Confusion Cognitive impairment
Systemic sclerosis (scleroderma)	Cranial and peripheral neuropathy Rarely cerebrovascular involvement (especially in the context of renal, heart, and pulmonary involvement)	Sclerotic skin Reynaud's phenomenon	Cognitive impairment
Sarcoidosis	Cranial neuropathy Meningeal involvement Seizures	Lung, skin, and eye manifestations Neuroendocrine involvement (in response to hypothalamic and pituitary involvement)	Cognitive impairment Psychosis Delirium
Celiac disease	Ataxia Headaches Encephalopathy Seizures Chorea	Chronic diarrhea Fatigue	Cognitive dysfunction Confusion

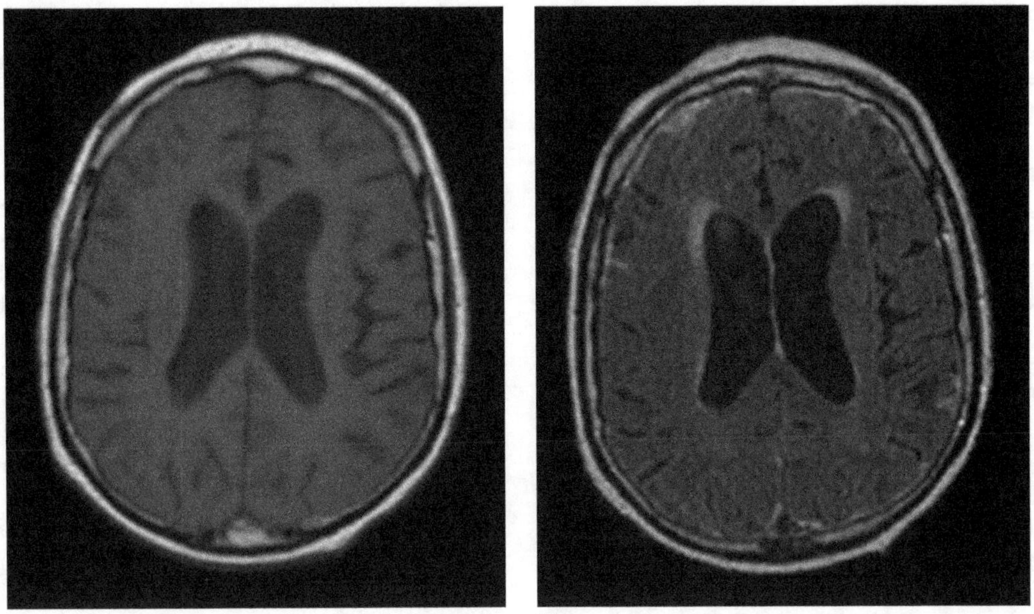

(a) (b)

Figure 14.1 MRI (**a**) T1-weighted image showing ventricular enlargement. (**b**) FLAIR image showing meningeal hyperintensity consistent with inflammation.

incontinence had resolved, and although gait remained apraxic, he could ambulate for 200 ft with a walker. He was then given mycophenolate, followed sequentially by azathioprine and methotrexate, to permit continuance of a low prednisone dose. One month after the start of treatment, CSF examination showed 2 WBCs/μL, predominantly lymphocytic, 3 RBCs/μL, protein 124 mg/dL, and glucose 44 mg/dL. After 5 months of treatment, the patient had normal cognition and gait. By 8 months, the P-ANCA titer had fallen to 1:40. A diagnosis of P-ANCA meningitis with hydrocephalus was reached for this case of reversible dementia due to a rheumatologic disease.

SLE

SLE is a chronic, multisystem autoimmune disease with the potential to affect any organ system. Prevalence rates of SLE are up to 120 cases per 100 000 [6–8]. Incidence rates of SLE in the Americas and Europe range from 2 to 8 per 100 000/year [9, 10], with peak incidence between ages 15 and 40 years and a female to male ratio of 6: 10 to 1 [11]. Traditionally, renal and lung involvement has been thought to be responsible for the greatest morbidity and mortality in SLE [12, 13]; however, with current medical therapies, involvement in these organ systems is now associated with increasingly favorable outcomes. Instead, neuropsychiatric manifestations have emerged as a major cause of morbidity in SLE [14–17].

In 1999, the American College of Rheumatology (ACR) developed a nomenclature system for 19 neuropsychiatric syndromes in SLE (NPSLE) [18], 12 of which are considered CNS manifestations (Table 14.2). These broad criteria encompass a range of psychiatric (e.g., mood disorders) and neurologic (e.g., stroke, seizure) syndromes, and prevalence studies using this nomenclature suggest that up to 80% of patients with SLE have at least one of these NPSLE syndromes [19, 20] and the majority of patients have more than one.

Table 14.2 Neuropsychiatric manifestations of SLE described by the American College of Rheumatology.

Central nervous system manifestations	Peripheral nervous system manifestations
Seizure disorders	Autonomic disorder
Cerebrovascular disease	Myasthenia gravis
Demyelinating syndrome	Neuropathy, cranial
Aseptic meningitis	Mononeuropathy, single or multiplex
Headache	Acute inflammatory demyelinating polyradiculoneuropathy
Movement disorder (chorea)	Plexopathy
Myelopathy	Polyneuropathy
Acute confusional state	
Anxiety disorder	
Cognitive dysfunction	
Mood disorder	
Psychosis	

Cognitive dysfunction has been observed to be the most common NPSLE manifestation in SLE, and if mild levels of cognitive impairment are included, prevalence rates reach 81% of persons with SLE. Using more conservative classification criteria of impairment, more moderate levels of cognitive impairment have been observed to affect approximately 50–66% of patients with SLE [19, 21]. Although severe cognitive impairment or dementia is relatively rare in SLE, studies have observed that this level of impairment occurs in approximately 6–8% of patients with SLE [19, 20].

The nature of cognitive impairment in SLE

Studies of SLE have observed impairment in almost any cognitive domain, but the most commonly affected include speed of information processing, attention, learning and recall, executive function, and visuospatial skills [22–29], suggesting predominant involvement of subcortical brain regions. In general, patients with SLE have been classified as having NPSLE after the onset of other NPSLE manifestations mentioned previously, and patients who have not had overt neuropsychiatric manifestations are classified as non-NPSLE. As might be expected, NPSLE patients demonstrate greater severity of cognitive impairment compared to non-NPSLE patients [23, 27, 30, 31]. However, several studies have observed that patients with non-NPSLE demonstrate more cognitive impairment than healthy matched peers [27, 29, 30, 32]. These studies suggest that in the absence of other overt neurological involvement, cognitive dysfunction may still be present in SLE, possibly heralding subtle brain involvement early in the disease course. It should be noted that some studies have not observed robust cognitive differences between non-NPSLE patients and controls [33, 34].

A number of approaches have been used to detect cognitive impairment in SLE, but the most commonly used assessment approach was developed by the ACR ad hoc committee in 1999 [18]. This expert committee assembled a 1 h neuropsychological battery that has since been validated and deemed reliable for use in SLE [21] (see Table 14.3).

Table 14.3 American College of Rheumatology-recommended neuropsychological assessment battery for use in systemic lupus erythematosus.

Cognitive domain	Measure	References
Executive function		
Response inhibition	Stroop Color–Word Interference Test	[177–180]
Verbal fluency	Phonemic Fluency Test	[181]
Sequencing/shifting	Trail Making Test Part B	[182]
Working memory	Letter–Number Sequencing Test	[183]
Processing speed	Digit Symbol Substitution Test	[183]
Verbal learning and recall	California Verbal Learning Test II	[184]
Nonverbal learning and recall	Rey–Osterrieth Complex Figure Test	[185, 186]
Semantic fluency	Animal Naming Test	[187]
"Premorbid" verbal ability	North American Adult Reading Test	[188]
Fine motor speed and manipulation	Finger tapping test	[189]

MRI findings in SLE

Both conventional and improved neuroimaging techniques have been used to study the associations between cognition and CNS involvement in SLE. Most of these studies have not included neuropsychological testing. Hyperintense WM lesions observed on conventional MRI are the most commonly observed neuroradiological findings in SLE, present in up to 70% of patients [35]. In general, these findings are more common among patients with antiphospholipid antibodies and manifestations of NPSLE, and WM changes have been associated with attentional dysfunction [36]. Additionally, cerebral atrophy has been observed in up to 12% of patients with SLE [37, 38]. Improved neuroimaging techniques have recently been used to examine correlations of brain abnormalities with cognitive dysfunction. One such technique that has shown promise in SLE is MR spectroscopy (MRS), with its capacity to measure WM choline (Ch) to creatine (Cre) ratios [39, 40], and diffusion tensor imaging (DTI) [41], which can examine specific WM tracts. An MRS study of frontal lobe WM in non-NPSLE, for example, demonstrated a correlation between increased Ch and measures of executive dysfunction and inattention, suggesting that immune-mediated myelinopathy may be an early pathogenic event in the cognitive dysfunction of SLE [52].

Mechanisms of cognitive decline in SLE

A broad range of factors have been studied in the context of cognitive decline in SLE. Autoantibody production, CV disease, inflammatory factors including cytokines, and other molecular and hormonal factors have all attracted attention as potential contributors to cognitive impairment and dementia.

Antiphospholipid antibodies (*aPL*)

SLE patients have a 7.9-fold increased risk for CVD [42], and the presence of aPLs is a recognized risk factor [43–47]. APLs include a wide and heterogeneous group of immunoglobulins; however, the majority of studies in SLE have focused on LAC, aCL, and more recently the presence of β2- glycoprotein 1. The laboratory classification of aPLs has evolved, and more recently, it has been suggested that aPL positivity be considered only when there is evidence of two subsequent positive tests assessed at least 12 weeks apart [4].

In SLE, the prevalence of aCL ranges from 12 to 30% [48–50], and the prevalence of LACs from 15 to 34% [51, 52]. The presence of aPL is one factor that is consistently associated with cognitive dysfunction in SLE [53–58]. Few studies have been conducted using the more recent and more conservative laboratory classification of persistent positivity of aPLs over time or incorporating the use of β2-glycoprotein 1. In one study of a large sample of SLE patients, aPL was associated with almost a twofold risk of cognitive dysfunction; and among those patients without other overt clinical manifestations of CNS involvement, aPL was associated with a threefold risk of cognitive dysfunction [59].

The cognitive impairment resulting from aPL can be quite severe and has been observed in case series and case reports to be predictive of the onset of marked cognitive impairment and dementia [60]. The use of specific drugs for prophylaxis of CV disease among patients who are aPL positive but who lack evidence of specific neuropsychiatric events is a topic of controversy, and results of studies using aspirin for the prevention of thrombotic events in people with aPL are mixed [61–63]. Among patients with evidence of thrombosis or other vascular pathology, the key clinical management approach is typically anticoagulation, especially when there is evidence of aPL-related clinical syndromes meeting criteria for antiphospholipid antibody syndrome (discussed in the following text).

Cross-reacting *N*-methyl-D-aspartate (NMDA) receptor antibodies

Recently, there has been significant enthusiasm regarding a specific autoantibody model of cognitive impairment in SLE, specifically cognitive impairment precipitated by cross-reacting anti-NMDA NR2 (anti-NR2) antibodies. Anti-NR2 antibodies appear to be present in 20–35% of patients with SLE [64–69] and produce glutamate excitotoxicity, neural injury, and cell death in mouse models [70, 71]. Behavioral studies find memory dysfunction in these mice, and pathological studies find neuronal loss in the hippocampus [70, 71] The anti-NR2 hypothesis has been tested in five clinical studies, and the majority have found no association between these antibodies and cognition in SLE [64, 67, 69, 72]. One study did find an association between anti-NR2 antibodies and memory function [67]. These studies all employed serum autoantibody markers to detect CNS processes, but it is unclear to what extent these antibodies are transported across the blood–brain barrier. One study did investigate the presence of anti-NR2 antibodies in the CSF and found associations with diffuse neuropsychiatric syndromes in SLE [73]. Ongoing work to better understand conditions that promote blood–brain barrier permeability in SLE is underway and may improve the understanding of the transport of anti-NR2 antibodies into the CNS. Such information would directly inform the use of therapies targeted at the NMDA receptor.

Other mechanisms under consideration

Other autoantibodies have long been studied as pathogenic mechanisms for cognitive impairment in SLE. The role of antiribosomal P antibodies has been a target of investigation, but no clear associations have been found between this autoantibody and cognition in SLE [74]. Inflammatory markers have also been under investigation as factors precipitating cognitive dysfunction, and one study observed an association between serum IL-6 [75] and C-reactive proteins [76]. Additionally, neuropeptide Y has also been implicated in clinical studies of cognition in SLE [77].

It is well known that SLE is characterized by accelerated cardiovascular and CV disease. This increased burden may be partially explained by the increased prevalence of traditional CV risk factors compared to non-SLE peers (e.g., tobacco use, hypertension, hyperlipidemia, obesity, and sedentary lifestyle) [78–81]. However, many studies also cite comparable rates of traditional CV risk factors compared to peers [79, 82]. Traditional risk factors do not fully explain the CV burden in SLE [42], and disease- and treatment-related factors must also be considered [83–85] (e.g., inflammation, chronic glucocorticoid use, etc).

Summary

SLE is often considered to be the prototypical autoimmune disease, and its neuropsychiatric manifestations are likely multifactorial in etiology. Although SLE is the rheumatologic condition whose cognitive and neuropsychiatric manifestations have received the most attention, the etiology of cognitive decline remains unclear. Through the ongoing study of large and diverse cohorts of SLE patients, a more standardized approach to the detection of cognitive decline, and advances in neuroimaging, it is likely that our understanding of these syndromes will be significantly improved.

Antiphospholipid syndrome and Sneddon's syndrome

The term antiphospholipid syndrome (APS) was coined to describe the clinical combination of the presence of aPL and a specific syndrome of arterial or venous thrombosis [86]. When APS occurs in the absence of SLE or other connective tissue disease, it is called primary APS. Primary APS occurs in 0.5–6% of the general population [87, 88]. Secondary APS is diagnosed when a patient has a diagnosis of another condition (most often SLE) and has aPL with evidence of hypercoagulability. Approximately 30% of patients with SLE have concomitant APS [87]. The average age at APS diagnosis is 34 with only 12% of patients diagnosed after age 50. The male to female ratio for primary APS is 1:3.5, and for secondary APS, it is 1:7 (more closely approximating the gender ratio for SLE) [49].

The primary clinical syndromes that can occur as a result of APS include thrombosis and pregnancy morbidity. Neurological manifestations of APS lead to the greatest morbidity and mortality. The most common and severe manifestation of APS is stroke, occurring in approximately 19% of patients, followed by transient ischemic attack in 11% [89, 90]. Other reported CNS sequelae have included migraine, cognitive dysfunction, seizures, chorea, transverse myelitis, psychosis, depression, and Guillain–Barré syndrome [91]. Rarely, patients can develop catastrophic APS, characterized by rapid development of multiple microthrombi in multiple organ systems (brain, kidney, lung, skin); mortality in catastrophic APS nears 50% [92].

Dementia is seen in less than 5% of patients with APS, but mild to moderate levels of cognitive dysfunction occur in 33–43%; these patients generally present with impairments in memory and learning, language, attention, and executive functions [93, 94]. In a study of 30 patients with APS-associated dementia, 47% of patients had primary APS, 30% had SLE, and 23% had characteristics of SLE [60]. Thirty-seven percent of this cohort had suffered a stroke, and 33% had Sneddon's syndrome (described in the following text). Notably, 37% did not present with other APS manifestations before to the diagnosis of dementia, suggesting that laboratory studies of aPL may be warranted among young individuals who present with unexplained cognitive impairment.

MRI findings in APS include multiple foci of WM hyperintensities, and occasionally, confluent areas of hyperintensity are observed [95]. MRS has shown a decreased ratio of *N*-acetylaspartate (NAA) to Cre and an increased Ch to Cre ratio [95]. The degree to which the MRS metabolic studies predict APS beyond MRI hyperintensities is unclear, but the use of NAA/ Cre ratios in SLE patients with APS may be a promising clinical method to quantify the course of neurological and neurobehavioral involvement [96].

Sneddon's syndrome is a related condition characterized by the development of CV disease (stroke and transient ischemic attacks) and concomitant livedo reticularis. The onset of CV disease occurs at a relatively young age, generally before age 45 [97]. Over 40% of those with Sneddon's syndrome have APS [98]. Neuroradiological findings suggest that Sneddon's syndrome presents with leukoaraiosis and lacunar infarcts [99] more frequently than primary APS, which is more typically characterized by larger arterial vascular lesions. The clinical course of Sneddon's syndrome is generally worse than APS, particularly with the recurrence of CV events. Greater than two-thirds of patients have cognitive impairment [100, 101], and cognition appears to deteriorate as CV events accumulate [102, 103]. Progressive cognitive decline and dementia in the absence of discrete events have also been reported in younger adults with Sneddon's syndrome [104, 105]. Clinical management of the neurologic aspects of Sneddon's syndrome is somewhat controversial, but anticoagulation remains the most commonly used treatment followed by other immunosuppressive drugs including glucocorticoids and cyclophosphamide [106].

Sjögren's syndrome

Sjögren's syndrome is a chronic autoimmune disorder characterized by lymphocytic infiltration of the exocrine glands, leading to the cardinal manifestation of dryness of the eyes, mouth, and other mucous membranes. The prevalence of Sjögren's syndrome ranges from 0.9 to 3.5%, and incidence from 3.9 to 5.3/100 000 [107]. Similar to other rheumatic conditions, Sjögren's syndrome affects significantly more women than men [108]. Secondary Sjögren's syndrome occurs when patients have a preexisting autoimmune disease, and the prevalence rates of Sjögren's syndrome secondary to rheumatoid arthritis and SLE approximate 25% [88]. Whereas peripheral nervous system manifestations have been described in up to 20% of patients with Sjögren's syndrome, CNS manifestations are less well understood. Reported frequencies of these complications range from 0.3 to 48% of patients [109, 110].

The CNS manifestations of Sjögren's syndrome include manifestations as diverse as transverse myelitis, meningoencephalitis, subarachnoid hemorrhage, cognitive deficits, psychiatric syndromes, and migraine [111]. Few studies have evaluated the cognitive consequences of Sjögren's syndrome using neuropsychological testing; however, existing studies have documented cognitive impairment in up to 50% of patients [112, 113]; and of these patients, approximately 27% exhibit moderate to severe cognitive dysfunction.

Little is known about the pathophysiology of cognitive decline in Sjögren's syndrome. Among patients with Sjögren's syndrome and SLE, the SLE-related mechanisms reviewed previously have been considered as possible etiological pathways. In primary Sjögren's syndrome, the pathogenesis is less clear, and CV manifestations are considered to play a lesser role in the development of cognitive decline. Some have suggested that immune vasculopathy is critical, given the observation of necrotizing vasculitis on pathological studies, particularly among patients testing positive for anti-Ro/SSA antibodies [114].

Conventional brain MRI studies have observed WM lesions and cerebral atrophy in patients with primary Sjögren's syndrome [115, 116]. DTI studies have observed reduced WM integrity, particularly in frontal regions, and these changes correlated with cognitive dysfunction [117]. Other imaging studies, using single-photon emission computed tomography (SPECT), found cortical hypoperfusion when compared to controls, and this hypoperfusion also correlated with cognitive dysfunction in a small sample of patients with primary Sjögren's syndrome [113].

There have been few randomized clinical trials to study specific treatments for CNS manifestations of Sjögren's syndrome. Systemic immunosuppressive treatment has generally been reserved for extraglandular manifestations including neurologic complications. Recently, large international cohorts of Sjögren's syndrome patients have been created for the purposes of better understanding this disorder and its manifestations. Specifically, the Sjögren's International Collaborative Clinical Alliance was funded under a National Institutes of Health (NIH) contract which began in 2003 and includes seven international sites [118].

Vasculitides

Inflammation directed against the walls of the blood vessel is called vasculitis, and this process produces one of three paths to vascular damage: (a) ischemia from swelling, fibrosis, and occlusion of the vessel lumen; (b) inflammation of the vessel wall causing weakening and the development of a rupture or aneurysm leading to hemorrhage; and (c) local and systemic inflammation accompanied by cytokine release and other inflammatory markers. Inflammation can often be detected through observation of edema and tenderness along a specific vessel (as in giant cell arteritis (GCA)), and in many patients secondary signs of inflammation are manifested as less specific constitutional symptoms. These conditions are relatively rare, and diagnosis of systemic vasculitis requires a combination of a consistent clinical phenotype, supportive serologic studies, exclusion of other diagnostic possibilities, and often biopsy of blood vessels disclosing inflammation. Angiographic evidence of abnormalities can also provide supportive evidence of vasculitis. The etiology of these diseases is generally unknown, but factors known to influence disease expression include race/ethnicity, genetic contributions (e.g., HLA and others), and environmental factors (e.g., smoking, drugs, UV light, etc).

Antineutrophil cytoplasmic antibody-associated vasculitides

One class of vasculitis includes those with serum evidence of antineutrophil cytoplasmic antibodies (ANCA), and these diseases are termed ANCA-associated vasculitides (AAV); specific diseases include Wegener's granulomatosis and the Churg–Strauss syndrome, among others. These syndromes are rare. As observed by an epidemiological study conducted in the 1990s of persons living in the United Kingdom, point prevalence rates of any of these primary systemic vasculitides approximated 145 per million; more males than females are affected, and risk increases with older age [119]. Wegener's granulomatosis typically presents with involvement of the upper respiratory tract and inflammatory lesions in the orbital and sinus regions. Pulmonary, renal, and peripheral nerve involvement may also occur, affecting 80%, 76%, and 58% of patients, respectively [88, 120]. Churg–Strauss syndrome is very rare, affecting approximately 2.4 persons per million. This condition is characterized by small vessel vasculitis and presents clinically with a prodromal phase of late-onset allergic rhinitis, followed by asthma, lung infiltrates, extravascular necrotizing granulomas, and hypereosinophilia. Cardiac complications are relatively common and are a major cause of mortality [121].

Cerebral vasculitis is relatively rare in the context of Wegener's granulomatosis or Churg–Strauss syndrome and is characterized by hemorrhagic CV events, particularly evident in the context of uncontrolled hypertension. Despite the variability in the presentation of neuropsychiatric manifestation, MRI studies of patients with Wegener's granulomatosis found evidence of WM lesions in 64%, basal ganglia involvement in 89%, and pontine involvement in 50% [122]. Case reports have documented a range of cognitive and psychiatric sequelae, including severe cognitive impairment [123] and disorientation [124]. One study of patients with either Wegener's granulomatosis or Churg–Strauss syndrome found neuropsychological impairment in 30%, particularly in the domains of memory, abstract reasoning, and attention [125]. A subset of these patients had brain MRI, and the majority of patients with cognitive decline also had multifocal WM lesions. Meningitis is a very rare P-ANCA manifestation [126, 127], and in the case presented previously, reversible dementia resulted primarily from hydrocephalus.

The clinical management of CNS involvement in these vasculitides typically involves the rapid quelling of inflammation. High-dose corticosteroids are commonly used, as are other immunosuppressant therapies including mycophenolate, azathioprine, cyclophosphamide, and rituximab.

Behcet's disease

Behcet's disease is another chronic inflammatory disorder that is also thought to be caused by an underlying vasculitis. Behcet's disease primarily occurs in younger adults between the ages of 25 and 30 and does not follow a preferential pattern for gender. The disease is more prevalent, however, in the eastern Mediterranean region, the Middle East, and East Asia, prompting the alternative name of Silk Road disease. Due to increased international recognition, prevalence rates appear to be increasing and range between 2.5/10 [5] in the northwestern Mediterranean regions and 1/10 [5] in Northern Europe, Central Europe, and the United States. Aphthous oral ulcers are typically the early and persisting clinical signs of Behcet's disease; skin lesions are also common, followed by other mucocutaneous involvement and ocular inflammation. The pathergy phenomenon is a diagnostic test considered to be specific to Behcet's disease and is found when a papule or pustule forms at the site of dermis puncture (typically in the forearm) [128].

CNS involvement is observed in approximately 5–13% of patients with Behcet's disease, or "neuro-Behcet's syndrome," and this disorder stems from vascular inflammation, resulting in various syndromes ranging from psychosis to vascular headache [128]. Neurological involvement is more common among men with Behcet's disease, and the male to female ratio is 4:1 [129]. Other CNS syndromes have been observed including a subacute brainstem syndrome characterized by cranial nerve findings, dysarthria, corticospinal tract dysfunction, and confusion. Progressive ataxia accompanied by cerebellar atrophy on MRI has also been observed [130]. Neuropsychiatric changes appear particularly common in Behcet's syndrome and may include euphoria, agitation, paranoia, and cognitive decline involving impaired learning and recall. Neuropsychological status has been observed in some cases to progressively decline independent of other neurological episodes [128].

Neuroimaging findings show inflammatory lesions with a predilection for the diencephalon, midbrain, and brainstem [128]. Cerebral hemispheric lesions are less common, and when present, they have almost always been associated with accompanying brainstem lesions. In some cases, brain lesions have had the appearance of a mass effect [131]. The lesions have also been observed to resolve after administration of corticosteroids [128]. SPECT studies have yielded evidence of hypoperfusion in the basal ganglia and frontal and temporal lobes, even among patients with normal MRI [132].

In general, neurological involvement in Behcet's disease is a significant cause of morbidity, with approximately 50% of patients becoming disabled within 10 years, most often due to problems in ambulation (45%) [128]. Cerebellar symptoms, a progressive course, and inflammatory CSF markers are factors related to a particularly poor prognosis [133, 134]. Currently, there are no controlled clinical trial data to guide the management of these complications of Behcet's disease. Corticosteroids and other immunosuppressive agents have been the most effective treatments for these manifestations in uncontrolled studies, case series, and case reports.

GCA

GCA is the most common primary vasculitis, affecting 15–25 per 100 000 of persons over the age of 50 years [135]. GCA primarily affects women and Caucasians, particularly those of Northern European descent [136]. HLA alleles, particularly specific variants of the HLA DR4 haplotype, are expressed in 60% of patients, suggesting a heritability of this disease [137].

GCA is characterized by granulomatous inflammation of the medium- and large-sized arteries of the head and neck, often leading to occlusion and ischemia. The external carotid system is most susceptible, and involvement of the optic nerve can lead to visual loss. The most common neurologic features are headache, amaurosis fugax, and neuro-ophthalmologic signs, and many patients also present with systemic symptoms including weight loss, fatigue, fever, and polymyalgia rheumatica. Two-thirds of patients with medium vessel involvement present with new-onset severe headaches, commonly located in temporal regions [138]. Scalp or temporal artery tenderness and jaw claudication are also common in medium vessel GCA. Large vessel involvement generally manifests as claudication in the arms, absent or asymmetrical pulses and blood pressure readings, and occasional tissue gangrene [139]. Aortic involvement is often not clinically detectable, but can lead to severe arterial dilation and aneurysm [140].

Thirty percent of patients present with neurological manifestations, including neuropathies (14%) and less commonly transient ischemic attacks and strokes (3–4%) that result from severe occlusion of carotid or vertebral arteries [141]. CV disease is probably the most common cause of early death in GCA [141]. Acutely, GCA has been observed to present as a confusional state. The etiology of mental status abnormalities in GCA is unclear but is hypothesized to result from vasculitic involvement of intracranial vessels, resulting in temporal or occipital lobe ischemia. Finally, vascular dementia due to multiple infarcts related to GCA has occasionally been described [142–144]. The clinical course of cognitive impairment is variable, and cognitive dysfunction has been observed to be responsive to corticosteroid treatment.

Comparable to the other vasculitides, treatment is largely empirical but typically involves high-dose intravenous or oral corticosteroids [145]. GCA-related cognitive disorders are another example of a steroid-responsive dementia syndrome, as a rapid resolution of symptoms can be observed after initiation of corticosteroids [145]. Anticoagulation has also been used in some cases, generally after evidence documents the formation of thrombi in the inflamed arteries [146]. Low-dose aspirin as prophylaxis has also been recommended [147].

Systemic sclerosis (scleroderma)

Systemic sclerosis is a multisystem autoimmune disease that confers serious risks for morbidity and mortality [148]. The two clinical types of this disease are diffuse cutaneous systemic sclerosis (dcSSc), with a more severe clinical course, and more limited cutaneous systemic sclerosis (lcSSc). dcSSC is an aggressive disease with major organ involvement in the first 3 years and a 10-year survival of approximately 84% [149]. Sclerotic skin is the primary manifestation of systemic sclerosis, along with severe secondary Raynaud's phenomenon related to vasospasm, and intimal proliferation in small vessels, leading to digital ulceration and ischemia.

Neurological symptoms are relatively uncommon but can include cranial and peripheral neuropathies. CV events are particularly rare and usually occur in the context of renal, heart, or pulmonary involvement [150, 151]. Despite the rarity of neurological and neuropsychiatric syndromes, MRI studies of patients with systemic sclerosis unselected for neurological status suggest the presence of WM lesions in approximately 36%, predominantly in the parietal (28%) and occipital (16%) regions. In another study, 52% of patients had lesions in the corticomedullary junction, 56% in the periventricular regions, 40% in the basal ganglia, and 40% in the pons [122]. As in many of these other systemic conditions, the clinical correlates of these MRI findings are unclear. Studies employing neuropsychological assessment show executive dysfunction, and it has been posited that cardiovascular reactivity plays a role in cognitive alterations of these patients [152]. Whereas specific therapies for neurological manifestations of systemic sclerosis have not been tested in controlled trials, immunosuppressive treatments are commonly used.

Sarcoidosis

Sarcoidosis is a granulomatous multisystem disorder of unknown etiology, although autoimmunity has been strongly implicated. Sarcoidosis can affect any part of the body, although lung, skin, and eye manifestations are the most common. The disease typically presents in the 30s and 40s and is more common among people of West African descent and North European Caucasians [153]. The prevalence in the United States is estimated at 40 per 100 000 [154], with annual incidence rates of 65.5 per 100 000 among African Americans and 10.9 per 100 000 in Caucasians [155]. Asymptomatic CNS involvement is suggested to occur in at least 10% of patients [156], as documented by postmortem histopathology.

Noncaseating granulomata, consisting of centrally organized macrophages and epithelioid cells encircled by lymphocytes, are the classic pathological features of sarcoidosis. Granuloma formation appears to be mediated by an interaction between CD4+ T cells and antigen-presenting cells, differentiation of CD4+ T cells into type 1 helper (T_H1) cells, and secretion of lymphocyte and macrophage-derived cytokines (interleukin-2, interferon gamma, and tumor necrosis factor alpha). Similar to systemic autoimmune conditions, a combination of genetic (in this case, HLA-B8, HLA-DRB1, and DQB1) and environmental factors (exposure to mold, metalworking, smoke exposure in firefighters and among those exposed to wood burning stoves, etc.) appear to be important in etiology [157].

Any part of the CNS can be affected by sarcoidosis. Cranial neuropathy appears to be the most common manifestation, affecting 50–75% of patients, followed by cognitive or behavioral manifestations in 20%, meningeal involvement in 10–20%, and seizures in 5–10% [157]. Many patients develop periventricular WM lesions that can mimic other conditions, including multiple sclerosis [158], and approximately 50% of neurosarcoidosis patients develop parenchymal brain disease resulting from granulomas [159]. Clinical manifestations are generally dictated by localization of lesions. For example, 10–15% of neurosarcoidosis patients develop neuroendocrine-related symptoms as a result of hypothalamic and pituitary involvement [160].

With respect to cognitive dysfunction and dementia, case reports of patients with neurosarcoidosis describe severe psychiatric manifestations including psychosis and delirium [161–163]. Aphasia, amnesia, and dementia have also been reported [164, 165].

MRI with gadolinium enhancement is important as part of the diagnostic evaluation of possible neurosarcoidosis. Involvement of the leptomeninges is the most common MRI finding, and perivascular lesions can also be seen in basal regions, midbrain structures, and the dura mater [157]. Positron emission tomography (PET) can show evidence of hyper- or hypometabolism related to sarcoidosis-related inflammation. Whole-body PET imaging with gallium-67 scanning can aid in the identification of lymph nodes with sarcoidosis involvement, but the sensitivity and specificity of this technique are not clear.

Although the procedure entails significant risk, the gold standard for the diagnosis of neurosarcoidosis is brain biopsy to seek evidence of noncaseating granulomata. In the absence of biopsy, other diagnostic criteria have been suggested, although a definite diagnosis may be difficult to reach. Probable neurosarcoidosis can be diagnosed when the clinical presentation is consistent with neurosarcoidosis, other mimickers have been excluded, and a therapeutic response has been observed to immunotherapy for 12 months [166]. As in other diseases for controlled trial evidence of treatment is lacking, therapy is largely empirical and employs the use of corticosteroids and other immunosuppressive drugs.

Celiac disease

Celiac disease is an autoimmune disorder caused by an adverse reaction to gliadin, a protein found in wheat, along with a similar reaction to related proteins in barley and rye. An inflammatory reaction in the gut is triggered when tissue transglutaminase enzyme modifies the triggered gliadin protein as it reacts with small bowel tissue. This process inhibits the absorption of nutrients, and small bowel involvement leads to symptoms including chronic diarrhea, failure to thrive (in children), and fatigue.

The prevalence of celiac disease is at least 1% of the population, and advances in screening have led to greater numbers of people being diagnosed with the disease who are mildly affected or even asymptomatic [167, 168]. The prevalence of neurological dysfunction resulting from celiac disease is unclear, but some reports suggest neurological dysfunction occurs in 10 to 23% of patients [169, 170]. The most common CNS manifestation among patients presenting to neurology subspecialty clinics is ataxia, occurring in up to 67% of patients, followed by encephalopathy in 36% of patients, and, less commonly, seizures and chorea (less than 3%) [169, 170].

"Gluten encephalopathy" has been used as a general term for patients with gluten sensitivity, headaches, and the presence of WM abnormalities on MRI. Initiation of a gluten-free diet has resulted in resolution of headaches, while WM lesions remained static [170]. Cerebral atrophy has also been observed among patients with celiac disease [171]. Hypoperfusion on PET imaging was observed in 73% of a small cohort of 11 patients with celiac disease who were not treated with a gluten-free diet, compared to 7% of healthy controls and 7% of celiac disease patients treated with dietary restriction [172]. Several studies have observed substantial cognitive deficits in small cohorts of patients with celiac disease [173].

The pathology of neurological involvement in celiac disease has been shown in some studies to be largely immune mediated, with evidence of diffuse infiltration of T lymphocytes in the WM and perivascular cuffing with inflammatory cells [174]. Diagnostically, the association between autoantibody production and neurologic dysfunction is unclear, with some patients showing serum antibody reactivity to one or more gangliosides, while other patients show no reactivity [169]. A proposed diagnostic schedule by Hadjivassiliou and colleagues included testing for gliadin, deamidated gliadin, and antitissue transglutaminase IgA and IgG antibodies, followed by duodenal biopsy to detect enteropathy or, in the absence of enteropathy, the identification of IgA deposits against tissue transglutaminase on the biopsy [174].

A lifelong gluten-free diet is the cornerstone of treatment of celiac disease. As it is very difficult to completely avoid gluten in the diet, some authors have suggested that a 100 mg/kg limit is reasonably safe for most patients, although there is some individual variability in tolerance at this level [175]. Other treatments under active exploration and development include enzyme supplements, engineered grains and pretreatment of flours, and neutralizing gluten antibodies [176].

Summary and conclusions

Each of the diseases and syndromes described previously is characterized by a broad range of clinical presentations and disparate neurological and cognitive sequelae, but they all share the presence of autoimmunity and a propensity to cause significant cognitive dysfunction and related disability in selected patients. It is clear that the cognitive manifestations of these rheumatologic conditions influence the development of disability by impacting activities of daily living, accelerating departure from the work force, and negatively impacting overall well-being. The majority of studies reviewed earlier have focused on patients with severe cognitive impairment and dementia, and it is likely that mild to moderate levels of cognitive impairment, possibly heralding more subtle brain involvement, remain undetected. For this reason, a more sensitive diagnostic workup involving neuropsychological testing may be warranted in patients presenting with cognitive impairment who do not meet criteria for dementia. Neuropsychological testing in these patients may facilitate the identification of specific patterns of cognitive impairment, assisting patient care and providing clues to pathophysiology. Additionally, neuropsychological status may also be an important indicator of the course of disease progression over time. Detecting milder levels of cognitive impairment provides the opportunity to detect preclinical predictors of disability for the purposes of intervention and prevention. This opportunity is often missed in patients whose cognitive status reaches the severity of dementia.

Neurologic complications in many of these diseases are rare, and our knowledge regarding diagnosis, clinical and neuroradiological presentation, and management is largely derived from case reports and case series. Even in SLE, which has received the most attention, a thorough understanding of specific neurobehavioral manifestations is lacking. It is clear that in order to move forward in our understanding of these manifestations, multinational cohorts that have the ability to amass a relatively large number of patients with these rarer conditions will be necessary to better understand the neurological complications. These investigative models are growing within communities related to several of these diseases [e.g., Sjogren's International Collaborative Clinical Alliance (SICCA), the Systemic Lupus Erythematosus International Collaborating Clinics (SLICC)] and will allow a better understanding of the epidemiology, clinical features, laboratory testing, neuroimaging characteristics, and optimal management of these challenging neurological and neurobehavioral disorders.

References

1 Julian L, Merluzzi NM, Mohr DC. The relationship among depression, subjective cognitive impairment, and neuropsychological performance in multiple sclerosis. *Mult Scler* 2007;**13**:81–86.

2 Leritz E, Brandt J, Minor M, Reis-Jensen F, Petri M. "Subcortical" cognitive impairment in patients with systemic lupus erythematosus. *J Int Neuropsychol Soc* 2000;**6**:821–825.

3 Solomon DH, Kavanaugh AJ, Schur PH. Evidence-based guidelines for the use of immunologic tests: antinuclear antibody testing. *Arthritis Rheum* 2002;**47**:434–444.

4 Giannakopoulos B, Passam F, Ioannou Y, Krilis SA. How we diagnose the antiphospholipid syndrome. *Blood* 2009;**113**:985–994.

5 Folstein MF, Folstein SE, McHugh PR. "Mini-mental State." A practical method for grading the cognitive status of patients for the clinician. *J Psychiatr Res* 1975;**12**:189–198.

6 Lawrence RC, Helmick CG, Arnett FC, et al. Estimates of the prevalence of arthritis and selected musculoskeletal disorders in the United States. *Arthritis Rheum* 1998;**41**:778–799.

7 Gabriel SE, Michaud K. Epidemiological studies in incidence, prevalence, mortality, and comorbidity of the rheumatic diseases. *Arthritis Res Ther* 2009;**11**:229.

8 Hochberg MC, Perlmutter DL, Medsger TA, et al. Prevalence of self-reported physician-diagnosed systemic lupus erythematosus in the USA. *Lupus* 1995;**4**:454–456.

9 Vilar MJ, Sato EI. Estimating the incidence of systemic lupus erythematosus in a tropical region (Natal, Brazil). *Lupus* 2002;**11**: 528–532.

10 Jimenez S, Cervera R, Font J, Ingelmo M. The epidemiology of systemic lupus erythematosus. *Clin Rev Allergy Immunol* 2003;**25**:3–12.

11 Lahita RG. The role of sex hormones in systemic lupus erythematosus. *Curr Opin Rheumatol* 1999;**11**:352–356.

12 Fessler BJ, Boumpas DT. Severe major organ involvement in systemic lupus erythematosus. Diagnosis and management. *Rheum Dis Clin North Am* 1995;**21**:81–98.

13 Boumpas DT, Austin HA, Fessler BJ, Balow JE, Klippel JH, Lockshin MD. Systemic lupus erythematosus: emerging concepts. Part 1: Renal, neuropsychiatric, cardiovascular, pulmonary, and hematologic disease. *Ann Intern Med* 1995;**122**:940–950.

14 Wong KL, Woo EK, Yu YL, Wong RW. Neurological manifestations of systemic lupus erythematosus: a prospective study. *Q J Med* 1991;**81**:857–870.

15 Kaell AT, Shetty M, Lee BC, Lockshin MD. The diversity of neurologic events in systemic lupus erythematosus. Prospective clinical and computed tomographic classification of 82 events in 71 patients. *Arch Neurol* 1986;**43**:273–276.

16 Sibley JT, Olszynski WP, Decoteau WE, Sundaram MB. The incidence and prognosis of central nervous system disease in systemic lupus erythematosus. *J Rheumatol* 1992;**19**:47–52.

17 Bluestein HG. Neuropsychiatric disorders in systemic lupus erythematosus. In: Lahita RG, ed. *Systemic Lupus Erythematosus.* New York: Wiley, 1987, 593–614.

18 No author. The American College of Rheumatology nomenclature and case definitions for neuropsychiatric lupus syndromes. *Arthritis Rheum* 1999; **42**:599–608.

19 Ainiala H, Loukkola J, Peltola J, Korpela M, Hietaharju A. The prevalence of neuropsychiatric syndromes in systemic lupus erythematosus. *Neurology* 2001;**57**:496–500.

20 Brey RL, Holliday SL, Saklad AR, et al. Neuropsychiatric syndromes in lupus: prevalence using standardized definitions. *Neurology* 2002;**58**:1214–1220.

21 Kozora E, Ellison MC, West S. Reliability and validity of the proposed American college of rheumatology neuropsychological battery for systemic lupus erythematosus. *Arthritis Rheum* 2004; **51**:810–818.

22 Brey RL. Neuropsychiatric lupus: clinical and imaging aspects. *Bull NYU Hosp Jt Dis* 2007;**65**:194–199.

23 Carbotte RM, Denburg SD, Denburg JA. Prevalence of cognitive impairment in systemic lupus erythematosus. *J Nerv Ment Dis* 1986;**174**:357–364.

24 Denburg SD, Carbotte RM, Denburg JA. Cognitive impairment in systemic lupus erythematosus: a neuropsychological study of individual and group deficits. *J Clin Exp Neuropsychol* 1987;**9**: 323–339.

25 Ginsburg KS, Wright EA, Larson MG, et al. A controlled study of the prevalence of cognitive dysfunction in randomly selected patients with systemic lupus erythematosus. *Arthritis Rheum* 1992; **35**:776–782.

26 Glanz BI, Slonim D, Urowitz MB, Gladman DD, Gough J, MacKinnon A. Pattern of neuropsychological dysfunction in inactive systemic lupus erythematosus. *Neuropsychiatry Neuropsychol Behav Neurol* 1997;**10**:232–238.

27 Hanly JG, Fisk JD, Sherwood G, Jones E, Jones JV, Eastwood B. Cognitive impairment in patients with systemic lupus erythematosus. *J Rheumatol* 1992;**19**:562–567.

28 Hay EM, Black D, Huddy A, et al. Psychiatric disorder and cognitive impairment in systemic lupus erythematosus. *Arthritis Rheum* 1992;**35**:411–416.

29 Kozora E, Thompson LL, West SG, Kotzin BL. Analysis of cognitive and psychological deficits in systemic lupus erythematosus patients without overt central nervous system disease. *Arthritis Rheum* 1996;**39**:2035–2045.

30 Wekking EM, Nossent JC, van Dam AP, Swaak AJ. Cognitive and emotional disturbances in systemic lupus erythematosus. *Psychother Psychosom* 1991;**55**:126–131.

31 Loukkola J, Laine M, Ainiala H, et al. Cognitive impairment in systemic lupus erythematosus and neuropsychiatric systemic lupus erythematosus: a population-based neuropsychological study. *J Clin Exp Neuropsychol* 2003;**25**:145–151.

32 Hay EM, Huddy A, Black D, et al. A prospective study of psychiatric disorder and cognitive function in systemic lupus erythematosus. *Ann Rheum Dis* 1994;**53**:298–303.

33 Kozora E, Arciniegas DB, Filley CM, et al. Cognitive and neurologic status in patients with systemic lupus erythematosus without major neuropsychiatric syndromes. *Arthritis Rheum* 2008;**59**: 1639–1646.

34 Mulherin D, Doherty E, O'Connell A, Bresnihan B. Assessment of cognitive function in patients with systemic lupus erythematosus. *Ir J Med Sci* 1993;**162**:9–12.

35 Appenzeller S, Faria AV, Li LM, Costallat LTL, Cendes F. Quantitative magnetic resonance imaging analyses and clinical significance of hyperintense white matter lesions in systemic lupus erythematosus patients. *Ann Neurol* 2008;**64**:635–643.

36 Kozora E, West SG, Kotzin BL, Julian L, Porter S, Bigler E. Magnetic resonance imaging abnormalities and cognitive deficits in systemic lupus erythematosus patients without overt central nervous system disease. *Arthritis Rheum* 1998;**41**:41–47.

37 Appenzeller S, Bonilha L, Rio PA, Min Li L, Costallat LT, Cendes F. Longitudinal analysis of gray and white matter loss in patients with systemic lupus erythematosus. *Neuroimage* 2007; **34**:694–701.

38 Appenzeller S, Rondina JM, Li LM, Costallat LT, Cendes F. Cerebral and corpus callosum atrophy in systemic lupus erythematosus. *Arthritis Rheum* 2005;**52**:2783–2789.

39 Brooks WM, Jung RE, Ford CC, Greinel EJ, Sibbitt WL, Jr. Relationship between neurometabolite derangement and neurocognitive dysfunction in systemic lupus erythematosus. *J Rheumatol* 1999;**26**:81–85.

40 Kozora E, Arciniegas DB, Filley CM, et al. Cognition, MRS neurometabolites, and MRI volumetrics in non-neuropsychiatric systemic lupus erythematosus: preliminary data. *Cogn Behav Neurol* 2005;**18**:159–162.

41 Julian L, Katz PP, Trupin L, et al. Cardiovascular disease, cognitive functioning, and depression in SLE: a study using diffusion tensor brain imaging *Arthritis Rheum* 2009;**60**:1581.

42 Esdaile JM, Abrahamowicz M, Grodzicky T, et al. Traditional Framingham risk factors fail to fully account for accelerated atherosclerosis in systemic lupus erythematosus. *Arthritis Rheum* 2001; **44**:2331–2337.

43 Sanna G, Bertolaccini ML, Cuadrado MJ, et al. Neuropsychiatric manifestations in systemic lupus erythematosus: prevalence and association with antiphospholipid antibodies. *J Rheumatol* 2003; **30**:985–992.

44 Chapman J, Rand JH, Brey RL, et al. Non-stroke neurological syndromes associated with antiphospholipid antibodies: evaluation of clinical and experimental studies. *Lupus* 2003;**12**:514–517.

45 Kandiah DA, Sali A, Sheng Y, et al. Current insights into the "antiphospholipid" syndrome: clinical, immunological, and molecular aspects. *Adv Immunol* 1998;**70**:507–563.

46 Wilson WA, Gharavi AE, Koike T, et al. International consensus statement on preliminary classification criteria for definite antiphospholipid syndrome: report of an international workshop. *Arthritis Rheum* 1999;**42**:1309–1311.

47 Mok CC, Lau CS, Wong RW. Neuropsychiatric manifestations and their clinical associations in Southern Chinese patients with systemic lupus erythematosus. *J Rheumatol* 2001;**28**:766–771.

48 Chakravarty KK, Al-Hillawi AH, Byron MA, Durkin CJ. Anticardiolipin antibody associated ischaemic strokes in elderly patients without systemic lupus erythematosus. *Age Ageing* 1990;**19**: 114–118.

49 Cervera R, Piette JC, Font J, et al. Antiphospholipid syndrome: clinical and immunologic manifestations and patterns of disease expression in a cohort of 1,000 patients. *Arthritis Rheum* 2002; **46**:1019–1027.

50 Merkel PA, Chang Y, Pierangeli SS, Convery K, Harris EN, Polisson RP. The prevalence and clinical associations of anticardiolipin antibodies in a large inception cohort of patients with connective tissue diseases. *Am J Med* 1996;**101**:576–583.

51 Cervera R, Khamashta MA, Font J, et al. Systemic lupus erythematosus: clinical and immunologic patterns of disease expression in a cohort of 1,000 patients. The European working party on systemic lupus erythematosus. *Medicine (Baltimore)* 1993;**72**: 113–124.

52 Filley CM, Kozora E, Brown MS, et al. White matter microstructure and cognition in non-neuropsychiatric systemic lupus erythematosus. *Cogn Behav Neurol* 2009; **22**:38–44.

53 Denburg SD, Carbotte RM, Denburg JA. Cognition and mood in systemic lupus erythematosus. Evaluation and pathogenesis. *Ann N Y Acad Sci* 1997;**823**:44–59.

54 Leritz E, Brandt J, Minor M, Reis-Jensen F, Petri M. Neuropsychological functioning and its relationship to antiphospholipid antibodies in patients with systemic lupus erythematosus. *J Clin Exp Neuropsychol* 2002;**24**:527–533.

55 Menon S, Jameson-Shortall E, Newman SP, Hall-Craggs MR, Chinn R, Isenberg DA. A longitudinal study of anticardiolipin antibody levels and cognitive functioning in systemic lupus erythematosus. *Arthritis Rheum* 1999;**42**:735–741.

56 Hanly JG, Hong C, Smith S, Fisk JD. A prospective analysis of cognitive function and anticardiolipin antibodies in systemic lupus erythematosus. *Arthritis Rheum* 1999;**42**:728–734.

57 Whitelaw DA, Spangenberg JJ, Rickman R, Hugo FH, Roberts M. The association between the antiphospholipid antibody syndrome and neuropsychological impairment in SLE. *Lupus* 1999;**8**:444–448.

58 Denburg SD, Denburg JA. Cognitive dysfunction and antiphospholipid antibodies in systemic lupus erythematosus. *Lupus* 2003;**12**: 883–890.

59 Denburg SD, Carbotte RM, Ginsberg JS, Denburg JA. The relationship of antiphospholipid antibodies to cognitive function in patients with systemic lupus erythematosus. *J Int Neuropsychol Soc* 1997; **3**:377–386.

60 Gomez-Puerta JA, Cervera R, Calvo LM, et al. Dementia associated with the antiphospholipid syndrome: clinical and radiological characteristics of 30 patients. *Rheumatology* 2005;**44**:95–99.

61 Hereng T, Lambert M, Hachulla E, et al. Influence of aspirin on the clinical outcomes of 103 anti-phospholipid antibodies-positive patients. *Lupus* 2008;**17**:11–15.

62 Erkan D, Harrison MJ, Levy R, et al. Aspirin for primary thrombosis prevention in the antiphospholipid syndrome: a randomized, double-blind, placebo-controlled trial in asymptomatic antiphospholipid antibody-positive individuals. *Arthritis Rheum* 2007; **56**:2382–2391.

63 Tektonidou MG, Laskari K, Panagiotakos DB, Moutsopoulos HM. Risk factors for thrombosis and primary thrombosis prevention in patients with systemic lupus erythematosus with or without antiphospholipid antibodies. *Arthritis Rheum* 2009;**56**:2382.

64 Harrison MJ, Ravdin LD, Lockshin MD. Relationship between serum NR2a antibodies and cognitive dysfunction in systemic lupus erythematosus. *Arthritis Rheum* 2006;**54**:2515–2522.

65 Husebye ES, Sthoeger ZM, Dayan M, et al. Autoantibodies to a NR2A peptide of the glutamate/NMDA receptor in sera of patients with systemic lupus erythematosus. *Ann Rheum Dis* 2005;**64**:1210–1213.

66 Sharma A, Isenberg D, Diamond B. Studies of human polyclonal and monoclonal antibodies binding to lupus autoantigens and cross-reactive antigens. *Rheumatology (Oxford)* 2003;**42**:453–463.

67 Omdal R, Brokstad K, Waterloo K, Koldingsnes W, Jonsson R, Mellgren SI. Neuropsychiatric disturbances in SLE are associated with antibodies against NMDA receptors. *Eur J Neurol* 2005;**12**: 392–398.

68 Hanly JG, Robichaud J, Fisk JD. Anti-NR2 glutamate receptor antibodies and cognitive function in systemic lupus erythematosus. *J Rheumatol* 2006;**33**:1553–1558.

69 Lapteva L, Nowak M, Yarboro CH, et al. Anti-N-methyl-D-aspartate receptor antibodies, cognitive dysfunction, and depression in systemic lupus erythematosus. *Arthritis Rheum* 2006;**54**:2505–2514.

70 DeGiorgio LA, Konstantinov KN, Lee SC, Hardin JA, Volpe BT, Diamond B. A subset of lupus anti-DNA antibodies cross-reacts with the NR2 glutamate receptor in systemic lupus erythematosus. *Nat Med* 2001;**7**:1189–1193.

71 Kowal C, DeGiorgio LA, Nakaoka T, et al. Cognition and immunity: antibody impairs memory. *Immunity* 2004;**21**:179–188.

72 Kozora E, West SG, Maier SF, et al. Antibodies against *N*-methyl-D-aspartate receptors in patients with systemic lupus erythematosus without major neuropsychiatric syndromes. *J Neurol Sci* 2010;**295**:87–91.

73 Yoshiyuki A, Tamiko Y, Shunsei H. Association of cerebrospinal fluid anti-NR2 glutamate receptor antibodies with diffuse neuropsychiatric systemic lupus erythematosus. *Arthritis Rheum* 2008; **58**:1130–1135.

74 Fotini BK, Antonella A, Ales A, et al. Accuracy of anti-ribosomal P protein antibody testing for the diagnosis of neuropsychiatric systemic lupus erythematosus: an international meta-analysis. *Arthritis Rheum* 2006;**54**:312–324.

75 Kozora E, Laudenslager M, Lemieux A, West SG. Inflammatory and hormonal measures predict neuropsychological functioning in systemic lupus erythematosus and rheumatoid arthritis patients. *J Int Neuropsychol Soc* 2001;**7**:745–754.

76 Shucard JL, Parrish J, Shucard DW, McCabe DC, Benedict RH, Ambrus J, Jr. Working memory and processing speed deficits in systemic lupus erythematosus as measured by the paced auditory serial addition test. *J Int Neuropsychol Soc* 2004;**10**:35–45.

77 Harle P, Straub RH, Wiest R, et al. Increase of sympathetic outflow measured by neuropeptide Y and decrease of the hypothalamic-pituitary-adrenal axis tone in patients with systemic lupus erythematosus and rheumatoid arthritis: another example of uncoupling of response systems. *Ann Rheum Dis* 2006;**65**:51–56.

78 Bessant R, Duncan R, Ambler G, et al. Prevalence of conventional and lupus-specific risk factors for cardiovascular disease in patients with systemic lupus erythematosus: A case-control study. *Arthritis Rheum* 2006;**55**:892–899.

79 Roman MJ, Shanker B-A, Davis A, et al. Prevalence and correlates of accelerated atherosclerosis in systemic lupus erythematosus. *N Engl J Med* 2003;**349**:2399–2406.

80 Asanuma Y, Oeser A, Shintani AK, et al. Premature coronary-artery atherosclerosis in systemic lupus erythematosus. *N Engl J Med* 2003; **349**:2407–2415.

81 Bruce IN, Urowitz MB, Gladman DD, Ibanez D, Steiner G. Risk factors for coronary heart disease in women with systemic lupus erythematosus: the Toronto Risk Factor Study. *Arthritis Rheum* 2003;**48**:3159–3167.

82 Frostegard J. SLE, atherosclerosis and cardiovascular disease. *J Intern Med* 2005;**257**:485–495.

83 Davis JM, 3rd, Maradit Kremers H, Crowson CS, et al. Glucocorticoids and cardiovascular events in rheumatoid arthritis: a population-based cohort study. *Arthritis Rheum* 2007;**56**:820–830.

84 Maxwell SR, Moots RJ, Kendall MJ. Corticosteroids: do they damage the cardiovascular system? *Postgrad Med J* 1994;**70**:863–870.

85 Nashel DJ. Is atherosclerosis a complication of long-term corticosteroid treatment? *Am J Med* 1986;**80**:925–929.

86 Hughes GRV, Harris NN, Gharavi AE. The anticardiolipin syndrome. *J Rheumatol* 1986;**13**:486–489.

87 Cohen D, Berger SP, Steup-Beekman GM, Bloemenkamp KWM, Bajema IM. Diagnosis and management of the antiphospholipid syndrome. *BMJ*;**340**:c2541.

88 Klippel JH, Crofford LJ, Stone JH, Weyand CM, eds. *Primer on the Rheumatic Diseases*, 12 ed. Atlanta, Georgia: Arthritis Foundation, 2001.

89 Cervera R, Boffa MC, Khamashta MA, Hughes GR. The Europhospholipid project: epidemiology of the antiphospholipid syndrome in Europe. *Lupus* 2009;**18**:889–893.

90 Cervera R, Khamashta MA, Hughes GR. The Euro-lupus project: epidemiology of systemic lupus erythematosus in Europe. *Lupus* 2009;**18**:869–874.

91 Kearon C, Kahn SR, Agnelli G, Goldhaber S, Raskob GE, Comerota AJ. Antithrombotic therapy for venous thromboembolic disease: American college of chest physicians evidence-based clinical practice guidelines (8th Edition). *Chest* 2008;**133**:454S–545S.

92 Miyakis S, Lockshin MD, Atsumi T, et al. International consensus statement on an update of the classification criteria for definite antiphospholipid syndrome (APS). *J Thromb Haemost* 2006;**4**:295–306.

93 Roldan JF, Brey RL. Neurologic manifestations of the antiphospholipid syndrome. *Curr Rheumatol Rep* 2007;**9**:109–115.

94 Erkan D, Kozora E, Lockshin MD. Cognitive dysfunction and white matter abnormalities in antiphospholipid syndrome. *Pathophysiology* 2011;**18**:93–102.

95 Liberato B, Levy RA. Antiphospholipid syndrome and cognition. *Clin Rev Allergy Immunol* 2007;**32**:188–191.

96 Appenzeller S, Li LM, Costallat LT, Cendes F. Evidence of reversible axonal dysfunction in systemic lupus erythematosus: a proton MRS study. *Brain* 2005;**128**:2933–2940.

97 Frances C, Piette JC. The mystery of Sneddon syndrome: relationship with antiphospholipid syndrome and systemic lupus erythematosus. *J Autoimmun* 2000;**15**:139–143.

98 Frances C, Papo T, Wechsler B, Laporte JL, Biousse V, Piette JC. Sneddon syndrome with or without antiphospholipid antibodies. A comparative study in 46 patients. *Medicine (Baltimore)* 1999;**78**: 209–219.

99 Fetoni V, Grisoli M, Salmaggi A, Carriero R, Girotti F. Clinical and neuroradiological aspects of Sneddon's syndrome and primary antiphospholipid antibody syndrome. A follow-up study. *Neurol Sci* 2000;**21**:157–164.

100 Adair JC, Digre KB, Swanda RM, et al. Sneddon's syndrome: a cause of cognitive decline in young adults. *Neuropsychiatry Neuropsychol Behav Neurol* 2001;**14**:197–204.

101 Geschwind DH, FitzPatrick M, Mischel PS, Cummings JL. Sneddon's syndrome is a thrombotic vasculopathy: neuropathologic and neuroradiologic evidence. *Neurology* 1995;**45**:557–560.

102 Tanne D, Hassin-Baer S. Neurologic manifestations of the antiphospholipid syndrome. *Curr Rheumatol Rep* 2001;**3**:286–292.

103 Weissenborn K, Ruckert N, Ehrenheim C, Schellong S, Goetz C, Lubach D. Neuropsychological deficits in patients with Sneddon's syndrome. *J Neurol* 1996;**243**:357–363.

104 Wright RA, Kokmen E. Gradually progressive dementia without discrete cerebrovascular events in a patient with Sneddon's syndrome. *Mayo Clin Proc* 1999;**74**:57–61.

105 Devuyst G, Sindic C, Laterre EC, Brucher JM. Neuropathological findings of a Sneddon's syndrome presenting with dementia not preceded by clinical cerebrovascular events. *Stroke* 1996;**27**:1008–1010.

106 Hannon PM, Kuo SH, Strutt AM, York MK, Kass JS. Improvement of neurological symptoms and memory and emotional status in a case of seronegative Sneddon syndrome with cyclophosphamide. *Clin Neurol Neurosurg*;**112**:544–547.

107 Binard A, Devauchelle-Pensec V, Fautrel B, Jousse S, Youinou P, Saraux A. Epidemiology of Sjogren's syndrome: where are we now? *Clin Exp Rheumatol* 2007;**25**:1–4.

108 Pillemer SR, Matteson EL, Jacobsson LT, et al. Incidence of physician-diagnosed primary Sjogren syndrome in residents of Olmsted County, Minnesota. *Mayo Clin Proc* 2001;**76**:593–599.

109 Soliotis FC, Mavragani CP, Moutsopoulos HM. Central nervous system involvement in Sjogren's syndrome. *Ann Rheum Dis* 2004;**63**:616–620.

110 Govoni M, Padovan M, Rizzo N, Trotta F. CNS involvement in primary Sjogren's syndrome: prevalence, clinical aspects, diagnostic assessment and therapeutic approach. *CNS Drugs* 2001;**15**:597–607.

111 Morgen K, McFarland HF, Pillemer SR. Central nervous system disease in primary Sjögren's syndrome: The role of magnetic resonance imaging. *Semin Arthritis Rheum* 2004;**34**:623–630.

112 Harboe E, Tjensvoll AB, Maroni S, et al. Neuropsychiatric syndromes in patients with systemic lupus erythematosus and primary Sjogren syndrome: a comparative population-based study. *Ann Rheum Dis* 2009;**68**:1541–1546.

113 Le Guern V, Belin C, Henegar C, et al. Cognitive function and 99mTc-ECD brain SPECT are significantly correlated in patients with primary Sjogren syndrome: a case-control study. *Ann Rheum Dis*;**69**:132–137.

114 de la Monte SM, Hutchins GM, Gupta PK. Polymorphous meningitis with atypical mononuclear cells in Sjogren's syndrome. *Ann Neurol* 1983;**14**:455–461.

115 Coates T, Slavotinek JP, Rischmueller M, et al. Cerebral white matter lesions in primary Sjogren's syndrome: a controlled study. *J Rheumatol* 1999;**26**:1301–1305.

116 Pierot L, Sauve C, Leger JM, et al. Asymptomatic cerebral involvement in Sjogren's syndrome: MRI findings of 15 cases. *Neuroradiology* 1993;**35**:378–380.

117 Segal BM, Mueller BA, Zhu X, et al. Disruption of brain white matter microstructure in primary Sjogren's syndrome: evidence from diffusion tensor imaging. *Rheumatology (Oxford)*. 2010;**49**: 1530–1539.

118 Daniels TE, Criswell LA, Shiboski C, et al. An early view of the international Sjogren's syndrome registry. *Arthritis Rheum* 2009;**61**:711–714.

119 Watts RA, Lane SE, Bentham G, Scott DG. Epidemiology of systemic vasculitis: a ten-year study in the United Kingdom. *Arthritis Rheum* 2000;**43**:414–419.

120 Hewins PM, Tervaert JWCMDP, Savage COSMDPF, Kallenberg CGMMDP. Is Wegener's granulomatosis an autoimmune disease? [Miscellaneous Article]. *Curr Opin Rheumatol* 2000;**12**:3–10.

121 Eustace JA, Nadasdy T, Choi M. The Churg Strauss syndrome. *J Am Soc Nephrol* 1999;**10**:2048–2055.

122 Joerg S, Sonja K, Juergen S, Stefan F, Angela G, Ulf M-L. Cerebral lesions in patients with connective tissue diseases and systemic vasculitides: are there specific patterns? *Ann N Y Acad Sci*; **1193**: 167–175.

123 McKeith IG. Neuropsychiatric symptoms in the course of Wegener's granulomatosis. *J Neurol Neurosurg Psychiatry* 1985;**48**:713–714.

124 Leitch DN, Heald A, Goodship TH. Wegener's granulomatosis: an unusual presentation. *Nephrol Dial Transplant* 1994;**9**:421–422.

125 Mattioli F, Capra R, Rovaris M, et al. Frequency and patterns of subclinical cognitive impairment in patients with ANCA-associated small vessel vasculitides. *J Neurol Sci* 2002;**195**:161–166.

126 Jacobi D, Maillot F, Hommet C, et al. P-ANCA cranial pachymeningitis: a case report. *Clin Rheumatol* 2005;**24**:174–177.
127 Horino T, Takao T, Taniguchi Y, Terada Y. Hypertrophic pachymeningitis with MPO-ANCA-positive vasculitis. *Clin Rheumatol* 2010;**29**:111–113.
128 Siva A, Saip S. The spectrum of nervous system involvement in Behçet's syndrome and its differential diagnosis. *J Neurol* 2009;**256**:513–529.
129 Siva A, Altintas A, Saip S. Behcet's syndrome and the nervous system. *Curr Opin Neurol* 2004;**17**:347–357.
130 Gardner RC, Schmahmann JD. Ataxia and cerebellar atrophy—a novel manifestation of neuro-Behcet disease? *Mov Disord* 2008; **23**:307–308.
131 Matsuo K, Yamada K, Nakajima K, Nakagawa M. Neuro-Behcet disease mimicking brain tumor. *AJNR Am J Neuroradiol* 2005; **26**:650–653.
132 Huang WS, Chiu PY, Kao A, Tsai CH, Lee CC. Decreased cerebral blood flow in neuro-Behcet's syndrome patients with neuropsychiatric manifestations and normal magnetic resonance imaging—a preliminary report. *J Neuroimaging* 2002;**12**:355–359.
133 Harper CM, Jr., O'Neill BP, O'Duffy JD, Forbes GS. Intracranial hypertension in Behcet's disease: demonstration of sinus occlusion with use of digital subtraction angiography. *Mayo Clin Proc* 1985; **60**:419–422.
134 Siva A, Kantarci OH, Saip S, et al. Behcet's disease: diagnostic and prognostic aspects of neurological involvement. *J Neurol* 2001; **248**:95–103.
135 Hunder GG. Epidemiology of giant-cell arteritis. *Cleve Clin J Med* 2002;**69** Suppl 2:SII79–82.
136 Fraser JA, Weyand CM, Newman NJ, Biousse V. The treatment of giant cell arteritis. *Rev Neurol Dis* 2008;**5**(3):140–152.
137 Barrier J, Bignon JD, Soulillou JP, Grolleau J. Increased prevalence of HLA-DR4 in giant-cell arteritis. *N Engl J Med* 1981;**305**:104–105.
138 Hayreh SS, Podhajsky PA, Raman R, Zimmerman B. Giant cell arteritis: validity and reliability of various diagnostic criteria. *Am J Ophthalmol* 1997;**123**:285–296.
139 Klein RG, Hunder GG, Stanson AW, Sheps SG. Large artery involvement in giant cell (temporal) arteritis. *Ann Intern Med* 1975;**83**:806–812.
140 Evans JM, O'Fallon WM, Hunder GG. Increased incidence of aortic aneurysm and dissection in giant cell (temporal) arteritis. A population-based study. *Ann Intern Med* 1995;**122**:502–507.
141 Gonzalez-Gay MA, Blanco R, Rodriguez-Valverde V, et al. Permanent visual loss and cerebrovascular accidents in giant cell arteritis: predictors and response to treatment. *Arthritis Rheum* 1998;**41**:1497–1504.
142 Caselli RJ, Hunder GG, Whisnant JP. Neurologic disease in biopsy-proven giant cell (temporal) arteritis. *Neurology* 1988;**38**:352–359.
143 Pascuzzi RM, Roos KL, Davis TE, Jr. Mental status abnormalities in temporal arteritis: a treatable cause of dementia in the elderly. *Arthritis Rheum* 1989;**32**:1308–1311.
144 Small P. Giant cell arteritis presenting as a bilateral stroke. *Arthritis Rheum* 1984;**27**:819–821.
145 Solans-Laque R, Bosch-Gil JA, Molina-Catenario CA, Ortega-Aznar A, Alvarez-Sabin J, Vilardell-Tarres M. Stroke and multi-infarct dementia as presenting symptoms of giant cell arteritis: report of 7 cases and review of the literature. *Medicine (Baltimore)* 2008;**87**:335–344.
146 Lee MS, Smith SD, Galor A, Hoffman GS. Antiplatelet and anticoagulant therapy in patients with giant cell arteritis. *Arthritis Rheum* 2006;**54**:3306–3309.
147 Nesher G, Berkun Y, Mates M, Baras M, Rubinow A, Sonnenblick M. Low-dose aspirin and prevention of cranial ischemic complications in giant cell arteritis. *Arthritis Rheum* 2004;**50**:1332–1337.
148 Denton CP, Black CM. Targeted therapy comes of age in scleroderma. *Trends Immunol* 2005;**26**:596–602.
149 Nihtyanova SI, Tang EC, Coghlan JG, Wells AU, Black CM, Denton CP. Improved survival in systemic sclerosis is associated with better ascertainment of internal organ disease: a retrospective cohort study. *QJM*;**103**:109–115.
150 Shah AA, Wigley FM. Often forgotten manifestations of systemic sclerosis. *Rheum Dis Clin N Am* 2008;**34**:221–238.
151 Estey E, Lieberman A, Pinto R, Meltzer M, Ransohoff J. Cerebral arteritis in scleroderma. *Stroke* 1979;**10**:595–597.
152 Giuliodori G, Fraticelli P, Bartolini M, et al. Cognitive and cerebral hemodynamic impairment in scleroderma patients. *Eur J Neurol* 2009;**16**:1285–1290.
153 Hunninghake GW, Costabel U, Ando M, et al. ATS/ERS/WASOG statement on sarcoidosis. American Thoracic Society/European Respiratory Society/World Association of Sarcoidosis and other Granulomatous Disorders. *Sarcoidosis Vasc Diffuse Lung Dis* 1999; **16**:149–173.
154 Hosoda Y, Sasagawa S, Yasuda N. Epidemiology of sarcoidosis: new frontiers to explore. *Curr Opin Pulm Med* 2002;**8**:424–428.
155 Rybicki BA, Major M, Popovich J, Jr., Maliarik MJ, Iannuzzi MC. Racial differences in sarcoidosis incidence: a 5-year study in a health maintenance organization. *Am J Epidemiol* 1997;**145**:234–241.
156 Nowak DA, Widenka DC. Neurosarcoidosis: a review of its intracranial manifestation. *J Neurol* 2001;**248**:363–372.
157 Terushkin VBS, Stern BJMD, Judson MAMD, et al. Neurosarcoidosis: presentations and management. *Neurologist* 2010;**16**:2–15.
158 Hoitsma E, Faber CG, Drent M, Sharma OP. Neurosarcoidosis: a clinical dilemma. *Lancet Neurol* 2004;**3**:397–407.
159 Powers WJ, Miller EM. Sarcoidosis mimicking glioma: case report and review of intracranial sarcoid mass lesions. *Neurology* 1981; **31**:907–910.
160 Murialdo G, Tamagno G. Endocrine aspects of neurosarcoidosis. *J Endocrinol Invest* 2002;**25**:650–662.
161 Hayashi T, Onodera J, Nagata T, Mochizuki H, Itoyama Y. A case of biopsy-proven sarcoid meningoencephalitis presented with hallucination, nominal aphasia and dementia. *Rinsho Shinkeigaku* 1995; **35**:1008–1011.
162 O'Brien GM, Baughman R, Broderick JP. Paranoid psychosis due to neurosarcoidosis. *Sarcoidosis* 1994;**11**:34–36.
163 Bourgeois JA, Maddock RJ, Rogers L, Greco CM, Mangrulkar RS, Saint S. Neurosarcoidosis and delirium. *Psychosomatics* 2005;**46**:148–150.
164 Willigers H, Koehler PJ. Amnesic syndrome caused by neurosarcoidosis. *Clin Neurol Neurosurg* 1993;**95**:131–135.
165 Friedman SH, Gould DJ. Neurosarcoidosis presenting as psychosis and dementia: a case report. *Int J Psychiatry Med* 2002;**32**:401–403.
166 Zajicek JP, Scolding NJ, Foster O, et al. Central nervous system sarcoidosis—diagnosis and management. *QJM* 1999;**92**:103–117.
167 Sanders DS, Patel D, Stephenson TJ, et al. A primary care cross-sectional study of undiagnosed adult celiac disease. *Eur J Gastroenterol Hepatol* 2003;**15**:407–413.

168 West J, Logan RF, Hill PG, et al. Seroprevalence, correlates, and characteristics of undetected coeliac disease in England. *Gut* 2003;**52**:960–965.

169 Briani C, Zara G, Alaedini A, et al. Neurological complications of celiac disease and autoimmune mechanisms: A prospective study. *J Neuroimmunol* 2008;**195**:171–175.

170 Hadjivassiliou M, Sanders DS, Grünewald RA, Woodroofe N, Boscolo S, Aeschlimann D. Gluten sensitivity: from gut to brain. *Lancet Neurol* 2010;**9**:318–330.

171 Collin P, Pirttila T, Nurmikko T, Somer H, Erila T, Keyrilainen O. Celiac disease, brain atrophy, and dementia. *Neurology* 1991;**41**: 372–375.

172 Addolorato G, Giuda DD, Rossi GD, et al. Regional cerebral hypoperfusion in patients with celiac disease. *Am J Med* 2004; **116**:312–317.

173 Hu WT, Murray JA, Greenaway MC, Parisi JE, Josephs KA. Cognitive impairment and celiac disease. *Arch Neurol* 2006; **63**:1440–1446.

174 Hadjivassiliou M, Grunewald RA, Kandler RH, et al. Neuropathy associated with gluten sensitivity. *J Neurol Neurosurg Psychiatry* 2006;**77**:1262–1266.

175 Collin P, Maki M, Kaukinen K. Safe gluten threshold for patients with celiac disease: some patients are more tolerant than others. *Am J Clin Nutr* 2007;**86**:260; author reply 260-261.

176 Schuppan D, Junker Y, Barisani D. Celiac disease: from pathogenesis to novel therapies. *Gastroenterology* 2009;**137**:1912–1933.

177 Stroop JR. Studies of interference in serial verbal reactions. *J Exp Psychol* 1935;**18**:643–662.

178 Golden CJ. *Stroop Color and Word Test*. Chicago, IL: Stoelting, 1978.

179 Trenerry MR, Crosson B, DeBoe J, Leber WR. *Stroop Neuropsychological Screening Test*. Florida: Psychological Assessment Resources, 1989.

180 Dodrill CB. A neuropsychological battery for epilepsy. *Epilepsia* 1978;**19**:611–623.

181 Spreen O, Strauss E. *A Compendium of Neuropsychological Tests: Administration, Norms, and Commentary*, Second ed. New York: Oxford University Press, 1998.

182 Army Individual Test Battery: *Manual of Directions and Scoring*. Washington, DC: War Department, Adjutant General's Office, 1944.

183 Wechsler D. *Wechsler Adult Intelligence Scale—Third Edition*. San Antonio: Psychological Corporation, 1997.

184 Delis D, Kramer J, Kaplan E, Ober B. *California Verbal Learning Test Manual: Second Edition, Adult Version*. San Antonio, TX: Psychological Corporation, 2000.

185 Rey A. *L'examen clinique in psychologie*. Paris: Presses Universitaires de France, 1964.

186 Corwin J, Bylsma FW. "Psychological examination of traumatic encephalopathy" by A. Rey and "The Complex Figure Copy Test" by P.A. Osterreith. *Clin Neuropsychol* 1993;**7**:3–21.

187 Spreen O, Benton AL. *Neurosensory Center Comprehensive Examination for Aphasia (NCCEA)*. Victoria: University of Victoria Neuropsychology Laboratory, 1977.

188 Blair JR, Spreen O. Predicting premorbid IQ: a revision of the national adult reading test. *Clin Neuropsychol* 1989;**3**:129–136.

189 Lezak MD. *Neuropsychological assessment (3rd edition)*. New York: Oxford University Press, 1995.

CHAPTER 15

Comprehensive management of the patient with an atypical dementia

Jennifer Merrilees[1], Cynthia Barton[1], Amy Kuo[2] and Robin Ketelle[1]
[1] University of California, San Francisco, San Francisco, CA, USA
[2] On Lok Lifeways, San Francisco, CA, USA

After the diagnosis

The management of a patient with an atypical dementia presents a variety of challenges to health-care providers. Such patients often have diverse symptoms and uncommon clinical presentations, which can lead to incorrect diagnoses and delay appropriate treatment. By the time a correct diagnosis is obtained, the family might have spent months or even years searching for answers from various providers. This can result in significant financial and emotional stress, leaving families closer to crisis with urgent need of resources. Health-care providers, therefore, need to be aware of these issues when managing atypical dementia patients and their families.

This chapter identifies issues pertinent to the management of patients diagnosed with an atypical dementia, although most topics discussed here are common to many dementias. Key considerations (functional changes, safety concerns, and psychosocial adjustments) for specific diseases and issues to consider for promoting caregiver health and coping are discussed. A partial list of resources for patients and families also is provided in Appendix 15.2.

Evaluating functional abilities

Functional skills are traditionally divided into two broad categories—instrumental activities of daily living (IADLs) and basic activities of daily living (ADLs). IADLs include complex tasks of managing finances, working, driving, providing childcare, managing medications, and household duties. ADLs encompass basic abilities of dressing, hygiene, walking, and eating. Each dementia syndrome has a variable impact on functional abilities. For example, the patient with dementia with Lewy bodies (DLB) might be unable to cook safely or manage bill paying due to visuospatial deficits and executive dysfunction rather than the short-term memory loss associated with typical Alzheimer's disease (AD). In most dementias, capacity for instrumental tasks is typically affected first, and basic skills are affected later in the disease course.

Changes in the patient's cognition, insight, and judgment create challenges in obtaining an accurate functional assessment [1]. For this reason, the majority of functional assessment scales rely on ratings by an informant (someone knowledgeable about the patient, typically a family member or caregiver). In atypical cases or when there is not an informant, direct observation of ADL performance may be helpful. Validated measures include the Assessment of Motor and Process Skills (AMPS) [1], the Kohlman Evaluation of Living Skills (KELS) [2], and the Texas Functional Living Scale [3].

Vulnerability and safety

Multiple issues contribute to a patient's vulnerability regarding safety issues, and it is necessary to periodically review risk factors as they can change over the course of the illness. Common concerns involve driving, communication, judgment and decision-making, and the impact of neuropsychiatric symptoms on personal and social conduct. Patient and caregivers might lack insight about potential hazards and can better prepare for the future with appropriate anticipatory education. Discussions often center on issues of maintaining patient autonomy while simultaneously ensuring safety. Table 15.1 lists common areas of concern along with examples of interventions.

Occupational issues for the patient and caregiver

Compromised work performance common in atypical dementias can occur for a variety of reasons. Patients with Huntington's disease (HD) might be unable to work due to emotional liability,

Non-Alzheimer's and Atypical Dementia, First Edition. Edited by Michael D. Geschwind and Caroline Racine Belkoura.
© 2016 John Wiley & Sons, Ltd. Published 2016 by John Wiley & Sons, Ltd.

Table 15.1 Safety concerns.

Risk areas	Suggested interventions
Legal and financial decision-making	1. Complete advance directive and power of attorney forms early in the disease while patient is able to articulate his or her wishes 2. Organize a family meeting perhaps facilitated by social worker or counselor 3. Refer family to financial advisor and/or attorney with expertise in legal and financial issues 4. Have patient carry only a limited amount of cash 5. Establish restrictions on the amount of money that can be withdrawn from bank accounts 6. Block junk mail and solicitations if patient is vulnerable to scams 7. Divert mail to a post office box to prevent delivery to the home 8. Use caregiver cell phone as primary phone number in order to prevent patient receiving calls at home 9. Maintain duplicates of driver's license, birth certificate, and/or passport 10. Conservatorship might be necessary
Driving	1. Determine whether patient should be evaluated with written/road testing. Follow local guidelines on whether reporting and testing are mandatory or voluntary (in the United States, rules vary by state: http://www.nhtsa.gov/people/injury/olddrive/OlderDriversBook/index.html) 2. Disable or sell the patient's car 3. Arrange transportation/rides for the patient
Social misconduct	1. Limit patient's access to the public, that is, go to restaurants during times that are less busy, position patient away from the public, and/or avoid heavily populated areas such as parks and shopping centers 2. Provide 1 : 1 supervision 3. Many families benefit from carrying business-size cards or letters from the provider containing a brief statement that the person suffers from a condition that affects their behavior and judgment. These cards and letters can be passed to others as a form of explanation for the patient's inappropriate behavior. See Appendix 15.1 for an example
Communication and comprehension deficits	1. Patient should wear MedicAlert® type of identification 2. Notes and signs might be helpful for the patient 3. Provide physical cuing in addition to verbal instructions 4. Provide a letter from the patient's provider and/or business-size cards with a brief explanation of how the illness affects communication and comprehension 5. Provide 1 : 1 supervision 6. Referral to speech therapist
Getting lost	1. Patient should wear a Safe Return®/MedicAlert® bracelet type of identification (http://www.alz.org/safetycenter/we_can_help_safety_medicalert_safereturn.asp) 2. Caregiver should have an up-to-date photograph of the patient that can be provided to authorities in the event patient becomes lost. A cell phone with camera is an easy way to maintain a current photograph

irritability, or depression, whereas patients with frontotemporal dementia (FTD) might have decreased performance secondary to social misconduct or executive dysfunction. The language and speech deficits common in progressive aphasias may interfere with comprehension and effective communication.

Patients with dementia often stop working much earlier than they intended. This has repercussions beyond income; non-working individuals no longer make contributions into social security and retirement plans and might lose employer-sponsored health insurance. Additionally, family caregivers might have to enter or return to the work force or, conversely, not be able to work due to their caregiving responsibilities. Some caregivers assume the responsibility of managing a business on the patient's behalf to maintain financial solvency and contractual obligations. Families sometimes deplete their savings or retirement accounts to cover the costs involved in caring for a family member with dementia.

Occupational concerns can be addressed during the initial evaluation. Patients and family members might not be aware of performance issues. In some cases, families prefer that the patient continue working out of a desire for income or concern about the effect of job loss on self-esteem. Some patients enjoy a supportive work environment in which colleagues cover for the patient's reduced work performance or have supervisors who are willing to make appropriate accommodations to allow the patient to perform modified duties. A realistic and pragmatic approach to employment is recommended, given that patients might be putting themselves, their families, and their employers or clients at legal and/or financial risk.

Providing assistance with a disability application or the retirement process might be necessary. Families will need to identify whether the patient is eligible for Social Security Disability Insurance (SSDI) and Supplemental Security Income (SSI) in the United States or equivalent in other countries. Health-care providers are typically asked by governmental support agencies to provide documentation of the patient's expected progressive deficits and reasons why certain work is not feasible. Health-care providers can also provide counseling resources to facilitate decision-making regarding family caregivers returning to work. In some situations, families might be eligible for medical leave in order to care for the patient. In some countries or US states, certain diagnoses allow for automatic disability.

When a patient's occupational capacity is compromised, it may be possible for them to contribute in volunteer or work-related tasks that match their functional level. For example, patients with rigid and obsessive habits (e.g., FTD) might be able to sort objects (and may excel at such tasks).

Managing motor symptoms

Gait instability and falls

Motor symptoms (e.g., poor balance, falls, coordination deficits, rigidity, slowed movements, and supranuclear gaze palsy) are early symptoms in some atypical dementias, and almost all the dementias are associated with some motor impairment near the end of the disease course. Due to the high prevalence of falls in atypical dementia conditions, safety and fall prevention must always be a primary concern. Home safety assessments should be performed to identify potential safety hazards in the home and appropriate safety modifications (e.g., safe footwear choices, flooring, nonskid rugs, and grab bars) should be implemented. One-to-one care might be required, especially in bathrooms. Electronic room monitors such as those used for infants can assess auditory or visual information, allowing caregivers to monitor the patient's activity in another room. Emergency notification systems (e.g., LifeAlert®) might also be necessary, either on the walls or worn by the patient. A variety of assistive devices can be used to help steady the gait. Four-wheeled walkers have been shown to provide increased stability to patients with gait problems [4, 5]. Patients with impulsivity might require one-to-one supervision and can also be encouraged to wear a safety helmet to prevent head injury. In a study of patients with Parkinson's disease, performing cognitive tasks while walking was associated with changes in stride and balance that increased the risk for falling [6], suggesting that multitasking while walking should be discouraged.

Exercise is an important component of maintaining strength and balance. Patients should be encouraged to work with a physical therapist or personal trainer and to exercise a few times per week (e.g., active cardiovascular exercise 30 min three times per week mixed with strength training). Additional measures, such as massage and gentle yoga, might improve range of motion, flexibility, and balance [7].

Dysphagia

Dysphagia (difficulty swallowing liquids, food, and/or saliva) is commonly associated with advanced stages of dementia. Consequences of dysphagia include weight loss (due to the difficulty in meeting caloric and nutritional requirements) and aspiration (the inhalation of food or fluid into the lungs) pneumonia. Managing dysphagia in conjunction with other disease symptoms can be challenging. For example, patients with behavioral variant frontotemporal dementia (bvFTD) often exhibit hyperorality, characterized by food craving, eating past satiety, consuming large amounts of food without proper swallowing techniques, and impulsivity. Hyperorality, alone, presents a risk for aspiration but becomes exceptionally hazardous when coupled with dysphagia.

The initial step in managing potential dysphagia is to obtain a swallowing evaluation by a speech (and swallowing) therapist to determine which mechanisms are contributing to swallowing deficits and outline strategies to minimize the risk of aspiration. Strategies often include modifying food and liquid choices, strict supervision at mealtimes, limiting distractions while eating, cutting up food in smaller pieces, proper positioning of the patient during feeding and drinking, limiting the amount of oral medications, and a schedule for checking weight (for more information, see http://youtu.be/H6ooxyGpj4o and http://youtu.be/6Fv9B4t9L8A).

Managing behavioral symptoms

Behavioral symptoms are very common in dementia and manifest in ways often specific to the type of dementia. For example, visual hallucinations are common early in DLB and Parkinson's disease with dementia (PDD) but might occur in late stages of AD and are uncommon in most other dementias. Management of problematic behaviors can be one of the most challenging aspects of caring for a patient with dementia. Employing an "Antecedent, Behavior, and Consequences (ABC)" method of assessment is helpful in the assessment and management of behavioral symptoms [8]. The "A" refers to the potential triggers for the behavior. Examples could include pain or environmental demands exceeding patient tolerance. The "B" refers to the behavior and should be described in specific terms. For example, "Walks up and stands uncomfortably close to strangers and touches their shoulders" is more specific than "is embarrassing in public." The "C" refers to consequences following the behavior. For example, did the response by the caregiver improve the behavior? An assessment of behavioral symptoms should always include identification of the onset of the behavior as abrupt changes might reflect medical illness (e.g., a urinary tract infection), pain, or side effect from medication, rather than an expected feature of advancing disease.

Generally, there are four categories of interventions designed to manage behavioral symptoms ranging from least restrictive to the most restrictive. The first, and least restrictive, type of intervention involves modifications to the patient's environment. Scheduling activities at a certain time of day more suitable to the patient's tolerance, removing visually disruptive objects from the house, and simplifying communication to enhance comprehension are examples of environmental modifications. The second type of intervention is behavioral modification.

Some examples include distraction from an inappropriate behavior toward a more acceptable activity or providing a reward for more acceptable behavior. The third category of intervention involves strategies internal to the caregiver, such as coaching the caregiver to accept that the behaviors are an expected feature of the disease. The fourth, and most restrictive, type of intervention involves chemical or physical restraints. Although medications might treat specific behavioral symptoms, there are many instances in which a medication is not appropriate, is ineffective, and/or is associated with negative side effects. Polypharmacy and the inappropriate use of medications often potentiate many behavioral symptoms [9]. Physical restraints frequently are associated with negative consequences for patients and should also be avoided whenever possible.

An individualized assessment of the behavior(s) and the creation of tailored interventions have the best chance of success at ameliorating the negative impact of symptoms. New models of care have been proposed and include dyadic interventions with patients and caregivers or referrals to experts in managing behavioral symptoms [10]. Setting appropriate and realistic goals is another critical feature. A reasonable goal might be a reduction in the severity of the behavior and/or the caregiver experiencing reduced levels of distress, rather than a goal of eliminating the behavior entirely. A frequent reassessment of behaviors and interventions (including medications) is required, as prior behaviors often will disappear over the course of the disease, whereas other new behaviors might arise that require different interventions.

Care across the disease trajectory

It is inevitable that families will require assistance to provide care. Formal (paid) and informal (unpaid and typically refers to care provided by family) support is usually needed and may include hiring caregivers from an agency, enrolling in adult day programs, or identifying facilities for placement. The majority of these services were established for frail elders, and finding a good "fit" for younger individuals or those with challenging physical or behavioral symptoms is often difficult. Working with a placement advisor or local disease associations to identify resources that can meet the needs of these populations may be helpful.

End-of-life care

The most common cause of death in atypical dementias is similar to those in other forms of dementia, usually complications related to aspiration and immobility. Problems with swallowing and movement occur earlier in many of the atypical dementias and therefore contribute to an earlier morbidity and mortality [11]. A discussion of end-of-life choices should occur early in the disease course to capitalize on the patient's ability to participate in decision-making. Establishing a durable power of attorney (DPOA) and identifying personal preferences are a critical first step in this process.

The introduction of a palliative approach to care can also be addressed with the patient and family at various times along the course of the illness [12]. A palliative approach covers everything from counseling to caregiver respite and attention to symptom management and thus may ensure a more peaceful passing by allowing families to avoid the psychological stress of involving emergency services at the time of death. Due to the complexity and rarity of some of these conditions, however, arranging palliative care can be a challenge [13].

Patients might not be deemed eligible for hospice care due to the differences between their conditions and more common dementias. The motor and behavioral components of HD, progressive supranuclear palsy (PSP), and corticobasal degeneration (CBD) might complicate the referral in that patients may still benefit from ongoing physical therapy for comfort reasons but also need concurrent hospice care. Providers should provide support and documentation to facilitate appropriate referrals. The National Hospice and Palliative Care Organization has a helpful website for resources (www.nhpco.org).

Autopsy decisions

Neuropathological diagnosis can be helpful to clinicians and family members after death in cases of atypical dementia. This diagnostic confirmation can serve as closure for family members who have struggled with the disease for years. For clinicians, it provides a determinative correlation between the clinical syndrome and specific neuropathological findings. Brain autopsy can be sensitively included in any end-of-life decision-making session with the family [14]. See videos about what is involved in, and the benefits are of, an autopsy: http://youtu.be/_yL2OlkuNSc and http://youtu.be/q1wXypAlAEQ).

Key considerations for the clinical management of atypical dementias

Atypical AD

Functional changes

Atypical AD refers to a disease in which memory loss is not the predominant deficit at presentation and/or when the disease occurs in people under the age of 65 (see Chapter 3 for review). This includes early-onset Alzheimer's disease (EOAD) affecting those under the age of 65, as well as patients in whom symptoms are associated with changes in the frontal or more posterior lobes—frontal variant AD (FAD) or posterior cortical atrophy (PCA).

The changes associated with these atypical dementias have particular implications for care. Patients with EOAD often have earlier and increased relative impairment in the domains of attention [15], language [16], and visuospatial abilities [17].

Because these deficits result in greater effects on working, driving, and other instrumental tasks, EOAD carries special significance for occupational and family issues. The executive deficits in the FAD patient produce more functional impairment than typical AD [18]. PCA has been associated with EOAD [17], and the significant visuospatial deficits impair basic function early in the disease. Patients may see several eye specialists before diagnosis; unfortunately, traditional visual aids are not helpful as it is not a problem with visual acuity.

The younger age of onset predicts an increased need for ADL assistance, and progression of EOAD is more rapid with higher rates of institutionalization than in typical AD [19]; therefore, careful attention to providing training to in-home caregivers or incorporating in-home help early may be necessary.

Safety concerns

The visual impairments associated with PCA and executive impairments in FAD put these individuals at particular risk for unsafe behaviors. Home safety evaluations are necessary to provide specific alterations to minimize risk and encourage independence.

Psychosocial adjustments

Patients with EOAD and their families are often contending with traditional midlife issues such as caring for aging parents, caring for children, and planning for retirement while also managing the symptoms of a neurodegenerative disease. FAD patients often have more neuropsychiatric symptoms, and caregivers report more stress than typical AD [18, 20]. Younger children might become the primary caregiver for a parent or might lose a parent at a critical time. Targeted support groups or referrals to individual therapists may provide more personalized family-oriented approach in these cases [21, 22]. Strategies for modifying the environment have been developed to assist in management (http://memory.ucsf.edu/caregiving/tips#safety).

Vascular dementia

Functional changes

Vascular dementia (VaD) refers to cognitive impairment from strokes and/or cerebrovascular disease (see Chapter 4). The degree of impairment depends on the extent of disease and specific regions affected, and interventions should be targeted to an individual's symptoms. For example, patients with a stroke or ischemic vascular disease in the frontal lobes might show behavioral impulsivity and need interventions to manage these issues, whereas someone with occipital involvement might need more visuospatial assistance. Motor impairment is common in VaD, tends to occur earlier in the disease process than in AD, and requires earlier intervention and activation of supportive services. Autonomic dysfunction (fatigue, urinary symptoms, constipation, and postural dizziness) is also common, leading to increased fall risk and a greater need for ADL and IADL assistance [23].

Patients with VaD typically have less anomia than patients with AD [24], and speech may be easier to understand [25]. They also have been reported to have preserved insight about their condition [26] and therefore might benefit from verbal activities and support groups.

Safety concerns

In VaD, impairments may be global or focal depending on the location of injury, so there is not one consistent functional profile [27]. Families often report more fluctuation in cognition than in AD [28], and this variability requires flexibility in approach. Deficits in attention, speed of processing, and executive function [29] may present specific safety concerns, especially in regard to driving and independent function. The frequency of gait and balance disorders in VaD increases the risk for falls [30]. Providers can consider referral for balance and gait training, encourage more ambulation, and assess for appropriateness of assistive devices.

Psychosocial adjustments

Although neuropsychiatric profiles in VaD overlap with other dementias, there is an increased risk of depression in VaD [31, 32]. Assessment and treatment of depression and other neuropsychiatric symptoms (e.g., anxiety), including therapy, support group, and medications, should be considered. Some studies report more sleep disturbance in patients with cortical VaD than in AD or subcortical VaD [33]. Attention to proper sleep hygiene including maintenance of day/night rhythms through a structured daily routine and minimizing daytime napping is important.

FTD (behavioral variant)

Functional changes

bvFTD presents with early and prominent changes in behavior, emotion, and personality (see Chapter 5). Compared to the other FTD subtypes and typical AD, bvFTD is associated with more severe and rapid impairment in functional abilities [34]. The loss of a job, inability to master new tasks, personality conflicts with coworkers or employers, and difficulty in keeping up with executive responsibilities are often some of the first signs of the illness. Function around the home often declines; patients might participate less with chores and exhibit a lower standard of personal hygiene and clothing selection while demonstrating little concern for these changes. Patients with profound apathy often exhibit a complete loss of concern or initiative in maintaining hygiene. FTD can occur concomitantly with ALS [35], causing a more rapid decline [11, 36].

Safety concerns

The ability to engage responsibly in certain activities typically is compromised in bvFTD. For example, driving skills, supervision of children, participation in finances, and legal planning are commonly affected. Due to loss of insight, patients typically do not acknowledge how troubling the behavioral changes are

Table 15.2 Assessment of caregiver health and coping.

Domain	Method
Caregiver strain	The Modified Caregiver Strain Index (CSI) from the Try This series at http://consultgerirn.org/resources [101]
Caregiver depression	Geriatric Depression Screen from the Try This series at http://consultgerirn.org/resources
Caregiver burden	Zarit Burden Interview (ZBI) [102]

to others nor do they show remorse for the negative consequences of their actions.

Psychosocial adjustments

Patients with bvFTD typically exhibit diminished empathy, increased self-centeredness, and apathy, with little or no insight into these changes. It can take several years from symptom onset to obtain a proper diagnosis [37]. Even with the diagnosis, families are often not able to get targeted assistance because of the lack of knowledge about the disorder [38, 39].

The disease has a negative impact on the quality of relationships. Although research suggests there is great variation among FTD caregivers in terms of their psychological well-being [40], FTD caregivers have described a diminished closeness, communication, and ability to get along with the patient with FTD [41] and often have anger and a sense of isolation [42]. FTD caregivers report lower marital satisfaction compared to AD caregivers [43]. FTD caregivers also report higher burden levels and lower levels of competency compared to caregivers of patients with AD [44, 45].

Semantic variant FTD

Functional changes

Semantic variant (SV) FTD is associated with bilateral anterior temporal lobe atrophy (left more than right) and manifests with fluent aphasia and a loss of word comprehension and semantic knowledge [46, 47] (see Chapter 5). Patients with predominantly left-sided disease often exhibit visual preoccupations (bright objects or shapes) and compulsions [48]. Other cognitive functions (episodic and visual memory, spatial abilities and navigation, and executive abilities) are typically spared [49, 50]. Function at home is often not affected in the earlier disease stages; although the patient might be unable to name a household object, they typically demonstrate correct use of the item [47].

When SV FTD predominantly affects the right temporal lobe, behavioral changes similar to bvFTD manifest. These changes include loss of empathy, insight, rigidity and adoption of compulsive routines, and constitutional complaints [48, 51, 52]. Patients might develop fixations and verbal compulsions (word games and puns) [48], often spending hours engaged in these activities while ignoring other responsibilities.

Safety concerns

Safety concerns for patients with semantic dementia relate to the progressive deficits in language, comprehension, and social comportment. Patients might develop parsimonious beliefs and develop compulsions for collecting things. In our clinical experience, communication deficits have placed patients in vulnerable situations when they are caught taking items without paying. Many patients have been unable to provide a coherent explanation for their actions, resulting in law enforcement becoming involved. Suggested interventions to prevent negative sequelae from these behaviors are provided in Table 15.1.

The adoption of rigid compulsions and food fads [50] create challenges in maintaining adequate weight and nutrition. Interventions include providing frequent meals, ready access to food, and altering one's expectations about the patients eating habits. Patients might also develop heightened somatic complaints. These sensations create challenges in identification of what is a real medical problem and what is not. In some cases, patients lose the ability to process important environmental cues, such as high temperatures and other painful stimuli. Examples include patients sitting in the sun without adequate protection or reaching for dishes from the oven without protective mitts.

In advanced stages, patients might be unable to distinguish food from nonfood items, mistakenly putting nonedible items in their mouth. They might no longer handle hazardous items safely. Locking up potential household dangers (e.g., knives, cleansers, and chemicals) is critical.

Psychosocial adjustments

Patients with right-sided brain disease lose the ability to read social cues and sometimes act inconsiderately [50]. These interpersonal and social changes can be a source of frustration, embarrassment, and helplessness for caregivers, who often benefit from counseling or participation with a support group and should be encouraged to seek respite from caregiving.

Lewy body disorders: DLB and PDD

Functional changes

Lewy body disorders (LBDs) (DLB and PDD) have prominent parkinsonism, autonomic dysfunction, fluctuating cognition, and frequent neuropsychiatric symptoms that can have an early negative impact on functional abilities [53, 54] (see Chapter 6). The extrapyramidal symptoms and autonomic dysfunction contribute to rigidity, gait instability, and syncope, increasing risk of falls and making care particularly demanding [23, 53]. In the early stages, patients with DLB have visuospatial, executive, and attention deficits [55] with a relative sparing of memory and language [56]; this often necessitates coaching and direction to carry out activities. Caregivers should be encouraged to use strategies, such as breaking tasks down into simple steps, removing distractions, and providing frequent rest breaks, as these individuals are particularly prone to daytime fatigue. Fluctuations in cognition and arousal are common and unpredictable, during which it may be difficult for patients to perform particular tasks. To the extent possible, important tasks should be performed during "optimal" periods of clarity. Occupational and physical therapy can both be helpful.

Safety concerns

Visuospatial and memory difficulties contribute to patients getting lost. Attention to lighting, bold signs, and barriers can aid in guiding the individual to proper paths. Refer to Table 15.1 for strategies.

Falls are a significant risk due to autonomic, gait, and balance dysfunction [23]. Interventions include safety evaluations at home, and physical therapy and exercise are appropriate while preserved memory allows participation. Assistive devices such as walkers can be helpful in maintaining safe ambulation.

Swallowing difficulty is common early in the disease and is not solely determined by severity of dementia or parkinsonism [53, 57]. Families need education about this early in the disease course, and patients should be referred for a formal swallowing evaluation, even at baseline evaluation. Changes in sleep patterns, including the occurrence of REM sleep behavior disorder (RBD), occur early in LBDs [53, 58] and often precede other symptoms by years or decades. These changes often result in diminished sleep for the caregiver. Interventions include psychopharmacological (i.e., clonazepam), daytime napping together, sleeping in separate bedrooms, or hiring a caregiver to supervise patient care needs at night allowing the family member to sleep uninterrupted.

Psychosocial adjustments

Common neuropsychiatric symptoms in LBDs include apathy, purposeless hyperactivity, depression, anxiety, and visual hallucinations [59]. These symptoms are often quite troublesome for patients and the caregivers, although the visual hallucinations are usually benign and nonthreatening. Delusions and hallucinations persist over the trajectory of the disease [60]. The Capgras misidentification syndrome, in which a spouse is thought by the patient to be an imposter, is particularly disturbing for spouse caregivers. Caregivers need reassurance that this is a symptom of the disease and is most successfully dealt with by not directly confronting the delusion but instead distracting the individual or redirecting the conversation. Caregivers of those with DLB are significantly more stressed than AD [54]; this may be due to functional impairment, isolation, behavioral symptoms, delays in obtaining the correct diagnosis, and/or limited access to resources [59, 61]. As the course of DLB may be rapid and the presence of autonomic dysfunction may predict poorer survival, early consideration of hospice and discussion of advanced directives should be encouraged [62].

CBD, corticobasal syndrome, and PSP

Functional changes

PSP and CBD/corticobasal syndrome (CBS) have effects on both motor and cognitive function (see Chapter 7). In addition, language and communication difficulties are common. These disorders pose unique challenges for caregivers. Functional decline in the motor domain may be more rapid than the decline in cognitive function, and therefore, physical exercise, physical therapy, and gait training may be employed as early interventions. Language and communication impairments might require attention and intervention earlier than in typical AD. Communication interventions including communication boards, computer-assisted devices, and notebooks for written communication may be helpful.

Safety concerns

Patients with CBD and PSP often have motor impairments that lead to frequent falls or household accidents. Fall prevention should be a high priority in their care. Impulsivity occurs frequently in PSP and increases fall risk. Swallowing problems emerge at any stage and should be assessed early.

Psychosocial adjustments

Depression is common in both PSP and CBD/CBS [63] and apathy is a hallmark of PSP [64]. Apathy can be misinterpreted as depression or might present concurrently with other behavioral symptoms. Realizing that apathy is a feature of the disease, rather than a willful emotional rejection or lack of interest, might help caregivers to cope with the behavior [64]. In PSP, pseudobulbar affect (PBA), uncontrollable laughing or crying, can be distressing for caregivers and patients alike, causing embarrassment. Caregivers might erroneously interpret the uncontrolled crying as a sign of depression. Medication such as the combination of dextromethorphan HBr and quinidine sulfate might be helpful in treating this symptom [65]. Language problems that occur in CBS have been associated with caregiver burden [66].

HD

Functional changes

Functional loss in HD results from a combination of motor, cognitive, and psychiatric symptoms [67, 68] (see Chapter 8). The earliest functional deficits in HD occur in occupational capacity, with 65.1% of patients reporting some loss in their ability to work (unable to continue with usual work, manage gainful employment, and/or engage in volunteer activities). At home, these individuals may be unable to manage finances, drive safely, supervise children, shop independently, perform household chores, or prepare meals [67]. Obsessive and compulsive behaviors occur in 20–50% of patients with HD [69], and those with higher severity of symptoms have lower functional capacity and greater duration of illness [70]. Early depressive symptoms are also associated with a more rapid functional decline [71]. Disruption in the sleep–wake cycle is a common problem, particularly in the later stages of disease with deleterious effects on the function and on quality of life factors for both the patient and the caregiver [72]. Motor symptoms typically involve chorea, bradykinesia, dystonia, and rigidity with varying impacts on disability [73]. Increased severity of motor symptoms is associated with decision to institutionalize, although psychosis and behavioral symptoms also contribute to this decision [74].

Safety concerns

The neuropsychiatric and cognitive manifestations of HD affect judgment and decision-making; thus, attention to safety concerns is critical. Patients with HD often exhibit irritability, anxiety, depression, disinhibition, aggression, and/or hostility [75–77]; they also typically underestimate their deficits in executive function and have overall impaired insight regarding their symptoms [78]. Perhaps due to a combination of their lack of insight and their impulsivity, patients with HD have an increased risk of suicide that is four to six times higher than the general population [79]. The highest risk periods are the time preceding predictive testing [80], immediately before receiving the formal diagnosis of HD, and in early disease stages characterized by diminished functional independence [81], mandating careful and consistent screening for depression and suicide risk.

A lower body mass index has been reported in early disease stages, which is independent of a hyperkinetic movement disorder [82]. Dysphagia (involuntary movements) and a hypermetabolic state create variable challenges in maintaining a healthy weight [83, 84]. The assistance of a speech therapist and dietician can be helpful in developing strategies for addressing weight loss. Multiple environmental strategies can be used to maintain adequate nutrition and safe swallowing [85].

Psychosocial adjustments

Adult family caregivers of patients with HD describe the emotional experience as "disintegration of the caregiver's life" and "the loss of life as it was." Additionally, spouses report distress over the loss of intimacy with their partners [86]. Caregivers often experience fatigue and loneliness and neglect their own needs as a result of their caregiving responsibilities [87, 88].

Emotional and ethical dilemmas exist regarding reproductive decision-making. Caregivers have expressed concern regarding the "ever-present shadow" of their children's risk for developing HD [86]; thus, genetic counseling is a critical part of care for patients and families. A review by Klitzman et al. provides sample questions and an interview guide for exploring reproductive decision-making in families at risk for HD [89].

Creutzfeldt–Jakob disease

Functional changes

In the early stages, patients usually are still relatively independent in their ADLs and can present with the following deficits (in descending order of frequency): cognitive, cerebellar, behavioral, constitutional, sensory, motor, and visual [90] (see Chapter 9). As the disease progresses, new symptoms can present abruptly as patients continue to lose cognitive and motor function. Mobility, bowel and bladder control, and the ability to communicate are eventually lost; and in the end stages of Creutzfeldt–Jakob disease (CJD), patients become bedbound, mute, and akinetic. With the loss of swallowing and gag mechanisms, the vast majority of CJD patients eventually succumb to aspiration pneumonia. Except for minor fluctuations, families generally should expect to see the same rate of decline as they observed early in the course, although periods of temporary stabilization occur. As with other dementias, if sudden, dramatic declines are seen, other causes such as secondary infection should be explored.

Safety concerns

New symptoms might present on a weekly if not daily basis; therefore, safety issues should be addressed in an anticipatory fashion. The involvement of hospice early in the disease course can help families plan ahead for safety, caregiving, and end-of-life needs, particularly as this disease usually progresses with great rapidity. With the overwhelming risk of aspiration pneumonia, it is recommended that CJD patients be evaluated frequently by a speech therapist. At a minimum, patients should have an early evaluation with instructions for managing worsening swallowing as the disease progresses. Families should be observant of when the patient experiences increased difficulty swallowing, excessive coughing during meals, and more obvious signs of choking. These can serve as helpful indicators of advancing disease. When aspiration risk increases, general precautions include having patients sit completely upright, either with their chins tucked or if this is not possible, then with their chins extended when food or drink is being placed in the mouth. As liquids go down more quickly and more likely to lead to aspiration, they might need to be thickened to a honey consistency using such products as Thicket®. Food might need to be cut in small pieces and eventually pureed. If there is difficulty consuming pills or tablets, they might be crushed (if allowable) in oatmeal, pudding, ice cream, or pureed foods to facilitate swallowing.

Caregivers should be reassured that the person-to-person transmissibility of CJD is extremely unlikely and has occurred only iatrogenically or through endocannibalism. Touching, kissing, and other forms of intimacy are not considered a risk for transmission; however, universal precautions should be applied when managing bodily fluids or secretions.

When dealing with invasive medical procedures, medical personnel should be informed that the patient has CJD so that appropriate precautions are utilized. For more information on managing patients with CJD, please see videos at http://www.youtube.com/playlist?list=PLD1F21FF7C31F8659. Affected individuals and any at-risk family members (from known genetic prion families or from families with CJD in whom genetic testing has not been performed) should refrain from donating blood products due to theoretical risk of transmission (although there is a real risk for variant CJD; Chapter 9).

Psychosocial adjustments

The experience of caregivers for patients with CJD is unique among the atypical dementias due to its rapid course. Median survival is approximately 5–7 months, and 90% of patients survive less than 1 year; thus, families have little or no time to adapt to both the logistical and psychological aspects of caring for their affected loved ones [90].

Caregiver health and coping

Family members provide the bulk of care for patients with dementia. Although caregiver responsibilities exist on a continuum, there is more to the experience than task-related responsibilities. Many atypical dementias manifest with less familiar symptoms (e.g., personality, behavioral, or psychiatric changes) than are associated with typical dementias, and therefore, it can be difficult to accept that the person has a neurodegenerative disorder. The abrupt entry into the caregiving role is associated with negative well-being for caregivers [91]. Several studies show evidence of caregiver dissatisfaction with resources for conditions such as FTD [38, 39], HD [92], and DLB [59]. Without resources targeting their specific needs, these caregivers face the danger of "falling through the net" [93].

Dementia caregiving exacts a physical and emotional toll on family caregivers [94, 95]. Specific factors have been associated with negative outcomes for the caregiver including younger age [96, 97], being female [98, 99], and poorer quality of the premorbid relationship [100]. It is important to note that dementia caregivers may ascribe positive benefits of caregiving. They may describe success and mastery in managing difficult situations and learning new skills. Caregivers may express satisfaction in helping their loved one. Despite this, providers should never underestimate the negative impact of dementia caregiving. Care of the patient with dementia requires an appraisal of how well the caregiver is managing and coping with the disease.

Assessment of the caregiver

A multitude of assessment scales exist for measuring caregivers' physical and emotional health, level of coping, caregiver burden, and distress. Although it is beyond the scope of this chapter to summarize them, Table 15.2 lists several measures that can be used in the clinical setting to objectively assess family caregiver burden. When problems are identified, the caregiver should be referred to appropriate resources, including counseling or support groups. Referrals typically incorporate interventions for the patient (e.g., participation at a day program) and for the caregiver (psychologist or support group to manage emotional stress and enhance coping skills).

Promoting healthy coping and adaptation for the caregiver

Of all the interventions for dementia family caregivers, education and support are consistently associated with positive outcomes [103, 104]. Interventions that are individually tailored, incorporate the patient, and are provided on an ongoing basis show the greatest benefit [105–107]. For the atypical dementias, however, resources can be limited, difficult to access, and may not target the caregiver's unique needs. A caregiver needing education about DLB might need to combine available resources to meet their individual needs (i.e., attend both an Alzheimer's and a Parkinson's disease support group). Day programs and long-term care facilities might not be adequately prepared to manage a younger, physically healthy person with dementia, and it can be difficult to locate appropriate services for these patients. Some caregivers are overwhelmed with inquiries from friends and other family members about how the patient is doing. Rather than responding to each inquiry, many caregivers find it easier to write a summary blog online. Table 15.3 suggests interventions for family caregivers.

Table 15.3 Resources for caregivers.

Needs	Suggested actions	How to locate
Respite from caregiving	1. Adult day program for the patient 2. Engage a companion or caretaker for the patient (paid position or by eliciting family members or friends) 3. Encourage a division and sharing of caregiving responsibilities among family members 4. Obtain in-patient or in-home respite care	1. Alzheimer's Association 2. Family Caregiver Alliance 3. Home Health Agencies 4. Bulletin boards and job advertisements
Caregiver coping	1. Psychologist or therapist for 1 : 1 counseling 2. Support groups	1. Review the caregiver's health insurance regarding coverage for psychological services
Caregiver physical health	1. Encourage the caregiver to engage in regular checkups with their provider 2. Encourage respite from caregiving 3. Encourage the caregiver to incorporate healthy and enjoyable activities into their schedule	
Managing patient symptoms	1. Education and information	1. Fact sheets and strategies (see 15.A.1) provided by the Alzheimer's Association and Family Caregiver Alliance 2. Consultation with experts 3. Local and national conferences
Communication and support	1. Encourage effective strategies for facilitating communication	1. CarePages are blogs that facilitate communication between family and friends during illness (http://www.carepages.com)

Summary

The atypical dementias are a set of heterogeneous conditions manifesting with a variety of symptoms sometimes overlapping, but often quite distinct from those seen in more common dementias such as AD. The patients and their families/caregivers face unique issues and concerns. This chapter has identified many of the special challenges faced by those with an atypical dementia. Further research will expand our knowledge about their experience and pave the way for the development of appropriate treatment and interventions for these patients and their families.

15.A.1 Example of business-style card

My companion has a brain disorder. Your patience is appreciated.

15.A.2 Resources for patients and families (some organizations are based in the United States, although most countries have equivalent organizations)

General resources

Alzheimer's Association: http://www.alz.org (1-800-272-3900)
Family Caregiver Alliance: https://caregiver.org
National Institute on Aging: www.nia.nih.gov

Resources for patients and families (by dementia type)

Alzheimer's disease

Video about early AD: http://www.hbo.com/alzheimers/index.html
http://www.nia.nih.gov/alzheimers (1-800-435-4380)
University of California, San Francisco (UCSF) Memory and Aging website with information about diagnosis, treatment, and caregiving: http://www.ucsf.edu
UCSF videos providing background on AD and caregiving for patients with dementia: https://www.youtube.com/user/UCSFMemoryandAging
Online videos about caregiving: http://www.videocaregiving.org/

Dementia with Lewy bodies

The Lewy Body Dementia Association: http://www.lbda.org/

FTD and subtypes

Association for Frontotemporal Dementia in the United States provides education and support: http://www.ftd-picks.org/
CurePSP in the United States provides support and information for PSP, CBD, and related disorders: http://www.psp.org/
US National Institute of Health (NIH) booklet on FTD; copies available free of charge: https://www.nia.nih.gov/alzheimers/publication/frontotemporal-disorders/introduction
University of California, San Francisco (UCSF) Memory and Aging website provides information about FTD and all clinical subtypes: http://memory.ucsf.edu/ftd/

HD

Huntington's Disease Society of America: www.hdsa.org
Stanford University HOPES website is a very informative website on basic and clinical aspects of HD: http://hopes.stanford.edu
European Huntington's Disease Network provides information in several languages: http://www.euro-hd.net/html/disease
International Huntington Association: www.huntington-assoc.com

CJD

University of California, San Francisco (UCSF) Memory and Aging Center provides information and videos on CJD—from introduction to the basic biology, caregiving, and the importance of autopsy
UCSF Medical Center Division of Infection Control provides information and protocols, including how to handle/disinfect the more infectious biohazards: http://infectioncontrol.ucsfmedicalcenter.org/infection-control-policy-manual
The CJD Foundation in the United States provides information for patients, families, medical professionals, funeral home directors, and more. They have a 24 h telephone support line. The site lists CJD other support organizations in the United States and other countries: www.cjdfoundation.org
The National Prion Disease Pathology Surveillance Center provides information and free brain autopsy service in the United States: www.cjdsurveillance.com
The European Union has an extensive prion disease surveillance and research network. Their website provides information on prion disease of humans and animals, including videos from prion meetings and conferences: www.neuroprion.org
The US Centers for Disease Control and Prevention (CDC) and the World Health Organization provide information and protocols regarding CJD: http://www.cdc.gov/ncidod/dvrd/cjd/qa_cjd_infection_control.htm

References

1 Fisher A editor. *Assessment of Motor and Process Skills*. 3rd ed. Fort Collins, CO: Three Star Press; 1999.
2 Kohlman-Thomson L. *KELS: Kohlman Evaluation of Living Skills*. 3rd ed. Bethesda, MD: American Occupational Therapy Association; 1992.
3 Cullum CM, Saine K, Chan LD, Martin-Cook K, Gray KF, Weiner MF. Performance-based instrument to assess functional capacity in dementia: the Texas Functional Living Scale. *Neuropsychiatry Neuropsychol Behav Neurol* 2001 Apr–Jun;**14**(2):103–8.
4 Kloos AD, Kegelmeyer DA, White SE, Kostyk SK. The impact of different types of assistive devices on gait measures and safety in Huntington's disease. *PLoS One* 2012;7(2):e30903.
5 Kegelmeyer DA, Parthasarathy S, Kostyk SK, White SE, Kloos AD. Assistive devices alter gait patterns in Parkinson disease: advantages of the four-wheeled walker. *Gait Posture* 2013 May;**38**(1):20–4.
6 LaPointe LL, Stierwalt JA, Maitland CG. Talking while walking: cognitive loading and injurious falls in Parkinson's disease. *Int J Speech Lang Pathol* 2010 Oct;**12**(5):455–9.

7 Raub JA. Psychophysiologic effects of Hatha Yoga on musculoskeletal and cardiopulmonary function: a literature review. *J Altern Complement Med* 2002 Dec;**8**(6):797–812.
8 Merrilees J. A model for management of behavioral symptoms in frontotemporal lobar degeneration. *Alzheimer Dis Assoc Disord* 2007 Oct–Dec;**21**(4):S64–9.
9 Beers MH. Explicit criteria for determining potentially inappropriate medication use by the elderly. An update. *Arch Intern Med* 1997 Jul 28;**157**(14):1531–6.
10 Barton C, Merrilees J, Ketelle R, Wilkins S, Miller B. Implementation of advanced practice nurse clinic for management of behavioral symptoms in dementia: a dyadic intervention (innovative practice). *Dementia* 2014 Sep;**13**:686–96.
11 Roberson ED, Hesse JH, Rose KD, Slama H, Johnson JK, Yaffe K, et al. Frontotemporal dementia progresses to death faster than Alzheimer disease. *Neurology* 2005 Sep 13;**65**(5):719–25.
12 Wolf-Klein G, Pekmezaris R, Chin L, Weiner J. Conceptualizing Alzheimer's disease as a terminal medical illness. *Am J Hosp Palliat Care* 2007 Feb–Mar;**24**(1):77–82.
13 Sachs GA, Shega JW, Cox-Hayley D. Barriers to excellent end-of-life care for patients with dementia. *J Gen Intern Med* 2004 Oct;**19**(10): 1057–63.
14 Sampson EL, Warren JD, Rossor MN. Young onset dementia. *Postgrad Med J* 2004 Mar;**80**(941):125–39.
15 Suribhatla S, Baillon S, Dennis M, Marudkar M, Muhammad S, Munro D, et al. Neuropsychological performance in early and late onset Alzheimer's disease: comparisons in a memory clinic population. *Int J Geriatr Psychiatry* 2004 Dec;**19**(12):1140–7.
16 Lawlor BA, Ryan TM, Schmeidler J, Mohs RC, Davis KL. Clinical symptoms associated with age at onset in Alzheimer's disease. *Am J Psychiatry* 1994 Nov;**151**(11):1646–9.
17 Migliaccio R, Agosta F, Rascovsky K, Karydas A, Bonasera S, Rabinovici GD, et al. Clinical syndromes associated with posterior atrophy: early age at onset AD spectrum. *Neurology* 2009 Nov 10; **73**(19):1571–8.
18 Swanberg MM, Tractenberg RE, Mohs R, Thal LJ, Cummings JL. Executive dysfunction in Alzheimer disease. *Arch Neurol* 2004 Apr;**61**(4):556–60.
19 Jacobs D, Sano M, Marder K, Bell K, Bylsma F, Lafleche G, et al. Age at onset of Alzheimer's disease: relation to pattern of cognitive dysfunction and rate of decline. *Neurology* 1994 Jul;**44**(7):1215–20.
20 Back-Madruga C, Boone KB, Briere J, Cummings JL, McPherson S, Fairbanks L, et al. Functional ability in executive variant Alzheimer's disease and typical Alzheimer's disease. *Clin Neuropsychol* 2002 Aug;**16**(3):331–40.
21 Barca ML, Thorsen K, Engedal K, Haugen PK, Johannessen A. Nobody asked me how I felt: experiences of adult children of persons with young-onset dementia. *Int Psychogeriatr* 2014 Jan **15**:1–10.
22 Millenaar JK, van Vliet D, Bakker C, Vernooij-Dassen MJ, Koopmans RT, Verhey FR, et al. The experiences and needs of children living with a parent with young onset dementia: results from the NeedYD study. *Int Psychogeriatr* 2013 Nov **14**:1–10.
23 Allan L, McKeith I, Ballard C, Kenny RA. The prevalence of autonomic symptoms in dementia and their association with physical activity, activities of daily living and quality of life. *Dement Geriatr Cogn Disord* 2006;**22**(3):230–7.
24 Baillon S, Muhommad S, Marudkar M, Suribhatla S, Dennis M, Spreadbury C, et al. Neuropsychological performance in Alzheimer's disease and vascular dementia: comparisons in a memory clinic population. *Int J Geriatr Psychiatry* 2003 Jul;**18**(7):602–8.
25 Powell AL, Cummings JL, Hill MA, Benson DF. Speech and language alterations in multi-infarct dementia. *Neurology* 1988 May;**38**(5):717–9.
26 Bathgate D, Snowden JS, Varma A, Blackshaw A, Neary D. Behaviour in frontotemporal dementia, Alzheimer's disease and vascular dementia. *Acta Neurol Scand* 2001 Jun;**103**(6):367–78.
27 Knopman DS. Dementia and cerebrovascular disease. *Mayo Clin Proc* 2006 Feb;**81**(2):223–30.
28 Vetter PH, Krauss S, Steiner O, Kropp P, Moller WD, Moises HW, et al. Vascular dementia versus dementia of Alzheimer's type: do they have differential effects on caregivers' burden? *J Gerontol B Psychol Sci Soc Sci* 1999 Mar;**54**(2):S93–8.
29 Desmond DW. The neuropsychology of vascular cognitive impairment: is there a specific cognitive deficit? *J Neurol Sci* 2004 Nov 15; **226**(1–2):3–7.
30 Allan L, Ballard CG, Burn DJ, Kenny RA. Prevalence and severity of gait disorders in Alzheimer's and non-Alzheimer's dementias. *J Am Geriatr Soc* 2005 Oct;**53**(10):1681–7.
31 Ballard C, Neill D, O'Brien J, McKeith IG, Ince P, Perry R. Anxiety, depression and psychosis in vascular dementia: prevalence and associations. *J Affect Disord* 2000 Aug;**59**(2):97–106.
32 Lyketsos CG, Lopez O, Jones B, Fitzpatrick AL, Breitner J, DeKosky S. Prevalence of neuropsychiatric symptoms in dementia and mild cognitive impairment: results from the cardiovascular health study. *JAMA* 2002 Sep 25;**288**(12):1475–83.
33 Fuh JL, Wang SJ, Cummings JL. Neuropsychiatric profiles in patients with Alzheimer's disease and vascular dementia. *J Neurol Neurosurg Psychiatry* 2005 Oct;**76**(10):1337–41.
34 Mioshi E, Hsieh S, Savage S, Hornberger M, Hodges JR. Clinical staging and disease progression in frontotemporal dementia. *Neurology* 2010 May 18;**74**(20):1591–7.
35 Ringholz GM, Greene SR. The relationship between amyotrophic lateral sclerosis and frontotemporal dementia. *Curr Neurol Neurosci Rep* 2006 Sep;**6**(5):387–92.
36 Olney RK, Murphy J, Forshew D, Garwood E, Miller BL, Langmore S, et al. The effects of executive and behavioral dysfunction on the course of ALS. *Neurology* 2005 Dec 13;**65**(11):1774–7.
37 Rosness TA, Haugen PK, Passant U, Engedal K. Frontotemporal dementia: a clinically complex diagnosis. *Int J Geriatr Psychiatry* 2008 Aug;**23**(8):837–42.
38 Diehl J, Forstl H, Jansen S, Kurz A. [Frontotemporal dementia: specific problems for caregivers]. *Z Gerontol Geriatr* 2004 Aug;**37**(4):301–6.
39 Rosness TA, Haugen PK, Engedal K. Support to family carers of patients with frontotemporal dementia. *Aging Ment Health* 2008 Jul;**12**(4):462–6.
40 Bristow M, Cook R, Erzinclioglu S, Hodges J. Stress, distress and mucosal immunity in carers of a partner with fronto-temporal dementia. *Aging Ment Health* 2008 Sep;**12**(5):595–604.
41 Riedijk S, Duivenvoorden H, Rosso S, Van Swieten J, Niermeijer M, Tibben A. Frontotemporal dementia: change of familial caregiver burden and partner relation in a Dutch cohort of 63 patients. *Dement Geriatr Cogn Disord* 2008;**26**(5):398–406.
42 Massimo L, Evans LK, Benner P. Caring for loved ones with frontotemporal degeneration: the lived experiences of spouses. *Geriatr Nurs* 2013 Jul–Aug;**34**(4):302–6.
43 Ascher EA, Sturm VE, Seider BH, Holley SR, Miller BL, Levenson RW. Relationship satisfaction and emotional language in

frontotemporal dementia and Alzheimer disease patients and spousal caregivers. *Alzheimer Dis Assoc Disord* 2010 Jan–Mar;**24**(1):49–55.

44 de Vugt ME, Riedijk SR, Aalten P, Tibben A, van Swieten JC, Verhey FR. Impact of behavioural problems on spousal caregivers: a comparison between Alzheimer's disease and frontotemporal dementia. *Dement Geriatr Cogn Disord* 2006;**22**(1):35–41.

45 Wong C, Merrilees J, Ketelle R, Barton C, Wallhagen M, Miller B. The experience of caregiving: differences between behavioral variant of frontotemporal dementia and Alzheimer disease. *Am J Geriatr Psychiatry* 2012 Aug;**20**(8):724–728.

46 Gorno-Tempini ML, Dronkers NF, Rankin KP, Ogar JM, Phengrasamy L, Rosen HJ, et al. Cognition and anatomy in three variants of primary progressive aphasia. *Ann Neurol* 2004 Mar;**55**(3): 335–46.

47 Hodges JR, Patterson K. Semantic dementia: a unique clinicopathological syndrome. *Lancet Neurol* 2007 Nov;**6**(11):1004–14.

48 Seeley WW, Bauer AM, Miller BL, Gorno-Tempini ML, Kramer JH, Weiner M, et al. The natural history of temporal variant frontotemporal dementia. *Neurology* 2005 Apr 26;**64**(8):1384–90.

49 Perry RJ, Hodges JR. Differentiating frontal and temporal variant frontotemporal dementia from Alzheimer's disease. *Neurology* 2000 Jun 27;**54**(12):2277–84.

50 Thompson SA, Patterson K, Hodges JR. Left/right asymmetry of atrophy in semantic dementia: behavioral-cognitive implications. *Neurology* 2003 Nov 11;**61**(9):1196–203.

51 Liu W, Miller BL, Kramer JH, Rankin K, Wyss-Coray C, Gearhart R, et al. Behavioral disorders in the frontal and temporal variants of frontotemporal dementia. *Neurology* 2004 Mar 9;**62**(5):742–8.

52 Nyatsanza S, Shetty T, Gregory C, Lough S, Dawson K, Hodges JR. A study of stereotypic behaviours in Alzheimer's disease and frontal and temporal variant frontotemporal dementia. *J Neurol Neurosurg Psychiatry* 2003 Oct;**74**(10):1398–402.

53 McKeith IG, Rowan E, Askew K, Naidu A, Allan L, Barnett N, et al. More severe functional impairment in dementia with Lewy bodies than Alzheimer disease is related to extrapyramidal motor dysfunction. *Am J Geriatr Psychiatry* 2006 Jul;**14**(7):582–8.

54 Ricci M, Guidoni SV, Sepe-Monti M, Bomboi G, Antonini G, Blundo C, et al. Clinical findings, functional abilities and caregiver distress in the early stage of dementia with Lewy bodies (DLB) and Alzheimer's disease (AD). *Arch Gerontol Geriatr* 2009 Sep–Oct;**49**(2):e101–4.

55 Crowell TA, Luis CA, Cox DE, Mullan M. Neuropsychological comparison of Alzheimer's disease and dementia with Lewy bodies. *Dement Geriatr Cogn Disord* 2007;**23**(2):120.

56 Tiraboschi P, Salmon DP, Hansen LA, Hofstetter RC, Thal LJ, Corey-Bloom J. What best differentiates Lewy body from Alzheimer's disease in early-stage dementia? *Brain* 2006 Mar;**129**(Pt 3):729–35.

57 Shinagawa S, Adachi H, Toyota Y, Mori T, Matsumoto I, Fukuhara R, et al. Characteristics of eating and swallowing problems in patients who have dementia with Lewy bodies. *Int Psychogeriatr* 2009 Jun;**21**(3):520–5.

58 Rongve A, Boeve BF, Aarsland D. Frequency and correlates of caregiver-reported sleep disturbances in a sample of persons with early dementia. *J Am Geriatr Soc* 2010 Mar;**58**(3):480–6.

59 Galvin JE, Duda JE, Kaufer DI, Lippa CF, Taylor A, Zarit SH. Lewy body dementia: the caregiver experience of clinical care. *Parkinsonism Relat Disord* 2010 Jul;**16**:388–92.

60 Ballard CG, O'Brien JT, Swann AG, Thompson P, Neill D, McKeith IG. The natural history of psychosis and depression in dementia with Lewy bodies and Alzheimer's disease: persistence and new cases over 1 year of follow-up. *J Clin Psychiatry* 2001 Jan;**62**(1):46–9.

61 Leggett AN, Zarit S, Taylor A, Galvin JE. Stress and burden among caregivers of patients with Lewy body dementia. *Gerontologist* 2011 Feb;**51**:76–85.

62 Stubendorff K, Aarsland D, Minthon L, Londos E. The impact of autonomic dysfunction on survival in patients with dementia with Lewy bodies and Parkinson's disease with dementia. *PLoS One* 2012;**7**(10):e45451.

63 Kertesz A, McMonagle P. Behavior and cognition in corticobasal degeneration and progressive supranuclear palsy. *J Neurol Sci* 2010 Feb 15;**289**(1–2):138–43.

64 Bak TH, Crawford LM, Berrios G, Hodges JR. Behavioural symptoms in progressive supranuclear palsy and frontotemporal dementia. *J Neurol Neurosurg Psychiatry* 2010 Sep;**81**(9):1057–9.

65 Rosen H. Dextromethorphan/quinidine sulfate for pseudobulbar affect. *Drugs Today* 2008 Sep;**44**(9):661–8.

66 Knutson KM, Zamboni G, Tierney MC, Grafman J. Neural correlates of caregiver burden in cortical basal syndrome and frontotemporal dementia. *Dement Geriatr Cogn Disord* 2008;**26**(5):467–74.

67 Beglinger LJ, O'Rourke JJ, Wang C, Langbehn DR, Duff K, Paulsen JS. Earliest functional declines in Huntington disease. *Psychiatry Res* 2010 Jul 30;**178**(2):414–8.

68 Rothlind JC, Bylsma FW, Peyser C, Folstein SE, Brandt J. Cognitive and motor correlates of everyday functioning in early Huntington's disease. *J Nerv Ment Dis* 1993 Mar;**181**(3):194–9.

69 Anderson KE, Louis ED, Stern Y, Marder KS. Cognitive correlates of obsessive and compulsive symptoms in Huntington's disease. *Am J Psychiatry* 2001 May;**158**(5):799–801.

70 Anderson KE, Gehl CR, Marder KS, Beglinger LJ, Paulsen JS. Comorbidities of obsessive and compulsive symptoms in Huntington's disease. *J Nerv Ment Dis* 2010 May;**198**(5):334–8.

71 Marder K, Zhao H, Myers RH, Cudkowicz M, Kayson E, Kieburtz K, et al. Rate of functional decline in Huntington's disease. *Neurology* 2000 Jan 25;**54**(2):452–8.

72 Goodman AO, Morton AJ, Barker RA. Identifying sleep disturbances in Huntington's disease using a simple disease-focused questionnaire. *PLoS Curr* 2005;**2**:RRN1189.

73 Phillips W, Shannon KM, Barker RA. The current clinical management of Huntington's disease. *Mov Disord* 2008 Aug 15;**23**(11): 1491–504.

74 Wheelock VL, Tempkin T, Marder K, Nance M, Myers RH, Zhao H, et al. Predictors of nursing home placement in Huntington disease. *Neurology* 2003 Mar 25;**60**(6):998–1001.

75 Kirkwood SC, Siemers E, Viken R, Hodes ME, Conneally PM, Christian JC, et al. Longitudinal personality changes among presymptomatic Huntington disease gene carriers. *Neuropsychiatry Neuropsychol Behav Neurol* 2002 Sep;**15**(3):192–7.

76 Paulsen JS, Nehl C, Hoth KF, Kanz JE, Benjamin M, Conybeare R, et al. Depression and stages of Huntington's disease. *J Neuropsychiatry Clin Neurosci* 2005 Fall;**17**(4):496–502.

77 Tabrizi SJ, Langbehn DR, Leavitt BR, Roos RA, Durr A, Craufurd D, et al. Biological and clinical manifestations of Huntington's disease in the longitudinal TRACK-HD study: cross-sectional analysis of baseline data. *Lancet Neurol* 2009 Sep;**8**(9):791–801.

78 Ho AK, Robbins AO, Barker RA. Huntington's disease patients have selective problems with insight. *Mov Disord* 2006 Mar;**21**(3):385–9.

79 Bindler L, Travers D, Millet B. [Suicide in Huntington's disease: a review]. *Rev Med Suisse* 2009 Mar 18;**5**(195):646–8.

80 Haw C, Harwood D, Hawton K. Dementia and suicidal behavior: a review of the literature. *Int Psychogeriatr* 2009 Jun;**21**(3):440–53.
81 Paulsen JS, Hoth KF, Nehl C, Stierman L. Critical periods of suicide risk in Huntington's disease. *Am J Psychiatry* 2005 Apr;**162**(4):725–31.
82 Djousse L, Knowlton B, Cupples LA, Marder K, Shoulson I, Myers RH. Weight loss in early stage of Huntington's disease. *Neurology* 2002 Nov 12;**59**(9):1325–30.
83 Hamilton JM, Wolfson T, Peavy GM, Jacobson MW, Corey-Bloom J. Rate and correlates of weight change in Huntington's disease. *J Neurol Neurosurg Psychiatry* 2004 Feb;**75**(2):209–12.
84 Robbins AO, Ho AK, Barker RA. Weight changes in Huntington's disease. *Eur J Neurol* 2006 Aug;**13**(8):e7.
85 Moskowitz CB, Marder K. Palliative care for people with late-stage Huntington's disease. *Neurol Clin* 2001 Nov;**19**(4):849–65.
86 Williams JK, Skirton H, Paulsen JS, Tripp-Reimer T, Jarmon L, McGonigal Kenney M, et al. The emotional experiences of family carers in Huntington disease. *J Adv Nurs* 2009 Apr;**65**(4):789–98.
87 Skirton H, Glendinning N. Using research to develop care for patients with Huntington's disease. *Br J Nurs* 1997 Jan 23–Feb 12; **6**(2):83–90.
88 Aubeeluck AV, Buchanan H, Stupple EJ. 'All the burden on all the carers': exploring quality of life with family caregivers of Huntington's disease patients. *Qual Life Res* 2012 Oct;**21**(8):1425–1435.
89 Klitzman R, Thorne D, Williamson J, Chung W, Marder K. Decision-making about reproductive choices among individuals at-risk for Huntington's disease. *J Genet Couns* 2007 Jun;**16**(3): 347–62.
90 Geschwind MD, Shu H, Haman A, Sejvar JJ, Miller BL. Rapidly progressive dementia. *Ann Neurol* 2008 Jul;**64**(1):97–108.
91 Gaugler JE, Zarit SH, Pearlin LI. The onset of dementia caregiving and its longitudinal implications. *Psychol Aging* 2003 Jun;**18**(2):171–80.
92 Skirton H, Williams JK, Jackson Barnette J, Paulsen JS. Huntington disease: families' experiences of healthcare services. *J Adv Nurs* 2010 Mar;**66**(3):500–10.
93 LoGiudice D, Hassett A. Uncommon dementia and the carer's perspective. *Int Psychogeriatr* 2005;**17** Suppl 1:S223–31.
94 Pinquart M, Sorensen S. Correlates of physical health of informal caregivers: a meta-analysis. *J Gerontol B Psychol Sci Soc Sci* 2007 Mar;**62**(2):P126–37.
95 Schulz R, Beach SR. Caregiving as a risk factor for mortality: the Caregiver Health Effects Study. *JAMA* 1999 Dec 15;**282**(23): 2215–9.
96 Croog SH, Sudilovsky A, Burleson JA, Baume RM. Vulnerability of husband and wife caregivers of Alzheimer disease patients to caregiving stressors. *Alzheimer Dis Assoc Disord* 2001 Oct–Dec;**15**(4): 201–10.
97 Freyne A, Kidd N, Coen R, Lawlor BA. Burden in carers of dementia patients: higher levels in carers of younger sufferers. *Int J Geriatr Psychiatry* 1999 Sep;**14**(9):784–8.
98 Robinson KM, Adkisson P, Weinrich S. Problem behaviour, caregiver reactions, and impact among caregivers of persons with Alzheimer's disease. *J Adv Nurs* 2001 Nov;**36**(4):573–82.
99 Torti, Jr, FM, Gwyther LP, Reed SD, Friedman JY, Schulman KA. A multi-national review of recent trends and reports in dementia caregiver burden. *Alzheimer Dis Assoc Disord* 2004 Apr–Jun;**18**(2): 99–109.
100 Beeson R, Horton-Deutsch S, Farran C, Neundorfer M. Loneliness and depression in caregivers of persons with Alzheimer's disease or related disorders. *Issues Ment Health Nurs* 2000 Dec;**21**(8):779–806.
101 Thornton M, Travis SS. Analysis of the reliability of the modified caregiver strain index. *J Gerontol B Psychol Sci Soc Sci* 2003 Mar;**58**(2):S127–32.
102 Zarit SH, Reever KE, Bach-Peterson J. Relatives of the impaired elderly: correlates of feelings of burden. *Gerontologist* 1980 Dec;**20**(6):649–55.
103 Callahan CM, Boustani MA, Unverzagt FW, Austrom MG, Damush TM, Perkins AJ, et al. Effectiveness of collaborative care for older adults with Alzheimer disease in primary care: a randomized controlled trial. *JAMA* 2006 May 10;**295**(18):2148–57.
104 Chodosh J, Mittman BS, Connor KI, Vassar SD, Lee ML, DeMonte RW, et al. Caring for patients with dementia: how good is the quality of care? Results from three health systems. *J Am Geriatr Soc* 2007 Aug;**55**(8):1260–8.
105 Connor KI, McNeese-Smith DK, Vickrey BG, van Servellen GM, Chang BL, Lee ML, et al. Determining care management activities associated with mastery and relationship strain for dementia caregivers. *J Am Geriatr Soc* 2008 May;**56**(5):891–7.
106 Pinquart M, Sorensen S. Helping caregivers of persons with dementia: which interventions work and how large are their effects? *Int Psychogeriatr* 2006 Dec;**18**(4):577–95.
107 Parker D, Mills S, Abbey J. Effectiveness of interventions that assist caregivers to support people with dementia living in the community: a systematic review. *Int J Evid Based Healthc* 2008 Jun;**6**(2):137–172.

Index

Non-Alzheimer's and Atypical Dementia, First Edition. Edited by Michael D. Geschwind and Caroline Racine Belkoura.
© 2016 John Wiley & Sons, Ltd. Published 2016 by John Wiley & Sons, Ltd.

www.ingramcontent.com/pod-product-compliance
Lightning Source LLC
LaVergne TN
LVHW082151200926
848484LV00008B/2137